PSYCHOLOGY
for Nurses

PSYCHOLOGY
for Nurses

M Basavanna MA DMP PhD
Professor of Psychology (Retired)
Sri Venkateswara University
Tirupati, Chittoor, Andhra Pradesh, India

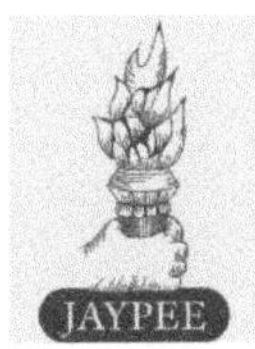

JAYPEE BROTHERS MEDICAL PUBLISHERS
The Health Sciences Publisher
New Delhi | London

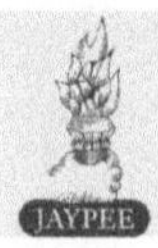

Jaypee Brothers Medical Publishers (P) Ltd

Headquarters
EMCA House
23/23-B, Ansari Road, Daryaganj
New Delhi 110 002, India
Landline: +91-11-23272143, +91-11-23272703
+91-11-23282021, +91-11-23245672
E-mail: jaypee@jaypeebrothers.com

Overseas Office
JP Medical Ltd.
83, Victoria Street, London
SW1H 0HW (UK)
Phone: +44-20 3170 8910
E-mail: info@jpmedpub.com

Corporate Office
Jaypee Brothers Medical Publishers (P) Ltd.
4838/24, Ansari Road, Daryaganj
New Delhi 110 002, India
Phone: +91-11-43574357
Fax: +91-11-43574314
E-mail: jaypee@jaypeebrothers.com

EU GPSR Authorised Representative
Logos Europe, 9 rue Nicolas Poussin
17000, La Rochelle, France
Phone: +33 (0) 6 67 93 73 78
E-mail: Contact@logoseurope.eu

Inquiries for bulk sales may be solicited at: jaypee@jaypeebrothers.com

Psychology for Nurses

First Edition: 2015, ***Reprint: 2025***

ISBN 978-93-5152-564-6

Printed in India

Dedicated to

My students who challenged me,
enriched me and loved me immensely
during the last 50 years
of my academic life

Preface

Although this book is titled as *Psychology for Nurses*, but it can be read by anybody who is interested in the science of psychology. After all, psychology will not be different for different people. It is the same for doctors, engineers or men in the street. Anyone can read and understand this text if only he/she is interested in the subject. The book is just an introduction to the science of psychology. Psychology is the scientific study of behavior and mental processes. It is a tough subject, but it is interesting, fascinating and challenging. It is interesting because it is about people, 'us' and 'others'. All of us are eager to know why we think and act the way we do and why others behave the way they do. It is challenging because, in spite of several centuries of hard work, what we know about the human mind and behavior is pretty little. But do not be discouraged, it is the fate of all sciences including physics and physiology. Physics does not know everything about the physical world and physiology has not completely unraveled the mysteries of the human body. So, it is not surprising that psychologists are struggling to understand the marvels of human mind. However, what little we know about mind and behavior is encouraging enough to prod us to move forward. Psychology promises to help you to understand others and yourself; not that you will be able to understand yourself and others fully with the existing knowledge of psychology. That is a difficult task and a distant dream. The complexities and contradictions of the human mind cannot be easily understood and explained. Psychology can only help you to take the first step toward that end. Toward this end, you will find a number of theories, research studies and isolated facts presented throughout this book. Study of these facts may help you to have a better understanding of your own thoughts, feelings and behaviors as well as those of others.

An American psychologist, Ross Stagner, has explained the goals of psychology succinctly. According to him, each individual lives in two worlds; an external world and an internal world. The external world consists of people who affect you in several ways. Their actions may help you or hurt you. Most of the time, you understand why they behave the way they do. But often you are perplexed by some of their actions, which may appear irrational and even bizarre. Sometimes their behavior is beneficial to you and at other times it is not. Some people are highly cooperative and others are violent. You have to understand these people and their actions—normal and abnormal, rational and irrational, good and bad—because you have to live with them. Having a fairly accurate knowledge of their behavior is necessary if you were to have a comfortable social life.

You also live in an internal world, the world of your own memories, thoughts, feelings, emotions, desires and aspirations. Even among these, you realize, some are good and some bad, some are rational and some crazy. To be at peace with yourself, you have to understand your internal world. Psychology, as the science of behavior and experience, tries to help you in understanding these two worlds.

As a nursing student, you will be in constant touch with people, mostly people who are suffering from one or the other ailments. You can see fear, pain and hope or expectation written on their face. Unless you feel with them, empathize with them and understand their inner world, you will not be effective as a nurse. Remember, the doctor treats the 'disease', but you treat the 'person' with a disease. Knowledge of psychology will go a long way in helping you undertake the task of caring for the patient. A special feature of your profession is that you confront death and disease everyday. In order to face such poignant situations you must be psychologically strong and healthy. It is hoped that knowledge of psychology will help you in this regard.

By the time you complete studying this book, you will have a fairly good view of contemporary psychology. An attempt is made here to introduce you to a broad, exciting field of knowledge, rich in its implications for life and living. It is not intended to make you a full-fledged psychologist but, the aim here is to help you to develop a scientific attitude toward human behavior. The text attempts to help you to ponder over questions such as: What are human beings? What do we know about them? What do we need to know? How to know? How to improve matters?

M Basavanna

Acknowledgments

Science is created by scientists and I am indebted to all those theorists and researchers whose works I have used in preparing this text. The scientists and their contributions are cited throughout the book and their publications are given in the bibliography. Interested students may look into these original works if they want to learn more about the specific topic that is cited in the text.

Writing is a solitary task. But converting the author's words into a finished book requires help from several sources. Many of my friends, colleagues and students generously spared their time and effort in preparing the book. They have read the draft and made valuable suggestions to improve the text. My special thanks are due to Dr Venkata Reddy, Gulbarga University, Gulbarga, Karnataka, India, and Dr Jayashankar Reddy and his faculty, Department of Psychology, CMR Institutions, Bengaluru, Karnataka, India. Ms Anusha and Ms Seema of Bengaluru, and Ms Vandhana of Chennai, who have reviewed the manuscript and offered constructive criticisms and supportive commentaries.

I am thankful to Shri Jitendar P Vij (Group Chairman), Mr Ankit Vij (Group President), Mr Tarun Duneja (Director–Publishing) and Mr Venugopal Vishnumurthy [General Manager–Sales and Marketing (South)], Bengaluru of M/s Jaypee Brothers Medical Publishers (P) Ltd, New Delhi, India, for their great support and endeavor in this project.

I am also thankful to other staff of M/s Jaypee Brothers Medical Publishers (P) Ltd, especially Mr Santhosh Kumar (Commissioning Editor), Mr Vasudev (Mangalore Branch In-Charge/Commissioning Editor), Ms Sajini SV (Team Head) and all staff of Bengaluru Branch who worked in this project and have helped me in more than one way in preparing the text. I am thankful to all others in the publication division of M/s Jaypee Brothers Medical Publishers (P) Ltd, who have taken extra care to make the text presentable.

Contents

To the Students

Psychology is a tough subject. Without concerted effort, it is difficult to comprehend the subject matter. You may follow the suggestions given below in reading the text. First familiarize yourself with the logic of the book's structure. Read the table of contents. It provides you with an overview of the topics covered and how the topics are interrelated. Go through the preface, which describes the features of the text. Concentrate on the key terms and concepts. If you do not understand them, ask the instructor to explain. Consult the glossary given at the end of the book or a dictionary of psychology. Familiarize yourself with the way citations to previous research are made. These are given by name(s) and date, typically set off in parentheses. Each of these names and dates refers to a book or research paper given in the bibliography at the end of the book.

Develop a study skill. Psychologists have devised several excellent techniques for improving study skills. One of which, called SQ3R (SQRRR), is briefly described here. The SQ3R includes five steps designated by the initials S-Q-R-R-R. The first letter S refers to the Survey, the Q to Question, the 3Rs refer to Read, Recite and Review respectively.

The first step is to survey the material in each chapter before reading it. Familiarize with chapter headings, chapter contents and the preview; it provides you with an overview of the major points of the Chapter. The next step is to question. Write down the questions for which you need answers when you complete reading the issues discussed in the Chapter. Questioning makes you an active learner and enhances your ability to understand and retain information. The third and the most crucial step is to read the material. Read the material carefully, actively and critically. While reading, try to get the answers for the questions you have formulated. You may find yourself coming up with new questions as you read along. The next step, recite, is the most unusual one. Here, you talk to yourself or a friend about what you have read. Try to answer the questions you have formulated. Psychological research has shown that communicating material to others and reciting it to yourself enhance your memory for the material and also the capacity for retrieval. The final step, review, consists of three processes: recite the material, recall it and think about it. Re-read the material; try to recall; test yourself; fill in the gaps. Reviewing is a prerequisite to learning and remembering the material. Reviewing is an active process in which you link together different pieces of information to create an overall picture.

Well, this is one way of studying. There are also others. For that matter, you may yourself have method of study. The important thing is when, where and how you study? Study the material in small chunks over several sessions instead of massing your study into one lengthy period. Remember all-night studying just before an examination is going to be less effective and a lot more tiring than employing a series of steady, regular study sessions. You should also choose a convenient place to study. It does not matter where it is as long as it has minimal distractions and is a place that you use only for studying. Identifying a special territory allows you to get into a right mood as soon as you begin. Study psychology with single-minded effort. It is worth the effort. The excitement, challenge and promise that psychology holds for you are significant.

M Basavanna

1 CHAPTER Introduction to Psychology

PREVIEW

The first chapter of the book introduces you to the origins and development of psychology as a scientific discipline. You will see here the trials and tribulations the discipline has undergone before it has reached the present state. Psychology did not exist in its present form, from the beginning. It has changed enormously through the years. The definition, the subject matter and the research methods employed to investigate the issues have evolved and are evolving even today. In the beginning, psychologists were not agreed upon what constitutes psychology, its definition, subject matter and the methodology. There were disagreements as to what psychology should study and how it should be studied. There were several approaches to the study and often these were referred to as Schools of Psychology. Each school with a leader and a group of followers emphasized a certain point of view. Thus, one group asserted that psychology should study the structure of consciousness, by analyzing the immediate experience into its constituent elements using the method of introspection. Another group thought that analysis of experience destroys the essence of experience and conscious experience should be studied as it occurs, as a whole. A third group emphasized the usefulness of psychological processes in life and living. A fourth group asserted that no one can observe consciousness or experience; all that we see is what people do, their behavior; if psychology were to be a science, its subject matter should be something objectively observable. Therefore, psychology should be the science of observable behavior. Even today, there is no complete concurrence of opinion as to what constitutes the subject matter of psychology. It is not surprising why psychologists disagree with each other. Psychology is a complex discipline that deals with an array of such diverse matters that are mind boggling. Look at some of the questions that modern psychologists are trying to answer: Why do people hate each other? Why do we make love? Why do we quarrel? Why do we help (or not help) in an emergency? Why some people are violent, can we reduce the incidence of violence? Why do we sleep and why do we dream? What is intelligence? Can intelligence be improved? What are the best methods of teaching and learning? Why do we forget what we learn? What are the causes of prejudice and discrimination? Why some people get addicted to drugs, alcohol or nicotine? Can we improve the productivity of industrial workers, the performance in sports and efficiency of military personnel? No one brand of psychology can answer all these questions. That is the reason why there are several varieties of psychologies and different kinds of psychologists. The diversity of the subject matter has led to the emergence of a number of subfields of psychology and each of the subfield is engaged in answering certain basic questions about behavior and experience. There are pure scientists engaged in studying the basic processes involved in behavior and experience. These are experimental psychologists, comparative psychologists, social psychologists, developmental psychologists, abnormal psychologists, so on and so forth. On the other hand, there are educational psychologists, industrial psychologists, clinical psychologists, and counseling psychologists who are applying the psychological insights to improve life and living.

This chapter presents information on several topics that are central to the understanding of psychology. It traces the way in which the meaning of the word psychology, its definition and the methods psychology uses to investigate its subject matter have evolved over the years. The chapter provides a brief history of the subject. Psychology has its roots in philosophy, physiology and physics. It has borrowed the subject matter from philosophy and its methodology from science. Therefore, you will be introduced to the origins of psychology within philosophy and within science. You will learn something about the founding fathers of the discipline. You will learn about the early laboratories of psychology, the first text books and the first students of psychology. You will also learn how these early students contributed to the development of psychology in their parts of the world. Psychology today is a sprawling discipline; it has several specialty areas. You will have a bird's eye view of the major areas of contemporary psychology. The differing approaches to psychological issues are presented to you in the section on contemporary perspectives. Note that in spite of the differing approaches to the study, there is a unifying thread that makes psychology a unified scientific discipline. Today, most psychologists hold that the field of psychology should be receptive to a variety of approaches and viewpoints.

Chapter Outline

INTRODUCTION

Psychology is a fascinating as well as a challenging branch of study in the family of sciences. It is fascinating because it concerns us, human beings, our behavior and experience. All of us are eager to know why we act as we do and why others behave the way they do. It is challenging because the complexities and contradictions of human behavior defy easy understanding and explanation in spite of serious theorizing and research for over hundreds of years. We have varieties of people around us. Some people are good and some are bad, some are kind and some others are cruel, some are logical and some others are illogical, some moral and several immoral, some cooperative and some others violently competitive. Why? There are no satisfactory answers. Human behavior has been and remains a mystery. Today, it seems that we know a great deal about everything else except ourselves. However, it is small satisfaction that over 500,000 psychologists hailing from various parts of the globe are engaged in the enterprise of unraveling the mystery of the human mind.

The scope of psychology is very vast; it studies myriad phenomena concerning the human experience and behavior. It is attempting to answer complex questions such as: How do we come to know the world around us? How do we acquire knowledge? What is learning? Where is the learned material stored? What is intelligence? Why do we hate some people and why do we love others? Why do we help people and sometimes, why we don't? Why some people suffer from mental disorders? What are the causes of psychological disturbances? Can we cure mental disorders? Why do some people commit suicide? Why do some get addicted to drugs? Why people are aggressive? Can we control terrorism? Why do we sleep, and why do we dream? Do dreams have meaning? By means of patient research, careful observation, imaginative hypothesizing, and constructive self-criticism, psychologists are trying to answer these and countless other questions. But before we proceed further, let us face the basic question: What is psychology?

DEFINITION OF PSYCHOLOGY

Psychology is such a complex discipline that defining it has not been that simple. Even if you define it today, tomorrow it may become inadequate. In fact, psychology is *not a thing*, it is *about a thing*. It is what a number of scientists and philosophers have created to fulfill the need to understand the mind and behavior of living organisms. Therefore, it has always been hard to define its theme and its boundaries. However, attempts have been made to define psychology and these have been changing over the years (Box 1.1). Literally, psychology means the study of the soul (psyche = soul, logy = study). But, psychology is not interested in the study of the soul. Only religion and theology are interested in the abstract concept of soul. During the early years of its existence, psychology was defined as the study of mind, or the science of mental life. It was thought that mind is reflected in one way or the other in processes such as, sensations, perceptions, memory, thinking, motivation, emotion and manifestation of personality

Box 1.1: Definitions of Psychology Down the Ages

1. Psychology is the study of immediate conscious experience. Its goal is to analyze consciousness into elements, discover the laws by which mental elements combine into more complex mental experiences. —**Wilhelm Wundt** (1874)
2. Psychology is the science of mental life, both of its phenomena and of their conditions. The phenomena are such things as we call feelings, desires, cognitions, reasonings, decisions, and the like. —**William James** (1890)
3. Psychology may be best and most comprehensively defined as the positive science of the conduct of living creatures. —**William McDougall** (1908)
4. All consciousness everywhere, normal or abnormal, human or animal, is the subject matter which the psychologist attempts to describe or explain; and no definition of his science is wholly acceptable which designates more or less than just this. —**James R Angell** (1910)
5. For the behaviorist, psychology is the division of the natural science which takes human behavior—the doings and sayings, both learned and unlearned—as its subject matter. —**John B Watson** (1919)
6. As a provisional definition of psychology, we may say that its problem is the scientific study of behavior of living creatures in their contact with the outer world. —**Kurt Koffka** (1925)
7. Conceived broadly, psychology seeks to discover the general laws which explain the behavior of living organisms. It attempts to identify, describe, and classify the several types of activity of which the animal, human or other, is capable. —**Arthur Gates** (1931)
8. What is man? To this question psychology seeks an answer. —**EG Boring** (1939)
9. Today, psychology is most commonly defined as "the science of behavior." Interestingly enough, however, the meaning of "behavior" is itself expanded, so that it takes in a good bit of what was formerly dealt with as experience....such private (subjective) processes as thinking are now dealt with as "internal behavior." —**NL Munn** (1951)
10. Psychology is usually defined as the scientific study of behavior. Its subject matter includes behavioral processes that are observable, such as gestures, speech, and physiological changes, and processes that can only be inferred such as thoughts and dreams. —**Kenneth Clark & George Miller** (1970)
11. Psychology is the study of behavior and experience. —**Stagner & Solley** (1970)
12. We will define psychology as the science that studies behavior and mental processes. —**ER Hilgard, RC Atkinson & RL Atkinson** (1975)
13. Psychology is the science of human and animal behavior; it includes the application of this science to human problems. —**CT Morgan, RA King, JR Weisz & J Schopler** (1986)
14. Psychology is the scientific study of behavior and mental processes. —**RS Feldman** (2002)
15. Psychology is the science of mental processes and behavior.—**SM Kosslyn & R Rosenberg** (2006)
16. Psychology is the scientific study of behavior and mind. —**JS Nairne** (2006)
17. Psychology is "the scientific study of behavior and mind." —**MW Passer & RE Smith** (2007)
18. Psychology is the science of behavior and mental processes. —**JS Nevid** (2007)

traits. At or around the same time, some pioneers asserted that psychology should engage in the analysis of consciousness. These early definitions were not acceptable to scientifically-oriented psychologists of the 20th century. They argued that mind and consciousness are abstract and subjective concepts that cannot be objectively observed; all that we observe is behavior; the mind, if there is one, manifests in the form of behavior; so, why not we simply study behavior? Not surprisingly, they asserted that psychology is or should be the science of behavior.

Behavior for these early scientists includes all that a person or an animal does. Behavior, unlike mind, can be observed, controlled, and manipulated. We have never seen or heard a mind, but we can see and hear behavior. More importantly, behavior can be objectively measured. Measurement is the heart of science. We can make inferences about the motives, feelings, attitudes, thoughts and other mental phenomena that underlie behavior from what people do and say. In this way, internal mental activities can be studied as they manifest themselves through what people do—*behavior*. In this approach, mind and subjective mental processes are not actually excluded from psychology; behavior is used as the avenue through which mind and other internal mental phenomena are studied.

Today, the majority of psychologists assert that psychology is the scientific study of behavior. Reviewing the definitions of psychology, one psychologist humorously observed: "Psychology lost its soul first, and then it lost its mind, further it lost its consciousness, somehow in the end, it is left with some behavior."

Actually, there is nothing wrong in including mind and mental processes in the definition of psychology. Although mind cannot be observed, it cannot be denied that mind exists and it mediates behavior. Mind can be considered as a hypothetical construct. After all, physicists do not observe gravity; still the concept of gravity is extensively used in physics. It is used as a hypothetical construct to explain certain phenomena in the physical world. Similarly, we can employ the concept of mind in psychology. We will miss a great deal in understanding human behavior if we do not take into consideration the existence of subjective mental activities. It is a healthy sign that modern psychologists do not hesitate to use the word mind in defining psychology as it can be seen in the last five definitions in the Box 1.1. Therefore, we can define psychology as the *scientific study of behavior and mental processes*. The definition has three important terms—scientific study, behavior and mental processes. Mental processes refer to what is happening within when you are seeing, hearing, remembering, thinking or making a decision. Behavior refers to what you do, your outwardly observable activities. It includes speech, facial expressions and physical movements of the various parts of the body. A particular behavior is often preceded by mental processes such as, seeing (perception) something. For example, when you see a speeding car on the road, you move away toward the footpath. Psychologists study mental processes and behavior using scientific method. Scientific method is the universal procedure used by scientists to establish facts. Psychologists, like scientists, logically develop certain ideas about the possible causes of mental and physical activities and then test the resulting ideas by collecting additional facts, which will either support the ideas or refute them. We will learn more about the scientific method as used in psychology in the next chapter.

A better way of understanding psychology is by examining what psychologists are doing. Psychology is a vibrant but sprawling discipline. The tremendous diversity of issues that psychologists are tackling may give the beginning student the impression that the so-called science of psychology is a collection of unrelated topics. Fortunately, it is not so. There is an undercurrent that binds all the provinces of psychology, as well as psychologists. As Feldman (1997) puts it, psychologists constitute a huge joint family in which members are engaged in diverse activities; they may not interact with each other on a day-to-day basis, but are related to one another in fundamental ways and meet on important occasions. Let us examine the various areas that the members of this huge joint family of psychologists are exploring.

MAJOR AREAS OF PSYCHOLOGY

Psychology is a vast field; the areas covered are many and varied. The American Psychological Association (APA), the premier body of psychologists in the United States of America, lists over 54 divisions, which represent the broad fields of specialization within contemporary psychology. Some of the major areas are outlined below.

Biopsychology

A few psychologists are studying the biological basis of behavior. They are interested in the structure and functions of the nervous system, digestive system, endocrine system and such other bodily organs and their functions. This area is called **biopsychology** or **physiological psychology**. Some biopsychologists are studying the effect of hormones on emotional behavior; some others are investigating the role of **neurotransmitters** in the causation of mental disorders; certain others may be interested in locating brain sites associated with pain, pleasure, eating and water intake. Biopsychology is an exciting area of study; you cannot be a good psychologist without the knowledge of physiology. In recent years, **behavioral neuroscience** has emerged as a separate discipline. This field concentrates on the study of the brain and hormonal processes that underlie behavior. Sometimes, **behavior genetics** and **evolutionary psychology** are grouped under behavioral neuroscience. A related area of study, **clinical neuropsychology**, combines the area of clinical psychology and biopsychology by focusing on the relationship between biological factors and psychological disorders.

Experimental Psychology

A substantial number of psychologists are engaged in studying the basic processes of sensation, perception, attention, learning, remembering, forgetting, thinking, problem solving, motivation and emotion. They work in laboratories experimenting with human and animal subjects. These are called experimental psychologists. In fact, experimental psychologist is misleading term. Experimental methods are used by several other psychologists other than experimental psychologists. For instance, biopsychologists, social psychologists, cognitive psychologists, to mention a few, make use of laboratory procedures. It is not the method which distinguishes **experimental psychology** from other fields. It is distinguished by what it studies. Experimental psychologists are engaged in understanding the fundamental causes of behavior. They do what is sometimes called the basic research. During the late 1950s and early 1960s, some researchers looked at the computer as a model for the way human mental processes work which, ultimately during the 1970s, lead to a prosperous branch of psychology called **cognitive psychology**. This branch which focuses on higher mental processes such as memory, thinking, reasoning, judging, problem solving, decision making and language acquisition is a subfield of experimental psychology. In short, cognitive psychology is engaged in the study of the nature of human information processing, that is, the way information is stored and operated internally.

Comparative Psychology

Scientists who study the behavior of non-human species are called comparative or animal psychologists. They study animal behavior in their natural habitat or in laboratory settings. The study includes genetics, brain processes, social behavior and evolutionary processes. Major advances in the area of learning, thinking and problem solving have been made by studying rats, cats, pigeons, monkeys and other animals in the laboratory. **Comparative psychology** is closely related to experimental psychology.

Developmental Psychology

Psychologists who are interested in the study of the development of behavior throughout life are called developmental psychologists. They try to understand complex behaviors by studying their beginnings and the orderly ways in which they change during lifetime. They study motor development, language development, social and emotional development, moral development, cognitive development and development of intelligence. Within **developmental psychology**, there are subfields such as child psychology, psychology of adolescence, adulthood and old age.

Personality Psychology

The scientific study of personality—its structure, dynamics, development and measurement—constitutes a very absorbing branch of psychology. Personality psychologists try to explain the factors contributing to consistency and change in peoples' behavior over time. They are also interested in determining the components of personality that differentiate the behavior of one person from another under similar conditions. Personality is both a developmental and social product and hence, it overlaps developmental psychology and social psychology.

Social Psychology

Human beings are social animals. We spend most of our life in the presence of others with whom we interact in a variety of ways and in different settings. Our actions, thoughts and feelings are affected by others. The primary focus of social psychology is on understanding how individuals are affected by other people. Social psychologists study the ways in which we perceive others and how these perceptions determine our behavior toward them. They investigate the dynamics of interpersonal relations, development of attitudes, prejudices and stereotypes. They also study diverse topics such as inter-group conflict, propaganda, persuasion, conformity, obedience, public opinion and the impact of media. **Cross cultural psychology** is an emerging subdivision of social psychology. It tries to determine similarities and differences of behavior in various cultures and ethnic groups.

Industrial-organizational Psychology

Social psychology has made inroads into industry and the result is the emergence of industrial-organizational psychology (I-O psychology). It is concerned with the behavior of people in the work context. I-O psychologists study issues concerning personnel selection and training, productivity, job-satisfaction, employee morale and motivation, industrial unrest and such other issues. Two subfields within I-O psychology, namely, organization behavior and managerial psychology are taught prominently in institutes of management offering MBA courses. Another related area is **consumer psychology**; consumer psychologists analyze people's buying behavior including the effect of packing and advertisement on buyers.

Abnormal Psychology

Abnormal psychology is the branch of psychology that is focused on dysfunctional behavior or mental maladjustment. Abnormal psychologists try to determine causes, consequences and treatment of psychological disorders. They are also engaged in distinguishing normality from abnormality, classification of mental disorders, estimating their prevalence and suggesting prevention strategies. Several offshoots of abnormal psychology that have shown tremendous progress in recent times are clinical psychology, counseling psychology, health psychology and community psychology.

Clinical Psychology

This branch attracts the largest number of psychologists all over the world. Most of the clinical psychologists work in mental hospitals, psychiatric clinics and community mental health centers. Generally, they work along with psychiatrists and other mental health professionals who are engaged in the diagnosis and treatment of mental disorders. There is some confusion in the minds of many people about the difference between clinical psychologists and psychiatrists. The clinical psychologist holds a degree in psychology (MA, MSc or PhD) with specialized training in clinical work for over two years. A psychiatrist is a medical doctor holding a degree in medicine (MBBS or MD) and a special degree or diploma from a psychiatric institution. As a consequence a psychiatrist can prescribe drugs, while a psychologist does not.

Counseling Psychology

The work of counseling psychologist is very much similar to that of a clinical psychologist. The difference is in the work setting; while a clinical psychologist works in a mental hospital dealing with problems of mental patients, the counseling psychologist works with relatively normal people with minor adjustment difficulties. Mostly, they work with high school and college students helping them to solve problems pertaining to personal-social adjustments and educational and vocational goals. Counseling psychologists make extensive use of psychological tests to measure intelligence, aptitudes, attitudes, interests and personality traits. They may offer psychotherapy to solve the problems of their clients. A number of people consult counselors to deal with familial and marital problems. Some business organizations, orphanages, rescue homes and prisons employ counseling psychologists.

Health Psychology

Health psychology is a recent specialty that studies the factors that influence well-being and illness as well as measures that can be taken to promote health and prevent illness. The study of stress and coping is an area of special interest for health psychologists. They are also engaged in exploring factors that influence pain perceptions and in developing psychological interventions to reduce people's suffering. Health psychologists may also engage in developing and evaluating health-promotion and disease-prevention programs.

Community Psychology

The area of **community psychology** is difficult to define because community psychologists are engaged in highly diverse activities. In general, they apply psychological insights to help solve (or prevent) social and personal problems of people in their natural settings. Problems that arise in homes, schools and work settings are hard to solve in a therapist's clinic. Therefore, the community psychologist goes to the place where problems occur, observes how the problems unfold naturally, design interventions to fit the setting and assesses the impact of those interventions. Community psychologists often serve as consultants to community mental health workers, police who work with trouble makers, departments of social service, school teachers and administrators. By first hand observation, the consultant can shed new light on a problem and help generate solutions.

Educational Psychology

An area that is closely related to counseling is educational psychology. Educational psychologists are engaged in developing effective teaching and learning methods. They are concerned with methods of motivating students, increasing academic achievement, creating favorable classroom climate, and establishing cordial teacher-student relationship. School psychology is a subfield of educational psychology. School psychologists work with primary and high school children focusing on their academic or/and emotional problems. One of their special jobs is to diagnose reading difficulties of children and trying to remedy them. They meet teachers, students, their parents and discuss the problems and suggest action to correct anomalies.

Evolutionary Psychology

One of the new areas that emerged in the late 1980s is **evolutionary psychology**, which seeks to explain how evolution shapes human behavior. Evolutionary psychologists, following Darwin, stress that through natural selection, human mental abilities and behavioral tendencies evolve along with changing body. They explain human social behavior as a product of evolutionary principles. For example, look at some of the issues that evolutionary psychologists are concerned within the context of mate selection. Why humans seek out a long-term bond with a mate? Why men prefer women who are somewhat younger than themselves, whereas women prefer somewhat older men? Why men attach greater importance than women to potential mate's physical attractiveness and domestic skills, whereas women place more importance than men to a potential mate's earning capacity, status and ambitiousness? Examine the explanation evolutionary psychologists give for polygamous tendency in men and the general monogamous tendency in women. According to one evolutionary viewpoint called sexual strategies theory, mating strategies and preferences reflect inherited tendencies, shaped over the ages in response to different types of adaptive problems that men and women faced. According to this viewpoint, men who had sex with more partners increased the likelihood of fathering more children. Men also take a woman's youthfulness and attractiveness as signs of fertility and capacity to live longer to bear more children. In contrast, women had little to gain and much to lose by mating with many men. Woman makes greater investment (costs) than men in having a child, and she wants a committed person to help her in raising the child. When a woman has multiple sex partners, she will be uncertain about which one is the father, thereby decreasing a male's willingness to commit resources to help the mother to raise the child. Therefore, women select a mate who is willing and able to commit time, energy, and other resources (food, shelter, protection, etc.). Through natural selection, the differing qualities that maximized men's and women's reproductive success eventually became part of their biological nature. Thus, men and women have become biologically predisposed to seek somewhat different qualities in a mate.

In addition to the above, several new areas have emerged in recent years. For example, **Environmental psychology** studies the relation between people and their living environments. **Forensic psychology** studies legal issues, such as the role of juries, credibility of witnesses, human errors in judgment, so on and so forth. Sport psychology investigates the factors affecting optimum performance in games, role of sports in maintaining mental and physical fitness and such other issues. Psychology of women includes a broad range of issues such as discrimination against women, violence against women, brain-size difference between men and women, the effect of sex hormones on behavior and such other feminine-related issues. **Psychometric methods** deal with problems of measurement in psychology. **Positive psychology** is a growing field that encourages greater exploration of human strengths, virtues and assets rather than weaknesses and deficits.

As you can see, the scope of modern psychology is very broad; it stretches from borders of medicine and the biological sciences to those of social sciences. To understand the causes of behavior more fully, psychologists examine them at different levels. At the biological level, they examine brain processes, the impact of hormones and the genetic factors. At the psychological level, our thoughts, emotions and motives are examined and at the environmental level, our physical and sociocultural environments are examined. You may wonder just how psychology's scope became so broad. It happened partly because it has its roots in such diverse disciplines as physics, physiology, and philosophy. As a consequence, during its evolution, psychology developed different ways of looking at human behavior. These divergent views led to the emergence of several **schools of psychology**. After some years, the schools faded and gave rise to certain approaches or perspectives to the study of psychology. The perspectives guided the theorizing and research in psychology. Generally, the perspectives are the driving forces in science. When a perspective is proposed, its assumptions are challenged, discussed and debated and in the light of new evidence the perspective may be revised; the revised point of view, the new perspective, may again be challenged by newer perspectives. It is a continuous activity in any scientific endeavor. Since, the schools and perspectives in psychology have their roots in the historical evolution of the discipline, it is necessary to have a peep into the history of psychology.

ORIGINS OF PSYCHOLOGY

Although it is generally held that psychology formally began in 1879 when Wilhelm Wundt, the German philosopher and physiologist, started the first psychological laboratory in Leipzig, it must be remembered that the psychological ideas were in the air from ancient times. Wundt's psychology was the offspring of the marriage between philosophy and physiology and that may be the reason why he called it physiological psychology—philosophical ideas studied according principles of science, especially physiology. Although psychology received its stuff from both philosophy and science, it must be remembered that psychology as a discipline with that name, before the middle of the 19th century, was a formal division not of science, but of philosophy. Of course, during the early period, there was no clear distinction between science and philosophy. Science was simply referred to as natural philosophy. For instance, Aristotle did not distinguish between rationalistic and empirical methods. It was only later that science and philosophy diverged and still later that philosophy became predominantly psychological, thus making psychology philosophical and not scientific. But these differences are artificial. Basically knowledge is one (Boring, 1950). However, it would be interesting to examine what it was within philosophical psychology that was married to physiology, which gave birth to physiological (experimental) psychology during Wundt's time.

Roots of Psychology within Philosophy

Philosophers have all along been asking questions about human phenomena such as: Who am I? Where did I come from? What am I doing? Where am I going? Why do I act as I do? Greek philosophers such as **Socrates, Plato & Aristotle** and several others had made significant statements about the nature of mind. For Socrates, the aim of all education was to help man to know the contents of his mind; it is exemplified by his dictum "know thyself." Aristotle said that the mind was a ***tabula rasa***, a blank tablet as yet unwritten on by experience, thus anticipating the school of empiricism of Hobbes and **Locke**. Aristotle laid down the basic principles of memory—similarity, contrast and contiguity—which are still actively influencing theoretical thinking about learning. He wrote on sensation, imagination and dreaming and hinted at the role of motivation and emotion on perception. More importantly, the best of the ancient thinkers have all along been thinking about the nature of the relationship between mind and body. Many early philosophers held that the mind is an immaterial entity not governed by physical laws and that body is matter that obeys physical laws. Their position was called **dualism**. The renowned French philosopher René Descartes (Fig. 1.1), who inaugurated the modern period of philosophy, was one such dualist (one who believes that the body and mind are two different entities obeying different sets of laws). Although different, he held, that body and mind interacted and influenced each other, a point of view called **interactionism**.

There were other dualists like the German philosopher **Leibniz**, who did not agree with Descartes' interactionism and proposed **psychophysical parallelism** (the view that mind and body are different and run parallel courses without interacting with each other, but giving the appearance of interaction). There were others who asserted that there was only one entity, either mind or body. Their view was called **monism**. Among monists, those who believed that only mind exists were called **idealists** and those who thought that only body (matter) exists were called **materialists**. A third group believed that mind and body were merely two sides of the same coin; this viewpoint was called **double aspectism** or double aspect monism. According to them, matter and consciousness were two inseparable aspects of everything in the universe. An important philosopher who proposed such a view was Spinoza. According to him anything happening to the body is experienced by the mind and emotions and thoughts influence the body.

One of the significant events that accelerated the emergence of psychology was the birth of British empiricism, which held that all knowledge was gained by sensory experience. Thomas Hobbes and John Locke (Fig. 1.2), the two eminent British

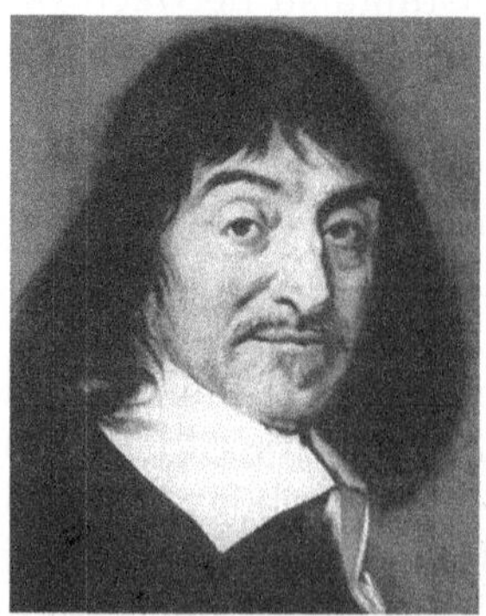

FIGURE 1.1: René Descartes

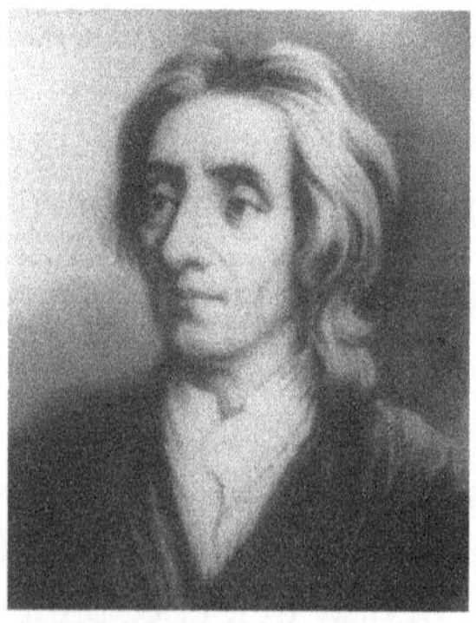

FIGURE 1.2: John Locke

thinkers, were the founders of **empiricism**. Both believed that mind was made up of sense-experience. Chronologically Hobbes began the school of empiricism, but **Locke** was its spiritual head. It seems Locke did not receive his inspiration from Hobbes. Locke held that mind in the beginning was a ***tabula rasa*** and sensory experience wrote on it. For him, mind was a product of experience and it was made up of ideas which were derived from sensory experience. The ideas were arranged and organized by the principles of association. This makes Locke one of the founders of **associationism**, a theory that played a significant role in the evolution of psychology.

Other British philosophers such as George Berkeley, David Hume, David Hartley, James Mill, John Stuart Mill & Alexander Bain extended the empiricistic-associationistic tradition within philosophical psychology. The mind postulated by British empiricists was a passive agent that simply represented physical experiences as mental images, recollections and associations; it only reflects cognitively what is occurring or what has occurred in the physical world. On the other hand, another group of philosophers, who espoused rationalism, postulated an active mind that not only transformed the sensory information to make it meaningful, but also could discover and understand principles and concepts not contained in sensory data. For a rationalist, mind is more than a collection of ideas derived from sensory experience and held together by laws of association. It is active and creative; it adds something to our mental experience that is not found in our physical experience. Spinoza, Leibniz, Hegel & Herbart were eminent rationalists. Herbart is considered a pioneer in educational psychology.

The philosophies of empiricism and rationalism pictured humans as either complex machines (products of experience) or highly rational beings operating in accordance with lofty, abstract principles. But they left something important from their analyses—the irrational aspect of humans. Those who stressed on the irrationality of humans came to be called as romantics. Generally romantics emphasized the inner, personal experience and distrusted both scientists and philosophers who pictured humans as products of either experience or as totally rational beings. Rousseau is considered the father of **romanticism**. He advised that people should trust their heart rather than the mind to guide them. Rousseau's influence can be seen in the works of 20th century psychologists such as Maslow & Rogers. Schopenhauer was also a romanticist who influenced Freud. Another group of philosophers who followed **existentialism** opposed both empiricism and rationalism. Existentialists stressed meaning in life, freedom of choice, subjective experience, personal responsibility and the uniqueness of the individual. **Kierkegaard** and **Nietzsche** were the first influential existentialists. According to Nietzsche, there are no universal truths, only individual perspectives. The only source of information for what is good or bad, desirable or undesirable, are individuals themselves. Nietzsche referred to humans, who had the courage to live in accordance with their own values, thus rising above conventional morality, supermen. The influence of romanticism and existentialism in modern psychology is seen in psychoanalysis and humanistic psychology.

Roots of Psychology within Physiology

Although philosophers have been spinning theories of mind, they did not say anything important about the body where the mind resides. It was left to the 19th century physiologists to discover the mechanisms by which we come to know the physical world; that is, how the empirical events come to be represented in consciousness. Everything from sense perception to motor reactions was studied in detail during the first half of 19th century and these path breaking discoveries led to the birth of experimental psychology. In 1811, **Sir Charles Bell** discovered that the sensory fibers of a mixed nerve enter the spinal cord at a posterior (dorsal) nerve root, whereas, the motor nerves of the same nerve leave the cord by an anterior (ventral) root. **François Magendie**, a French physiologist made the same discovery later in 1822. This fact of anatomical and functional discreteness of sensory and motor nerves came to be known as the **Bell-Magendie law**. This was an important discovery in physiology. It established the fact that conduction in a nerve normally occurs in only one direction (the law of forward direction in the nervous system). The law is basal to the conception of reflex action and the reflex act.

The next important discovery was the division of the sensory fibers into kinds. **Johannes Müller** (Fig. 1.3), the German physiologist in 1826 discovered that there are five kinds of nerves, one for each of the five senses and each containing a characteristic energy and when they are stimulated a characteristic sensation results. That is, each nerve responds in its own characteristic way no matter how it is stimulated. For example, whatever the stimuli applied to the eye-light, pressure, electricity—all cause visual sensations only. This has come to be known as the **doctrine of specific nerve energies**. Müller formulated ten laws the central one of which states that we are directly aware, not of objects, but of our nerves themselves; that is to say, the nerves are intermediaries between the perceived objects and the mind and thus impose their own characteristics on the mind. However, Müller was worried over the question of whether the characteristic of the nerve itself or the site in the brain where the nerve terminated accounts for specificity. He concluded that the nerve is responsible,

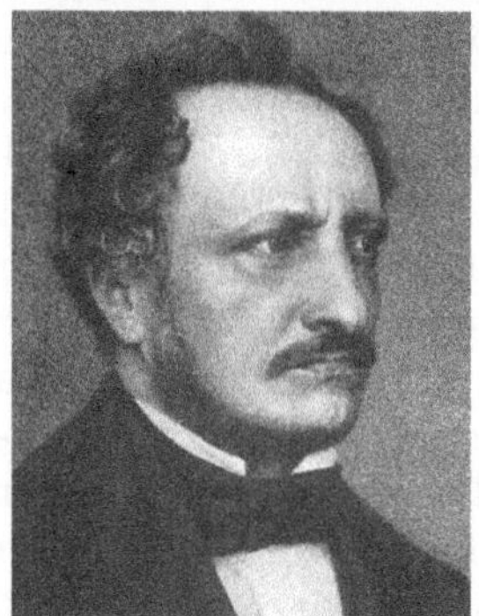

FIGURE 1.3: Johannes Müller

but subsequent research demonstrated that the brain site is the determinant. Müller anticipated a close relationship between physiology and psychology. He said that nobody can be a psychologist, unless he first becomes a physiologist (*nemo psychologus nisi physiologus*).

Müllerian theory was extended by **Helmholtz** (Fig. 1.4), another great German physiologist, who demonstrated that there are specific qualitative differences within a single sense modality; that is to say that there are specific fiber energies. For example, Helmholtz stated in his famous *trichromatic theory of color vision* that there are specific fibers that when stimulated give rise to different color sensations; one for red, one for green and a third for violet.

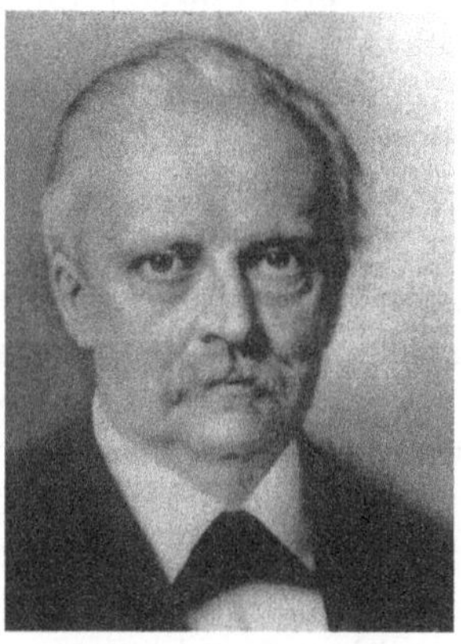

FIGURE 1.4: Helmholtz

This was corroborated by Thomas Young and the theory is often called Young-Helmholtz theory of color vision. Ewald Hering & Christine Ladd-Franklin proposed alternative theories of color. Later, fiber specificity was shown in other senses—hearing, touch, smell and taste.

Helmholtz, a student of Müller, was an eminent figure in the history of science. His contributions to science are many and varied. He proposed the theory of conservation of energy, measured the velocity of nerve impulse and offered a theory of audition, in addition to his theory of color vision, and differentiated between sensation and perception. His work moved physiology closer to psychology thus paving the way for the emergence of experimental psychology.

Around the same time, tremendous progress was witnessed in the area of neurophysiology. Du Bois Reymond demonstrated the electrical nature of nerve impulse; Bernstein described the nerve impulse as a wave of negativity; Marshall Hall, extending the early work of Robert Whytt, described reflex action. It was also in 1850 that Fechner was toying with the idea of his psychophysics. Also young Wundt, who was around 18 years must have been a witness to all these advances. But before we take up the work of Wundt, we have to familiarize ourselves with other advances in physiology especially brain physiology.

BRAIN PHYSIOLOGY

Like several other theories, the views pertaining to brain functions started with wrong assumptions. From ancient times people were interested in determining the site within the body where mind is situated. Early thinkers located mind in various parts of the body. Aristotle located mind (soul) in the heart; so did the Egyptians. Pythagoras thought of the brain as the seat of the mind; Plato also thought on the same lines. Descartes located the mind in the entire body. It was Franz Joseph Gall who firmly believed that brain is the seat of the mind. He was the founder of a theory called phrenology.

PHRENOLOGY

Gall argued that the mental faculties are housed in specific areas of the brain, and depending on whether a faculty is well developed or underdeveloped in the brain, there would be a protrusion or depression respectively on the corresponding part of the skull, and by examining the bumps and depressions on the exterior of the skull, one can determine the strength or weakness of a person's mental faculties. Gall and his student Spurzheim divided the skull into 37 patches, each one associated with a specific faculty. Such an analysis was named phrenology, and it became very popular at that time because it provided an opportunity for the objective analysis of the human mind. It strengthened the idea of faculty psychology—the belief that the mind consists of several mental powers or faculties proposed by the Scottish philosopher Thomas Reid. Phrenology was ridiculed and derided by both physiologists and philosophers. Physiologists did not find any evidence to show that the conformation of the exterior of the skull corresponds to the conformation of its interior. Philosophers objected to the division of the unitary mind into faculties. However, ridiculous phrenology might be; it served psychology in certain ways. It made brain the "organ of mind" and suggested that different parts of the brain have different physiological and perhaps psychophysiological functions, thus leading to localization of brain functions. Although the theory was basically wrong, it was enough right to stimulate the right type of scientific research.

Localization of Brain Functions

French physiologist **Pierre Flourens** is the most important figure in the advancement of brain physiology. Chronologically Luigi Roland (after whom central fissure of the cerebrum is named) is the first person to have engaged in the study of the anatomy and pathology of the brain. But he was unconvincing in his experimental procedures and often incorrect in his conclusions. Flourens was precise in his technique, clear in exposition and right in his conclusions. Using the method of extirpation or ablation of specific areas of brain in animals, he showed that cerebrum is the seat of perception, intelligence and the will; the function of cerebellum is the coordination of movements of locomotion; the medulla oblongata is the organ of conservation, the vital knot that is essential to the life of the organism including the nervous system; the corpora quadrigemina function for seeing; the function of the cord is conduction and the function of nerves is excitation. **Flourens** also demonstrated that in spite of the diversity of structure and functions (action proper), the nervous system acts as unit (action commune); there is a community of reaction. Thus, he anticipated one century earlier Franz & Lashley's conception of equipotentiality and mass action and the Gestalt view that cerebrum acts as a whole.

In 1861, **Paul Broca**, using clinical methods, announced the localization of center for speech at the base of the third frontal convolution of the left cerebral hemisphere. The area has come to be called **Broca's area**. In 1870, Gustav Fritsch & Eduard Hitzig discovered the motor areas in the cerebral cortex and David Ferrier fixed the visual center in the occipital lobe. By the end of the century, hearing was localized in the temporal lobes and somesthetic sensation in the post-central region, back of the motor area. The areas of taste and smell were uncertain. So, there was a good deal of localization of functions on the cortex as the phrenologists had maintained, but never was a mental function found where Gall had said it was.

Birth of Psychophysics

As we have seen, while the philosophers were developing the theory of mind, the nature of consciousness, experience and awareness, physiologists were locating the organs of the mind, investigating the bodily processes that produce conscious experience. It was shown that conscious experiences (the sensations) were triggered by brain processes. But how are the two, mental sensations and the bodily (sensory) processes related? It was left to two persons, **Weber** and **Fechner**, to find out the answer and develop an area of psychology called **psychophysics**.

German physiologist Ernst Heinrich Weber, using a two-point threshold and **just noticeable difference (jnd)**, was the first to demonstrate the systematic relationship between stimulation and sensation. He showed that jnds correspond to a constant proportion of a standard stimulus. This has been called **Weber's law**. He determined the **two-point threshold** for various parts of the body by observing the smallest distance between two points of stimulation that would be reported as two points. Working with weights, he determined how much heavier or lighter than a standard a weight must be before it is reported as being heavier or lighter than the standard weight. This sensation of difference was called just noticeable difference. Thus, Weber's law was the first statement of the systematic relationship between physical stimulation and a psychological experience. Weber was a physiologist and was not interested in psychology. It was Gustav Theodor Fechner (Fig. 1.5), who realized the implication of Weber's work to psychology. He expanded Weber's findings by showing that jnds are related to stimulation in a geometric fashion. Fechner, although a physicist, was a philosopher by nature,

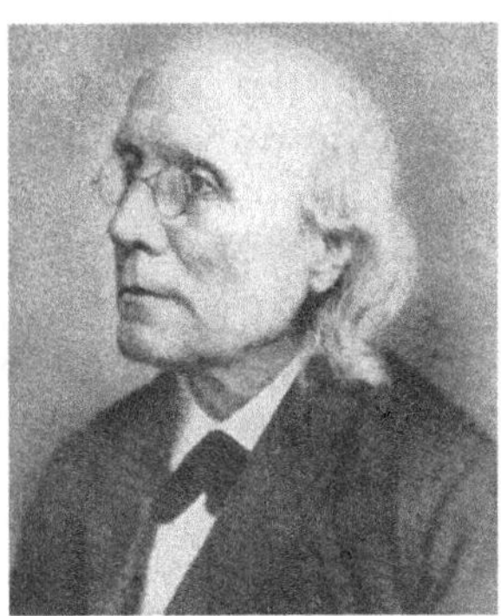

FIGURE 1.5: Fechner

and wanted to suggest a solution to the mind-body problem in a way that would satisfy materialistic scientists of his day. He thought that a systematic relation between bodily and mental experiences could be demonstrated if a person were asked to report changes in sensations as a physical stimulus was systematically varied. This way he came to hypothesize that for mental sensations to change arithmetically, the physical stimulus would have to change geometrically. In testing these ideas, Fechner created psychophysics—the study of the functional relationship between mind and body. Since, it is impossible for one person to study the entire psychophysics, Fechner restricted himself to study the relation between sensation and stimulus. The results of his studies culminated in the enunciation of the famous *psychophysical law*. The law can be mathematically stated as $S = c \log R$, where S is sensation, R is stimulus (Reiz in German), and c is constant. He derived the equation starting from the Weber's law: $\Delta R/R = c$, where ΔR is the minimum change in R that could be detected; that is, the minimum change in physical stimulation necessary to cause a person to experience a *jnd* and R is the stimulus and c is a constant.

Fechner's claim to greatness in psychology does not, however, derive from his law. The important thing he accomplished was the development of a set of new methods of measurement in psychology. These are the now famous psychophysical methods: the method of average error, the method of limits and the method of constant stimuli that are used to determine **absolute limen, difference limen** and several other important constants. Several people recognize Fechner as the founder of psychology. The famous historian of psychology EG Boring (1950) writes: "Fechner, because of what he did and the time at which he did it, set experimental psychology off upon the course which it had followed."

Birth of Experimental Psychology

So, by about 1860, the stage was set for the emergence of experimental psychology and the honor of inaugurating the discipline goes to **Wilhelm Wundt** (Fig. 1.6), a professor of philosophy at the Leipzig University, Germany. Wundt collected the diverse achievements in the various areas of science and philosophy, synthesized them into a unified scientific discipline and organized it around certain constructs, theories and methods, thus giving rise to the discipline of experimental psychology.

Wundt's contribution to psychology was amazing. He wrote a textbook of experimental psychology, started the first official psychological laboratory in 1879, directed an array of research, founded a journal to publish the research and expounded a system of psychology. Wundt dominated experimental psychology for three decades. Leipzig became the Mecca of

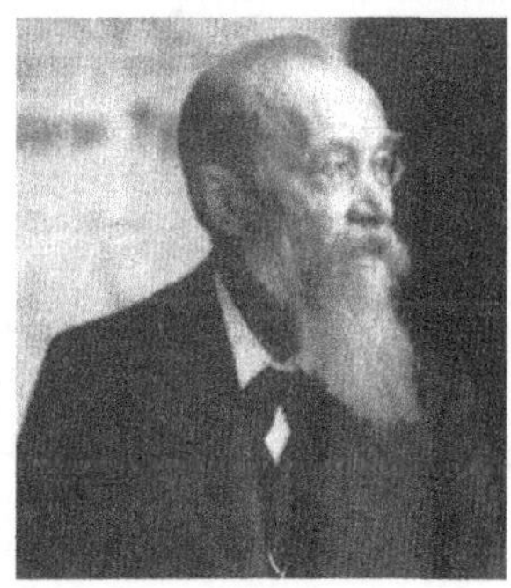

FIGURE 1.6: Wilhelm Wundt

psychology. People from all over the world came to study with Wundt. Almost all of them went back and founded laboratories in their countries and became great psychologists in their own right. During his stay at Leipzig, Wundt supervised 186 doctoral theses (70 in philosophy and 116 in psychology).

According to Wundt, the subject matter of psychology was immediate experience, the method was introspection and the problem of psychology was the analysis of conscious process into elements, determination of the manner of connection of these elements and the determination of the laws of their connection. The goal of psychology was the analysis of mind into simple qualities such as sensations, images, feelings and the determination of their ordered multiplicity. Thus, Wundt's psychology was introspective, sensationistic, elementistic and associationistic. This brand of psychology continued as a school called structuralism for some time in the United States under the leadership of Titchener an eminent student of Wundt. But it did not survive for long.

Psychology after Wundt

Wundt's system of psychology did not survive in its original form for long. His system was referred to as psychology of contents because of its concern with the contents of the mind. Objections to this kind of psychology came from many directions. In fact, almost all the later developments in psychology were founded as protests against one or the other characteristic of Wundt's psychology. There were people like Franz Brentano who opposed the exclusive emphasis on structure and insisted with considerable vigor that the outstanding characteristics of conscious mind are its active processes and not its passive contents. Sensing and not sensations, thinking and not ideas, imaging and not images and similar acts (processes), **Brentano** argued, should be the proper subject matter of psychology. This line of thinking led to what came to be known as **act psychology**, which in turn led to the emergence of **Gestalt psychology**. Wundt held that higher mental processes cannot be studied experimentally. But, one of the students of Wundt, Oswald Kulpe, demonstrated that thinking could be studied in the laboratory and also suggested that there were imageless thoughts. **Ebbinghaus** demonstrated that learning and memory can be studied objectively in the laboratory. Thus, strong differences of opinion about what psychology should study and how it should do it, paved the way for the emergence of several **schools of psychology**—groups of like-minded psychologists formed around influential teachers who argued for one viewpoint or another (Table 1.1).These

Table 1.1: Schools of Psychology

Name of school	*App. date*	*Significant individuals*	*Main emphasis*
Psychology of content associationism	1879	Wilhelm Wundt	Immediate experience
Structuralism	1893	EB Titchener	Immediate experience
Psychoanalysis	1895	Sigmund Freud	Unconscious motivation; sex and aggression
Functionalism	1896	W James, John Dewey, JR Angell, H Carr	Adaptive value of mind
Gestalt psychology	1912	Max Wertheimer, W Kohler, Kurt Koffka	Study of experience as a whole
Behaviorism	1913	IP Pavlov, JB Watson, CL Hull, BF Skinner	Study of observable behavior

schools of psychology set the direction for much of research in psychology during the early years of 20th century. Let us review some of these schools of psychology.

Gestalt Psychology

The first organized German protest to Wundt's psychology came in the form of Gestalt psychology, which was founded by Max Wertheimer (Fig. 1.7) and his colleagues Wolfgang Kohler (Fig. 1.8), Kurt Koffka (Fig. 1.9). These pioneers opposed the idea of dissecting the mind into elements. They asserted that analysis destroys the very essence of conscious experience, namely, its wholeness. The German word *Gestalt* means "form" or "configuration" and the

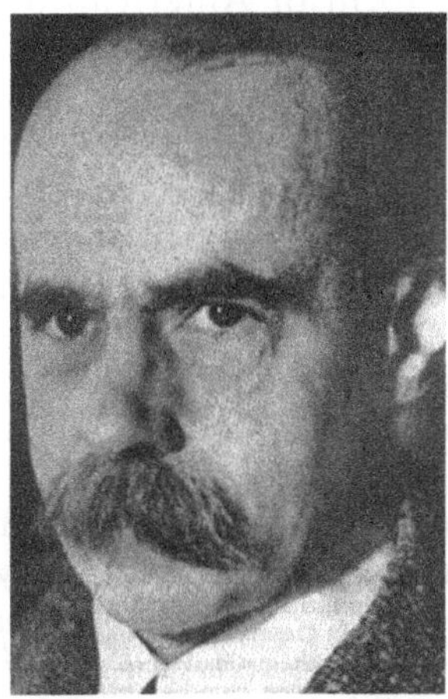

FIGURE 1.7: Max Wertheimer

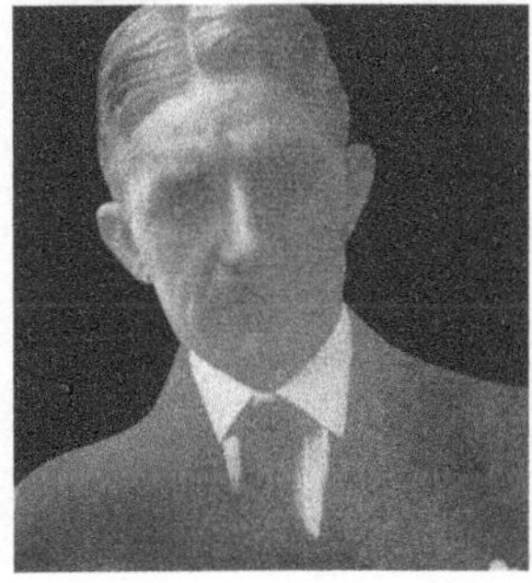

FIGURE 1.8: Wolfgang Kohler

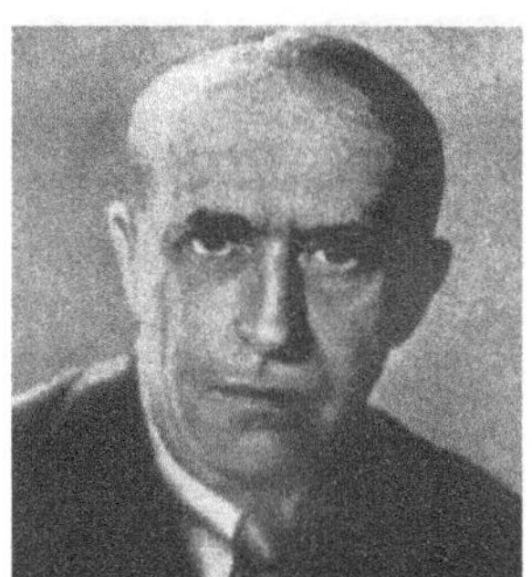

FIGURE 1.9: Kurt Koffka

Gestalt psychologists maintained that the conscious experience should be thought of as resulting from the whole pattern of sensory activities and the relationships and organizations within this pattern and not by the compounding of elements. The contribution of Gestalt psychologists toward our understanding of perception, learning and thinking is phenomenal. You will learn more about Gestalt psychology in later chapters on perception, learning and thinking.

Functionalism

American protest to Wundt's system took the form of **functionalism**, another influential school of psychology. The origins of functional school can be traced to **William James** (Fig. 1.10), the great Harvard professor of philosophy, who is recognized as the father of psychology in America. His book, *The Principles of Psychology* (1890), marks the beginning of psychology in the Americas.

The first formal psychological laboratory was set up at Johns Hopkins University in 1883 by Stanley Hall, who was a student of both James & Wundt. Within a few years, most of the major universities in the USA had psychology laboratories and departments. Functionalism as a school of thought was started by John Dewey, James R Angell (Fig. 1.11) & Harvey Carr (Fig. 1.12) at the University of Chicago. Functional psychology may be regarded as the psychology of mental operations in contrast

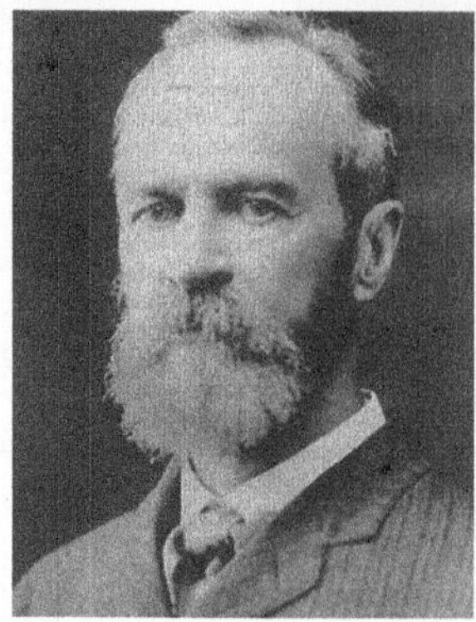

FIGURE 1.10: William James

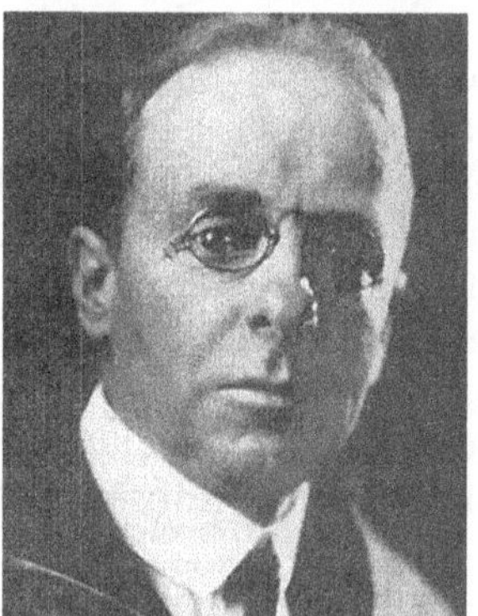

FIGURE 1.11: JR Angell

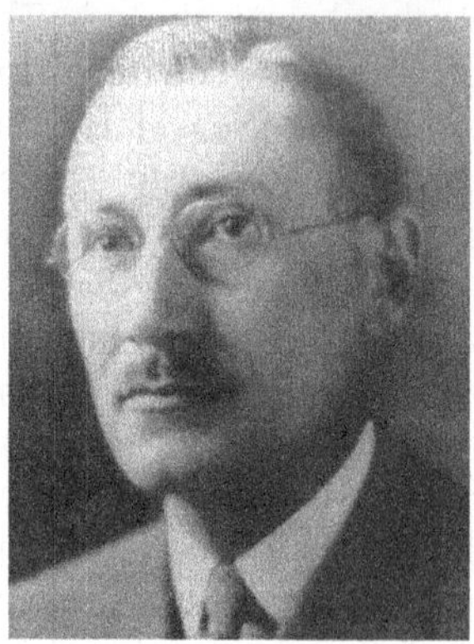

FIGURE 1.12: H Carr

to Wundt's psychology of mental contents. It emphasized the fundamental utilities of mind. Functional psychologists were interested in the adaptive aspects of mind; that is, the mind enabling the individual to adjust to the changing environment. They investigated the ways in which learning, remembering, thinking, problem solving, and motivation help people adapt to their environment, instead of limiting themselves to the description and analysis of the mind. In short, they were interested in studying the functions of mind. Functionalists were influenced by Darwin's theory of evolution and proposed that there was a link between humans and nonhuman animals. This insight led them to believe that the study of animals could provide clues to human behavior, which in turn led to the emergence of animal psychology.

Behaviorism

A radical form of American opposition to Wundt's system came in the form of **behaviorism**. The proponent of this school, **JB Watson** (Fig. 1.13), rejected the concept of mind itself and insisted that psychology was a branch of natural science, and it should study only observable behavior. He emphasized that most of human behavior is learned and made the Pavlov's conditioning model the corner-stone of his stimulus-response psychology.

Watson was a radical environmentalist and argued that the goal of psychology was to predict and control behavior by determining how behavior was related to environmental events. America produced

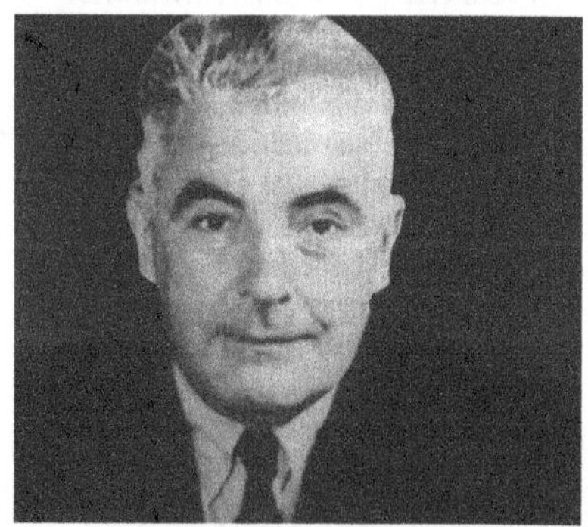

FIGURE 1.13: JB Watson

a great array of behaviorists such as **EL Thorndike, CL Hull & BF Skinner**, all of whom rejected the idea that psychology should study unseen phenomena, such as mind, mental processes, or consciousness. Some of them acknowledged that mental processes probably exist, but they thought it was neither necessary nor useful to focus on them. Instead they asserted that to understand behavior, we should study behavior. The behaviorists' emphasis on controlled, objective observation of behavior had a deep and lasting impact on 20th century psychology. You will learn more about it in the chapter on learning.

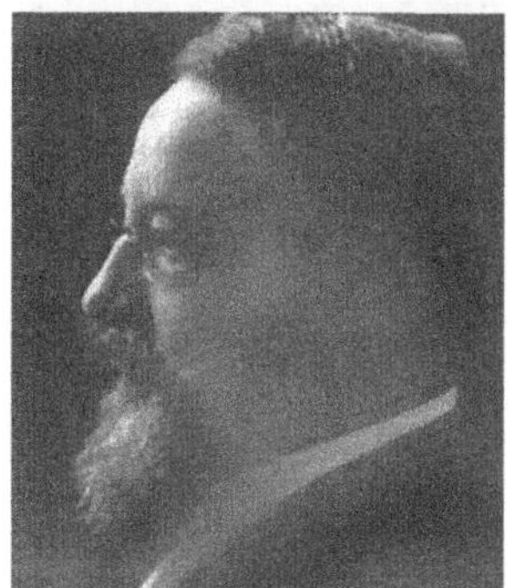

FIGURE 1.14: EB Titchener

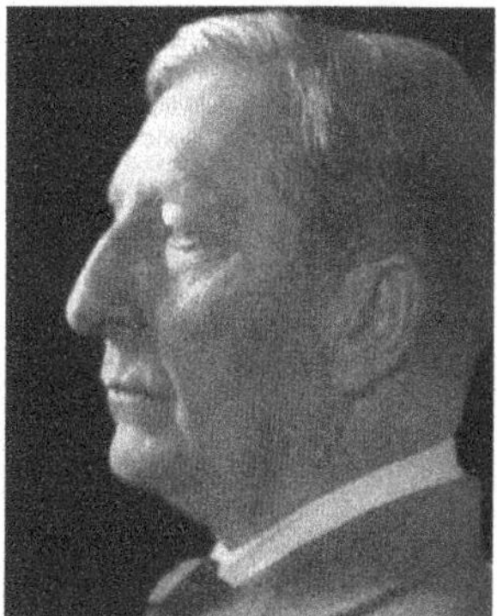

FIGURE 1.15: W McDougall

Structuralism

The third American school of psychology, structuralism, was not a protest but an elaboration of Wundt's psychology. Its founder was a British student of Wundt, **Edward B Titchener** (Fig. 1.14), who stood firm by Wundt's ideology and taught German psychology, as propounded by his teacher, in Cornell University to American students. Structuralism, however did not survive in its original form. Titchener was a great experimental psychologist and as such, he influenced the growth of experimental tradition in the United States of America.

Purposivism

British psychologist, **William McDougall** (Fig. 1.15), agreed with Watson in defining psychology as the study of behavior, but insisted that purposive behavior should constitute the subject matter of psychology. McDougall made **instincts**, the innate patterns of behavior, the cornerstone of his theory and said that all behavior was goal directed. His system is also called **hormic psychology** because of its emphasis on the goal-directed nature of behavior. McDougal was a great social psychologist; he wrote the first textbook of social psychology, which has been published and republished an innumerable number of times.

Psychoanalysis

A very influential school of psychology that had nothing to do with the mainstream psychology of Wundt or James is **psychoanalysis** founded by **Sigmund Freud** (Fig. 1.16), a Viennese psychiatrist. Freud asserted that behavior is controlled by unconscious instincts and made unconscious motivation cornerstone of his theory. He emphasized the role of sex and aggression as prime determiners of conscious behavior.

Freud was probably the most criticized scientist in the world. But Freud was a genius and his ideas have revolutionized the thinking and theorizing of many psychologists all over the world and today **psychoanalysis** continues to survive as psychodynamic approach within psychology. We will come across Freud's teachings in several chapters later in this book.

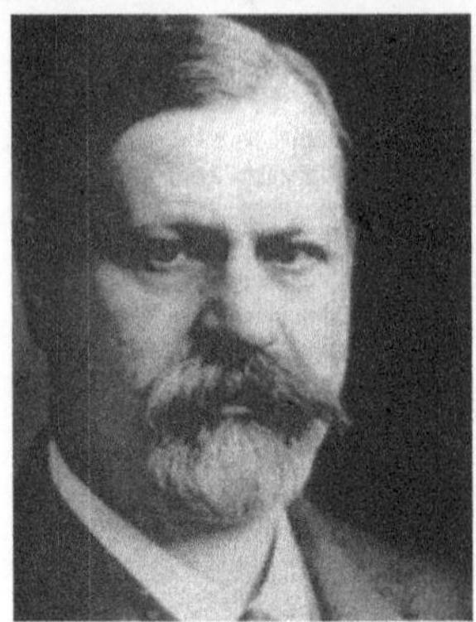

FIGURE 1.16: Sigmund Freud

CONTEMPORARY PERSPECTIVES

Today, the discoveries made by the early schools of psychology have become part of the general store of psychological knowledge, but the schools as such have disappeared. Of course, behaviorism and psychoanalysis are still active in modified forms. Along with these two, several other ways of looking at human behavior and experience, called perspectives or approaches, have emerged during the last several years. Each of these broad perspectives emphasizes different aspects of behavior and experience. A review of these perspectives will help us to understand the later chapters of this book. What perspective a psychologist follows depends on his or her area of interest and also the personal inclination of the scientist. Certain perspectives are more suitable to study some aspects of behavior than others. We shall have a brief preview of some of the major perspectives in contemporary psychology in the following paragraphs.

Biological Perspective

All said and done, there cannot be a mind without the body. Therefore, there is a small but powerful group of psychologists who emphasize the role of the body or biology in determining behavior. These people who follow biological perspective naturally try to relate behavior and experience to the functions of the body. For example, they are interested in knowing the neurological bases of behavior, determining sites of the brain that are associated with specific psychological functions, the impact of hormones on behavior, bodily changes during emotions, the mechanisms of heredity, so on and so forth. Biological psychology, which is also often called **physiological psychology** or **behavioral neuroscience**, has made enormous progress in recent times especially with the modern technological advancements. Two leaders of biological psychology, KS Lashley and DO Hebb, have studied the role of the brain in learning, memory and perception. The studies of biological bases have led to the discovery of **neurotransmitters**. Neurotransmitters, chemicals released at the synapses, help communication between the nerve cells. The study of the role of these chemicals in determining behavior, especially deviant behavior, is an exciting area of behavioral neuroscience. Today, using computer aided brain-imaging techniques and brain wave recording procedures, it has become possible to watch live brain processes during perceiving, learning, remembering, thinking, problem solving and emotional states such as fear or anger and motivational states such as hunger, thirst and sex.

Behavioral neuroscience has led to the emergence of new disciplines such as **cognitive neuroscience** (the study of brain activities underlying higher mental processes such as attending, reasoning, problem solving, and so forth); **behavior genetics** (the study of behavior as influenced by genetic endowment); and evolutionary psychology, the discipline that tries to investigate the effect of evolution on behavior. Psychologists who subscribe to biological perspective have made major contributions to the understanding and betterment of human living ranging from developing of certain drugs to cure mental disorders to brain surgery.

Behavioral Perspective

The origins of behavioral perspective can be traced back to British empiricism of John Locke & Russian reflexology of **Ivan Pavlov**, but the real impetus to its emergence came from JB Watson. Watson banished all subjective concepts such as mind, experience, and consciousness from the purview of psychology and insisted that psychology should study what is observable and measurable—behavior. All that we engage in from the time we are born till we die is behavior. We eat, drink, talk, sing, laugh, fight, make love, sleep, and engage in a myriad of activities; these are behaviors which can be objectively observed, measured, controlled, manipulated and predicted. Why not study these activities without bothering about what is going on within the organism? That is exactly what Watson said and did. He revolutionized psychology in America with his brand of psychology that has come to be called behaviorism. He maintained that only by studying what people do, we can have an objective science of psychology. Thus, Watson helped shape the course of psychology during the first half of 20th century. He believed that one could gain a complete understanding of behavior by studying and modifying the environment in which people live. He asserted that by properly controlling a person's environment, one could elicit any desired sort of behavior. This belief is reflected in one of his very famous statements: "Give me a dozen healthy infants, well-formed and my own specified world to bring them up in and I will guarantee to take any one at random and train him to become any type of specialist I might select—a doctor, lawyer, artist, merchant-chief and yes, even beggar-man and thief, regardless of his talents, penchants, tendencies, abilities, vocations and race of his ancestors (Watson, 1924)." As you can see, Watson was an extreme environmentalist.

Later, behaviorism prospered under the leadership of an eminent Harvard psychologist, **Skinner**, who also asserted that the real causes of behavior reside in the environment and not within the individual. He maintained that "No account of what is happening inside the human body, no matter how complete, will explain the origins of human behavior (Skinner, 1989)." Further he asserted: "A person does not act upon the world, the world acts upon him (Skinner, 1971)." Skinner studied the stimuli that elicit behavioral responses, the reinforcements (rewards and punishments) that maintain or extinguish these responses and the modifications in behavior obtained by changing the reinforcements. He never bothered about any mental process that intervened between the stimulus and response. Because Skinner took such an extreme position regarding the determiners of behavior, his system has come to be called radical behaviorism.

Most of the experiments conducted by behaviorists were on animals and they believed that whatever principles operate in animal learning holds good for humans as well. The contributions of behaviorists made in the area of learning and the application of learning principles to various aspects of human living are unparalleled in the history of psychology. Behaviorism challenged the assumptions of all other psychological perspectives and dominated American psychology for several years. However, the influence of radical behaviorism faded after 1970 with the advent of cognitive psychology, which brought back to psychology the mental processes. Still, the impact of behaviorism continues to be felt in several areas of modern psychology, especially in the field of learning and its application to the treatment of psychological disorders.

Cognitive Perspective

Cognitive approach to the study of human behavior considers the S-R psychology of behaviorists too narrow. To think of human activities solely in terms of stimulus input and response output may be adequate to explain simple forms of behavior, but it is insufficient to understand several complex psychological phenomena such as attending, remembering, thinking, reasoning, problem solving and information processing. In fact, the word cognition is derived from the Latin root *cogitare* which means "to think." Naturally, cognitive perspective examines the mind and how the mental activities influence behavior. According to cognitive psychologists, people think and plan the course of action in terms of remembered information; people are not merely passive receivers of stimuli; the human mind actively processes the information it receives and converts it into new ideas. Cognitive psychologists focus on the processes that enable people to know, understand and think about the world. They try to explain how people process information and how their ways of thinking about the world influence their behavior. Cognitive psychology today is as influential as was behaviorism during the first half of the 20th century.

Cognitive psychology has several subspecialties. For instance, **cognitive behaviorism** proposes that our learning experiences and the environment determine our expectations and thinking pattern and in turn our thoughts determine our behavior. Another area is **cognitive neuroscience**, which with the help of sophisticated brain-imaging techniques and electrical recording devices, studies brain activities when people are engaged in thinking, remembering, planning, learning language, acquiring knowledge and information processing in the laboratory. Modern information technology and computer technology have had a great impact on the development of cognitive perspective.

Psychodynamic Perspective

While behaviorists thought that all behaviors are learned, cognitivists asserted that behavior is determined by the way people think and process information, the psychodynamic perspective believes that it is our unsatisfied wishes, which are stored at the dark corners of the mind, that impel us to do what we do. As we have seen earlier, it was **Sigmund Freud**, who propounded this line of thinking. According to Freud, most of our behavior is determined by a set of innate urges that are repressed and unconscious. He argued that humans have evolved from animal ancestry; they share with them several urges that cannot be satisfied directly in the civilized society, these desires are pushed into the unconscious mind, these repressed desires do not keep quiet and they remain active and will be trying to find gratification. But the conscious forces do not permit the expression of the repressed desires. These unfulfilled wishes try to manifest themselves in indirect fashion and influence our behavior.

According to Freud, mind is like an iceberg a large portion of which is invisible and a small portion only is visible. The invisible part is the unconscious and the visible portion the conscious. The role of the conscious mind in determining behavior is minimal and it is the unconscious that plays a major role in determining human behavior. The most important unconscious urges that shape human behavior are sex and aggression, which are not easily satisfied in society and hence pushed into the unconscious mind from where they exert immense pressure on human behavior. Freud's theory, called psychoanalysis, is one of the most controversial but influential psychological theories of 20th century, especially in the areas of personality, psychopathology, and psychotherapy. Several of Freud's views were not acceptable to his own associates and some of them developed modified versions of the theory and others such as **Alfred Adler** and **Carl Jung** proposed alternative theories. All these theories are grouped under **psychodynamic perspective** and because the ongoing conflicts within the human mind are dynamic in nature (active, energetic and driving) the approach is named psychodynamic.

Humanistic Perspective

Among the several perspectives we have discussed so far, behaviorism and psychodynamic were the two most powerful forces that were dominant during the first fifty years of the last century. Psychoanalysts viewed man as an animal driven by unconscious urges and behaviorism made him a machine controlled and manipulated by external forces. Both these views were not acceptable to a group of psychologists. Therefore, a "third force" emerged within psychology and came to be known as **humanistic psychology**. Two important leaders of this humanistic perspective, **Carl Rogers** and **Abraham Maslow**, emphasized that man is neither an animal, nor a machine; he is endowed with certain special characteristics not found either in animals or machines; man is a *human being*. Human beings are capable of choosing their life's goal; they have free will, they are capable of personal growth and self-actualization. Humanists believe that man is intrinsically good. Given freedom he becomes what he can become and can lead a rich and satisfying life. Thus, the humanists emphasize the positive and noble side of human beings. This approach in modern times has led to the development of the *positive psychology movement* whose emphasis is on human strengths, fulfillment and optimal living.

Humanistic ideology has come to be applied in various walks of life, such as industry, education, family living, and psychotherapy. Humanistic perspective has evolved as a reaction against dehumanizing, technological and societal forces. It has been influenced by existential thinking and **phenomenology**. It emphasizes the importance of subjective experience, especially man's view of himself—his **self-concept**, self-fulfillment in addition to positive human qualities such as altruism, love, value orientation and cordial interpersonal relationships. Thus, humanistic psychology stresses the role of psychology in enriching people's lives and making human life worth living.

Sociocultural Perspective

We are social beings. We live in a society, and each society is characterized by a culture. The word **culture** refers to the enduring set of values, beliefs and traditions that are shared by all members of society and passed on from one generation to the next. All societies develop their own **social norms**, which are a set of unwritten rules that specify what behavior is acceptable and expected for members of the group. Social norms prescribe how we have to dress, talk, walk and respond to elders. These rules are internalized by all of us through a process called socialization. This is what is implied by the statement: "Be a Roman when you are in Rome." Naturally, our behavior is influenced by the cultural group to which we belong. The subfield of psychology, which studies the ways in which social environment and cultural learning influence human behavior is called cultural psychology. This field (also called cross-cultural psychology) examines how culture is transmitted to its members and studies the similarities and differences among members belonging to diverse cultures. A large group of psychologists emphasize the importance of the social setting in shaping our behavior and these psychologists are following the **sociocultural perspective**.

For example, some cross-cultural psychologists have differentiated cultures based on the extent to which they emphasize individualism versus collectivism (Triandis, 2001). Most industrialized societies in North America and Europe promote **individualism** in which greater emphasis is placed on personal goals, achievements and personal identity. In contrast, several countries in Asia, Africa and South America nurture **collectivism** in which individual needs are subordinated to those of the society and personal identity is defined largely by social ties that bind one to family and the group. This difference is said to be the result of social learning experiences that begin during childhood. It is found that Japanese schools encourage children to work in groups, while American children are made to work on individual assignments. It is found that in some cultures love is an essential prerequisite to enter into marriage, whereas in others love is viewed as irrelevant and it is the family that determines whom you marry.

UNIFYING FEATURES AMONG THE PERSPECTIVES

When you review the differing perspectives in the study of humans, there is a possibility for you to think of psychology as a divided house. Fortunately, it is not so. Humans are the most complex and mysterious organisms in the universe. It is not possible to explain human behavior and experience in terms of a simple, single formula. An individual's behavior may have to be examined from different angles. That is what is implied in the existence of various perspectives. What perspective one adopts depends on the area of his or her interest. For example, one who is interested in studying learning and memory may search for the neural basis for these phenomena (biological approach). Another may investigate how stimulus and response are connected under the conditions of reward and punishment (behavioristic approach). A cognitive psychologist may look at memory in terms of information processing procedure (how information is received, coded, stored and retrieved). A person following psychodynamic perspective may consider forgetting as an instance of repression. The humanist may examine the value of meaningfulness, significance and personal relevance of the learning material in understanding the process of forgetting. The important thing to remember is that each approach offers a somewhat different explanation of the same behavior and each makes a substantial contribution to our understanding of the total person. So, one should not go with the idea that psychology is a fragmented discipline consisting of a series of separate, unrelated, subject areas that lack cohesion. In spite of the apparent disparity among the various topics and perspectives, psychology is more unified in terms of the links between the various areas and perspectives. As mentioned earlier, psychology is a joint family of members engaged in different professions; they always meet during lunch and dinner.

We close this chapter with a mention of the major developments in the field of psychology over the years and the people who contributed to these developments in Table 1.2.

Table 1.2: Landmarks in the History of Psychology

Year	*Landmarks*
1860	Fechner publishes *Elements of Psychophysics*
1878	Stanley Hall receives the first PhD in psychology
1879	Wundt establishes the first laboratory in psychology at Leipzig
1883	Stanley Hall establishes first laboratory at Johns Hopkins University
1887	Stanley Hall starts the *American Journal of Psychology*
1890	William James publishes *Principles of Psychology*
1892	Stanley Hall starts *American Psychological Association*
1896	Lightner Witmer establishes the first psychological clinic
1900	Sigmund Freud publishes *Interpretation of Dreams*
1905	Alfred Binet & Theodore Simon develop the first test of intelligence
1908	Pavlov's work on conditioning is published in an *American Journal*
1909	Freud & Jung visit the United States
1910	Wertheimer and colleagues begin work in Gestalt psychology
1913	Watson publishes *Psychology as the Behaviorist Views it*
1930s	Karl Lashley, Donald Hebb & Roger Sperry fosters psychobiology
1950s	GA Miller inaugurates cognitive psychology
1960s	Maslow & Rogers initiate humanistic psychology movement

Chapter Summary

Psychology is defined as the scientific study of behavior and mental processes. Behavior refers to observable activities of an organism while mental processes refer to inner psychological activities that cannot be objectively observed but are inferred from observed behavior. In the early years, psychology was considered as the subject that studies mind. Later, students of psychology were not happy with the concept of mind that could not be objectively observed and instead concentrated on behavior that can be seen and manipulated as scientists did. Thus, psychology became the science of behavior. But toward the latter part of 20th century, especially with the advent of cognitive psychology, psychologists realized that mind or mental activities cannot be dispensed from psychology. Human beings think, plan, solve problems, make judgments, learn, remember and recall information. These are essential aspects of human living and psychology cannot ignore them. Therefore, today the importance of higher mental processes is appreciated in understanding human behavior, and psychologists are not averse to use the concept of mind and conscious experience.

Modern psychology is a vast area consisting of a number of branches and specializations.. There are so many branches of psychology that one wonders whether psychology is a single unified discipline. According to Sigmund Koch (1993), psychology is not a single discipline; it is a collection of studies of varied cast. Look at the major branches of psychology: biopsychology, experimental psychology, comparative psychology, developmental psychology, personality psychology, social psychology, industrial/organizational psychology, abnormal psychology, clinical psychology, counseling psychology, health psychology, community psychology, educational psychology and evolutionary psychology. In addition, there are some special branches, such as sport psychology, forensic psychology, school psychology, geropsychology, and feminine psychology, rehabilitation psychology, consumer psychology, environmental psychology and military psychology.

The roots of psychology can be traced to philosophy, physiology, medicine and physics. Psychology broadly can be described as the offspring of British philosophy and German physiology. As is well known, the birth of psychology as an independent experimental science occurred at Leipzig University, Germany, under the leadership of Wilhelm Wundt in 1879. Wundt was interested in the analysis of conscious experience into its constituent elements using the method of introspection. This view of psychology was opposed by other thinkers, which led to the emergence of several schools of psychology. William James was responsible for the development of psychology in the Americas. The early American psychologists, under the influence James & Darwinism, were interested in the application of psychology for a better living. This approach came to be called the school of functionalism. Another group of psychologists wanted psychology to be a branch of natural science and made observable behavior the subject of psychology. The work of these people under the leadership of Watson gave rise to behaviorism. In America, there was one devoted student of Wundt, EB Titchener, who was not swayed by the American trend toward functionalism or behaviorism. He propagated his mentor's ideas; he and his followers developed a school of psychology that came to be known as structuralism. In Germany, a group of psychologists did not agree with Wundt's analysis of conscious experience and emphasized the holistic nature of experience. The work of this group, under the leadership of Max Wertheimer, developed into Gestalt psychology. The greatest influence on psychology came from medicine in the form of Freud's psychoanalysis. Freud emphasized the irrational nature of mind under the influence of unconscious forces.

Toward the mid 20th century, most of these schools got absorbed into the mainstream psychology. Today, there are no schools of psychology; there are only certain broad perspectives that offer distinct outlooks and emphasize different factors in explaining human behavior and experience. Contemporary psychologists have embraced five major perspectives: biological perspective that views behavior from the perspective of the biological functioning; psychodynamic perspective which asserts that behavior is motivated by inner unconscious forces over which the person has no knowledge or control; cognitive perspective which examines the ways in which people think and understand the world around them; behavioral perspective, which concentrates on the observable behavior; and humanistic perspective which believes that people know what they are doing and why they are doing and they are trying to become what they can become. As you can see, each of these perspectives emphasizes different aspects and mental processes and each provides certain insights into the working of human psyche from somewhat different angles.

You may wonder why so many perspectives. The answer is simple. Psychology today is diverse, but psychology has almost always been diverse. In psychology's long history, there has never been a time when all psychologists accepted a single paradigm. What distinguishes modern psychology from psychology during the period when schools existed is the current relatively peaceful coexistence of psychologists holding dissimilar views. When schools flourished there was disagreement bordering on hostility among the members of rival schools. Today, the schools are gone and the spirit of eclecticism prevails. Psychologists today choose from diverse sources those ideas and techniques that are most effective in dealing with a problem. In fact, remnants of all the schools and methodologies are found in contemporary psychology.

Contd...

Contd...

Human behavior is very complex. There are no simple answers to questions that psychology encounters; definitely there are no final answers. Science's ability to answer certain questions is unequaled, but there are crucial questions that science cannot answer. There are no final truths even in science. According to Popper, the eminent philosopher of science, the highest status that a scientific explanation can have is "not yet disconfirmed." All explanations, even scientific explanations, will eventually be found to be false; the search for truth is unending. In psychology, there is no one truth; there is no "one principle" that explains everything about human behavior. Psychology is not a place for people with a low tolerance for ambiguity. The diverse and sometimes conflicting viewpoints that characterize contemporary psychology will undoubtedly continue to characterize psychology in the future. There is growing recognition that psychology must be as diverse as the humans whose behavior it tries to explain. For those looking for the "one truth", this state of affairs is distressing. For those willing to ponder several truths, psychology is and will continue to be an exciting field (Hergenhahn, 2001).

CHAPTER 2 Research Methods in Psychology

PREVIEW

This chapter will tell you about some of the procedures psychologists employ to observe, explain and predict behavior and mental processes. The procedure they use is often called the scientific method. Scientific method is a multistep procedure that generates accurate knowledge. It is a method of developing knowledge based on evaluating evidence gathered from careful observation and experimentation. The first step in scientific method is the observation of the event (behavior or experience) in which the scientist is interested. See the regularity with which it occurs. The second step is to ask a question: Why did it occur? What might have caused it? Then formulate a tentative answer to the question. In scientific terms, the tentative answer is called the hypothesis. The final step is to test the hypothesis by collection of relevant information (data). You may say: Why should I bother about scientific method, when I am not interested in conducting research? Even if you are not interested in becoming a researcher, it is good to know the scientific method. It helps you to inculcate an objective, scientific attitude toward issues of life. You will not be swayed by popular opinions and faulty assumptions. If you have a scientific attitude, you ask questions, ask for evidence and think about the pros and cons instead of blindly accepting what is presented to you.

Every day in your life, you face problems, which have to be solved and you have to do so according to systematic procedure. Take for example, an advertisement in the media, which proclaims that use of a particular cream makes your skin fair within seven days. You should not blindly accept it. Ask whether it is true. Ask your friends who used it whether it really works. You may yourself use it and see whether the claim is true. Nowadays several drugs are introduced into the market; they are proclaimed as miracle cures for certain complaints. Should you blindly accept the claim and start prescribing the drug? If you do so, you are not a critical thinker. You should question the authenticity of the claim; ask whether the claim is true; study the literature pertaining to the drug; try to evaluate its effectiveness. That is scientific attitude. According to American psychologist George Kelly, every human being is a scientist; knowingly or unknowingly people use the scientific method. Suppose you meet a person for the first time and you assume that he is honest. You just do not keep quiet after that. You watch the behavior of the person in several situations and try to find out whether your assumption about him/her is correct. Based on the information, either you accept your assumption or reject it. Here you are following the scientific method.

Scientists have not descended from heaven. They are as human as you are. They are scientists primarily because they follow well-established procedures to generate knowledge. As scientists, psychologists follow the same scientific methodology to answer questions pertaining to behavior and experience, as the chemist uses to explain the chemical properties of matter. Psychologists are awfully skeptical; they do not accept anything on its face value. They question everything. They ask: What is it? How does it work? Why does it work the way it does? Their objective is to observe, describe, explain, predict and control behavior and mental activities. That is, they start with a question (a problem), formulate a tentative answer to the question (hypothesis), gather evidence, test the hypothesis and draw conclusions. In this chapter, you will have a brief review of the procedures psychologists use to investigate questions pertaining to human behavior and mental functions.

Chapter Outline

INTRODUCTION

Psychology is a complex subject of study. Psychologists are expected to explain several intriguing facets of human living, and answer puzzling questions and solve intricate problems pertaining to human behavior and experience. Some questions are simple and many are not that easy. For example, psychologists may be called upon to answer questions like: What are the effective methods of teaching school children? Should children be punished when they disobey? Why some people get addicted to drugs? What are the factors leading to marital conflict? Are leaders born or made? What are the causes of industrial unrest and how to resolve them? Why people fight with each other and what are the causes of aggression? What is stress and what are its effects on human organism? What are the causes of mental disorders and which are the effective methods to cure them? Why do we help others in an emergency, or why do we not help? We need answers to these questions. These and several other questions pertaining to our life have been fairly satisfactorily answered by psychologists. How do they get relevant information (data) concerning these issues and how do they process the information, so that they can provide credible answers to these questions? This chapter deals with methods psychologists employ in answering questions pertaining to behavior.

SCIENTIFIC METHOD

Like all other scientists, psychologists rely on the scientific method to unravel the mysteries of the human mind. **Scientific method** is the procedure used by all scientists including psychologists to understand and explain the universe in which they live. Translating the scientific method into action is what is called research. But before we proceed further in understanding research methodology, we must face a question that is often asked by students of introductory psychology: Why should we bother about research methods when we know that we are not going to undertake research? True, many of you may not become researchers, but still it is necessary that you should know about science and the scientific method. Whether you realize it or not, we are all bombarded by science most of the time in our lives. When you hear about a new cure for a disease, when you are persuaded to buy one product over another and when you read about opinion polls on political issues, you are being exposed to science. In order to deal with your world rationally, you must be able to analyze critically the information thrown at you and be able to separate scientifically verified facts from unverified conjectures. A study of scientific method helps you to cultivate a scientific attitude towards all that happens around you.

According to American psychologist George Kelly (1955), all human beings are scientists. Humans are curious and like to have explanations for the things that occur around them. Suppose you see a student who shoots and kills several of his classmates, you need an explanation for his behavior. Why did he do so? Is it because he was biologically predisposed to be violent? Is it because he was reared in an abusive and aggressive home environment? Or is it the result of watching violence in television or movies? We need explanations to this and similar events that occur abundantly around us, and we do come up with explanations. But our explanations are not based on accurate information obtained through objective observation.

Generally, our conclusions are based on hearsay, conjecture, anecdotal evidence or unverified sources of information. In most cases, our explanations are made on the spot with little attention given to ensuring the accuracy of information. Often, our explanations reflect personal opinions and biases. To make matters worse, there is a human tendency to look for information that will confirm prior beliefs and assumptions and ignore information that does not conform to those beliefs and assumptions (known as confirmation bias). We simply develop an explanation and, satisfied with its plausibility, adopt it as correct. We do not consider exploring whether our explanation is correct or whether there might be other better explanations. Unfounded, but commonly accepted explanations for behavior can have undesirable consequences on our social life. To avoid the trap of easy, untested explanations for our behavior, we need to abandon informal, unsystematic approach and adopt an approach that has been proved to provide explanations that are accurate. This approach is called the scientific method. An explanation developed through scientific method is called the **scientific explanation**.

Scientific explanations differ from other types of explanations such as the ones based on common sense or faith in several ways. Scientific explanations are based on empirical evidence; that is, based on objective observations made under controlled conditions. These are testable or verifiable and made with minimum number of assumptions (parsimonious). Specific predictions can be made about what should occur under conditions not yet observed. These explanations are rational in that they follow the rules of logic. Scientific explanations are general and can be applied to situations other than those under which they were derived. Finally, scientific explanations are tentative and entertain the possibility that they are faulty. Remember Newton's views of the universe had to be replaced when new evidence showed that some of his predictions were wrong. Scientific explanations are rigorously evaluated for consistency and with known principles, for their parsimony, and for generality.

Steps in Scientific Research

Whatever be the area of their interest, the scientists including psychologists follow the scientific method as the principal route for obtaining information about their subject matter. The scientific method is not just a means of obtaining knowledge; it is a way of examining the universe. An individual who subscribes to this method analyzes the problem carefully, defines its components, obtains required information, proposes a solution to the problem, and subjects the solution to rigorous testing. Scientific method is a way to gather facts that will lead to the formulation, and validation of a theory. It provides the general framework within which scientists operate. But to answer questions and to test the hypothesis the scientific method must be translated into a workable research study. The research process goes through several crucial steps. We review here briefly the steps psychologists take in conducting research.

The first step in research is to state the problem, which one wants to investigate. The problems do not fall from the sky. One has to observe nature, in our context human behavior; study the published research literature in scientific journals; discuss with senior researchers and experts in the concerned area. Formulating the problem is the most important step in the research process. The problem is generally stated in the form of a question such as: What is the effect of *X* on *Y*? The question must be stated in such a way that it can be answered. Suppose your question is: Is there life after death? It is a bad question; it cannot be answered. On the other hand, assume that your question is: Does punishment improve learning? This is a good question; it can be answered. You have observed people reporting their dreams. So, you may ask the question: Why do people dream? You can think of finding an answer to the question. It is not enough if the question is just answerable. It must be an important question. Researching a question involves quite a bit of time, effort and money. Answering a question is important when it can be applied to improve human living, when it leads to more important research questions and enriches our knowledge about human behavior.

Once the question has been stated, the next step is to develop an explanation to the observed phenomenon. The explanation you develop is called, a **theory** in scientific terminology. Giving a precise definition to the concept of theory has always been a headache to scientists. For our purpose, it is enough to define a theory as a set of assumptions or a broad explanation about an observed phenomenon. Theories provide a framework for understanding the relationships among a set of otherwise unorganized facts and principles. Theories vary both in their breadth and the particular level of details they employ. For example, a theory might seek to explain and predict as broad a phenomenon as learning in general. Or a narrow theory might attempt to predict the effect of meaning on learning. Psychologists establish formal and focused theories based on careful study of published research literature as well as their own understanding of the field of interest. You will come across several theories in this book, such as theories of personality, theories of psychotherapy, theories of learning and theories of aggression.

The third step in scientific research is to devise a way of testing the theory. For this purpose, a hypothesis is derived from the theory. According to Kerlinger (1973), "A hypothesis is a conjectural statement between two or more variables." It is a suggested answer to the question. It is a prediction stated in a way that allows it to be tested. A hypothesis helps to test the validity of the theory. Suppose the problem you are interested is: What is the effect of reward on learning? Then, the hypothesis could be: *Reward improves learning*. Theories and hypotheses help psychologists ask suitable questions. But how are the questions answered? The answers come from research. Research is the systematic inquiry, whose aim is to generate new knowledge. In short, research process proceeds through the following steps:

1. Asking questions about a phenomenon or event based on observation or careful study of relevant literature.
2. Formulating a tentative theory.
3. Deriving a testable hypothesis.
4. Collecting the necessary information (the data).
5. Analyzing the data.
6. Drawing conclusions.
7. Reporting the findings in scientific journals.
8. Building a theory to generate new hypotheses which are tested by further research.

An important thing to keep in mind is the scientific attitude. Insatiable curiosity, constant questioning, skepticism, seeking evidence and open-mindedness to change beliefs in the light of evidence, these are the basic components of the scientific attitude.

VARIABLES

Before we move further, it is necessary to clarify the meaning of the term variable, which is the most often used word in psychological research. We saw the use of the term in Kerlinger's definition of hypothesis (a hypothesis is a conjectural statement between two or more variables). All scientists including psychologists are engaged in studying the relations among variables. Then, what is a variable? A **variable** is anything that varies; it is anything that can take at least two values. A variable which takes only one value is a **constant**. A physicist relates heat to expansion of bodies. Here amount of heat is one variable (independent variable) and the amount of expansion is another variable (dependent variable). A psychologist may be interested in relating intelligence to school achievement. Here intelligence and school achievement are variables. One important issue in psychological studies is the measurement of variables. For example, how to measure intelligence and school achievement? For purposes of measurement, psychologists provide operational definitions to the variables. The **operational definition** is one where the variable is translated into a set of operations that can be observed and measured. For example, intelligence may operationally be defined as the number of arithmetic, verbal or spatial problems one solves, and school achievement in terms of the marks one obtains in the final examination. Variables are classified into several categories such as independent variables, dependent variables, stimulus variables, response variables, continuous variables, discrete variables, dichotomous variables and organismic variables and so forth. You will know about them later in this chapter.

Measuring Variables

Measurement is the heart of science and psychologists engage in measuring behavioral variables in several ways. Although measurement of psychological concepts is very difficult, psychologists have designed highly complex techniques to measure the behavior of living organisms. Some hard-headed scientists even make fun of psychological measurements. However, psychology has in its arsenal several special ways of measurement. Psychologists measure behavior through direct observation, self-reports of the participants and reports of others about the participants. They make use of psychological tests, physiological measures and questionnaires to gather information about people. Administering psychological tests is one of the straightforward methods of gathering useful information from subjects. The tests are important research tools in contemporary psychology. There are tests to measure abilities, aptitudes, interests, attitudes, values, personality traits and several other variables. A test is a standardized tool designed to measure objectively one or more aspects of total personality by means of samples of verbal or nonverbal responses. We can collect large amounts of information about people with less effort through tests. A careful analysis of test data relates variations in test scores to variations among people. The accuracy of the information gathered from self-reports and questionnaires are often doubtful. But psychologists make use of ingenious statistical procedures to estimate the reliability and validity of the data obtained from self-reports, reports of informants, questionnaires and psychological tests.

TYPES OF RESEARCH

Psychological research can be broadly divided into three categories such as descriptive research, correlational research and experimental research. The type of research method one uses depends on the problem that is being investigated.

Descriptive Research

Descriptive research is often called non-experimental research. The objective here is to observe behavior of subjects in their natural setting. Description of phenomena is the major goal of all sciences. Observation of animal and human behavior as it occurs in the natural settings provides useful information, which can be employed to test hypothesis. Careful observation helps to delineate variables and the potential relationships among them, which can be tested later experimentally. Naturalistic observation, survey research and case study are the major methodologies of descriptive research.

Naturalistic Observation

Observation of activities of human beings or animals in the natural environment can be a rich source of information for behavior scientists. Here, the researcher simply observes some naturally occurring behavior without intervening in the situation. In **naturalistic observation**, the researcher remains a passive observer and does not engage in controlling or manipulating any variable as it is done in experimental research. He/She simply records the behavior as it occurs. For example, one may observe the mating behavior of animals in the forest, the behavior of school children in the playground, shoppers in a mall, factory workers in the assembly line, behavior of college students in a classroom, participants in a court proceeding, people who are watching a film or a cricket match. The well-known Swiss psychologist Jean Piaget propounded a very influential theory of cognitive development by observing children, especially his own children.

Making an observation in the natural environment is not an easy task. Although unintended, the mere act of observing may disturb the behavior of the participants. In order to avoid this difficulty, the researchers may make unobtrusive observation. For example, one may make use of a one-way mirror to observe children's social behavior in a nursery school. Often, it is not easy to remain hidden. Therefore, it is better to habituate the participants to the presence of the observer. Habituation involves gradually introducing the observer to the environment. Eventually, the participants may take the presence of the observer as normal and may ignore his or her presence. Investigators who engage in naturalistic observation must be given special training to simply observe and record what is happening. Otherwise, there is the danger of their substituting anecdotes for genuine behavior or interpreting behavior instead of simply describing it. Every effort must be made to avoid the tendency toward anthropomorphism—interpreting animal behavior from a human angle.

Naturalistic observation has its advantages as well as disadvantages. On the positive side, the observations made here are genuine, devoid of the artificiality of the laboratory setting. However, because observations made are descriptive, one cannot establish causal relationships between behavioral components. Further, naturalistic observation is time consuming. Often, the observer may have to travel long distances in difficult terrain, especially when observing animal behavior.

Survey Research

The best possible way of finding out what people think, feel and act is to ask them. That is exactly, what is done in **survey research**. Surveys are a widely used research technique. Surveys are conducted to determine political opinions, religious beliefs, consumer preferences, health care needs, social attitudes and several such behaviors. The first step in the survey is the designing of a questionnaire or writing unambiguous questions to be asked. The second step is the selection of a proper sample. Both these—designing a questionnaire and selecting a representative sample—are technical matters and have to be made according to established procedures. A questionnaire is more than just a collection of questions. Constructing questionnaire involves more than sitting down and writing a set of items. It involves several steps including assessing its **reliability** and **validity**. Sampling the subjects of study is a crucial task in survey research. Because the results of the survey are to be generalized to a large group of people (population), care must be taken to see that the sample represents the population. Biased samples lead to incorrect conclusions. Sampling techniques include **simple random sampling** and **stratified random sampling**. The sample should be large enough to be representative of the population. When the questionnaire and the sample are ready, the next step is to administer the questionnaire, which can be done in several ways. The people may be seen personally or contacted by phone or they are sent questionnaires by post. Questionnaire may also be delivered via e-mail or posted on the internet. After collecting the data, appropriate statistical methods may be used to analyze the data; the results must be interpreted carefully and reported accurately.

Study of attitudes is an important research area of social psychology and attitude scale construction has been a specialized task. Pioneers in social psychology such as LL Thurstone, Likert, Bogardus and several others have developed special techniques to survey social attitudes. During 1940 to 1950, American biologist Alfred Kinsey conducted a survey of sexual behavior patterns among American men and women, which is considered a classic study in that field. Modern political opinion polls have used survey research to predict the outcome of elections accurately and also to determine the popularity or otherwise of political leaders.

There are several drawbacks in survey research. People may not want to give information; they may give wrong information; sometimes, they may give information they think the researcher wants to hear or the opposite of it. Finally, not everyone you approach will fill in the questionnaire and return it. Survey data cannot be used to draw conclusions about cause and effect. In spite of limitations, surveys provide data that can be used to formulate or test a hypothesis.

Case Study

Case study is an in-depth, intensive investigation of an individual, a group of people or an event. It is an important non-experimental research methodology that has often led to path-breaking discoveries in science. Sigmund Freud developed his entire system by studying a few cases. Physiologist Paul Broca identified the speech center in the brain using clinical case study. Exhaustive case studies have been undertaken by Henry Murray and his associates at the Harvard Psychological Clinic. Case studies may include interviews, conferences, conversations, observation of behavior and administering psychological tests and questionnaires. Case study is a time honored procedure in medicine and psychiatry. It may often provide basal data for developing a suitable hypothesis for further investigation.

The case study method appears deceptively simple; in fact it is not. Unless the researcher is a well-trained observer, there are possibilities of coming to wrong conclusions. The researcher must be thoroughly familiar with the existing theoretical knowledge of the concerned field. The subjective bias is a constant threat to the objective data gathering. There is the danger that the observer might develop a false sense of certainty about the conclusion arrived at. It is hazardous to generalize the conclusions of one or two case studies to the general population. Because there is no manipulation of independent variables, one cannot determine the causes of behavior observed in the case study. At best, the researcher can speculate about causes.

Correlational Research

The main purpose of scientific research is establishing a relationship among variables. For example, we may need answers to questions such as: Are wealthy people happy? Is intelligence related to academic achievement? How are height and weight related? In answering such questions, researchers try to determine the magnitude of the relationship between wealth and happiness, intelligence and academic achievement, and height and weight using **correlational research.** When we have scores on two variables obtained from the same group of subjects, we can determine the extent of the relationship between the two variables using a statistical measure called **correlation.** Suppose we have measured the heights and weights of 30 college students. Then, we can determine the relationship between height and weight by calculating the **correlation coefficient**. The correlation coefficient called "*r*" varies between *+1.00* and *–1.00*. If the two variables are perfectly related (correlated), that is, the increase in one is associated with an increase in the other, then the *r* will be *+1.00*. On the other hand, if the increase in one is associated with a decrease in the other, then the *r* will be *–1.00*. If there is no relationship between the two variables, then the coefficient will be zero. The degree of relationship is indicated by the extent to which the value of *r* approaches *1.00* plus or minus. So, if the *r* is *+0.50*, there is a good relation between height and weight; if it is *+0.20* or less, the two are not well related and if it is zero, then it means that the two are not related at all.

One of the advantages of correlation is that if we know the correlation between two variables, say x and y and the value of x, then we can predict the value of y. Another important thing to be remembered is that correlation does not imply causation. Just because x and y are correlated, we cannot say x causes y or vice versa. There may or may not be a causal relationship. The two variables simply co-exist and co-vary. Causal relationship can be established by experimental research. However, correlation is an important statistic and is extensively used by psychologists. The most often used correlation coefficient r is called Pearson product-moment correlation, named after the British statistician, Karl Pearson who propounded it. There are various other varieties of correlation, all of them derived from the basic product-moment correlation, such as Spearman rank difference correlation, tetrachoric correlation, biserial correlation, point biserial correlation and phi coefficient. In addition, there are two other types called multiple correlation and partial correlation. It is necessary that a student of psychology is familiar with the various types of correlation coefficients.

Although correlational research does not help establish a causal relationship between variables, it offers several other benefits. One is that it can help establish whether the relationships observed in the study can be generalized to the outside world. Secondly, correlational research indicates to relationships that can be later studied experimentally. Thirdly, when it is unethical to manipulate a variable experimentally, correlational research becomes very handy. Finally, correlational data allow us to make predictions. In fact, correlational research has led to the growth of a thrilling branch of psychometrics called factor analysis, which has helped psychologists to determine the factors that constitute intelligence, personality and several other psychological concepts.

Experimental Research

In experimental research, the primary focus is upon establishing cause and effect relationship among variables. Certain variables are controlled or manipulated and their effects on some other variables are examined. In an experiment, the conditions required to study a problem are created by the experimenter, who deliberately makes a change in those conditions in order to observe the effects of change. The change that is deliberately made in a condition is called experimental manipulation. The variable, which is selected and manipulated by the experimenter for the purpose of producing the observable changes in some aspect of behavior is called the **independent variable (IV)**. The behavior that is expected to change as a result of experimental manipulation of the independent variable is called the **dependent variable (DV)**. In all experiments, there is at least one IV and one DV. A research hypothesis predicts how a DV depends on the manipulation of the IV. The most important first step in any research is the restatement of the hypothesis in a way that will permit it to be tested. Here comes the importance of defining variables operationally. The variables are defined in such a way that they can be observed and measured.

Let us illustrate the steps involved in experimental research with a fictitious example. Suppose a pharmaceutical company has developed a drug that is believed to improve the memory power of college students and wants to ascertain whether the drug produces the claimed change. A psychologist is recruited to study the effect of the drug. Let us say the drug is named Memorex. How does the psychologist proceed to establish the claimed effect of the drug? Now, the first thing one must be clear about is the problem, the research question. Here, the question before the researcher is: Does Memorex improve memory? The next step is to frame the question in the form of a hypothesis. It can be stated in one of two ways:

1. Memorex does not improve memory. In research parlance this is called a **null hypothesis** or hypothesis of no difference.
2. Memorex improves memory; this is called the research hypothesis or simply the alternative hypothesis.

Here, the independent variable is the drug which may systematically be varied by the experimenter; that is, the experimenter administers the drug or does not administer the drug or administers a *placebo*. It means that the researcher varies the independent variable in three ways. These are called experimental treatments. The dependent variable in the experiment is memory, which the researcher has to measure in some way. He must choose, among various measures of memory, one that is convenient. Let us say he chooses memorizing of nonsense syllables as the measure of memory (nonsense syllables are extensively used in psychological experiments to study memory). These are ordinarily groups of three letters that do not convey any meaning; for example, MEB, DEV, KUD, etc. These nonsense syllables are presented to a learner using a memory drum—an apparatus that exposes the material to the subject (the learner) systematically for a specified duration. The number of trials the subject requires to learn a list of (say, 15) nonsense syllables is determined. After some lapse of time (say, 48 hours) the subject is tested again with the same list and the number of trials taken is recorded. Suppose the learner took 12 trials in the first testing and took 6 trials in the second session, we can easily determine the memory power using the formula 6/12 multiplied by 100, which is actually 50; that is, after 48 hours, the learner has saved 50 percent of the material. This way the researcher operationalizes memory power.

When these preliminary activities are decided, the investigator chooses a research design that is suitable for his problem. A research design is simply a plan of action for solving the problem. There are several of them out of which one that is suitable is chosen. Let us say that our researcher has chosen the following design. He selects at random three groups of college students. The first group of subjects is administered Memorex and their memory is tested as detailed above. This group is called the **experimental group**. The second group is not administered Memorex and their memory is tested. This is called the **control group**. The third group is given a *placebo*—a pill that looks like Memorex, but actually is an inert substance that has no effect whatever. This is a second control group (often called *placebo* group). Now, if the average memory score of the first group is substantially higher than those of the two control groups, it can be concluded that the drug in fact has improved memory; that is, it has produced the desired effect. If the researcher has put up a null hypothesis, he rejects it. On the other hand, if he had put up research hypothesis, he accepts it.

Selection of Subjects

Before we go further, some other important points must be made clear. The first one is regarding the selection of subjects. We said in the beginning that the subjects were selected at random. What does it mean? Remember that our researcher wants to study the effect of the drug on college students. He cannot study all college students. The number of college students available to him is called the **population**. A subset of the population, called **sample**, has to be drawn from the population for the study. And this sample must be representative of the population. Only then, it is possible to draw valid conclusions about a population after studying a sample. This can be achieved by drawing a random sample. A **random sample** is one that reflects the important characteristics of the population. Sampling theory is a branch of statistics. We need not worry about it here. For our purpose, it is enough to know how a simple random sample is selected. A random sample is one in which every member of the population has an equal opportunity of being selected to participate in the study. The simplest way of obtaining a random sample is to assign serial numbers to all the available members, write the numbers on slips of papers, put them into a box, shuffle well and draw the numbers one at a time, till we get the required number for the sample. An important thing here is to put back the slip back into the box before picking the next slip. This is called **sampling with replacement**. Sampling without replacement will not yield a random sample. Let us say our researcher has drawn three samples following the same procedure.

The second point to understand is why a second control group (the *placebo* group) was used. This was done to control an extraneous variable. You see, sometimes the mere fact of knowing that one is taking a drug—not the effect of the drug—may produce a change in behavior. Therefore, the members of the second control group take a pill that looks like the drug administered to the experimental group, but actually, it is an inert substance. This procedure rules out the effect of the knowledge factor (an extraneous variable) on behavior change.

The third point is that the groups must be tested under similar conditions. This means that the researcher has to control the effect of extraneous variables. The **extraneous variables** are those variables that may affect the behavior you are investigating, the effects in which you are not interested. Our researcher for example has already controlled one extraneous variable—the effect of the knowledge that one has taken a drug—by using the *placebo* group. The other extraneous variables may be the time of the day when the test is administered, the experimental set up, the apparatus used, the way instructions are given, the sex of the experimenter, the **experimenter bias**, and so forth. To identify a causal relationship between IV and DV, the effect of extraneous variables must be controlled. One way of controlling them is to hold them constant for all the subjects. If these variables do not vary over the course of your experiment, they cannot cause uncontrolled variation in your dependent variable.

The last step refers to the magnitude of the average difference that must show up to conclude that the IV has in fact produced a significant effect in the DV and that the difference is not a chance difference. This can be done by testing the significance of difference between the means using one of the measures from inferential statistics. A ***F-test*** or ***t-test*** is used for this purpose. You will know about these tests when you undertake psychological research. We close this section by drawing your attention to three crucial processes involved in the experimental method. First, it should be possible to manipulate at least one independent variable. Second, it should be possible to measure the changes in the dependent variable as objectively as possible. Third, it should be possible to control the extraneous variables. Any true experiment should satisfy these three conditions.

Strengths and Limitations of Experimental Research

The strength of experimental research is that it enables us to identify and describe causal relationships. Correlational research does not share this ability. In spite of this power, experimental research suffers from certain handicaps. An important limitation of experimental research is that you are not permitted to manipulate certain independent variables. Suppose you are interested in establishing the causal relationship between stress and heart attack. You cannot vary the amount of stress to determine the level at which it triggers an attack. You cannot do it; it is unethical. The second limitation pertains to control of extraneous variables. By controlling all extraneous variables, you create an artificial condition, an unnatural environment. As a consequence, you cannot generalize your experimental conclusions to real life situations where all these extraneous variables are operating.

RESEARCH SETTINGS

Researches are conducted either in the laboratory or in a field setting. The setting (one chooses) depends on the nature of the problem, the convenience, costs and ethical considerations. The term laboratory here is used in a broad sense. It need not have to be a specially designed room with several equipments. It can be a formal laboratory, a classroom, a room in the library or a corner of the union building. In contrast, the field experiment is conducted in the natural setting where the behavior occurs.

Laboratory Setting

Laboratory is an ideal place to conduct an experiment. An experiment by definition is observation under controlled conditions. It is easy to control the extraneous variables and manipulate the independent variable in a laboratory. Complete control over all extraneous variables may not be possible even in a laboratory, but still laboratory affords more control over the research situation than does the field setting. Unfortunately, controlling all the extraneous variables makes the laboratory situation artificial, thus making it difficult to generalize the results outside the laboratory. If it is essential to control all the extraneous variables and still not lose the generalizability, one may consider using simulation. In **simulation**, the researcher re-creates (as closely as possible) a real world situation in the laboratory. Researchers choose simulation when it is unethical to study in the real world. For example, if you are interested in studying how juries make decisions in court, you cannot stealthily overhear their conversation. Instead you can conduct a jury simulation study and analyze the deliberations of the simulated juries. Carefully designed and executed simulation increases the chances of generalizing results in the real world.

Field Setting

As you have seen, experiments afford an opportunity to make observations under controlled conditions. However, in gaining control over variables you lose a degree of generality of the results. Also, there is a lack of realism in laboratory work. In order to obviate these limitations, some investigators employ a field setting to conduct their research. A field experiment is one that is conducted outside the laboratory in the participants' natural environment (the field). It is just like a laboratory experiment except that it is conducted outside the laboratory. In field experiment also the investigator manipulates the independent variable systematically and measures the dependent variable.

Let us examine a field experiment conducted to support the Schachter-Singer cognitive theory of emotion. The authors of the theory had demonstrated with a laboratory experiment that human emotions were jointly determined by a non-specific kind of physiological arousal and its interpretation based on environmental cues (see chapter 10). Supporting evidence to the theory was offered by an imaginative and interesting field study conducted by Dutton & Aron (1974). The investigators posted a young and attractive college-aged woman at the end of a swaying, 450-foot suspension bridge across a deep canyon. The pretty woman posed as though she was conducting a survey and asked the men who were crossing the bridge a series of questions. She told the men that, if they were interested in the results of the survey, they could contact her over the phone after a week and gave them her phone number. In another condition, an attractive young woman stood at the end of a strong bridge built across a shallow stream 10 feet below and asked the men who were crossing the bridge similar questions, and also gave her phone number.

Surprisingly, there were big differences in the nature of responses the men gave under the two conditions. The men who had crossed the dangerous bridge showed enormous interest in ringing the woman for information, while not many from the second condition evinced any interest in the event. The interpretation of the results was as follows: the men who crossed the dangerous bridge were highly physiologically aroused and were searching for a reason for their arousal. When they saw the attractive woman, the arousal was attributed to her presence. In short, they interpreted the emotion as sex-related. In fact, in answering the survey questions, they had exhibited a good deal of sexual imagery. No such things were observed in the reactions of the men crossing the stable bridge over the shallow stream because there was no heightened arousal and need to interpret it. Consistent with the Schachter-Singer theory, the members of the first group were labeling their arousal based on environmental cues.

The field experiment mentioned above has all the features of a true experiment: the independent variable (arousal level) was systematically manipulated; the dependent variable (labeling of the emotion) was measured and causal relation was established. Because field experiments are conducted in the real world, the results can be easily generalized to the real world.

INTERNAL AND EXTERNAL VALIDITY

Whatever the general design of research, experimental or non-experimental, the researcher must carefully focus on two important attributes in the study: internal and external validity. **Internal validity** refers to the ability of the research design to test the hypothesis adequately. In an experiment, it means demonstrating that variation in the independent variable has actually caused the observed changes in the dependent variable. In correlational research, it means showing changes in the value of the first variable relate solely to changes in the values of the second variable and not to changes in other extraneous variables that may have varied with the first variable. Results from experimental designs, low in internal validity, are likely to be unreliable. A serious threat to internal validity comes from confounding. **Confounding** exists in a design when two variables are linked in such a way that the effects of one cannot be separated from the effects of the other. **External validity** is the ability of a research design to produce results that apply beyond the sample and the situation within which the data were collected. That is, would the results be similar with other types of participants (children, adults, elderly people) and with different tasks (learning music, sports, etc.)? Results from designs low in external validity have little generality when applied directly to real world situations. Confounding variables occur in both experimental and correlational designs, but they are far more likely to be a problem in the latter, in which strict control over extraneous variables is usually lacking. Researchers have identified several sources of confounding that may affect internal and external validities.

Apart from confounding variable, there are several other factors that threaten internal validity. One of them is **demand characteristics**. The cues offered by the investigator (consciously or unconsciously) to the subjects about the problem, hypothesis or the purpose of the experiment and what the participants think is expected of them during the experiment are called demand characteristics. The human participant in any study does not passively respond to what the researcher has created. The participant assesses the researcher and experimental situation. Based on the assessment, he/she draws inferences about what the experiment is about. The participants may pay attention to certain cues, and form hypotheses that are irrelevant to the experiment at hand and begin to behave in a manner consistent with those hypotheses. Obviously, this vitiates the results. A researcher must be aware of demand characteristics and take steps to avoid them or at least to decrease their impact.

Another threat to internal validity comes from the experimenter himself. This problem has been studied extensively by Rosenthal (1976) under the title **experimenter bias**. When the behavior of the researcher influences the results of the experiment, experimenter bias is operating. Experimenter bias stems from two sources: **expectancy effects** and uneven treatment of subjects across the experiment. When the experimenter has preconceived ideas about the capacities of the participants, expectancy effects emerge. For example, if the experimenter believes that the subjects are incapable of learning, he may treat them in such a way as to have that expectation fulfilled. This phenomenon is often called **self-fulfilling prophesy** or Rosenthal effect. The experimenter expectancy effects can be minimized by using the **double blind procedure**, in which both the participants and experimenter are kept blind as to which experimental condition the participant is in.

External validity can be determined by replication of the experiment. **Replication** is the act of repeating a study to find out whether the original findings can be duplicated when conducted on different participants and different tasks. For example, the classical studies conducted by Darley & Latané (1968) on helping behavior were replicated successfully in Canada, Israel, Japan and the United States (see Chapter 12) using different situations and different participants. Often cross-cultural replications are undertaken to see the extent of generalizability. If later studies consistently fail to replicate the original results of earlier studies, it can be safely said that the results of the original study may have been flawed or the finding was a fluke.

Although it is necessary to achieve a high degree of both internal and external validity in research, in practice it is noticed that steps taken to increase one type of validity tend to decrease the other. For example, a tightly controlled laboratory experiment may exhibit high degree of internal validity, but its results may not generalize to other samples and situations (external validity is reduced). One may have to bring about a compromise on the relative amounts of internal and external validity in research. In basic research, the emphasis is more on internal validity, whereas in applied research the emphasis is relatively more on external validity. These issues must be carefully considered at the time of designing research.

EX POST FACTO RESEARCH

Two basic requirements of a true experiment are that the participants are assigned randomly to experimental and control groups and the independent variable is systematically varied. But in actual practice, it is not always possible or even desirable to achieve these two conditions. There are several instances, when we have to study the effect of an independent variable that has already occurred. Under such circumstances, the researchers use **ex post facto research**. Kerlinger (1973) defines *ex post facto* research as "systematic empirical enquiry in which the scientist does not have direct control of independent variables because their manifestations have already occurred or because they are inherently not manipulable. Inferences about relations among variables are made, without direct interventions, from concomitant variation of independent and dependent variables."

Suppose you are interested in the relation between gender and aggressiveness in children. You can measure aggressiveness of a sample of boys and girls and test the significance of the difference between the means of the two sexes. Suppose the mean of boys is significantly higher than the mean of girls, then, you conclude that boys are more aggressive than girls. Your conclusion may or may not be valid. Of course there is the relationship between sex and aggression. This evidence is not sufficient to draw such a conclusion. The real question is: Is the demonstrated relationship really, between sex and aggression? Since many other variables are correlated with sex, it might have been one or more of these variables that produced the difference between the aggressiveness scores of the two sexes. Note, in the above illustration, the independent variable (sex) is not manipulated (it cannot be manipulated), and the subjects are not randomly assigned. The subjects assign themselves to groups on the basis of characteristics other than those in which the investigator is interested. The subjects and treatments come, as it were, already assigned to the groups.

The *ex post facto* procedures have three major weaknesses:

1. The inability to manipulate independent variables.
2. The lack of power to randomize either the subjects or the treatments.
3. The risk of improper interpretation because of confounding.

Ex post facto research is an instance of correlation research in which it is not possible to establish causal relationship between variables. In spite of the inherent weaknesses, a large proportion of research in anthropology, sociology, education and political science has been *ex post facto*. Even in psychology, a substantial portion of studies, perhaps half or more than half, are *ex post facto*. For example, a path-breaking research in the field of personality, "The Authoritarian Personality study," undertaken by Adorno and colleagues in Stanford University was basically *ex post facto*.

There is a great deal more to psychological research than what is presented briefly here. There are several do's and don'ts. You need not worry about the details, unless you are planning to engage in research. For now, it is enough to know briefly how psychological research is undertaken. But, before ending the chapter, it is necessary to familiarize with the statistical procedures used in the analysis and interpretation of data and to take note of certain ethical principles that are followed in psychological research.

STATISTICAL METHODS IN RESEARCH

Psychological research often involves collection of a large number of measurements. It is difficult to make much sense out of the data (information collected) by looking at the individual score of each participant. The data have to be organized and summarized. For this purpose, psychological researchers make use of **statistics**. Statistics is a branch of mathematics, which deals with collecting, classifying and analyzing data. Psychologists make extensive use of two areas of statistics: descriptive statistics and inferential statistics. **Descriptive statistics** deals with methods used to describe, organize and summarize data using **measures of central tendency**, **measures of variability** (also called **measures of dispersion**) and measures of correlation. **Inferential statistics** include procedures used to make inferences about the population from sample data, based on the principles of probability theory. Let us briefly familiarize with these two areas of statistics.

Descriptive Statistics

Measures of Central Tendency

The best known measures of central tendency are mean, median and mode. The mean is the arithmetical average of a set of scores. It is obtained by calculating the sum of the scores and dividing by the number of scores (the number of scores is generally indicated by the letter N). The median is the middle most score when the scores are arranged in the increasing order. The mode is the most frequent score in the distribution of scores. Let us say a teacher has conducted a language test on a group of 20 students, 10 boys and 10 girls. The obtained scores for the students and the calculation of mean, median and mode is shown below.

The formula for calculating mean is:

$$M = \bar{X} = \frac{\sum X}{N}$$

Scores of boys: 3, 3, 4, 4, 5, 5, 5, 6, 7, 8.
Mean = 50/10 = 5.
Scores of girls: 2, 3, 4, 5, 5, 6, 7, 8, 0, 10.
Mean = 50/10 = 5.
Median for boys: (5 + 5)/2 = 5 (midpoint of two middle score is divided by 2).
Median for girls: (5 + 6)/2 = 5.5.
Mode for boys: 5.
Mode for girls: 5.

The mean and other measures of central tendency summarize the data. They are the representatives of the scores. The scores generally cluster around these values. The most often used measure of central tendency in research is the mean. Although the mean is an excellent summary of the data, it can be misleading. For example, the means for boys and the girls are the same (5). Are there no differences between the two sets of scores? The scores of boys are more homogenous than those of girls. The girls' scores vary relatively more than that of boys. To know the extent of variation among the scores we calculate the measures of variability or measures of dispersion.

Measures of Variability

The measures of variability tell us the extent to which the scores differ from one another. There are four measures of variability, namely, the **range**, the **quartile deviation (QD)**, the average deviation (AD) and the **standard deviation (SD)**. The range is the difference between the highest and the lowest values in the distribution of scores. So, for boys the range is 8 – 3 = 5. For girls, it is 10 – 2 = 8. The variability is more for girls than boys. The range thus gives a rough idea of the spread of scores. The standard deviation is the most often used measure of dispersion in research. It is calculated by:

1. Finding the deviation (difference) of each score from the mean.
2. Squaring those deviations.
3. Finding the mean of the squared deviations.
4. Finding the square root of the resulting value.

Let us see how SD is calculated from the scores of boys in the example above. The formula for calculating the standard deviation is:

$$SD = \sigma = \sqrt{\frac{\Sigma x^2}{N}}$$

where, x = X – M (X = score and M = mean).

Deviations (x): 3 – 5 = –2; 3 – 5 = – 2; 4 – 5 = –1; 4 – 5 = –1; 5 – 5 = 0; 5 – 5 = 0; 5 – 5 = 0; 6 – 5 = 1; 7 – 5 = 2; 8 – 5 = 3.

Sum of squared deviations (x's) divided by N: 4 + 4 + 1 + 1 + 0 + 0 + 0 + 1 + 4 + 9 = 24/10 = 2.4.

SD = Square root of 2.4 = 1.549.

The SD for girls = 2.302 (you calculate the SD for girls).

You see the two values are different indicating the variability of scores. Whether these two values are significantly different is another matter, which is to be decided by inferential statistics.

Inferential Statistics

Inferential statistics are based on the laws of probability. Researchers use these to decide whether the difference between observations can be attributed to chance or to some other factor (experimental treatment). For example, whether the difference between the two SD's (or the lack of difference between the two means) above is due to chance or is it true difference can be decided by using inferential statistics. These are also used to decide whether the data obtained from a sample are representative of some larger population. The details of these are beyond the scope of this chapter and therefore, we will not proceed further to discuss them. But if you find the chance probability is extremely low, then your findings can be considered statistically significant. In most psychological studies, the probability that an outcome is due to chance must be lower than 0.05 (5%) for the outcome to be accepted as statistically significant.

ETHICAL PRINCIPLES IN RESEARCH

Since psychological experiments are conducted on living beings, there are possibilities that the participants (subjects) are exposed to painful or embarrassing conditions. Often, the subjects are not informed about the real purpose of the study or they are misinformed. In order to avoid any endangering predicaments to the subjects, the American Psychological Association (APA) issued a set of guidelines to researchers in 1953, which is being revised from time to time. The recent revision, published in 2002, has suggested the following ethical principles to be followed by all researchers.

Summary of 2002 APA Ethical Principles

1. The participants must be protected from all sorts of physical or psychological harm.
2. The participants' right to privacy regarding their behavior should be safeguarded.
3. The participants must be assured that their participation in research is completely voluntary and they are free to terminate it at any time.

4. The participants must necessarily be informed about the nature of the experiment prior to their participation in it.
5. Reasonable efforts must be made to avoid offering excessive or inappropriate financial and other inducements for research participation.
6. Deception shall be used only when it is essential and with the approval of an authorized institutional review board.

The most important ethical principle followed by all psychological researchers is **informed consent**. That is, prior to participating in an experiment, the participants sign a document affirming that they have been told about the basic nature of the investigation and are aware of what their participation will involve. Furthermore, the participants are given a **debriefing** immediately after the experiment. It means that the participants receive an explanation for the study and the procedures involved when the deception was used. However, informed consent and debriefing are not required when the experiments involve minimal risk.

Chapter Summary

Psychology is a science. In people's minds, the term science has an aura around it. There is no need for such a hallowed outlook toward science. Many persons, both layman and scientists alike, doubt whether psychology is a science at all because of its lack of precision in its procedures and lack of generalizability of its principles. In fact, what makes a given discipline a science has little to do with the definitiveness of its findings or the precision of its laws. It rests upon whether the practitioners adhere to the accepted canons of the scientific method. Psychology is a science because it follows scientific procedures in studying human behavior and experience.

Scientific method has certain established steps that are followed by all scientists. Broadly, research starts with a well-defined problem in the context of a theory. The second step is to formulate a hypothesis, which is a tentative answer to the problem. Then a definite procedure is determined to test the hypothesis. The next step is to collect the data which are analyzed to see whether it supports the hypothesis or rejects it. The final step is to incorporate the findings into the theory and make modifications in the theory, if necessary, in the light of the new findings.

In this chapter, you have learnt about the various research methods that psychologists use. Generally, the methods include case study, the survey method, naturalistic observation, the correlation method and the experimental method. In the case study, the researcher interviews or observes an individual or a group. The survey method involves interviewing or administration of questionnaires to obtain information from a sample of subjects. In the naturalistic observation, the researcher observes behavior where it occurs naturally. In correlational studies statistical procedures are used to determine the existing relationship between variables. In the experimental method, the researcher manipulates one or more independent variables and observes their effects on one or more dependent variables. Experiments are conducted to establish cause and effect relationships between independent and dependent variables. Experiments may be conducted in the field setting or in the laboratory. Often the manipulation of variable is not possible. Under such conditions, the researcher follows the correlational method. Correlation does not imply causation. It only tells that the variables are related. On several occasions, researchers study the effect of a variable after it has already occurred. For example, one may be interested in the behavior of people after a fire or flood has occurred. Such procedures are called *ex post facto* research.

Statistics is an essential tool in behavioral research. Psychologists use two types of statistical procedures: descriptive statistics and inferential statistics. Descriptive statistics are used to summarize the characteristics of the data. Measures of central tendency such as the mean or median are used to identify the typical score in a distribution and the measures of variability such as range or standard deviation are used to determine the dispersion of scores in the distribution. Inferential statistics are based on the laws of probability and these allow the researcher to determine whether his findings reflect a chance occurrence; that is, they help the researcher to know whether the observed differences between two groups are real or are due to chance.

Research psychologists are required to adhere to certain ethical principles while conducting research, whether on humans or animals. They have to protect and promote the dignity of the human subjects. They are precluded from using methods that may harm the participants. In human research, key issues are the use of informed consent, the participant's right to

Contd...

Contd...

privacy, potential risks to participants and the use of deception. Researchers are required to treat the animals humanely and the risks to which they are exposed must be justified by the potential importance of the research.

The purpose of this chapter is not to make you a researcher. Research may not be your cup of tea. It is enough if it helps you to develop a scientific attitude. Such an attitude fosters in you curiosity, skepticism and open-mindedness. You have to develop the habit of asking questions. People around you make all sorts of claims. The media bombards with all sorts of information; it tries to influence you especially through advertisements. You should not fall a prey to propaganda. In each case, you must ask for evidence and find out whether the claims are supported by facts. That means you have a scientific attitude.

3 CHAPTER Biological Foundations of Behavior

PREVIEW

We have seen in the first chapter that psychology has had its roots in philosophy and physiology. Philosophers discussed extensively about the structure and functions of the mind and physiologists studied the anatomy and physiology of the body and its parts. It is unfortunate that the early thinkers considered the body and mind as two independent entities and studied them separately. Today, people think of the whole organism, not its body or mind. They believe that it is not possible to think of mind without the body or the body without mind. It is often said that the concept of body or of mind is only an academic abstraction. One cannot exist without the other and the two are systemically related. Today, there is a growing tendency to look upon the individual as an organized system who should not be analyzed into body and mind. Body and mind are the two sides of the same coin. In spite of all this talk, the fact remains that the exact nature of the relationship between body and mind is still an unsettled issue. We need not go very deep into the mind-body relationship. Whatever be the relationship between body and mind, there is research evidence to show that many of our behaviors arise from the activities of the brain—not just mundane things such as breathing, heart rate, temperature and coordinated movements of the body, but also our inner thoughts and intimate feelings as well. Every time you think, act or feel, the activities in your brain play crucial, if not primary role. It is believed that psychological disorders such as schizophrenia or depression have their roots in the functioning of the brain. There are glaring instances in which brain impairment has produced psychological disturbances as is seen in the case of organic mental syndromes such as delirium, senile dementia and Alzheimer's disease. Therefore, it is necessary for every psychology student to have an understanding of how physiology influences psychological activities. Try to remember (in chapter one) what Johannes Müller, the father of physiology, said with regard to the relation between physiology and psychology: "One cannot be psychologist without being a physiologist."

In this chapter, we discuss certain structures and functions of the body, especially the brain, the nervous system and the endocrine system so far as they are related to psychological functions. The human brain is regarded as the most remarkable feat of engineering ever achieved. Brain is a living super-computer, which is far more elegant than any machine that a modern scientist could hope to create. In fact, it may be wrong to compare the brain to a computer. However, complicated computer may be, it is after all the creation of the human brain. You should not equate the creator with his or her creation. The human brain, along with the rest of the nervous system, provides solutions to the problems created by the constantly changing and sometimes hostile environment, both physical and social.

You have learned that psychologists who are interested in the study of the biological bases of behavior and mental processes are called physiological psychologists, biopsychologists, or psychobiologists. The new name to this branch of knowledge is behavioral neuroscience. Without going into the details of neuroscience, we shall study in this chapter, the structure and working of the basic units of the nervous system, the nerve cell or neuron. We then examine the workings of the two major divisions of the nervous system: the central nervous system comprised of the brain and the spinal cord and the peripheral nervous system, which connects the central nervous system to various parts of the body such as sense organs, muscles and glands. Of special interest to psychologists is that branch of the peripheral system called autonomous nervous system. We will also discuss elements of endocrinology and genetics. As you read through the book, you will realize how important the knowledge of biology is in understanding human behavior, thought, feeling and motivation.

Chapter Outline

The human organism is a psychophysical system. The psychical and the physical part of the system cannot be separated. Body and mind are two sides of the same coin; one cannot exist without the other; separating them is merely academic. Philosophers have always been discussing the way in which body and mind are related and have offered several theories about the relationship between the two. Some of them advocated that only body exists. Others said only mind exists. Another group asserted that both exist. Among the latter group, some said that body and mind interact and others proposed that they run in parallel course without interacting. Still another group of philosophers said that the two are aspects of the same phenomenon. There is a joke about mind-body relationship. It appears that after listening to a series of lengthy lectures from a learned teacher on mind-body relationship, one student stood up and asked: Sir, "What is mind?" The teacher replied: "No body!" Then, the student asked "What is a body?" The teacher replied "Never mind!" Although humorous, the conversation throws some light on the present state of mind-body relationship. However, the fact remains that psychology and physiology are intimately related. Therefore, it is necessary that a student of psychology is acquainted with elementary physiology, especially with the area pertaining to brain and nervous system. The brain and the nervous system control our behavior—our movements, hopes, aspirations, emotions, perceptions, learning—and the very awareness that we are human beings. Because of its importance, an interdisciplinary science called neuroscience has emerged in recent years. As a group, neuroscientists include neurologists, zoologists, medical experts, computer scientists and psychologists. Psychologists who study the biological structures and functions underlying behavior are often called biopsychologists, behavioral neuroscientists or physiological psychologists.

Several aspects of behavior and experience cannot be understood without the knowledge of biological processes underlying them. Our nervous system, sense organs, endocrine system, and muscles help us to understand and adjust to our environment. Our understanding (perception) depends on sensory reception of the stimulus and its interpretation by the brain. Large chunks of our behavior are triggered by needs such as hunger, thirst, sex and avoidance of pain; how we walk, talk, think, solve problems and plan our activities are controlled by our brain. Our emotions such as fear, anger, grief and love are mediated by complex neurophysiological functions.

In this chapter, we deal with the biological structures of the body, especially the brain and nervous system that are of interest to biopsychologists. First, we learn about the building blocks of the nervous system called the **neurons**—their structure and functions. Later, we deal with the various subdivisions of the nervous system. Finally, we discuss elements of endocrinology and genetics. As you read through the book, you will realize that our understanding of human behavior cannot be complete without the knowledge of the fundamentals of the brain and the nervous system.

NEURONS

Neurons are the basic units, the building blocks of the nervous system. These are specialized cells, which transmit the nerve impulses throughout the brain and body. It is estimated that there are as many as 100 or even 200 billion neurons in the brain alone (there may be a trillion neurons in the body). Like all other cells of the human body, the neuron has a **cell body**, which contains the **nucleus** (Fig. 3.1). The nucleus contains the inherited substance that determines how the cell functions. All activities of the brain hinge on the working of neurons. There are three types of neurons:

1. **Sensory neurons** that respond to input from the sense organs.

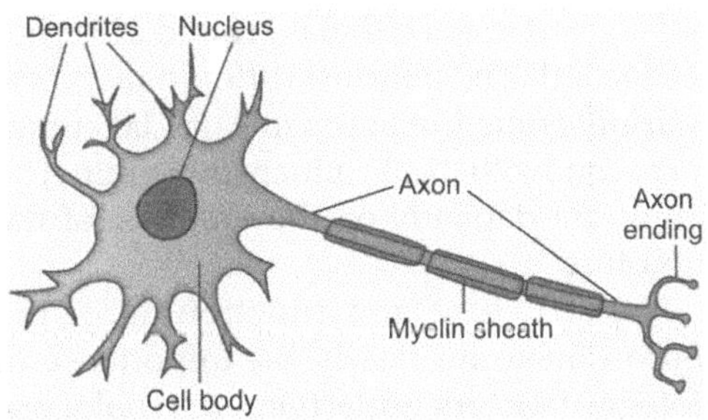

FIGURE 3.1: Neuron

2. **Motor neurons** that send signals to the muscles to control movements.
3. **Interneurons** that are connecting neurons, which stand between sensory and motor neurons.

Most of the neurons in the brain are interneurons and most of them are connected to other interneurons. Interneurons are also called internuncial neurons. As a specialized structure that communicates with other cells, the neuron consists of two more parts: the dendrites and the axon.

Dendrites are short fibers projecting from one side of the cell body. They receive messages from the axons of other neurons. The **axon** is a single, slim, long fiber extending from the other side of the cell body. The axon carries messages to other neurons, muscles and glands. The length of axon varies from a few millimeters to about a meter. Normally, nerve impulses move in one direction only, from dendrites through the cell body and along the axon to the dendrites or the cell body of the next neuron, or to a muscle or gland. A nerve is a bundle of axons belonging to hundreds or thousands of neurons. Although each neuron has only a single axon, most axons divide into small branches called terminals. At the end of the terminals are **terminal buttons** (or boutons or axon endings), little knob-like structures that release certain chemicals called **neurotransmitters** that help in the transmission of messages to other neuronal cells.

Axons have a protective covering called the **myelin sheath**. Myelin sheath serves to increase the velocity with which the nerve impulses travel through the axon and prevent messages from short circuiting with one another. The axons that carry emergency messages generally have the maximum covering of myelin. In certain diseases, such as multiple sclerosis, the myelin sheath degenerates exposing the axon that is normally covered. This condition may produce a kind of short-circuiting causing disturbance in the passage of messages between the brain and muscles, which in turn may give rise to symptoms such as visual disturbances, difficulty in walking and difficulty in muscular coordination.

Generally, nerve impulses move in one direction—from dendrite to the cell body to the axon. But in some instances certain chemicals travel through the neuron in the opposite direction carrying some nourishments (nutrients) to the nucleus. When such movement of chemicals in the reverse direction is disturbed, the neuron may die from starvation causing a disease called **amyotrophic lateral sclerosis (ALS)**. Rabies is also caused by the reverse flow of rabies virus along the axon.

Nerve Impulse

The formation and transmission of nerve impulses are the products of complex electrochemical processes. The thin cell membrane is not equally permeable to different types of electrically charged ions that float in the protoplasm of the cell and the liquid surrounding it. During the resting state of a neuron, the cell membrane keeps out positively charged sodium ions and allows in potassium ions and chloride ions. As a consequence, there is a small electrical potential across the membrane. The inside of the cell is slightly more negative than the outside. This is its **resting potential**. When stimulated, the electrical potential is reduced and the cell membrane allows the sodium ions to enter the cell. Now the outside of the cell membrane is negative with respect to the inside. This change influences adjacent part of the axon, allowing the inflow of sodium ions. This process of quick changes from negative to positive and vice versa along the axon is the nerve impulse. This electrical shift takes just a millisecond (one-thousandth of a second). That is why often a nerve impulse is referred to as a wave of negativity. The nerve impulse is also called **action potential** in contrast to the resting potential. In short, for a neuron to function properly, sodium and potassium ions must enter and leave the membrane at just the right rate. Certain drugs that alter the transit system can decrease or prevent neural transmission.

The action potential obeys an **all-or-none law**. That is, either the action potentials occur at a uniform and maximum intensity or they do not occur at all. Just after the action potential has passed, the neuron cannot be stimulated immediately whatever the strength of the stimulus. It becomes temporarily inactive. This phase is called the **absolute refractory period**. This is followed by a stage when only a very strong stimulus may be required to fire the neuron. This is called the **relative refractory period**. However, with the passage of time, the neuron is ready to be fired. Since, the nerve impulse is generated a new at each stage along the neuron, it does not diminish in size during transmission. In the myelinated fibers, the conduction of nerve impulses is faster. The myelin sheath insulating the fiber is interrupted approximately 2 millimeter by constrictions called *nodes*, where the sheath is thin or absent. Because the nerve impulse jumps from node to node, its velocity is increased. These electrochemical events occur too quickly. There is also variation in the velocity of nerve impulse among neurons; it depends on the diameter of the nerve and thickness of the myelin sheath. The longer and thicker fibers can carry messages at a speed that is around 225 miles per second. The neurons differ in their rate of firing. Some fire at the rate of 1,000 times per second, others at a much lower rate. The firing rate depends on the intensity of the stimulus.

The structure and functioning of the neuron illustrate clearly the importance of biological factors underlying psychological phenomena. Our understanding of the universe around us, how we perceive, learn, remember, think, plan and make decision have been enriched by the discoveries made by neuroscientists about the neuron.

Synaptic Transmission

We have learnt so far how an action potential is conducted within a neuron. But what happens to a nerve impulse when it reaches the terminal point of an axon? How is it transferred to the next neuron? The neurons are not structurally connected; there is a gap between one neuron and the other. How is the gap between the neurons bridged for the transmission of nerve impulse to cross over? The gap between any two neurons is called the *synaptic cleft* (Fig. 3.2). When a nerve impulse comes to the end of a neuron and reaches the end button, the *synaptic vesicles* within the button release a chemical that helps in the transmission. These chemicals called neurotransmitters carry the message across the synaptic cleft to the dendrite of a receiver neuron. The chemical mode of transmission of nerve impulse between neurons is completely different from the way in which transmission takes place within the neuron. The movement of impulses within the neuron is electrical in nature, while it occurs through chemical means between neurons. The neurotransmitters carry messages across the synaptic cleft like a boat carrying passengers across a river.

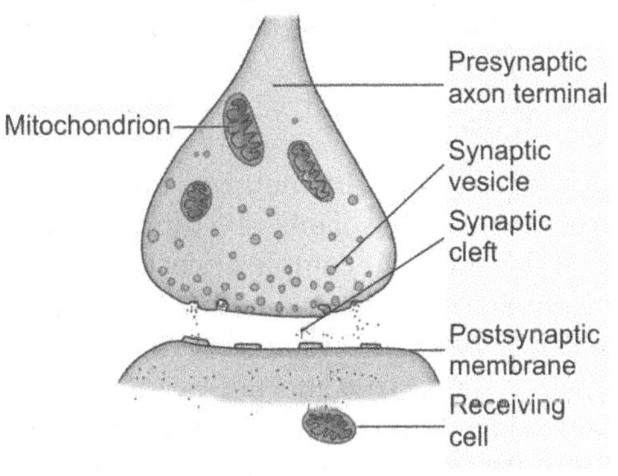

FIGURE 3.2: Synapse

Neurotransmitters

There are a number of neurotransmitters, and not all receiver neurons are capable of using the chemical message carried by a particular neurotransmitter. Each neurotransmitter can fit into a specific site on the receiving neuron. It is only when a neurotransmitter fits into a receptor site (a specific area of the membrane that is sensitive to a specific neurotransmitter) that successful communication is possible. When there is such a fit, the chemical message is delivered. There are two types of messages: excitatory and inhibitory. Excitatory message enables the receiving neuron to fire. Then an action potential will travel down the axon of the receiving neuron. Inhibitory message prevents the likelihood that the receiving neuron will fire.

The effect of neurotransmitters on behavior is tremendous. An abundance or deficit of a neurotransmitter can produce several behavioral problems. So far, some 50 neurotransmitters have been identified. Among them acetylcholine (ACh), norepinephrine (noradrenalin), gamma-aminobutyric acid (GABA), dopamine (DA), serotonin, and endorphin have been extensively studied (Table 3.1).

Acetylcholine (ACh) is found throughout the nervous system. It transmits messages relating to skeletal muscles (controlling all movements). There is growing evidence that ACh is related to memorization processes. It is also believed that decreased production of ACh is related to Alzheimer's disease. **Norepinephrine** is a hormone secreted by the adrenal medulla. It is a catecholamine that functions both like an excitatory and inhibitory neurotransmitter. It is found in some cells in the brainstem and on some sites of the sympathetic nervous system. It is believed to control learning, memory, wakefulness, and eating. Gamma-aminobutyric acid (GABA) is primarily an inhibitory neurotransmitter

Table 3.1: Major Neurotransmitters and Their Functions

Name of neurotransmitter	Major functions	Symptoms and disorders
Acetylcholine (ACh)	Excitatory at synapse, muscle control; memory	Alzheimer disease (shortage), delusions (shortage); convulsions, spasms, tremors (excess)
Dopamine (DA)	Excitatory; involved in emotional arousal, learning, memory, thinking, pain or pleasure, voluntary movement	Parkinson's disease; schizophrenia (excess); depression (shortage); attention deficit and hyperactivity disorder (shortage)
Norepinephrine (NE)	Excitatory and inhibitory; controls learning, memory, eating, wakefulness and dreaming	Depression (shortage); anxiety, panic, headache; schizophrenia (excess) distractibility (shortage)
Epinephrine	Orientation toward stimuli	Depression (shortage); arousal or apprehension (excess)
Serotonin	Inhibitory or excitatory; regulates mood, sleep, eating and arousal	Obsessive-compulsive disorder (excess); insomnia, depression (shortage); lack of motivation (excess)
Gamma-aminobutyric acid (GABA)	Inhibitory in motor system	Anxiety, epilepsy, sluggish, Huntington's disease (shortage) Lack of motivation (excess)
Endorphins	Inhibit transmission of pain impulses	Insensitivity (excess) or hypersensitivity (shortage) to pain

found in the brain and spinal cord. It is believed to moderate eating, sleeping and aggressive behavior. It also plays an important role in the way the brain inhibits anxiety in stressful situations. **Dopamine** is another catecholamine found in the brain, which functions both like an excitatory and inhibitory transmitter depending on the pathways and the properties of the postsynaptic receptors. It is implicated in a number of functions such as movement, attention and learning. Parkinson's disease is said to be due to dopamine deficiency in the brain. It also causes certain muscle disorders. Overproduction of dopamine seems to be a factor in the causation of schizophrenia and some other mental disorders. **Serotonin** functions both as an inhibitory or excitatory neurotransmitter. Found in the brain and spinal cord, it controls mood, arousal, sleep and eating. It is also involved in producing pleasure and pain. A great deal has been said about the serotonin's role in affective disorders, especially depression and bipolar disorders. **Endorphins** are inhibitory transmitters found in the brain and spinal cord. They inhibit transmission of pain impulses. Oversupply of endorphins produces insensitivity to pain and undersupply, hypersensitivity. They are implicated in the production of pleasurable feelings and appetite.

NERVOUS SYSTEM

As we have seen, the neurons are complex structures capable of intricate functions. If so, what should be the complexity of the nervous system that comprises some 100 to 200 billion neurons? Nervous system, its structure and functions, is a true marvel existing in the universe; it defies all human understanding. We are told that a single neuron may be connected to some 80,000 other neurons. The total number of connections in the nervous system is mind-boggling; some investigators have estimated it to be in the neighborhood of one quadrillion (1,000,000,000,000,000) and some others say it is still higher. In spite of its complexity, it is surprising that the nervous system functions quite systematically, logically and elegantly.

Basically, we can think of the entire nervous system as made up of three types of neurons: sensory neurons, motor neurons and interneurons. The sensory neurons bring messages from the sense organs to the spinal cord and to the brain. The motor neurons carry the orders of the brain through the cord to various organs of the body. The interneurons perform the associative functions within the nervous system; they link the input and output functions. The number of interneurons is more than the other two types put together. For example, when you hear the voice of your favorite singer, the interneuron helps you to recognize it by linking the sensory information with the memory of the picture of the person singing, which is stored somewhere in the brain. In fact, the interneurons explain the complexity of our higher mental processes.

Organization of the Nervous System

The nervous system is like a highly organized, well-coordinated corporation. It works as a unit. Any division is for academic purposes. It is broadly divided into several interrelated subsystems. It is customarily divided into two parts: the peripheral nervous system and central nervous system (Fig. 3.3). The **central nervous system (CNS)** includes all the nerves in the brain and the spinal cord. The **peripheral nervous system (PNS)** consists of the nerves branching out of the brain and spinal cord and reaches out to other parts of the body. The PNS is further divided into the somatic system and the autonomic nervous system. The **somatic system** is involved in the control of voluntary movements and carrying information from and to the sense organs. They convey to us the sensation of pain, pressure and temperature. All the voluntary muscular movements, our walking, talking, handling things and the involuntary adjustments we make in balancing the body are controlled by the somatic nerves. The **autonomic nervous system (ANS)** is concerned with the functioning of vital organs, such as the heart, lungs, glands and blood vessels. The autonomic nervous system plays a very important role in determining human behavior and will be discussed in a later section.

The central nervous system (CNS) consists of the brain and the spinal cord. The CNS is the highly evolved structure, which distinguishes human beings from all other living beings. Given below is a brief account of the various parts of CNS.

Spinal Cord

The **spinal cord** consists of nerve fibers running from various parts of the body to the

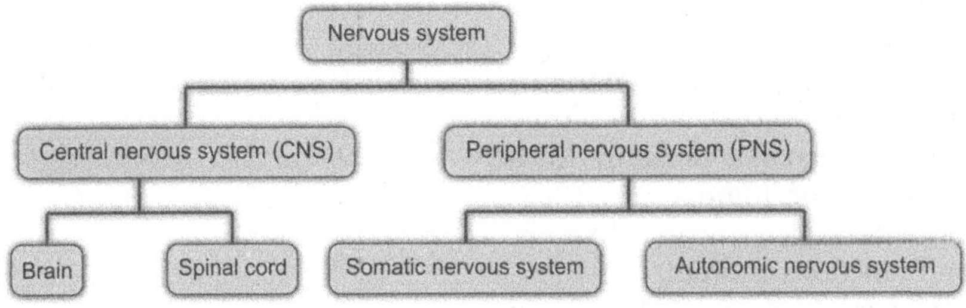

FIGURE 3.3: Divisions of nervous system

brain and back. It is about the thickness of a pencil (about 1 inch in diameter and about 17 inches in length) in an adult human being. The spinal cord runs through the bony spinal vertebrae, which protects it. The sensory nerves enter the cord from the back side (dorsal roots) and the motor nerves exit it from the front side (ventral roots). The main function of the cord is transmitting of the messages between the brain and the various parts of the body. It also controls some simple stimulus-response sequences called spinal reflexes without much involvement of the brain. Reflexes are involuntary, automatic responses to incoming stimuli. For example, the closing of your eyelid instantaneously when some foreign substance is about to strike your eye is a reflex action.

Brain

The **brain** is the most complex structure in the known universe and remains a challenge to all those who are engaged in studying it. It is the soft, spongy, wrinkled, pinkish-grey substance mostly consisting of protein, fat and fluid located in the hard bony protective case called the skull. It only weighs about 3 pounds (2 percent of the body weight), but consumes about 25 percent of oxygen, and 70 percent of glucose in the body. The brain, which is also called encephalon, works without rest all through your life and when it takes rest, it is death! In spite of innumerable impediments, the neuroscientists have made a lot of headway in unraveling this biological marvel, the brain, using techniques developed due to the great advances in science and technology. The complex procedures such as electroencephalography (EEG), computerized axial tomography (CAT), magnetic resonance imaging (MRI) and positron-emission tomography (PET) have made it possible to watch live the structure and functions of brain.

During embryonic development, the brain evolves into three separate portions called the hindbrain, the midbrain and the forebrain. The hindbrain differentiates into two parts called metencephalon and myelencephalon. The metencephalon includes the cerebellum and the pons, the myelencephalon includes medulla oblongata. The midbrain develops into tectum and tegmentum. Tectum consists of inferior and superior colliculi; the tegmentum contains the red nucleus, the substantia nigra and the nuclei and roots of oculomotor nerve (the third cranial nerve). The forebrain is subdivides into the telencephalon and diencephalon. The telencephalon (also called the end brain) develops into the cerebral cortex, the basal ganglia and the limbic system. The diencephalon becomes the thalamus and the hypothalamus. We shall study these three parts of the brain in some detail.

Hindbrain

From the evolutionary perspective, **hindbrain** is the most primitive part of the brain. It includes the medulla, pons and cerebellum (Fig. 3.4). As the spinal cord enters the skull, it enlarges into a structure called the **brainstem** which is the life-support system. The brainstem is the part of the brain left when both cerebrum and cerebellum are excluded. From the evolutionary point of view, the brainstem is the oldest and the most primitive part of the brain. The brainstem consists of structures

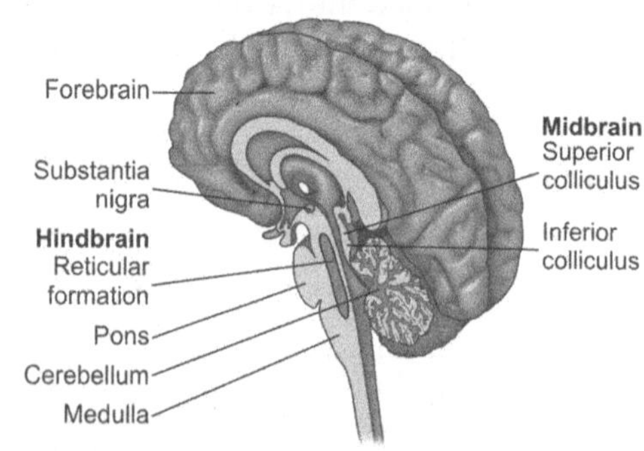

FIGURE 3.4: Hindbrain and midbrain

that are involved in the regulation of all vital functions of the body. The brainstem includes the **medulla oblongata** and the **pons**. The medulla (oblongata) is the first structure above the spinal cord; it controls the vital functions such as heart rate, respiration, appetite, body temperature and fluid balance. The medulla also contains all the ascending (sensory) and descending (motor) nerves that connect the body with higher brain structures. Damage to the medulla usually results in death. Appropriately, it has been called the 'vital knot'.

On the ventral side of the brainstem, just above the medulla, there is a rounded prominence called the pons. In Latin, 'pons' means 'bridge' and it carries nerve impulses between higher and lower levels of the nervous system. The **pons** connects the two halves of the cerebellum. It also transmits motor information, coordinating muscles and integrating movements between the right and left halves of the body. It has a cluster of neurons that help regulate sleep. Like the medulla, pons control several vital functions and damage to the pons can cause death.

Attached to the rear of the brainstem, slightly above the medulla and behind the pons, is the so-called "little brain" the cerebellum. It is called little brain because it just looks like a miniature brain. The **cerebellum** is involved in the regulation of motor coordination. Complex activities, such as walking, talking, writing, cycling and driving automobiles, seem to be programmed into the cerebellum and occur automatically without our consciously planning each step. Any damage to cerebellum results in uncoordinated movements. For instance, when one takes too much of alcohol, there is a depression in cerebellar activity leading to a wobbling movement that is characteristic of drunkenness. In addition to muscular movement coordination, it is also believed that the cerebellum plays a role in learning and remembering.

Midbrain

The **midbrain** is located just above the hindbrain (refer Fig. 3.4). It consists of a group of sensory and motor neurons. The sensory portion of the midbrain contains important relay centers for visual and auditory systems. The motor neurons in the midbrain control eye movements.

A very important part of the midbrain, extending from the medulla through the pons, is the **reticular formation**. It extends from the hindbrain up into the lower parts of the forebrain. Since, it appears like a net (reticulum) under microscope, it is called reticular formation. Reticular formation consists of groups of nerve cells that activate other parts of the brain to produce general bodily arousal. It plays an important role in regulating consciousness, attention and sleep. If somebody taps your door when you are asleep, it is this part that arouses you. It acts like a watchman; alerts higher brain centers that messages are coming; it may either block messages or allow them to go forward. Reticular formation has two parts: an ascending part and a descending part. The ascending part sends messages to higher regions of the brain to alert them and the descending part may either admit or block out sensory input. It can be said that the reticular system acts like a "consciousness switch," which turns on or off signals to various parts of the brain involved in consciousness maintenance. In this way, it plays an important role in the attention process. When a number of messages enter the nervous system at the same time, reticular formation decides which of them should be allowed to enter depending on its importance. When we are asleep, it filters out background stimuli and allows us to sleep without disturbance.

Forebrain

From the evolutionary point of view, the **forebrain** is the most advanced, highly evolved part of the brain. Its major structure is the cerebrum. It also includes important structures such as the thalamus, hypothalamus and the limbic system (Fig. 3.5).

Thalamus: Just above the midbrain (brainstem), there are two egg-shaped structures called the **thalamus**. One part of the thalamus acts as a relay station for information coming from sensory receptors and directs them to appropriate areas of the cerebrum. The other part plays an important role in the regulation of sleep. This region of the thalamus is considered as a part of the limbic system. When there is damage to an individual's thalamus, he/she may experience perceptual confusion. It is reported that among schizophrenics there are specific damages in their thalamus and as a consequence they experience garbled sensory experience causing confusion and hallucinations.

Hypothalamus: Just below the thalamus, there is a small (size of a fingertip) structure, consisting of tiny groups of neurons, called **hypothalamus** (the word means under the thalamus). In spite of its size, the hypothalamus plays a cardinal role in the regulation of many aspects of emotion and motivation, including sexual behavior, eating, drinking, sleeping, aggression and temperature regulation. It maintains a steady internal environment for the body (homeostasis). Damage to specific areas of hypothalamus may disrupt some or all of the above functions. The hypothalamus also plays an important role in the functioning of the endocrine system. Because of its connection with the pituitary gland, the hypothalamus controls many hormonal secretions that are involved in sexual behavior, metabolism and reactions to stress. Some researchers of the brain suggest that certain areas of the hypothalamus regulate the experience of pleasure and displeasure.

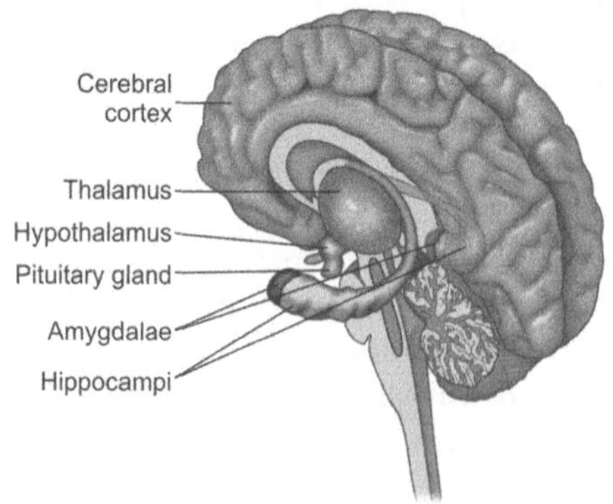

FIGURE 3.5: Forebrain

Limbic system: Lying deep within the cerebral hemispheres, there is a set of structures collectively called the **limbic system**. The limbic system is involved in coordinating behaviors necessary to satisfy motivational and emotional urges that arise in the hypothalamus. Two important structures of the limbic system are hippocampus (the term is derived from Greek hippokampos, which means sea horse) and amygdala (in Greek, almond). The **hippocampus** is involved in forming and retrieving memories. Damage to hippocampus causes memory disturbances especially for recent events. The **amygdala** is believed to organize motivational and emotional behavior patterns, especially those relating to fear and aggression. Hippocampus and amygdala play crucial roles as bridges between CNS and PNS. Stimulation of the amygdala is necessary for hippocampus's creation of emotional memories. It has been demonstrated that stimulation of certain areas of the amygdala produces aggression or fear in animals depending on the area stimulated. Just like the hypothalamus, the limbic system also contains areas that are implicated in the reward and punishment functions of motive.

Cerebrum: The outermost layer of the brain is called the cerebrum or cerebral cortex. It is the most prominent structure of the brain consisting of two hemispheres separated by the longitudinal fissure below which are the three **cerebral commissures** connecting the two halves. The inner core of the cerebrum is composed of white matter made up of myelinated fibers and the grey basal ganglia. The outer covering, the **cerebral cortex** (Fig. 3.6), is made up entirely of grey matter. From the evolutionary point of view, the cerebral cortex is the most advanced and the recent part of the brain. For this reason, often it is called the new brain. Cerebral cortex is not necessary for survival like the brainstem. Some lower animals like fish and amphibians have no cerebral cortex. The cortical tissues are found only among mammals. In humans, the cerebrum constitutes 80 percent of brain tissue. In fact, it is this portion of the brain that distinguishes humans from other organisms and enables them to think, plan and evaluate their actions.

The cerebrum consists of wrinkled, folded, rippled, convoluted and unmyelinated mass of grey cells. About 75 percent of the total cortical surface lies within canyon-like folds called **fissures**. Three of these fissures are important landmarks based on which the cortex is divided into lobes. The large **longitudinal fissure** divides the cerebrum lengthwise into left and right hemispheres. Within each hemisphere, a **central fissure** divides the cerebrum into the front and rear halves and the third one, the **lateral fissure**, runs front to rear along the side of the brain. The central fissure marks off the **frontal lobe**. The part of the cerebrum below the lateral fissure is called the **temporal lobe**. The area behind the central fissure is called the **parietal lobe** and at the back of the brain is the **occipital lobe**.

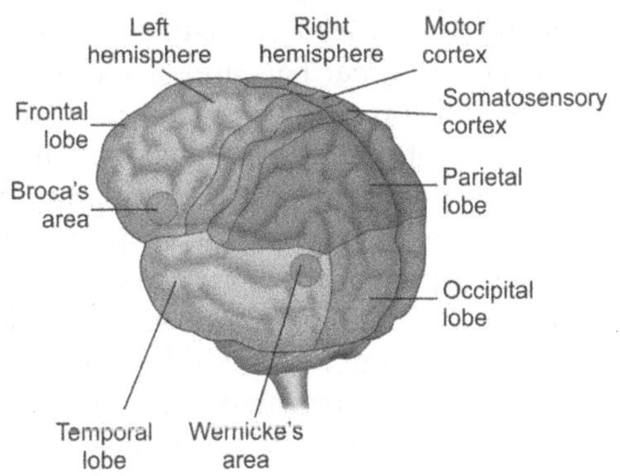

FIGURE 3.6: Cerebral cortex

Each lobe controls a specific function. In fact, one way of dividing the cerebrum is by considering the functions associated with a given area. Three major areas have been discovered. Roughly, we may think of some cortical areas to be largely sensory in function receiving messages from the sense organs. Others, called motor areas, are largely concerned with bodily movements. The third large area, called the association cortex, is engaged in higher mental functions such as learning, remembering, imagining and thinking. In addition, there are certain areas that are specifically controlling speech comprehension and speech production.

Although we talk about these areas as though they are separate and independent, we must remember that mostly behavior is influenced simultaneously by several structures and areas within the brain. Even within a given area, additional subdivisions exist. Further, when certain area is impaired, the unimpaired area may take over the functions that were earlier handled by the impaired area. Brain is extraordinarily adaptable. Having this in mind, let us learn about the functions of the cortical areas mentioned above.

Cortical Areas and Their Functions

Motor Area

The **motor area** (cortex) lies at the rear of the frontal lobe just adjacent to the central fissure. It controls all the voluntary movements (more than 600) of the body, the movements of the muscles, joints and tendons. Researchers have identified the amount and relative location of the cortical tissue associated with movement in the specific parts of the human body (Fig. 3.7).

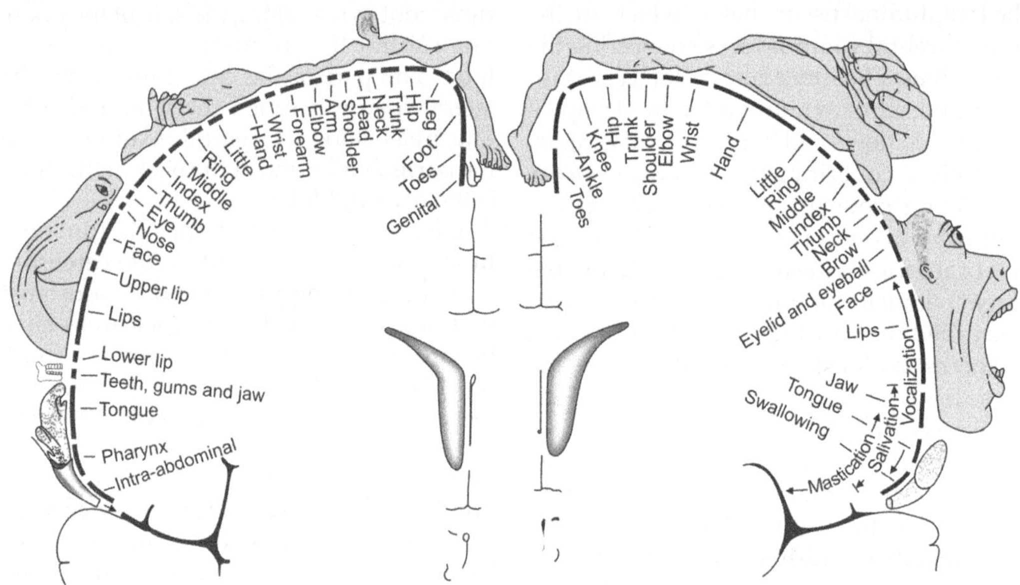

FIGURE 3.7: Motor and somatosensory cortexes

In the Figure 3.7, the specific body areas are represented in approximately upside down form. For example, movement of the toes is regulated by the part near the top of the head and movements of the mouth and tongue by the part near the bottom of the area toward the side of the brain. The amount of cortex devoted to each part of the body depends on the complexity of the movement carried out by that part. For example, the amount of cortical tissue devoted to the fingers that carry out precise and delicate movements is far greater than that devoted to the torso, whose movements are gross and imprecise, even though the torso is much larger than the fingers. When a particular point in the motor area is electrically stimulated, movements occur in the muscles governed by that part of the cortex. Because the nerve tracts from the motor area cross over at the level of the medulla, each hemisphere controls the movement of the opposite side of the body. Hence, damage to the right motor cortex produces paralysis in the left side of the body and vice versa.

Sensory Areas

There are specific areas of the cortex that receive input from different sense receptors. With the exception of taste and smell, at least one specific area has been identified for each of the senses. Sensory areas of cortex include three regions, one for the body sensations, and another for vision, and a third for audition.

Somatosensory area: The area that corresponds primarily to body sensations, including touch and pressure is called somatosensory area. This area is located at the front portion of the parietal lobe, just behind the motor area, separated from it by the central fissure. Electrical stimulation of this area gives rise to sensory experiences as though a part of the body was touched or moved. Temperature, pressure, touch, pain and experience of body balance and movements are represented in this area. As with the motor area, the amount of brain tissue allotted to a particular location on the body determines the degree of sensitivity of that location. The greater the space allotted within the cortex, the more sensitive that area of the body. Sensations from fingers are allotted proportionally more space than those from feet and toes. As in the case of motor area, each side of the body sends sensory input to the opposite hemisphere. Like the motor cortex, somatosensory strip is also organized in the upside down fashion with lower extremities represented high on the area and face down low. Any impairment or injury to somatosensory cortex produces impairment of sensations pertaining to that area, but surprisingly seldom results in complete loss of sensation.

Visual area: The primary sensory area for vision is located at the rear of the occipital lobe. Messages from the eyes are received, analyzed, integrated and converted into meaningful sights. Each eye sends messages to both the hemispheres. Stimulation of **visual area** electrically produces the experience of flashes of light or color. Also a particular area of the retina in the eye is related to a particular area in the visual cortex and of course, more space in the cortex is given to comparatively more sensitive portions of the retina.

Auditory area: An area located in the surface of the temporal lobe at the side of each hemisphere is responsible for the sense of hearing. When the **auditory area** is electrically stimulated, we will hear a humming or clicking sound. It is also reported that specific locations in the auditory area respond to specific pitches. As in the case of vision, each ear sends messages to the auditory areas of both the hemispheres. Surprisingly, the loss of one temporal lobe has very little effect on hearing.

Speech Centers

Two areas located in different lobes of the left hemisphere are involved in our verbal behavior. **Broca's area**, named after a French physiologist Paul Broca who discovered it, is located in the frontal lobe (for all right-handed individuals, it is located in the inferior frontal gyrus of the left hemisphere; for the left-handed individuals, it is still generally located in the left hemisphere, although on occasion it is found in the corresponding area on the right hemisphere). Broca's area is mainly involved in language processing (speech production). It works in concert with the motor cortex that controls the muscles used in speech. **Wernicke's area** is located in the left temporal lobe for all right-handed persons and the majority of left-handed persons. It is primarily involved in language reception and processing. However, the two areas function cooperatively when we converse with others. They help us in understanding what others are saying and in expressing our thoughts and ideas in words. Damage to Broca's area disrupts a person's ability to speak, but leaves intact the ability to understand what others are saying. He/She can comprehend speech, but cannot express in words. People with impairment in the Wernicke's area cannot understand written or spoken words. However, one should note that language reception and production are complex functions. It is now known that several areas, such as arcuate fasciculus (that connects Broca's area and Wernicke's area), neighboring regions of the auditory cortex and the many interconnections with the frontal lobes, work in combination with Broca's and Wernicke's areas in language processing.

Association Area

There are large areas of cerebral cortex that, when electrically stimulated, do not produce any sensory experience or motor response. For this reason, these regions are sometimes referred to as "silent areas." These are the **association areas** that are involved in higher mental processes such as perception, learning, thinking and reasoning. The inputs from more than one sense organ are integrated here. Damage to specific sites in the association area impairs the ability to perceive, understand, speak, think, plan out the action and to solve problems. The association area increases dramatically as we move up the brain ladder from lower organisms to human beings. Among humans it occupies approximately 75 percent of the area in the cerebrum. This is the reason why humans are far superior to animals in their cognitive functions.

Frontal Lobe

The portion of the cerebral cortex lying in front of the precentral gyrus is called **frontal lobe** (refer Fig. 3.6). It is believed to be the most important area of the brain that distinguishes humans from all other animals. Some people regard the entire period of human evolutionary existence as the 'age of frontal lobe'. This part of the brain hardly exists in mammals such as rats. It is estimated to occupy 3.5 percent of the cerebrum in cats, 7 percent in dogs, 17 percent in chimpanzees, but 29 percent in humans. The frontal lobes contain the sites that are supposed to be involved in the control of distinctly human qualities such as self-awareness, planning a course of action, taking initiative and responsibility. They are also believed to be regulating emotional experiences such as feelings of happiness, sadness and disgust. It is recently reported that an area of frontal lobe known as **prefrontal cortex** is the seat of executive ability—goal setting, planning, judgment and impulse control. However, it should be remembered that our knowledge of the frontal lobe is limited and it is still a less known part of the brain.

Lateralization of Cerebral Hemispheres

We have seen that the brain is divided into two hemispheres. The two halves are connected by a broad white band of myelinated nerve fibers called the corpus callosum. Each hemisphere controls the side of the body opposite to its location. Although the two hemispheres normally act in concert, there are significant differences between the two. There appears to be relatively greater localization of a function in one hemisphere or the other. This dominance of one hemisphere regarding a specific function is known as **lateralization**. The proof for this comes from the studies conducted on people suffering from brain injuries. From such studies it has been found that speech is localized in the left hemisphere and mathematical and logical abilities in the right hemisphere. When there is damage to Broca's area or Wernicke's area, the person suffers from a speech disorder known as aphasia, impairment in the ability to communicate using words. When the right hemisphere is affected, there will be failure to perceive spatial relations. The person may not recognize a familiar face or he/she may forget a well-traveled route. It appears that mental imagery, the capacity to perceive and understand spatial relations, music and artistic abilities are also localized in the right hemisphere. However, it is good to remember that the differences are not large and the lateralization varies from person to person.

Split-brain Studies

The most dramatic evidence for the differential functioning of the two halves of the brain comes from the **split-brain studies** (Figs 3.8A to C) conducted by Roger Sperry, the Nobel Prize winning scientist and his associates. Sperry studied some patients whose corpus callosum has been severed for the purpose of controlling epileptic seizures. In Sperry's experiments, the split-brain subjects were asked to focus on a fixation point, a dot on the center of a screen, while slides containing visual stimuli (words, pictures, and so on) were flashed very briefly to the left or right side of the fixation point. When words were flashed to the right of the visual field, the subject described it because the information has reached the

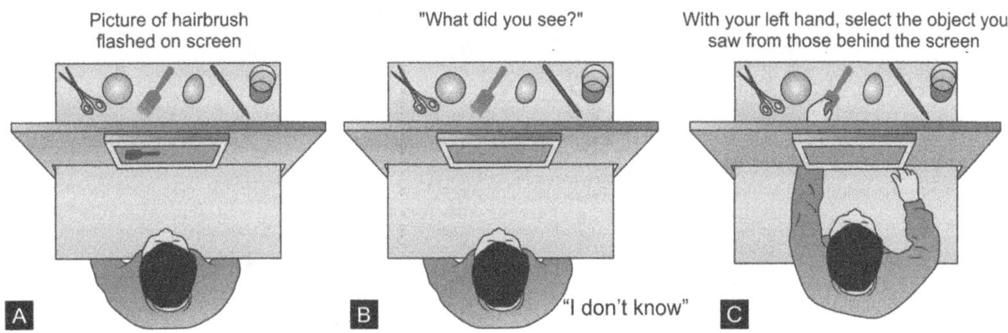

FIGURES 3.8A to C: Split-brain studies. In the experiment depicted above, a split-brain patient focuses on the fixation point in the center of the screen. **A.** A picture of a hairbrush is briefly projected to the left side of the visual field, thus sending the information to the right hemisphere; **B.** The patient is asked to report what he saw. He cannot name the object; **C.** He is then asked to select the object he saw and he quickly finds it with his left hand (*Courtesy:* Passer and Smith, 2007).

language sensitive left hemisphere. Subjects even wrote down what they saw with their right hand, which is controlled by the left hemisphere. But if the words were flashed to the left side of the visual field, sending the information to the right hemisphere, the subjects could not describe what they saw. If a picture of an object (a pencil) was flashed to the right hemisphere and the left hand was allowed to touch different objects including a pencil kept behind a screen, the subject would immediately select the pencil, but could not name it. However, if the pencil was transferred to the right hand, the person could immediately name it. In other words, until the object was transferred to the right hand, the left hemisphere had no knowledge of what the right hemisphere was experiencing. The split-brain researches have unequivocally established the fact that the two hemispheres possess different abilities. Recent studies have shown that the right hemisphere is superior to the left in the recognition of visual patterns.

The split brain researches have led some psychologists to speculate that the self-consciousness that is based on the linguistic memories of the past, resides in the left hemisphere, and that the right hemisphere is generally unconscious, but achieves consciousness by communicating with the left hemisphere across the corpus callosum.

Autonomic Nervous System

We noted earlier that the autonomic nervous system (ANS) is one of the two divisions of peripheral nervous system. The ANS regulates the functions of vital organs that keep us alive. It controls the functioning of endocrine glands, and the smooth muscles that comprise the heart, blood vessels and the lining of the stomach and intestines. The **smooth muscles** are so named because they do not have the striated appearance characteristic of the **skeletal muscles**. The somatic nervous system controls the striated muscles. The ANS is largely concerned with involuntary functions such as digestion, respiration and blood circulation. These activities are not under our conscious control and occur even when we are asleep or unconscious.

The ANS is divided into two parts: the **sympathetic nervous system (SNS)** and the **parasympathetic nervous system (PNS)**. The two divisions (Fig. 3.9) are mostly antagonistic in their activities; the SNS is generally excitatory and the PNS inhibitory.

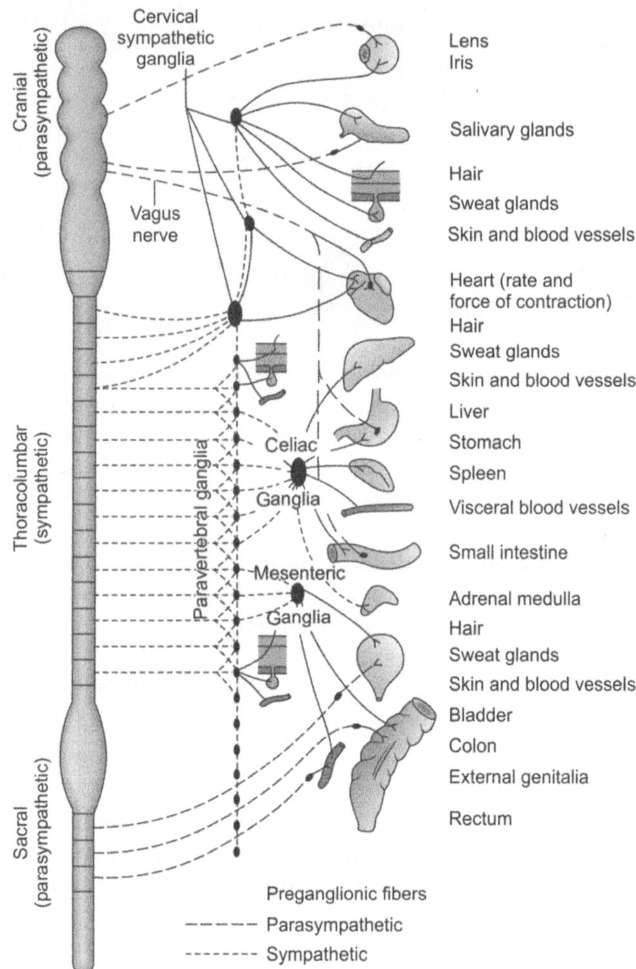

FIGURE 3.9: Autonomic nervous system

The SNS prepares the organism to face an emergency or stressful situation; it acts as a unit engaging all of the organism's resources to face the threat. For example, when you face a threat, the SNS helps you to confront the enemy by providing extra energy. The heart pumps more blood to muscles, dilates your pupils (so that you can see well), digestive activities are slowed down (so that blood flows toward muscles) and the respiration rate is accelerated (so that more oxygen is available to the body). These activities are often referred to as "fight or flight" responses. On the other hand, the PNS is active during quiet and restful periods in contrast to SNS. The PNS is engaged in energy-conservation and protective activities. It calms down the body after the emergency is over; the heart rate comes down and digestion is resumed. PNS helps to get the organism back to a state of equilibrium. In short, the sympathetic division serves energy expending (catabolic) functions, and the parasympathetic division the energy building (anabolic) functions. Sometime, the two divisions work cooperatively; for instance, during sexual activity of the male, the arousal (erection) is controlled by PNS and ejaculation (orgasm) by SNS.

ENDOCRINE SYSTEM

The nervous system interacts with two other systems, namely, the endocrine system and the immune system. The interactions between these three systems have major implications for the psychological well-being of individuals. The **endocrine system** is a chemical communication network. The endocrine system secretes several chemicals called **hormones** that circulate through the blood stream sending messages to the nervous system and thereby affecting growth and functioning of several organs of the body. Hormones operate like neurotransmitters sending chemical messages. The endocrine system is closely tied to the hypothalamus, which stimulates the pituitary gland to release other hormones, including growth hormone.

The endocrine system consists of several ductless glands that produce different kinds of hormones (Fig. 3.10). The major endocrine glands are the pituitary, adrenal, thyroid and sex glands (testis in males and ovaries in females). Pineal body and pancreas are other endocrine glands. Among them, the **pituitary gland** (also called hypophysis) is the most important one. Often it is called the "master gland" because it controls the functioning of all other glands. The pituitary is located near the hypothalamus and is regulated by it. It produces the largest number of hormones. The pituitary consists of two independently functioning parts, namely, anterior pituitary (adenohypophysis) and posterior pituitary (neurohypophysis).

Anterior pituitary secretes several important hormones: the **somatotropic hormone**, which regulates growth, the **adrenocorticotropic hormone (ACTH)**,

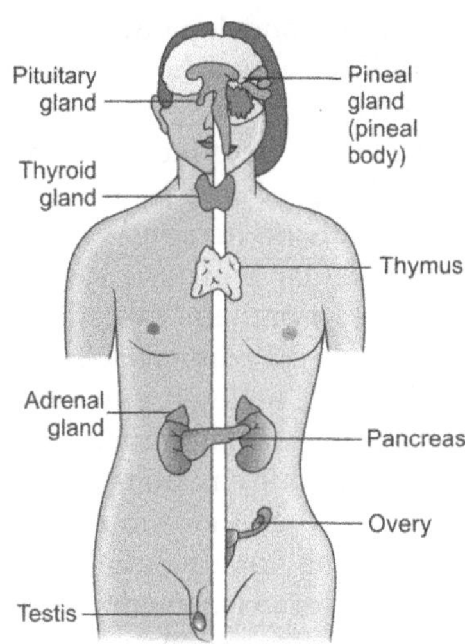

FIGURE 3.10: Endocrine system

which controls the functioning of adrenal cortex, the **thyrotropic hormone (TH)**, which has control over the functioning of the thyroid gland, a group of **gonadotropic hormones (GTH)** including **follicle-stimulating hormone (FSH)**, which stimulates the development of ovarian follicles in the female and spermatogenesis in the male, **luteinizing hormone (LH)** also called **interstitial cell-stimulating hormone (ICSH)**, which along with FSH stimulates secretion of estrogens and ovulation and **lactogenic hormone** (prolactin or luteotropic hormone), which controls milk production in the mature mammary glands. The posterior lobe of pituitary secretes the **antidiuretic hormone (ADH)**. ADH is also called **vasopressin,** which works as part of the system that maintains water balance in the body and oxytocin, which induces uterine contractions, controls milk-ejection from the mammary glands and blood pressure.

The **adrenal glands** are twin structures situated just above the kidneys. Adrenal has two parts: adrenal cortex and adrenal medulla. The **adrenal medulla** secretes mostly **adrenalin** (also called epinephrine), some amount of **noradrenalin** (also called norepinephrine) and **dopamine.** The **adrenal cortex** produces several hormones including glucocorticoids, the mineral corticoids, and sex hormones. The effect of adrenalin is similar to that produced by the stimulation of the sympathetic nervous system. It acts upon the reticular activating system, which excites the sympathetic system, which in turn stimulates the adrenals to secrete more adrenalin. Thus, a closed circuit is formed maintaining emotional arousal. That is the reason why a strong emotional state does not subside even when the stimulus causing it is removed. The noradrenalin prepares the organism to meet an emergency. It stimulates the pituitary to release ADH. These hormones (steroids) promote the release of sugar stored in the liver thus, providing the extra energy for action. The noradrenalin also works like a neurotransmitter.

The thyroid gland, situated at the base of the neck, secretes **thyroxin**, which controls the metabolic rate. Excessive secretion of thyroxin produces hyperthyroidism and deficiency results in hypothyroidism. Among the sex glands, the testes in the male produce **testosterone** and the ovaries in the female **estrogen**. These are involved in the physical development of reproductive organs, sex characteristics of the respective sexes, and their sexual behavior. Pancreas secretes insulin, which is an essential component of proper metabolism. Pineal body, a small endocrine gland situated in the brain, produces the hormone called melatonin, which is involved in regulating sleep-wake cycles. Insulin also regulates the concentration of glucose (sugar) in the blood.

IMMUNE SYSTEM

The nervous system, the endocrines, and the immune system interact to protect us from dangerous foreign substances called the **antigens**. When bacteria, viruses, and many other chemicals with antigenic properties enter the body, the immune system destroys them by creating **antibodies**. The nervous, endocrine, and immune systems are all parts of a communication network, which underlies every mental and physical activity. Candace Pert, an expert neuroscientist working in this area, has appropriately called the network "bodymind." There are indications that immune cells can actually produce hormones and neurotransmitters, thus having direct influence on brain and endocrine system. It is also found that psychological factors, such as stress, pessimistic thinking, and depression, reduce immune functioning, whereas effective stress management skills, optimistic outlook, sense of humor, and social support help preserve immunity (Passer & Smith, 2007).

GENETIC INFLUENCE ON BEHAVIOR

The study of biological foundations of behavior will be incomplete without some knowledge of behavior genetics. The field of behavior genetics deals with the inheritance of behavior characteristics. We know that we inherit several physical characteristics such as height, weight, body structure, color of hair and eyes. But have we also inherited psychological characteristics such as intelligence, emotionality and temperament? Behavior geneticists are interested in the degree to which these psychological features are transmitted from parents to children. The old heredity versus environment (nature versus nurture) issue is irrelevant even today. All behaviors are dependent on the interaction between heredity and environment. Today, researchers are interested in determining how heredity limits human potential and to what extent environmental conditions change the inherited potential.

Life starts in the form of a zygote, which is the result of union of two cells, i.e. the egg from the mother and the sperm from the father. The egg and the sperm carry the material of heredity within their nuclei the material of heredity called the chromosome. The **chromosome** is a double stranded and tightly coiled molecule of **deoxyribonucleic acid (DNA)**. All the hereditary information is encoded in various combinations of four nucleotide bases (adenine, thymine, guanine and cytosine—ATGC) that occur throughout the chromosome. The specific arrangement of these ATGC bases on the chromosome creates the specific commands for every characteristic and function of the human body.

Every cell of the human body contains 46 chromosomes. During conception, the human offspring receives 23 chromosomes from the father and 23 from the mother. The 46 chromosomes form into 23 pairs. These are duplicated by a process called mitotic cell division as the individual grows. The DNA portion of the chromosome contains **genes**, which are the ultimate carriers of heredity. Within each chromosome, the corresponding genes coming from parents occur in matched pairs. One important characteristic of some genes is that they may be dominant or recessive. If both members of a gene pair are dominant, the characteristic carried by the gene will manifest in the offspring. If one of the gene pair is dominant and the other recessive, the offspring will show the trait carried by the dominant gene. If both genes are recessive, the trait carried by the recessive gene will appear in the offspring. In human beings, brown eyes are dominant over blue eyes. A child will have blue eyes only when it receives recessive genes for blue eyes from both parents. If both parents are brown eyed, they can still have a blue eyed child when both parents contribute recessive gene for blue eyes. Baldness, hemophilia and albinism are carried by recessive genes. All genes do not follow the dominant-recessive pattern. Most human traits are created by the combined effect of a number of genes. This phenomenon is known as **polygenic transmission**.

Of the 23 pairs of chromosomes, 22 pairs are called **autosomes** and the 23rd pairs called **sex chromosome**. In the normal female, the 23rd pair is XX and in the normal male XY. The X chromosome is the female determining chromosome, the Y male determining. If during conception, the offspring has received the X from the father, it will be female child. If it receives the Y from the father, then it will be a male. Because the mother has only XX chromosomes, she does not have a role in the sex determination of the child.

The specific genetic makeup of an individual is called **genotype** and his/her observable characteristics the **phenotype**. Genotype is present from conception and all of it may not manifest as phenotype. The phenotype may be affected by other genes and by the environment. The work of geneticists in the **Human Genome Project** has revolutionized our understanding of the human genetic endowment. The genetic structure in all the 23 pairs of chromosomes has been mapped. The investigators have virtually disassembled the genes on each chromosome and studied the specific sequence of substances (ATGC). The Genome Project has thrown several exciting results. It has shown that there are about 30,000 genes rather than the previously estimated 100,000. The location and structure of more than 80 genes that contribute to hereditary diseases have been identified. It has been shown that gene interactions are more complicated than what was formerly believed and single gene manipulation cannot solve the complex problem such as schizophrenia.

Chromosomal Anomalies

Several abnormalities or anomalies of chromosomes have been noticed. Sometimes, part of the chromosome may be lost during cell division. There may be loss of one chromosome or the addition of one or more chromosome. On rare occasions, a female child may be born with only one X chromosome instead of the normal XX pair. Such females suffer from a condition known as **Turner's syndrome**; these females are marked by short stature and webbed neck. Often the ovary is missing and such girls do not develop sexually and may exhibit certain cognitive deficits. Sometimes males are found to have an extra X chromosome; that is, they have XXY instead of the normal XY pair. These males suffer from a condition called **Klinefelter's syndrome**; they are physically male, but possess marked feminine features such as enlarged breasts. Their penises and testicles are unusually small and generally sperms are not produced. Some men are born with an extra Y chromosome, that is, they have XYY instead of XY; these men are unusually tall, highly aggressive, mature sexually very early and may exhibit more than normal sexual drive. They are often referred to as 'super male'. Still another anomaly of the X chromosome, called **fragile X syndrome**, is found among both men and women. Men will have large ears and large testicles and are marked by poor speech and mental retardation. Afflicted women are often subclinical (producing effects that are not detectable by the usual clinical tests). Abnormalities of autosomes are also often noticed. For example, an extra chromosome in pair 21, called **trisomy 21**, is noticed in **Down's syndrome** (mongolism is the old name). The condition is marked by features such as flat skull, stubby fingers, a fissured tongue, unusual pattern of skin folds and mental deficiency.

Behavior Genetics

Behavior genetics as an area of study is interested in investigating how heredity and environment interact in influencing behavior. Behavior geneticists estimate the relative contributions of heredity and environment in three ways: studying family and kinship, adoption studies and study of twins.

Studies of Family and Kinship

Degree of relatedness to one another in a family depends on genetic similarity. Children get half of their genetic material from each parent. Therefore, the probability of sharing any particular gene with one of the parents is 0.50 (50%). Brothers and sisters also have 0.50 probability of sharing the same gene with one another since they get their genetic material from the same parents. With a grandparent the probability is 0.25, for half-siblings it is 0.25 and for first cousins it is 0.125. These facts about genetic similarity give us a basis for studying the role of genetic factors in the determination of physical and psychological characteristics. If a characteristic has a high concordance (co-occurrence) rate in people who are more closely related to one another, then it points to a possible genetic contribution, particularly, if the people have lived in different environments. Thus, knowing the level of genetic similarity among family members provides a basis for estimating the relative contributions of heredity and environment to a physical or behavioral characteristic. Many studies have shown that the more people are similar genetically, the more similar they are likely to be psychologically, although the level of similarity depends on the trait in question.

Adoption Studies

In **adoption studies**, people who were adopted early in life are compared on some characteristic with both their biological parents with whom they share the genetic endowment and with their adoptive parents, with whom they share no genes. If adopted children are more similar to biological parents (with whom they share 50% genes) than to adoptive parents (with whom they share a common environment, but no genes), a genetic influence is indicated. If they are more similar to their adoptive parents than to their biological parents, environmental factors are judged to be more important for that particular characteristic. For example, adopted children who were diagnosed to be schizophrenic were identified. Then the investigators examined the backgrounds of biological as well as adoptive parents and their relatives for signs of schizophrenia in the two sets of families. The researchers found that 12 percent of biological family members had been diagnosed as schizophrenics compared with only 3 percent among the members of adoptive family members suggesting that there is a hereditary link.

Twin Studies

Another important method of determining the relative role of heredity and environment on behavior involves the study of twins. There are two types of twins: monozygotic (identical) twins and dizygotic (fraternal) twins. **Monozygotic twins** come from a single egg and sperm as a result of a division of a fertilized cell (zygote) and as a consequence, they share the same heredity. It is estimated that one in 250 births results in monozygotic (identical) twins. On the other hand, **dizygotic twins** result from two eggs fertilized by two sperms. They are like two siblings and share only half of the genes. One in 150 births result in dizygotic twins. Identical twins are always of the same sex, while fraternal twins may belong, to same or different sex.

Geneticists have compared identical twins raised in the same environment (heredity and environment both same) with identical twins reared apart (heredity same, but environment different). They also compared sets of identical and fraternal twins who were separated very early in life and raised in different environments, thus eliminating environmental similarity. Identical twins tended to be more similar to one another than were fraternal twins even when they were separated early in life and reared in different environments. On the other hand, identical twins reared together tended to be more similar than identical twins reared apart indicating that environment also produces some difference. Several characteristics including intelligence, personality traits and certain psychological disorders have significant genetic basis. Adopted children were found to be more similar to their biological parents than to their adoptive parents on these characteristics.

While estimating the contribution of genetic factors to behavior, geneticists have realized that heredity and environment are not really separate determinants; instead, they operate as a single integrated system. Gene expression is influenced on a daily basis by the environment. Two children of equal intelligence may exhibit intelligence quotient (IQ) difference as great as 16 to 20 points, if one is raised in an impoverished and the other in an enriched environment. High or low environmental stress may inhibit or encourage gene manifestation.

Gene Manipulation

Recent technological advances have enabled scientists not only to map the human genome, but also to duplicate and modify the gene structure; they have learned to repair dysfunctional genes. These advances promise new methods of treating some mental disorders. Psychologists are attempting to apply gene-manipulating procedures in the area of learning, remembering, emotion and motivation. They have learnt to alter a specific gene, in a rat, in such a way that it prevents the animal from carrying out its normal function. This is called *knockout procedure* because that particular function of the gene is knocked out and its effect on behavior is studied. For example, researchers may insert a genetic material that prevents neurons from responding to a particular neurotransmitter and observe its effect on learning. They can even insert a new gene into an animal during embryonic period and study its effect on behavior. This is called the *knockin procedure*. Gene manipulation procedures in future may enable us to alter genes to prevent schizophrenia or depression.

Chapter Summary

In this chapter, we discussed the biological bases of behavior, especially the role of the brain and nervous system. The branch of psychology that seeks to study the neural bases of behavior is physiological psychology or biopsychology. In recent years, with the help of advances in the area of brain imaging technology, biopsychology (also called behavioral neuroscience) has come to play an important role in understanding human behavior.

To understand the role of the brain and nervous system as determiners of behavior, it is necessary to have some knowledge of nerve cell (neuron), the connection between neurons (synapses), the nature of nerve impulse, and the chemicals (neurotransmitters) that play an important role in facilitating or impeding the transmission of nerve impulses at the synapse. The neurons are the building blocks of the nervous system. It is estimated that there are some 100 billion or more neurons in the human brain. Neurons are the information carriers of the nervous system. The information in the form electrical nerve impulse passes from one neuron to another through a complex network consisting of axons, dendrites and the synapses. The synapses are the areas of functional contact between neurons. The boutons at the end of axon release neurotransmitters that help in the transmission or inhibition of the nerve impulse at the synapse.

The nervous system is divided into two parts: central nervous system, consisting of brain, spinal cord, and peripheral system. The peripheral nervous system has two parts: somatic nervous system and autonomic nervous system. The autonomic nervous system is divided into sympathetic division and parasympathetic division.

The spinal cord and the brain, control and regulate vital bodily functions such as breathing. The brain is divided into three parts such as hindbrain, midbrain and forebrain. The hindbrain consists of the structures of the brainstem (pons and medulla) that support vital functions, and cerebellum that is involved in motor coordination. The midbrain consists of the reticular formation, which plays a vital role in consciousness, attention and sleep. Forebrain is the most advanced part of the brain; it consists of the thalamus, hypothalamus, the limbic system and the cerebrum. The thalamus is the brain's sensory switch board; it organizes the inputs from sense organs and sends them to appropriate centers of the brain. The hypothalamus plays a major role in many aspects of motivation and emotion, in addition to temperature regulation, sleeping, eating, water intake, aggression and sex. The limbic system helps to coordinate behaviors needed to satisfy motivational and emotional urges that arise in the hypothalamus. Two important structures of the limbic system are hippocampus and amygdala. The hippocampus is involved in memorization. Amygdala organizes motivational and emotional activities, especially those involved in fear and anger. Amygdala, like the hypothalamus, is involved in reward and punishment functions.

The major structure of the forebrain is the cerebrum. The outer portion of the forebrain has a thin covering called the cerebral cortex. The cerebral cortex is the crowning achievement of evolution. It is not vital for survival like the brainstem, but it is essential for human functioning; without cerebral cortex, people may live like vegetables. Most of the cortical surface lies within canyon-like folds called fissures. There are three important fissures. The longitudinal fissure divides the cortex into two halves, the left and right cerebral hemispheres. The central fissure divides the cortex into front and rear halves. The third one called lateral fissure, runs from front to rear along the side of the brain. On the basis of the fissures as landmarks, the brain is divided into two hemispheres (left and right hemispheres connected by corpus callosum) and four lobes, the frontal, temporal, parietal and occipital lobes. Each of the lobe is associated with particular sensory and motor functions. The frontal lobes are the most important, but least understood part of the human brain; they are supposed to be the sites of human qualities such as self-awareness, planning, and initiative. The two hemispheres are specialized to perform somewhat different functions; broadly, the left processes language and the right is involved in pattern recognition and spatial abilities.

In addition to brain and nervous system, we have learnt some elementary knowledge about the endocrine system and the effects of hormones they produce. The hormones, the chemical messengers, travel in the bloodstream and affect bodily organs, psychological functions and development of the person. The nervous system, endocrine system, and the immune system have extensive neural and chemical means of communication and are capable of affecting and being affected by each other. We have also discussed certain rudimentary facts about genetics that shed light on the relative importance of heredity and environment in the development of human behavior. Behavior geneticists study how genetic and environmental factors influence the development of body and mind.

4 CHAPTER Sensation and Perception

PREVIEW

The fundamental aim of all living beings is to survive in the world. For survival, they have to understand the environment, both physical and social. We have to know the world we live in. Without the accurate knowledge of our environment, which consists of objects, events and people, it is difficult to survive. Life is a continuous process of adjusting or adapting to the changing environment. But then, how do we get to know the environment? How do we acquire the knowledge about the world? Philosophers from times immemorial have been discussing the issue of the nature of knowledge and the way knowledge is acquired. This pursuit has given rise to a branch of philosophy called epistemology. One group of philosophers says that we get our knowledge through our senses and the other says that we acquire knowledge through thinking and reasoning. The former are called empiricists (Aristotle and his followers) and the latter rationalists (Plato and his followers). Without going into the details of empiricism and rationalism, let us accept that knowledge comes to us through both the channels; most of it comes through senses and some of it through thinking and reasoning. We shall discuss in this chapter the acquisition of knowledge through the senses and take up learning, thinking and reasoning in later chapters.

Senses, it is often said, are the royal roads to knowledge. True, we come to know the world around us through seeing, hearing, touching, smelling and tasting. It appears simple. But what happens when you say "I see something?" The answer is not that simple. For example, when you say "This is a book," what is happening to you or within you? Let us see. When you say that you see a book, the following processes occur: Light falls on the book (you cannot see the book in darkness); the book absorbs some light rays and reflects some light rays; the reflected light rays fall on the retina; in the retina some physical and chemical changes take place; these changes are converted into neural impulses; the neural impulses move through the optic nerve and reach the visual areas in the brain in the occipital lobe, where it is identified and interpreted as a "book." You see, this is a highly complicated process. When you say you see something, psychologists identify two important processes: sensation and perception. Sensation is the process by which physical stimuli impinging on the sense organs are converted into neural impulses that the brain uses to create your experience of seeing, hearing, smelling, tasting, touching and so on. Perception is the process by which the brain identifies, organizes, integrates and interprets sensory impressions to create meaningful representations of the objects in the world. When you see a book, your eyes send a pattern of neural impulses to the brain; this is sensation. These impulses are interpreted as "book" based on your past experience and knowledge stored: this is perception. Actually, it is very difficult to say where sensation ends and perception begins; the two merge in such a way that it is difficult to demarcate boundaries between the two and as a consequence, some psychologists prefer to use the term sense-perception to refer to the process. Whatever the complexities, the fact remains that most of all knowledge has its origin in our perceptions. Thank nature that it has given us specialized sensors that allow the brain to convert the many kinds of energy into the common language of nerve impulses and it has given us a brain that can take all this input—often from more than one sense—and construct our perceptual experiences. Sensation and perception are the basis of our existence as sentient, conscious organisms.

We are not sure of all the intricate psychological and neurological processes involved in sensation and perception. The area still remains a challenge. The world we perceive is complex; it is full of gorgeous colors, complex corners and shades, melodious sounds, fragrant smells and enticing tastes. How we differentiate this multitude of physical stimuli is still an enigma. You will have a brief introduction to the mysterious processes underlying sensation and perception in the following pages.

Chapter Outline

We live in a wonderful world around us. It is full of beautiful sights, melodious sounds, enticing smells, welcoming aromas and soothing touches. How do we experience these phenomena? All the information about the world around us comes to us through our senses—the eyes, ears, nose, tongue and skin among others. Most of all that we know comes to us through our senses. In this chapter, we discuss the ways in which our body takes in the information about the environment through its senses and analyzes, interprets and makes the information meaningful; we explore the complex processes of sensation and perception. These are the two fundamental topics in psychology whose understanding is essential for understanding the causes of behavior and experience. Without the knowledge of sensation and perception, we cannot answer questions such as: How do we distinguish red from green, one face from another, music from noise, hot from cold, pain from pleasure, soft from hard, and the beautiful from the ugly and a host of other questions.

Sensation is the process in which sense organs receive stimuli from the environment, translate them into nerve impulses and send them to the brain. **Perception** involves the sorting out, analysis, interpretation and integration of stimulus information reaching the brain. Although perception is regarded as a higher mental process beyond sensation, it is difficult to say where sensation ends and perception begins. Sensation and perception blend together so completely that it is not easy to separate the two. Nevertheless, psychologists do distinguish between sensation and perception on several grounds. For them, perception is an active and creative process; it adds to or subtracts from sensory impressions certain elements. For instance, the same sensory input may be interpreted differently by different people and by the same person at different occasions. Perception selects and organizes sensory inputs and attaches meaning to them; it goes beyond sensation. These points will become clear as we proceed further in the chapter.

SENSORY PROCESSES

You have been told in your school that there are five senses: vision, audition, smell (olfaction), taste (gestation) and touch. True, these are our basic senses. But today, we know there are more than five senses. For instance, there are more than one sensibilities within skin; we are not only sensitive to touch but, to several other stimuli such as temperature, pressure and pain; these are different skin sensations. The ear is not only sensitive to sound but also to body balance, its position and movement (vestibular sense).

The joints, tendons and muscles are sensitive to coordination and movements of limbs (kinesthetic sense). There are receptors in the brain that monitor the chemical composition of blood. Psychologists believe that there are more than a dozen different senses, all of which are interrelated.

Different kinds of stimuli activate different sense receptors. A stimulus is some form of energy that produces a response in a sense organ. Light is the energy for eye, sound for ear, certain chemicals for smell and the taste. A stimulus can vary in strength (intensity) and it must be of a known magnitude to produce a response in the sense organ. The lowest amount of intensity necessary to be noticed by a sense organ is called the **absolute threshold**. Psychologists have determined the absolute thresholds for the major senses of humans. The approximate estimates in common man's terminology are given in Table 4.1.

Just as there must be a certain minimum amount of stimulus intensity to evoke a sensory experience, so there must be a certain difference in intensity between two stimuli before they can be distinguished from each other. The minimum intensity difference necessary to distinguish the two is called **difference limen** or **just noticeable difference (jnd)**. An area of psychology called **psychophysics**, studies the relations between the physical characteristics of stimuli and sensory capabilities.

Table 4.1: Approximate Absolute Thresholds for Different Senses

Senses	*Absolute threshold*
Vision	A candle light seen at 30 miles on a dark clear night
Audition	The ticking of a watch at 20 feet under quiet conditions
Taste	One teaspoon full of sugar in 2 gallons of water
Smell	One drop of perfume diffused in a three-room apartment
Touch	A wing of a fly falling on the cheek from a distance of 1 centimeter

SENSORY SYSTEMS

We come to know the environment around us through our senses. The knowing is the function of the brain. But the brain cannot directly *"know"* the environment whose language is in terms of light, sound, chemicals and mechanical pressures. These stimuli must be translated into a language that can be understood by the brain. The translation is done by the **sensory receptors**—the sensitive nerve endings in each sense organ. The conversion of the physical energy of the stimulus into neural activity is called **transduction**. Thus, starting with the transduction process at the receptor, physical energy results in a pattern of nerve impulses, which are interpreted (known) by the brain. The interpreting and understanding of the sensory input by the brain is what is called perception. Before we deal with perception, it is necessary to understand the structure and functioning of sense organs.

Eye and Vision

Eyes are our windows to the world—its beautiful sceneries, colors and so many other things including the faces of your loved ones. The stimulus for the eye is light, which is a form of electromagnetic radiation with wave-like properties. Electromagnetic waves are measured and classified in terms of wavelength. The entire range of wavelengths is called the electromagnetic spectrum out of which only a small portion is visible and that is called the **visible spectrum** (Fig. 4.1). Wavelengths are measured in billionths of a meter or nanometers (nm) and the visible spectrum extends from about 380 to 780 nanometers.

Human Eye

You may be familiar with the structure and function of the human eye. The main

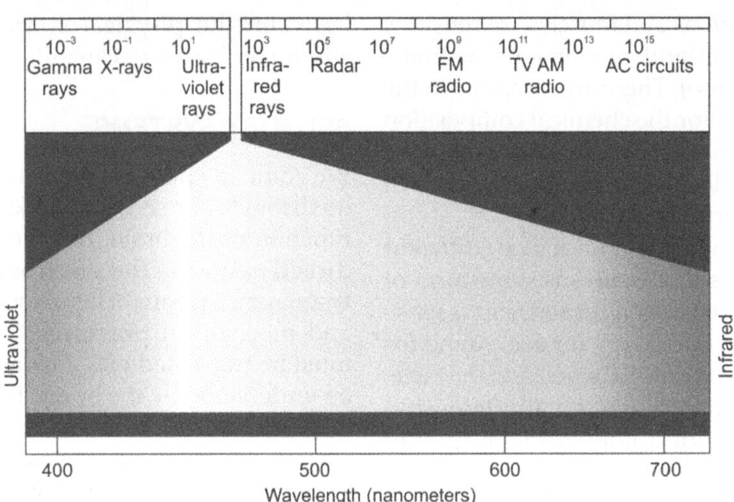

FIGURE 4.1: Visible spectrum (AC, alternating current; AM, amplitude modulation; FM, frequency modulation; TV, television).

structures of the human eye are shown in the Figure 4.2.

The light enters the eye through the cornea, a transparent protective structure of the eye. The amount of light entering the eye is regulated by the pupil situated behind the cornea. The pupil is surrounded by muscles of the iris. The size of pupillary opening is controlled by iris, either by dilating or constricting thus, controlling the amount of light entering the eye. Behind the pupil, there is the lens; it is an elastic structure that becomes thinner to focus on distant objects and thicker to focus on nearby objects. Just as the lens of a camera focuses the image on the film, so the living lens of the eye focuses the image on the **retina**. The retina is a multi-layered light-sensitive tissue at the rear of the liquid filled eye ball (vitreous humor). The image on the retina is upside down, but the brain reverses it as we see.

Our ability to see objects clearly depends on the functioning of the lens. Because of some anatomical or/and physiological defects, the lens may focus the object seen in front of the retina or behind. When one has difficulty in seeing far away objects (nearsightedness or myopia), the image is focused in front of the retina. If one has difficulty in seeing nearby objects (farsightedness or hyperopia), the image is focused behind the retina. These conditions can be corrected by using eye glasses or contact lenses.

Retina

The retina (meaning network), situated at the back of the eyeball, is actually an extension of the brain. It consists of three main layers: the **rods** and **cones**, the **bipolar cells** and the **ganglion cells**. The rods and cones, named

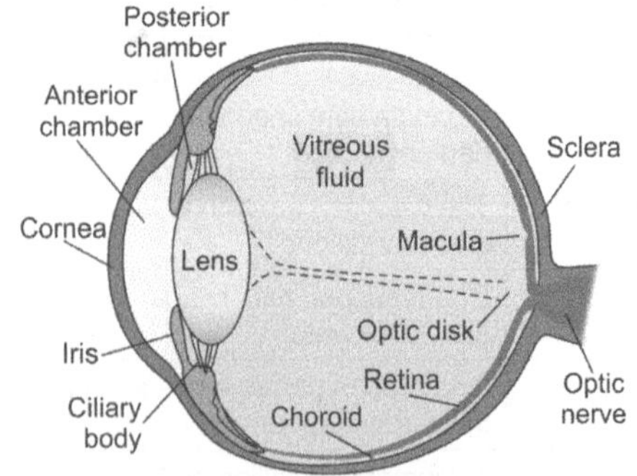

FIGURE 4.2: Human eye

so because of their shapes (Fig. 4.3), are the photosensitive elements (photoreceptors) of the retina. The rods are cylindrical in shape and the cones tapered and conical. It is estimated that there are about 120 million rods and about 5 million cones in the human eye. The rods are sensitive to black and white and the cones to colors.

The rods and cones are distributed unevenly in the retina; the rods are found throughout the retina except the fovea and the cones are most numerous in the fovea. The **fovea** is the most sensitive part of the retina. Visual acuity or sharpness is greatest at the fovea and it is this part we use when we want to see anything clearly. As we move from the center of the retina toward its periphery, the concentration of cones gets reduced and the periphery contains only rods. Generally, cones are active in bright light or daylight and rods in dim light.

The rods and cones send their messages to the brain through bipolar and the ganglion cells. The rods and cones have synaptic connections with bipolar cells, which in turn synapse with ganglion cells. The axons of the ganglion cell fibers form the **optic nerve**, which carries the nerve impulses to the brain. The axons of the ganglion cells in the optic nerve reach the lateral geniculate body of the thalamus; then fibers from the lateral geniculate cells carry nerve impulses to the primary visual area in the occipital lobe at the back of the brain. It is curious to note that the rods and cones, the photoreceptor cells that convert light into nerve impulses (transduction) form the rear layer of the retina. The light has to pass through the lens, the liquids of the eyeball, penetrate through the network of blood vessels, and the bipolar and ganglion cells before reaching the photoreceptors. The optic nerve exits through the back of the eye creating a **blind spot** (optic disk) in the retina. The blind spot lacks rods and cones. Ordinarily, we are unaware of the blind spot because our perceptual system fills in the missing part of the visual field.

The way in which the rods and cones are connected to the bipolar cells account for both the greater importance of rods in dim light and our greater ability to see fine details in bright illumination, when the cones are most active.

Visual Transduction

The visual transduction process, the conversion of light energy to nerve impulses, takes place in the retina. Rods and cones in the retina translate light waves into nerve impulses

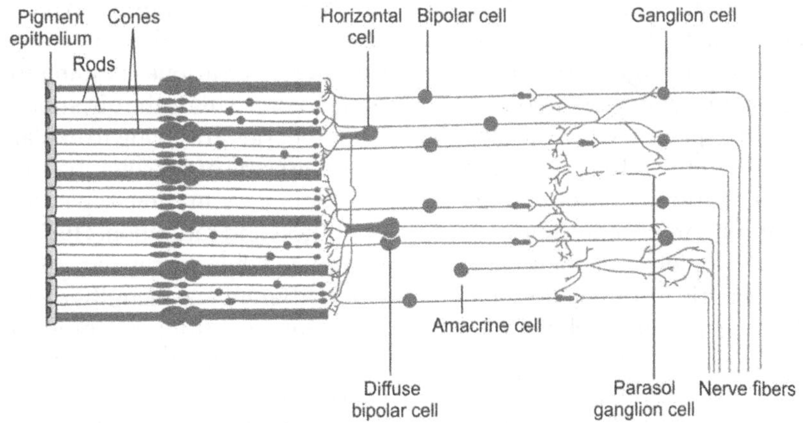

FIGURE 4.3: Structure of retina

through the action of protein molecules called photopigments. When light (electromagnetic energy) strikes the photopigments, some of the energy is absorbed by the pigments and chemical changes occur, which initiate the chain of events involved in seeing. Absorption of light energy causes the pigment molecules to change their shape and this process creates electrical energy. Following the shape change, a series of electrical events occurs, which results in a receptor potential. Through a series of further electrical steps involving several cells of the retina, electrical activity is passed from the rods and cones to the ganglion cells. The electrical events that have traveled across the retina generate nerve impulses in the ganglion cells (which form the optic nerve) and are conveyed to the brain. If a stimulus triggers nerve responses at each of the three levels (rod or cone, bipolar cell, and ganglion cell), the message is instantaneously sent to the visual relay station in the thalamus and then on to the visual cortex of the brain.

Dark Adaptation

Suppose you enter a theater to see a morning show a bit late, you cannot see anything around you. If you wait for a brief time, you gradually start seeing things around you much better. In fact, after about 30 minutes, you are about 100,000 times more sensitive to light than you are during full daylight. This process is called **dark adaptation**, the gradual increase in brightness sensitivity that occurs over time under conditions of low illumination. The speed at which adaptation occurs is a result of the rate of change in the chemical composition of rods and cones. After absorbing light, photoreceptors (rods and cones) are depleted of their pigment molecules for a period of time. If you are in bright light, a large portion of photopigments will be depleted. During dark adaptation, the photopigment molecules are regenerated and the sensitivity of the receptor increases. The cones reach their greatest level of adaptation in just a few minutes, while the rods take 15 minutes to reach the maximum level. That is why light adaptation (the process of adjusting to bright light after exposure to dim light; remember what happens when you come out of a theater after watching a morning show) occurs much faster, taking only a minute or so.

Color Vision

We are blessed with a colorful world. We can see and enjoy innumerable objects that vary in color. The sight of bright green paddy fields, the soothing blue sky, dazzling lovely flowers, delightful rainbow and several colorful things around us make life worth living. But how do we experience the colors? We do not know everything about the phenomenon of color vision, but what little we know itself is thrilling. Color sensation depends on the wavelength of light. Although the range of wavelength we are sensitive is small in comparison with the entire electromagnetic spectrum, the little portion to which we can respond allows us a great variety in sensing the world. It becomes amply clear when you realize the number and nature of colors you can distinguish. You will be surprised to know that a normal human eye is so wonderfully attuned to color vision that it can recognize more than seven million color variations. Are there really so many colors in the universe or are they produced by various combinations of some basic colors? This is the question that several color theories are trying to explain. We shall examine some of the color theories a bit later.

Colors vary in three separate ways: hue, brightness and saturation. **Hue** refers to what is implied when we say red, green, yellow or blue. Different wavelengths of light produce sensations of different colors. **Brightness** (lightness) depends on the amplitude (the energy of the light source) of the light wave and to some extent upon the wavelength. The third dimension along which colors vary is **saturation**, which refers to the apparent purity of the color. Highly saturated colors appear to be pure hues, without any gray. Colors of low saturation appear closer to grey. Saturation depends on the complexity of the light wave. Different combinations of values on these three dimensions produce the incredibly rich range of colors and highly complicated processes underlie our ability to see these visual phenomena.

There are some people who cannot experience one or the other colors. They are color blind people. There are three kinds of color blindness: red-green, yellow-blue and total color blindness. In red-green variety, which is the most prevalent, everything including the grass appears yellow. In yellow-blue type, people cannot differentiate between yellow and blue; this is a rare type. The total color blindness is the rarest type and for these people everything appears black and white. People who are color blind in only one of the color systems (either red-green or yellow-blue) are called **dichromats** and those who are sensitive to only black and white (totally color blind) are called **monochromats**. Approximately, one in 50 men and one in 5,000 women are found to be color blind, that is, they cannot see either red-green or yellow-blue or both. Normal people who can see all the colors are called **trichromats**.

Another interesting phenomenon concerning color sensation is the **afterimage**, especially negative afterimage. For example, if you look at a green patch steadily for 20 seconds and then transfer your gaze to a gray background, you will see a red patch on the gray background. Similarly, if you look at a yellow patch for 20 seconds and change your gaze, you will see blue on the gray background. Red-green and yellow-blue are called complementary colors and looking at one of them will produce the experience of its complementary. What is the explanation for the occurrence of afterimages and color blindness? During the past 200 years, there have been several attempts to explain these and other issues pertaining to color experience. Among them, two important theories: the trichromatic theory and the opponent process theory have tried to answer the questions we raised above, of course, in different ways. Let us see what these theories have got to say.

Trichromatic theory of color vision: According to the trichromatic theory, proposed by an English physicist Thomas Young & German scientist Hermann Helmholtz, there are three kinds of color receptors (cones) in the retina, each of which is most sensitive to wavelengths corresponding to either blue, green or red. Any color in the visible spectrum can be obtained by some combination of these three wavelengths, through the **additive color mixture** (mixing of color lights, not pigments). The theory could not explain satisfactorily certain other color phenomena such as color blindness and color afterimages. For instance, examine how people see yellow. According to the **Young-Helmholtz trichromatic theory**, yellow is produced by the activity of red and green receptors. But people with red-green color blindness (those who cannot see either red or green) are able to see yellow. How is it possible? Similarly, the experience of color afterimages is not satisfactorily explained by the theory. Therefore, an alternative theory, the opponent process theory, was advanced.

Opponent process theory of color vision: Opponent process theory, proposed by a German physiologist Ewald Hering, assumes that there are three types of cones each of which responds in two ways. One type of receptor responds to red-green, the second type to yellow-blue and the third type to black-white. Red, yellow and white cause a tearing down (catabolic) process in their respective receptors and green, blue, and black cause a building up (anabolic) process in their respective receptors. If both colors to which a receptor is sensitive are experienced simultaneously, the anabolic and catabolic processes are canceled out and the sensation of gray results. If one color to which a receptor is sensitive is experienced, its corresponding process is depleted, leaving only its opposite to produce an afterimage. Hering's theory also explains why individuals who are red-green blind can still see yellow and why the inability to see red is usually accompanied by an inability to see green.

Ever since the two theories were advanced, there has been a lively debate between those accepting Young-Helmholtz theory and those accepting Hering's. The matter is far from being settled. Today, investigators believe that Young-Helmholtz theory is correct in assuming that there are neural cells sensitive to red, green and blue, and Hering's theory is correct in asserting that there are neural processes beyond the retina that should be taken into account to explain color sensations. Researchers today hold on to a *dual process theory*, which combines the trichromatic and opponent process theories, to account for color transduction process. There are also several other theories of color vision, old and new, such as Ladd-Franklin's evolutionary theory, Edwin Land's retinex theory, which need not concern us here.

Ear and Audition

The ear is second only to the eye as a channel of information about the world around us. We learn great many things by hearing; we acquire information and impart knowledge through speech for which hearing is essential. In addition, we receive many important signals and cues through hearing—the ringing of a door bell, the siren of a fire-engine, the footsteps of an approaching person and the chiming of a clock. We derive one of the great pleasures of life by listening to music.

The stimuli for audition are sound waves, a form of mechanical energy—the pressure changes among the air molecules brought about by a vibrating object. Sound travels through the air waves. In fact, what we call sound is actually pressure waves in air, water or some other conducting medium. The sound waves have two characteristics: frequency and amplitude. The frequency is the number of sound waves or cycles per second [hertz (Hz) is the recent technical name for cycles per second (cps); one Hz equals one cps]. Frequency is related to the pitch of the sound (pitch is the characteristic that makes sound high or low). The higher the frequency (Hz), the higher is the perceived pitch. Normal human beings are capable of detecting sound frequencies from 20 to 20,000 Hz. Amplitude refers to the vertical size of the sound waves—that is, the amount of compression and expansion of the molecules in the conducting medium. Amplitude determines the perceived loudness or intensity of the sound (Fig. 4.4).

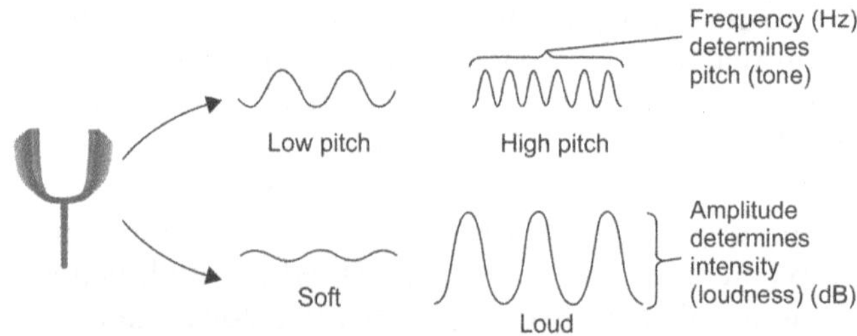

FIGURE 4.4: Auditory stimuli

Differences in amplitude are expressed as **decibels (dB)**. Decibel is the measure of the physical pressure that occurs at the eardrum. The absolute threshold for hearing is arbitrarily designated as 0 decibels and each increase of 10 decibels represents a tenfold increase in loudness; that is, a sound 10 times louder than the threshold sound is 10 dB; a sound 100 times louder than threshold level is 20 dB and one that is 1000 times louder is 30 dB and so on. For example, a whisper is 20 dB, sound of sewing machine is 60 dB and lawn mower sound is 90 dB, rock music 120 dB. Any sound over 80 dB can damage the ear if exposed for 8 hours or more, any sound of 140 dB can damage hearing after a single exposure and 160 dB sounds can break the eardrum on the spot.

Human Ear

The organ of hearing is the ear (Fig. 4.5). It is divided into three major parts: the external ear, the middle ear and the inner ear. The external ear consisting of pinna (the fleshy outer part of the ear), which collects the sound waves and sends them to the middle ear through the small air filled auditory canal (also called the external auditory meatus). The middle ear, the air filled space between the eardrum and the cochlea, contains the ossicles (three small bony structures called malleus, incus and stapes); the ossicles transmit the mechanical energy to the inner ear through the **oval window**. The inner ear contains the most important organ of hearing, the cochlea, where the physical energy is converted into neural impulses (the process of transduction) and the organs of balance (the **semicircular canals**).

The **pinna** collects the physical energy (the sound waves), which travels through the auditory canal and reaches the eardrum. The eardrum called **tympanic membrane** is a thin and flexible membrane stretched across the inner end of the **external auditory meatus** (the auditory canal). The tympanic membrane vibrates in response to the sound waves and these vibrations move the **ossicles** (the three tiny bones) and thus the physical energy changes reach the cochlea in the inner ear. The ossicles (**malleus**, **incus** and **stapes**, also called the *hammer*, the *anvil* and the *stirrup*, respectively, because of their resemblance to the latter objects) amplify the sound waves before sending them to the cochlea.

Cochlea

The **cochlea** is a coiled, snail-shaped, bony structure consisting of three fluid-filled canals

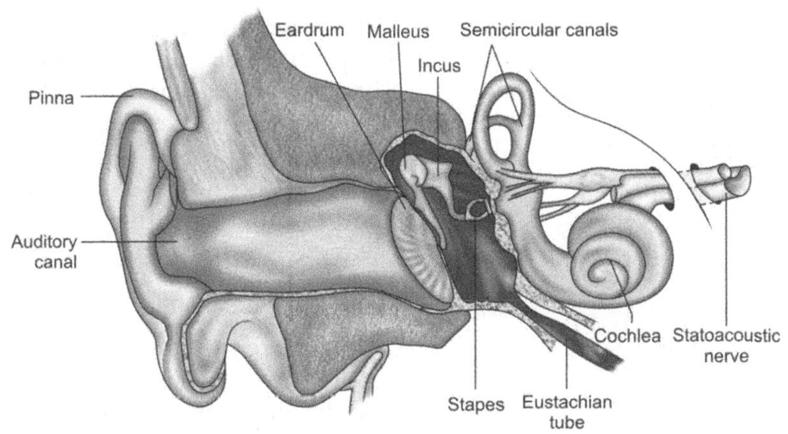

FIGURE 4.5: Structure of ear

spiraling around together and separated from one another by membranes. The three canals are called the vestibular canal (scala vestibuli), the cochlear canal (cochlear duct or scala media) and the tympanic canal (scala tympani). The first and second canals are separated by the **Reissner's membrane** and the second and third by **basilar membrane** (Fig. 4.6).

As the ossicles move back and forth, one of them, the stapes, presses on the membranous oval window and the sound waves move into the cochlea. In this way, when changes in air pressure move the ossicles, waves are set up in the fluid that fills the canals of the cochlea. The waves in the cochlea reach the **organ of Corti**, which lies on the basilar membrane. The pressure waves in the cochlear canals produce bending movements of fine, hair-like processes on the end of the hair cells of the organ of Corti. When these hair-like processes are bent, receptor potentials are initiated, thus starting the process by which nerve impulses are generated. The hair cells synapse with the neurons of the auditory nerve, which in turn sends impulses via an auditory relay station in the thalamus to the auditory centers in the temporal lobe of the brain. In summary, then, the bending of the hair cell fibers is the event that is responsible in the auditory system for the transduction of mechanical energy (air pressure variations caused by sound waves) into nerve impulses.

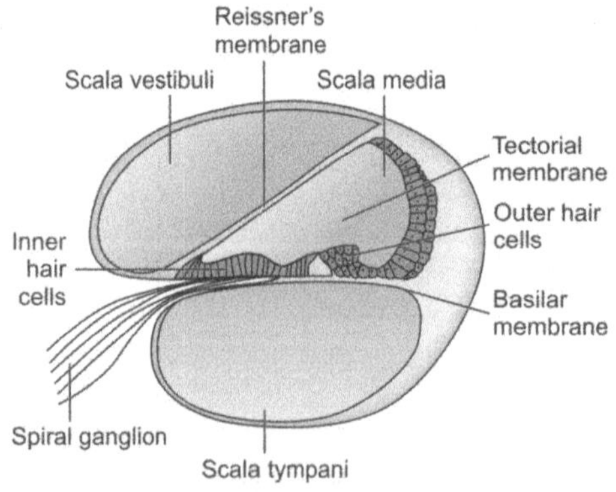

FIGURE 4.6: Structure of cochlea

The pitch, loudness and timbre in the sound system are analogues of hue, brightness and saturation in color vision. The pitch depends on the frequency of sound waves (CPS or Hz). The loudness (intensity of the sound) depends on the amplitude of the sound wave. The timbre is the component of sound, which helps us to differentiate the sound of one musical instrument from the other and the voice of one person from another.

In short, remember that sound waves travel through the fluid-filled cochlea and cause the basilar membrane to vibrate and activate the hair cells in the organ of Corti, which are connected to the auditory nerve. The nerve reaches the auditory centers in the brain and we have the experience of sound. But the question is: How does a small structure such as the organ of Corti, which is less than the size of a pea, help us to differentiate thousands of different tones and how do we discriminate varying pitches and loudness? Several theories have been proposed to answer these questions. We are told that loudness is determined by the total number of fibers firing and by the stimulation of certain high threshold fibers. Pitch is explained by two theories: the place theory and the frequency theory.

Theories of Hearing

The **place theory** says that the experience of pitch depends on the place at which the basilar membrane is stimulated. The area of the membrane nearer to the oval window is most sensitive to high-frequency waves and the part nearer to the cochlea's inner end is most sensitive to low-frequency waves. The **frequency theory** states that the nerve impulses sent to the brain match the frequency of the sound waves. Both the theories are partially correct. It is found that at low frequencies, the frequency theory holds good, and at higher frequencies, the place theory. The physical basis of timbre—the tonal quality that enables us to distinguish the sounds of different musical instruments and voices of different people depend on the pattern of harmonics. In fact, not much is known about the **afferent code** (the pattern of firings of nerve fibers corresponding to external stimuli) for timbre. There are several other minor theories of hearing, but none of them have adequately explained the complex phenomenon of hearing. Already one Nobel Prize has been awarded to Georg von Bekesy in 1961 for his work for coding pitch and more than one such prize is waiting for someone who can give an adequate picture of the brain mechanisms involved in the audition.

Hearing Loss

A large number of people suffer from hearing loss. Exposure to loud sounds may result in deafness. It is reported that in the United States some 20 million people suffer from hearing impairment. There are two types of hearing loss: conduction deafness and nerve deafness. **Conduction deafness** involves problems with the mechanical system that transmits sound waves to the cochlea. For example, a damaged tympanic membrane or inadequate functioning of the ossicles impairs the capacity of the ear to transmit vibrations. **Nerve deafness** is caused by damage to the receptors within the inner ear or to the auditory nerve itself. Repeated exposure to loud sounds of a particular frequency can eventually cause the loss of hair cells at a particular point on the basilar membrane, thereby causing deafness to that frequency. Even without any damage to the auditory system, many people develop some hearing loss as they grow old. Eventually, it appears that about 10 percent of people have some degree of auditory impairment. Minor hearing loss (especially conduction loss) can be treated with hearing aids. Deafness caused by damage to the hair cells is often treated by cochlear implant.

Sense of Smell

From the point of view of evolution, **olfaction** or the sense of smell is the most primitive of the senses. Olfaction is of immense importance for subhuman species. The social and sexual activities of several animals are regulated by the sense of smell. Some animals mark their territory using their urine just like humans putting fence around their living space. In fish, the entire brain is engaged in olfaction. In dogs, the olfactory cortex occupies about one-third of the area of the brain as contrasted with one-twentieth of this area in humans. Now, you can understand why police dogs are used in the detection of crime and in several other activities. Although humans are not as good as animals in detecting odors, they have enough ability to distinguish more than ten thousand separate smells. Women appear to have a keener sense of smell; it has been shown that they can identify their babies solely on the basis of smell just a few hours after birth. It has been found that women who live together for an extended period of time tend to menstruate around the same time. This phenomenon, known as **menstrual synchrony**, is believed to be mediated by the smell of some **pheromones** (chemicals found in natural body scents) secreted by them. Experiments have demonstrated that humans have the ability to distinguish males from females based on smell alone. Human beings are found to have a good memory for smells. Experiments have shown that substances present in the underarm secretions of young women can increase the women's sexual attractiveness to men. Scientists have also shown that male sweat can relax women.

Our knowledge of olfaction, although inadequate, is beginning to emerge slowly. Today, we know that smell is a chemical sense that starts working when molecules of some substance enter the nasal cavity and stimulate the cells (the smell receptors) in the **olfactory epithelium**. It is estimated that humans have about 40 million olfactory receptors (dogs have about a billion). More than one thousand separate receptor cells have been identified so far. Each of these cells is specialized to respond to a specific group of odors. The change in these receptor cells is transmitted to the brain where it is recognized as a separate smell. According to one theory, there are four basic odors: acid, fragrant, burnt and caprylic, which when mixed in right proportion accounts for all the odors. The importance of olfaction is suggested by the fact that the olfactory epithelium of each nasal cavity is directly connected (without synapses) to the **olfactory bulbs** of the brain, just below the frontal lobes. The bulbs in turn are connected to olfactory cortex on the inside of the temporal lobes and extend to the neighboring cortex. The exact nature of the neural connections mediating smell is still a matter of conjecture.

SENSE OF TASTE

Gustation or sense of taste and olfaction are called chemical senses because for both the stimuli are chemical molecules emitted by substances. In fact, the two senses are so intertwined that sometimes they are referred to as common chemical sense. It is not strange because you cannot enjoy your food when smell and taste are separated. You know also the food "tastes" bad when you have a stuffy nose. In fact, taste experience is a combination of smell, touch and temperature. Even sight is sometimes important because what you eat must also look good.

The receptors for taste are specialized cells located in the **taste buds** (humans have about 9 to 10 thousand of them) distributed differently on the tongue. There are four primary taste receptors: one for sweet, one for sour, one for salt, and the fourth one for bitter. Receptors for sweet are concentrated at the tip of the tongue, salt on the tip and sides, sour along the sides and bitter at the back; the central area of the tongue is relatively insensitive to taste. A few gustatory receptors are also found on the roof and the back of the mouth; they enable people without tongue to experience taste. When food is put into the mouth, it mixes with saliva forming a chemical compound, which in turn stimulates the receptor cells. The taste is the result of complex activity of neural fibers. People differ with regard to their ability to smell and taste things. Some people who are highly sensitive to taste are referred to as "supertasters". For them, sweets appear to be sweeter. Surprisingly, supertasters are more likely to be women than men. A person with an acute chemical sense may be employed by coffee board to sort and grade different varieties of coffee for marketing; it is a well-paid job.

SKIN SENSES

Most people do not realize the importance of skin senses. From the evolutionary perspective, the skin is the first sense modality to evolve and probably the last to disintegrate. One may survive without eyes, without ears and also without the chemical senses. But no one can survive without the sense of touch. The skin is often referred to as a "giant sense organ" that covers the body (Morgan et al, 1986). It is the largest organ of the human body; weighing between 6 to 10 pounds and covering about two square yards (Passer & Smith, 2007). Skin senses not only help us to avoid the dangers of extreme temperature and pain, they are also the source of the many pleasures of life including sex.

In fact, what we generally refer to as touch is not one sense, but made up of more than at least four sensations—touch or pressure, temperature (made up of two senses, warmth and cold) and pain. The skin can also tell us much more than these; we can identify objects by touching. Helen Keller, we are told, could recognize people by touching their faces. The skin is not uniformly sensitive; it is sensitive at some points and not so at others (punctate sensitivity). Also the points that are most sensitive to touch, warmth, cold and pain are distributed differently. In spite of its importance, it is surprising that we do not know the exact number and nature of skin receptors. A number of skin receptors have been identified (Fig. 4.7) and are implicated to mediate one or the other of the skin senses. For instance, it is believed that **Meissner's corpuscles** serve the pressure sense in the hairless parts of the body (for example, the palm of the hand), **basket nerve endings** (situated at the base of hair follicles) do the same thing for the roots of hairs and **pacinian corpuscles** are receptors for deep pressure.

We are told that there are some "cold fibers" and "warm fibers" that mediate cold and warm sensations. Certain **free nerve endings** (nerve cells beneath the skin surface that resemble bare tree branches) are found to be involved in pain sensation. All the skin receptors send their messages to the somatosensory cortex in the brain where they are interpreted. The amount of somatosensory cortex devoted to each area of the body is related to the sensitivity of that part; for instance, fingers, lips, nose, cheek and tip of the tongue occupy more space on the cortex compared to the arms, legs, and trunk because the former parts are more sensitive than the latter. The skin senses collectively are called **cutaneous senses**.

KINESTHETIC SENSE

The sensory system called **kinesthesis** provides us with information pertaining to the position and movement of the body parts. The receptors for kinesthesis are nerve endings located in muscles, joints and tendons. Position and movement are detected by receptors in joints; receptors in muscles and tendons inform us whether a muscle is stretched or contracted. Kinesthetic sense helps us to walk, climb, reach for objects, grasp, manipulate and maintain a posture and several other voluntary movements. It would be very difficult to make coordinated movements without the feedback provided by kinesthesis.

VESTIBULAR SENSE

Cooperating with kinesthesis is the **vestibular sense**, which informs us with the total body position in relation to gravity and with movement of the body as a whole. The movement of the body parts in relation to each other and to the objects in the environment is the function of kinesthesis

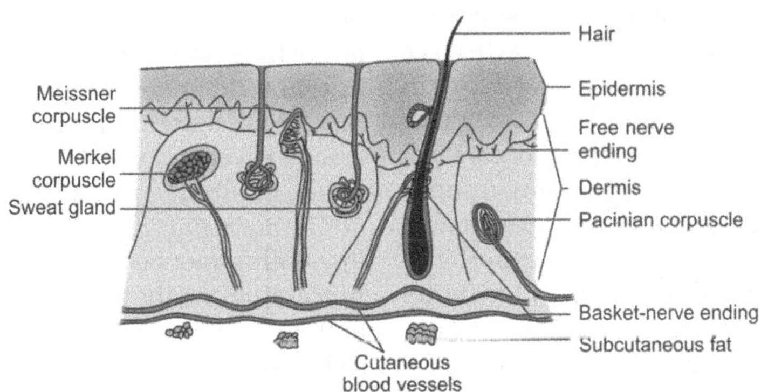

FIGURE 4.7: Skin receptors

and the movement of the body as a whole—its orientation in space, moving forward, backward, etc., is the responsibility of the vestibular sense. The vestibular receptors are located in the inner ear. There are two systems: the **semicircular canals** and the **vestibular sacs**. The first system consists of three semicircular canals (refer Fig. 4.5), each roughly perpendicular to the others, lying in three planes (left-right, backward-forward and up-down). These canals are filled with a fluid and lined with hair-like cells that function as receptors. When the head is moved, the fluid in the appropriate canal moves, stimulating the hair cells and sending messages to the brain. The second system, the vestibular sacs, located at the base of the semicircular canals, also contain hair cells that respond to the position of the body and inform us whether we are upright or tilted at an angle. The cutaneous, kinesthetic and vestibular senses are collectively called somatosenses or **somesthetic senses**.

PERCEPTUAL PROCESSES

Perceptual processes give coherence, unity and meaning to sensory input. The term perception covers the entire sequence of events starting from the presentation of physical stimulus to the sense organs, to the phenomenological experiencing of the stimulus. It includes the physical, physiological, neurological, sensory, cognitive, motivational and affective components. What is perceived is not determined by the physical stimulation of a sensory receptor alone; it is an organized, complex experience dependent upon a host of other factors. It is whatever that is experienced by a person, the experience of the world. In short, perception includes nearly every aspect of psychology.

The sensory input provides only the raw material for experience. The stimuli received by the sense organs are light, sound waves and pressure or chemical molecules. These are translated into a language that the brain can understand, the language of nerve impulses (transduction). The brain analyzes and reconstructs these messages and compares them with previously stored information, such as how things look, smell, taste or feel. This matching of new information with already stored information enables us to recognize the stimulus and give it meaning. This is conscious, perceptual experience. Our experiences are not simply a one to one reflection of stimuli impinging upon the sense organs. Same sensory input may be experienced differently by different people and the same person differently at different times. For example, suppose two persons, one a friend of yours and another a stranger, are standing in front of you. The sensory inputs sent to the brain about the two persons are more or less similar. But you recognize one of them as your friend and the other as a stranger. This depends on a number of central processes. When the brain receives the message, the higher brain centers are consulted and the message is compared with the available information in the memory store to determine whether the person has been seen earlier and if so where and when. Thus, perception is an active, creative process in which raw sensory data are organized and made meaningful. At any given time, we are bombarded by a number of stimuli, but we do not notice all of them. We ignore quite a few of them and attend only to what we want to notice. Often, we may notice several things that are not there. So, perception is a thrilling area of psychology and you will realize it as you read through next pages.

The brain engages in two types of activities in creating our perception: the **bottom-up processing** and the **top-down processing**. In bottom-up processing the brain recognizes individual elements of the stimulus and then combines them into a unified whole. In the top-down processing, the sensory input is interpreted in the light of our previous knowledge stored in the brain—that is, in terms of our concepts, ideas, values and expectations. When you read a printed sentence in this book, your visual system is following the bottom-up processing. That is, the feature detectors in the visual system analyze the elements in each letter of every word and then recombine them into a visual perception of letters and words. When you interpret the words and sentences constructed by the bottom-up processing, you are making use of top-down processing; that is, you are making use of your accumulated knowledge about the meaning of words and sentences. Our motives and expectations play an important role in top-down processing.

With this preliminary knowledge of perceptual processes, we now move on to various features and characteristics of perception. Most of the work in the area of perception pertains to visual perception. However, whatever is said about visual perception also applies to other areas such as auditory perception, tactile perception and other areas with slight modification.

Attention and Perception

One obvious feature of all of our perceptions is that they are selective. Although we are bombarded by innumerable number of stimuli at any given time, we do not notice all of them. If we notice all of them, our mind will be overloaded. Somehow, our brain selects those stimuli that are important and ignores others until a change in a particular stimulus makes it important for us to take note of it. This focal activity of the consciousness is called **attention**. Attention involves two processes:

1. It focuses on certain stimuli.
2. It filters out all other incoming information.

We cannot attend to more than one activity at a time. But we can shift our attention rapidly between two tasks, giving the appearance of divided attention. However, there is evidence that stimuli to which we are not attending are still registered in some form in our nervous system. Recently, scientists have coined the term *inattentional blindness* to refer to the failure of unattended stimuli to register in consciousness.

Determinants of Attention

Several factors determine why we attend to a certain stimulus among a number of competing stimuli. Attention is strongly influenced by stimulus factors as well as personal characteristics of the person attending. The stimulus characteristics that are important in gaining attention are size, intensity, color, contrast, novelty, repetition and movement of the stimulus. That is, other things being similar, we notice stimuli that are big, strong, unusual, different or moving. These factors are used by advertisers to attract the attention of potential customers. Personal factors such as motives, interests and expectations also influence the selection of stimuli. When you are hungry you notice restaurants rather than other shops in a street. We are also sensitive to stimuli that are threatening.

Perceptual Organization

When we look at the world around us, we see things as falling into groups. We see trees, buildings and people as separate from each other. But what our visual receptor is conveying to us is an array of varying intensities and frequencies of light energy. Yet, we perceive objects as separate and belonging to certain categories. That is due to some kind of organization imposed by our nervous system on our perception. These principles of perceptual organization have been extensively studied by Gestalt psychologists.

Gestalt Principles of Perceptual Organization

Figure-ground organization: During the early part of 20th century, Gestalt psychologists studied the processes operating in perceptual organization. The fundamental principle of perception according to them is that when we look outside, the perceptual field gets itself organized into a figure and a background. That is, there is a tendency to see certain stimuli as objects (figure) on a background. The figure appears to be well defined, more solid and tends to be slightly in front of the background. Very often, when the usual cues to distinguish figure from ground are absent, the figure and ground are reversible as can be seen in the case of vase-face figure (Fig. 4.8) and the book figure (Fig. 4.9). If you concentrate on the white portion of the figure, you will see a vase on the black background; if you concentrate on the black portion, you will see profiles of two people (facing each other) on the white background. You will also notice that when you continuously gaze at faces, after some time, it automatically becomes the vase and vice versa. The same processes operate in the case of book figure. Sometimes the figure looks like an open book and gradually it shifts to a closed book. These figures are called reversible figures. Two more reversible figures are also given (Figs 4.10 and 4.11). Watch them carefully and experience what happens.

The principle of figure-ground organization also occurs in auditory perception. For example, you may hear the melody played

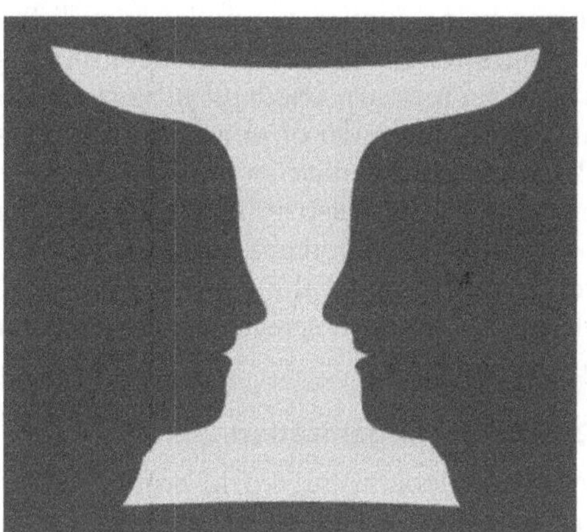

FIGURE 4.8: Vase-face figure

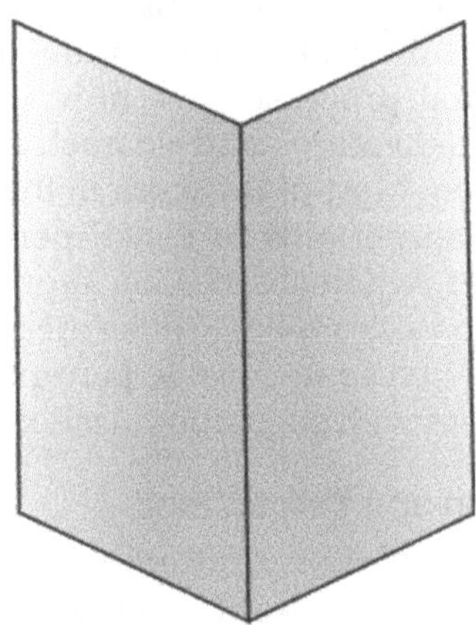

FIGURE 4.9: Book figure

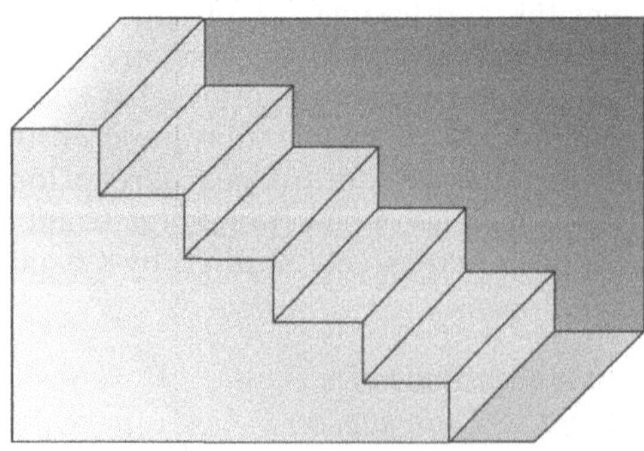

FIGURE 4.10: Staircase illusion

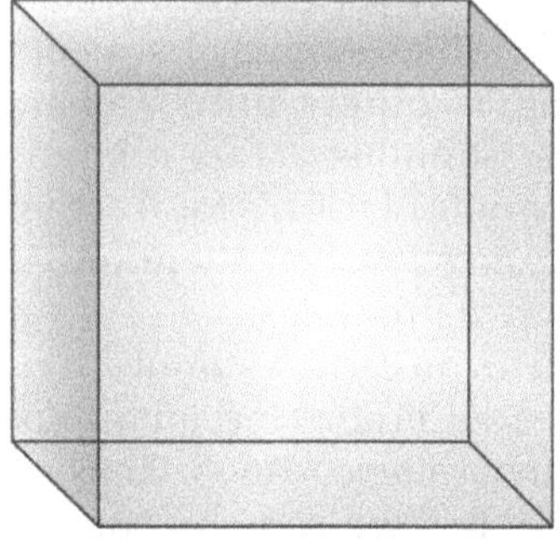

FIGURE 4.11: Necker cube

by violin against the background of other instruments in an orchestra. What is seen as figure depends upon several factors such as your interest, needs, expectations and so on.

Form perception: When we look at the world outside, we tend to perceive objects there as organized into patterns or groups. How does the organization take place? Gestalt psychologists have studied intensively the process of perceptual organization. They emphasized that the organized perceptual experience has properties, which cannot be understood by the analysis of the experience into its components. The experience must be considered as a whole and it should not be analyzed into its constituent parts. They asserted that the whole is more than the sum of the parts. This is the main theme of Gestalt psychology. According to Gestaltists, what is perceived has its own new properties; and these properties emerge from the organization. Organization in perception helps us to perceive forms or objects. If there has been no perceptual organization, we would not have seen books, trees, faces; instead we would see disconnected sensations. Gestalt psychologists have suggested that we group and interpret stimuli according to certain laws of organization such as the law of similarity, proximity, continuity and closure. These laws are illustrated in the Figures 4.12A to D.

The law of proximity or nearness states that elements, which are nearer to each other in space or time tend to be perceived as belonging together or forming an organized group. For example, in Figure 4.12A, we see six pairs of vertical lines instead of twelve single lines. The law of similarity states that elements that are similar are perceived as belonging to a group (refer Fig. 4.12B). Here, we tend to see XX as a pair, not XI or IX and proximity is ignored. The law of continuity says that we see elements together as they form a continuous line or pattern. For example, in the Figure 4.12D, we see the curved line cutting across the straight line and not as though the curved line becoming straight at the intersection point. The law of closure asserts that we tend to close the gaps in an incomplete figure to make it appear as a whole. In Figure 4.12C the brackets are pulled together, filling the intervening space in the act of closure; and in Figure 4.13, the left hand drawing is seen as a circle (or an ellipse) with gaps in it, and the central drawing is seen as a square (or rectangle) with gaps in it and not simply as disconnected lines. Similarly, in the last drawing, people see a man on horseback and not disconnected lines. The phenomenon of closure makes our perceived world of form more complete than the sensory stimulation that is presented.

Although the examples we have given pertain to vision, the same principles of grouping apply to other senses also. The rhythm we perceive in music is because of grouping according to proximity in time and the similarity in accents. Each of the above principles demonstrates how humans organize parts into wholes. The laws demonstrate the basic Gestalt assumption that

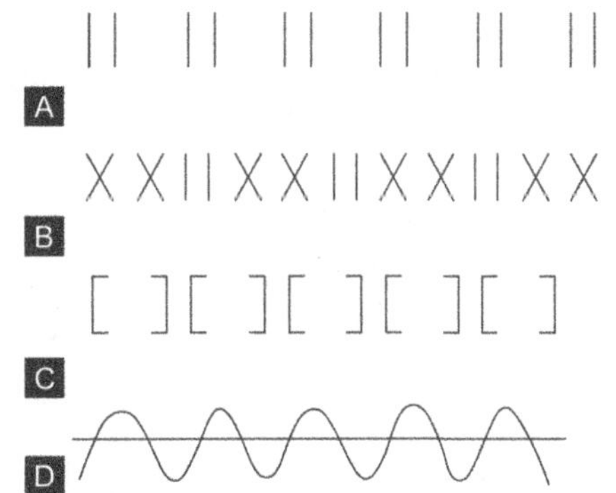

FIGURES 4.12A to D: Gestalt principles of perceptual organization. **A.** Proximity; **B.** Similarity; **C.** Closure; **D.** Continuation.

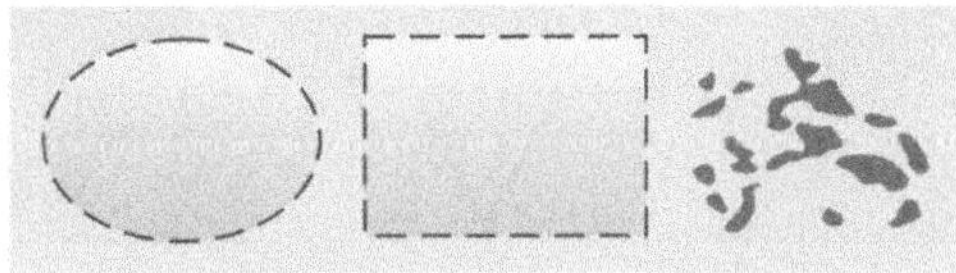

FIGURE 4.13: Principle of closure

the whole is more than the sum of the parts. In short, these laws show that the perceived organization has properties of its own that are not simply the result of adding together the elements of individual sensations.

Contours in visual form perception: We can separate forms from the background in our visual perception because of the contours. Contour is the outline of an object or a figure. Contours are formed whenever there is a marked difference in the brightness or color of the background. A white sheet of paper appears uniform. When you draw a vertical line in the middle of the sheet, the sheet is divided into two parts. Here you perceive a contour. Contours give shape to objects by marking one object off from the other or by marking an object from the background. While differences in energy level of light across the retina produce a contour, there are instances when contours are seen in the absence of any energy difference. This is called subjective contour. For example, in Figure 4.14, you see the contour of the upright triangle, even though there are no energy changes across its perceived borders except in the corners. Note that the three angles forming the corners of the inverted triangle do not produce a subjective contour.

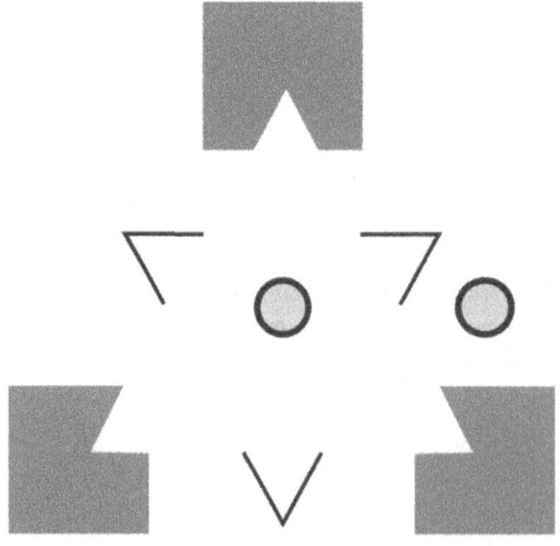

FIGURE 4.14: Subjective contour

In short, perception can be seen as an attempt to make sense of the stimulus input, to search for an acceptable interpretation of the sensory information based on our previous knowledge, and experience. In this sense, perception can be considered as a form of hypothesis testing. When we see something, we form an opinion about it (a hypothesis) and then test whether our opinion is right or not in the light of the data we have stored in the brain.

Perceptual Constancy

Suppose a familiar friend of yours is walking toward you. As he walks toward you, actually his image as formed on your retina becomes bigger and bigger. Do you wonder why he is bloating in size as he approaches you? No, you do not; you will see no change in his size or height in spite of the changes in the physical stimulus characteristics. This phenomenon is called **perceptual constancy**. Perceptual constancy refers to a phenomenon in which the size and shape of familiar objects or persons remain constant in spite of the changes in their appearance in the physical environment. This phenomenon helps us to recognize familiar objects in their original size and shape under varying conditions. In our day to day life, we experience several forms of perceptual constancies. The example of seeing your friend as not increasing in size is called **size constancy**. Suppose you see a round plate on the dining table from a distance. The physical stimulus of the plate that falls on your retina is oval in shape, but still you see the plate as circular. This is an example of **shape constancy**. Because of **brightness constancy**, a white towel in a dark room is seen as white and coal in bright light appears black although there is a change in illumination, the amount of light falling on the towel or coal. Similarly, a blue car appears blue whether you look at it in bright sunlight, in dim illumination or under a yellow street light. This is because of **color constancy**.

One of the dramatic illustrations of perceptual constancy is in the area of person perception. You see your mother as unvarying in height, size and shape for several years although several changes have taken place in her; she appears the same person to you. Because of perceptual constancy, we see a stable world around us; we perceive objects as enduring, as being the same as when we saw them last. The constancy phenomenon has some survival value. Suppose you see a wild elephant at a distance; it looks like small toy. But you still recognize it in its original size and avoid confronting it. A speeding truck at a distance appears very small; still you do not mistake it for a toy!

Depth Perception

The images of objects from the external world falling on the retina are flat and two-dimensional. But we see the world in three dimensions. We see certain things as being farther away and some as nearer to us. How do these experiences occur is a fascinating aspect of perception. The ability to see the world in three dimensions and to perceive distance is known as **depth perception** or space perception. The brain converts the two-dimensional images into three-dimensional pictures using two sets of cues called binocular cues and monocular cues.

Binocular cues occur because we have two eyes. One of the binocular depth cues comes from binocular disparity. **Binocular disparity** refers to the fact that each eye sees a slightly different image. This discrepancy between the two images in the two eyes is used by the brain to produce depth perception. This phenomenon can be seen when you look through a stereoscope (such as a *View master*). In a stereoscope, two flat pictures are presented one in front of each eye. The brain combines the two images to yield an experience of depth. The depth appears very real and you will see the objects as though they are set up on a stage.

The second binocular cue is **convergence**. When you focus on a nearby object, the two eyes turn inward (converge). The information provided by the muscles involved in turning the eyes is used by the brain to suggest that you are either seeing a nearby object or far away object. This does not mean that people with one eye cannot experience depth. The cues that help one-eyed people to perceive depth and distance are called **monocular cues**. Artists make use of monocular cues in their paintings to give us a three-dimensional experience. They use cues such as light and shadow, clearness, linear perspective, relative size, texture, interposition and motion parallax. All these except motion parallax are illustrated in the Figure 4.15 below.

The pattern of light and shadows on an object is an important cue that produces an experience of depth. In general, when an object is relatively clearer, we think it is nearer to us. In clear daylight, a distant tree appears nearer than on a hazy day; the haze in the atmosphere blurs the details and we see only

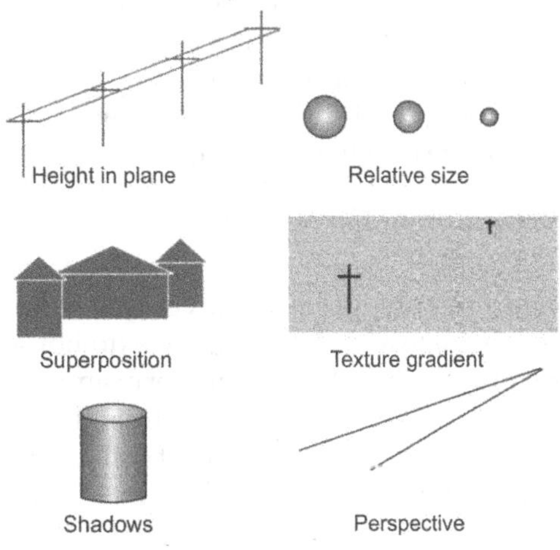

FIGURE 4.15: Monocular cues

larger features. When we see details clearly, the object appears to be nearer; when we see only the outline, we think the object is farther away. When you stand between railroad track and look farther, the rails appear to converge near the horizon and the distances between wooden planks appear to become smaller and smaller, thus giving an experience of depth. This is an example of linear perspective. When we see an object partially covering another object, the covered object appears to be farther away than the covering object. This is an instance of interposition or superposition. Gradient of texture provides a striking instance for depth perception. Look at the picture titled texture gradient. The regions closest to us appears to have a coarse texture and many details; as the distance increases, the texture becomes finer and finer. This continuous gradation in texture gives the eye and brain information that can be used to create an experience of depth.

Sometimes the movement of the objects works as cues for depth perception. For example, when you are in a moving train, the nearby objects (trees, telephone poles, etc.) move on a direction opposite to train's movement, but the distant objects appear to move in the same direction. Also, the nearer objects appear to move speedily in the opposite direction, while the far away ones move comparatively slowly. This phenomenon called **motion parallax** provides us with information, which helps us to judge depth and distance.

Perception of Movement

Movement perception is a strange phenomenon. We see movement where there is none and sometimes, we do not see movement when there is one. For example, in a movie, you see movement, although what is happening is the projection of still pictures at a known speed. All that is necessary to produce a movement experience is to move a stimulus across the retina under optimal conditions. The illusion of movement can be produced in the laboratory using the phi phenomenon apparatus (a stroboscope) as was done by Gestalt psychologist Max Wertheimer. Here, a light is briefly flashed in the darkness and then a few milliseconds later, another light is flashed nearby. If the timing and the distance between the two lights is just right and if the process is continued for a while, you will see the first light as moving from one place to another, thus producing an apparent movement, which looks like real movement. You must have seen stroboscopic movement in advertising. For example, you have witnessed strings of successively illuminated lights on a building that seem to move endlessly or that spell out some messages. It is the same stroboscopic movement principle that is used in motion pictures. The film you watch consists of a series of still pictures (called frames) projected on the screen in rapid succession with dark intervals in between. When the speed of projection of frames is 24 frames per second, you will have an illusion of smooth movement.

Perceptual Illusions

Illusions are false perceptions; they are compelling, but incorrect perceptions. These are intriguing, but delightful visual experiences, which provide information about how perceptual processes work under normal conditions. There are several physical stimuli that consistently produce errors in perception especially in the field of visual perception. In illusions, we select a perceptual hypothesis that is in fact wrong. Optical illusions have intrigued psychologists for long. Examine the geometrical illusions given in the figure in page 88 (Figs 4.16A to J) for an understanding of how illusions are produced.

In the Muller-Lyer illusion, the two lines appear unequal although physically the two are equal. Similarly, the vertical line appears longer than the horizontal line in the

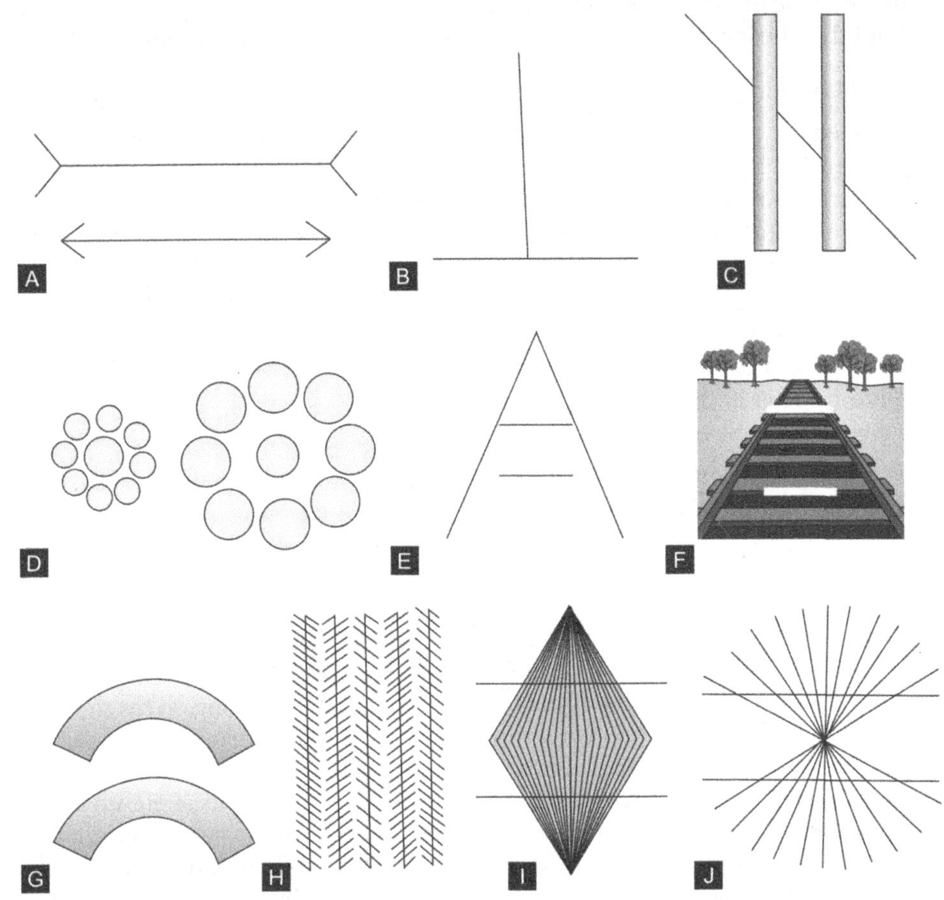

FIGURES 4.16A to J: Illusions. **A.** Muller-Lyer; **B.** Horizontal-vertical; **C.** Poggendorff; **D.** Ebbinghaus; **E.** Ponzo illusion-a; **F.** Ponzo illusion-b; **G.** Jastrow; **H.** Zollner; **I.** Hering; **J.** Helmholtz.

horizontal-vertical illusion. In Poggendorff illusion, the continuous line seems to be misplaced where it is partially obscured. In Ebbinghaus illusion, the two inner circles appear unequal, but actually they are equal. In Ponzo illusion, the two equal horizontal lines placed over two converging lines appear to be unequal in length. In Jastrow illusion, the upper of the two equal-sized ring sectors placed one above the other seems to be smaller. In Zollner illusion, the vertical lines are parallel, but do not appear so. Similarly, in Helmholtz and in Hering illusions, the lines are parallel, but do not appear so.

Illusion is not misperception or a trick; it is a perception. Illusions demonstrate that what we perceive often depends upon psychophysiological processes that go far beyond the stimulus input. Perceptual processes have done their work to produce the illusions. One of the intriguing phenomenon for which we do not have a satisfactory explanation is the moon illusion. The moon at the horizon appears bigger than when it is above your head. The moon does not change its size as it moves up; still you perceive the change in size. What causes the moon illusion? Although several explanations have been offered, none of them reveal the whole truth about the illusion.

Perceptual Learning

The phenomena of perceptual organization, constancy, illusion and perception of depth and of movement have all been demonstrated in the laboratory. But why do they occur? The answers given are not convincing. The major unanswered issue in psychology is whether we are endowed by birth the capacity to perceive the world as it is, or do we *learn* to perceive it. This is the age-old *nature-nurture controversy*. Several philosophers such as Descartes & Kant held that we are born with the capacity to perceive our environment. These are called nativists. Others such as Locke & Berkeley asserted that we learn the ways of perceiving the world through experience. These are called empiricists. Even eminent physiologists such as Helmholtz & Hering held opposing views. Hering was a nativist and Helmholtz an empiricist. Modern psychologists have found experimental evidence for both views. Eleanor Gibson (Gibson and Walk, 1960) presented enough evidence to show that young children are capable of depth perception through the now famous **visual cliff** (Fig. 4.17) experiment. It is shown that even animals are capable of depth perception. Today, psychologists believe that sensory and perceptual development is a product of both biological (hereditary) and experiential components. Your genes program biological development, but environmental experience can influence this development. Researchers have studied people who were accidentally blinded, and later learned to read braille. It was found that the area of the somatosensory cortex that is devoted to the finger tips gradually enlarged over time borrowing neighboring neurons to increase its sensitivity.

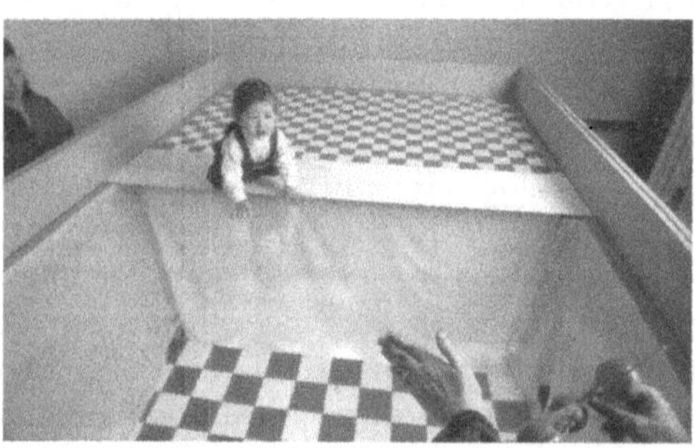

FIGURE 4.17: Visual cliff

The phenomenon of perceptual learning was demonstrated by George Stratton in 1896. You know that when light passes through the lens of the eye, the image formed on the retina is inverted (reversed); the right is left and the up is down. Stratton wore a special set of glasses that undid the natural reversion of the visual image; he saw the world upside down. The ground was at the top, his feet were up; he had to put on his hat from the bottom up; he had to reach to his left to touch something on his right. Stratton was terribly disoriented for some time. But gradually he adapted to his inverted world and by the end of eighth day he was able to reach for objects and walk around successfully. When he removed the inverting lenses, again there was disorientation, which became alright after a few days.

In addition to the above, there is experimental evidence to show that an individual's likes and dislikes, interest and values, expectations and motivational states influence perception. What appears ugly to one may appear to be attractive to another. The smell of fish may be nauseating to one, but it may be inviting to the other. People who are hungry, thirsty or sexually aroused are likely to perceive objects in the environment differently from those who are not. Therefore, some researchers think that perception is a function of perceiving individual; that is, perception to some extent depends on the individual's wishes, desires, motives, feelings, interests, values and past experience. This is especially, so when the stimulus environment is ambiguous and several interpretations are possible.

Cross cultural research has demonstrated that cultural environment often influences perception. For example, all of us see the lines in Muller-Lyer figure as unequal. This is because we live in "carpentered" environment, which has many corners and square shapes, inward-facing lines, and outward-facing lines. Living here, we have learned that inward-facing lines occur when the corners are closer and outward-facing lines occur when they are farther away. But people in other cultures who live in rounded environments see the lines in the Muller-Lyer figure as of equal length.

The evidence from cross-cultural studies, experiments on sensory deprivation in animals and humans and observations of congenitally blind people whose sight was restored suggest that biological and psychological factors interact in complex ways in determining what we perceive. Some of perceptual abilities are present at birth, but experience plays a crucial role in their normal development. Thus, perception is biopsychological process and we can learn more about it only when we examine the process from biological, psychological and environmental angles.

Extrasensory Perception

Before ending this chapter, something must be said about one of the most controversial areas known as extrasensory perception. The problem raised here is simple. If so many factors other than sensory stimuli influence perception, is it not possible to have a perception without any sensory stimulation at all? People who investigate extrasensory perception (sometimes called **psi phenomena**) are called parapsychologists; the most prominent among them was JB Rhine of Duke University. The phenomena parapsychologists investigate are two: **extrasensory perception (ESP)** and **psychokinesis (PK)**.

ESP includes three phenomena: **telepathy** referring to the transference of thoughts or ideas from one person to another without the actual involvement of any sensory channel; **clairvoyance**, which literally means "clear seeing" refers to the perception of objects or events without any sensory mediation whatsoever; and **precognition**, which refers to the perception of a future event. Psychokinesis refers to the capacity of an individual to move an object by mental operations without direct intervention or influencing of physical events (it is often called *parakinesis*).

Parapsychology is a highly controversial area and a majority of psychologists are skeptical about the existence of psi and some of them do not even accept it as a branch of psychology. However, there are some who believe that there is enough evidence to accept certain forms of ESP.

Chapter Summary

Sensation and perception are processes that enable us to understand the world around us. Each of our sense organs has a receptor and nerve fibers leading from this receptor to the brain or spinal cord. The physical energy falling on the receptor is converted into nerve impulses (transduction) corresponding to events in the environment. In vision, light passes through the cornea and lens and is focused on the retina. The receptors for vision are the rods and cones in the retina. Cones are active in bright light and rods in dim light. Transduction in the visual system occurs in the photosensitive elements in the rods and cones and the nerve impulses reach the brain through the optic nerve. Sensation of color (hue) depends on the wavelength of light. Brightness is determined by the intensity of light. The saturation depends on the degree to which the color is diluted by white light. Color sensation is explained by several theories. The trichromatic theory postulates three varieties of cones and the opponent process theory postulates four types of cells.

Contd...

Contd...

The physical stimuli for hearing are waves of pressure moving through the air and impinging on the eardrum. The waves create the vibrations in the ossicles (three small bones in the middle ear); these vibrations enter the cochlea through the oval window; the waves of the fluid of the cochlear canals produce bending movements of the fine hair like processes on the ends of the hair cells of the organ of Corti. The bending of the hair-cell fibers is the event responsible for transduction in the ear. The frequency of sound waves is related to pitch, the intensity of the sound waves to the loudness and the complexity of the sound waves to timbre (tonal quality).

Smell and taste are chemical senses. The receptors for smell respond to volatile chemical substances. The receptors for taste are specialized cells grouped together in clusters known as taste buds. When these are stimulated by chemicals dissolved in liquids, one or the other taste quality is produced. Evidence suggests that there are four taste qualities: salty, sour, sweet and bitter. According to one theory, there are four basic odors (acid, fragrant, burnt and caprylic), which when mixed in right proportion accounts for all the odors. There is no agreement about this view.

There are at least four skin senses: pressure, cold, warmth and pain. The stimulus for touch is a gradient of pressure on the skin or bending of the skin hairs. Experience of cold and warmth are produced by changes in the normal gradient of skin temperature, that is, by changes in the difference between the temperature on the skin surface and the temperature of the blood circulating beneath it. The cold and warmth receptors are specialized free nerve endings. The stimulus for pain seems to be an event which damages bodily tissues in some way. The receptors for pain are free nerve endings specialized in some way to respond to noxious stimulation. Pain gates in the central nervous system seem to block the transmission of pain signals and thus reduce the amount of pain perceived (see gate-control theory of pain in Chapter 14).

In addition to the eight senses mentioned above, there are two body senses: kinesthesis and vestibular sense. Kinesthesis provides us with information about the movement of body parts and their position in relation to each other. The receptors for kinesthesis are nerve endings in muscles, tendons and joints. Vestibular sense provides us information about the balance and position of our body in space. The vestibular sense receptors are located in the semicircular canals and vestibular sacs in the inner ear.

Perception is the process by which we take sensory input and organize it in ways that allow us to form a meaningful representation of the world around us. Perception is selective and controlled by attentional processes. Attention is an active process in which we focus on certain stimuli while blocking out others. Perception makes use of a combination of two processes: bottom-up processing in which individual stimulus fragments are combined into a perception and top-down processing in which existing knowledge and perceptual schemes are applied to interpret stimuli.

Gestalt psychologists have advanced our knowledge of perception through several principles of perceptual organization, including figure-ground organization and the laws of similarity, proximity, continuity and closure. An important perceptual organization is perceptual constancy, which allows us to recognize familiar stimuli in their original state under changing conditions. We respond to actual color, size, shape, brightness and not to the perceived attributes. Although the picture formed on the retina is flat, we are capable perceiving the world in three dimensions. This is possible because of two sets cues: monocular cues such as linear perspective, relative size, height, interposition, shadows, texture, clarity, motion parallax and binocular cues such as convergence of the eyes and retinal disparity. The basis of the perception of movement is an absolute movement of a stimulus across the retina or relative movement of an object in relation to its background. Often the experience of movement can be produced where there is no actual movement as seen in the case of phi phenomenon or apparent movement (stroboscopic movement like the one we experience in a movie).

Illusions are erroneous perceptions. They may be regarded as incorrect perceptual hypotheses. Perceptual constancies produce many illusions including the moon illusion and variety of other context-produced illusions.

Whether our capacity to perceive the world as we do is inborn or acquired has not yet been completely resolved. There is research evidence to show that the perceptual capacity is inherited; there is also enough proof to show that several perceptual phenomena are acquired. Perceptual development involves both physical maturation and learning. Although many aspects of perceptual experiences are constant across cultures, there appears to be some impact of culture in the perception of pictures and illusions. Some areas of perception, such as ESP are steeped in controversy.

5 CHAPTER

Fundamentals of Learning

PREVIEW

Learning is the most highly researched concept in psychology. The number of books and journal articles devoted to learning is legion. It is not surprising that so many people are interested in the area of learning and perception; the two are the fundamental processes that underlie all behavior and mental activities. Learning is an adaptive process. Our capacity to learn helps us to adapt to the demands of the environment. We are continuously modifying and adjusting our behavior in the face of environmental demands. The fact that all of us are engaged in learning something or the other most of the time, during our lifetime, is never doubted. But the question is: What is learning? What happens when you learn something? What happens to the material after it has been learned? Does the material learned remain in the mind permanently or disappear with lapse of time? What is forgetting? Is anything forgotten at all? Is there only one kind of learning or are there several varieties of learning. For example, is learning to drive a car the same as learning a passage from Shakespeare? When you sing your national anthem, do you know what line you are singing? One psychologist said that there are only two types of learning, another three types and still another eight types. Which is true? These and several other questions are haunting psychologists even today.

Psychologists are not in agreement upon what exactly is learning and not even on the definition of learning. The simplest definition that is generally offered by most people is that learning is "change brought about by experience." American psychologist Gregory Kimble (1961) has elaborated on this idea and defined learning as "a relatively permanent change in behavioral potentiality that occurs as a result of reinforced practice." This definition has four components: learning is a relatively permanent change, not temporary change brought about by habituation, fatigue, satiation, disease and the like. Learning is a potentiality to respond, which means that it may not manifest till the need arises; it may remain dormant or latent. Learning has to be reinforced, otherwise it will become extinct. Finally, the response must be practiced, repeated for it to survive. Not all these components are accepted by all thinkers in the area of learning. Some of the best brains in psychology have proposed different explanations of learning. Thorndike, Pavlov, Watson, Skinner, Bandura and the cognitive psychologists have interpreted learning differently and as a result, there are more than a dozen theories of learning. Behaviorists like Skinner emphasized reinforcement, but Guthrie did not think neither reinforcement nor repeated practice is necessary for learning to occur. His theory is often called "one-trial learning." Once a response is made, it is learnt. Contemporary cognitive psychologists look at learning from the information processing angle. While behaviorists explain learning in terms of external stimuli and responses, cognitive and social-learning theorists argue that mental activities—the thoughts and expectations—are crucial for understanding learning. So, the last word about the nature of learning is still to come.

You do not have to be unduly concerned about the theoretical controversies about learning. Also, you should not think that psychologists are all confused and have done nothing to help us understand the mechanisms involved in learning. The researches in this field have brought to light several significant insights about learning that have proved to be useful in several walks of life. Psychologists have suggested better and effective methods of teaching and learning. They have introduced the idea of programmed learning and devised teaching machines to implement it. Practical suggestions regarding how to study and how to remember and use the learned material have been offered. Regardless of the theoretical controversies, research on learning has allowed psychologists to make important contributions to the areas of education and psychotherapy (treatment of psychological disorders). There are various other suggestions that will be helpful to you in solving your day-to-day problems.

Chapter Outline

Learning is the key concept in psychology without which most of behavior and experience cannot be understood or explained. In order to realize its importance imagine for a while that you have lost all that you have learnt during your lifetime. What will happen? You will not know who you are, not even your name; you cannot understand the language people are speaking to you; you do not recognize the faces of people around you including your loved ones. In short, you cannot make out anything about the world around you. You will only be a bundle of muscles and nerves, just like a newborn child.

An infant in the cradle is helpless. He must be fed, bathed, dressed, cleaned and be looked after. But with the passage of time, when the infant grows up to be an adult, he /she will be capable of engaging in several complex activities. He can read, write, speak and understand a language, go to school and college, acquire a degree; take up an occupation, drive a vehicle, make love, marry, have children and interact with people and the environment. Between the time of birth and adulthood, great many changes take place in behavior. Most of these changes are products of learning. Learning plays an important role in the acquisition of the language we speak, our habits, beliefs, customs, ways of living, attitudes, opinions, goals, perceptions and in short, our personality. Naturally, learning is one of the most important areas of study in contemporary psychology and a great deal of theory and research has appeared about it.

But then, what is learning? The dictionaries say that learning is gaining knowledge or acquiring some skill through experience or study, or by being taught. Psychologists are not happy with this definition, because of the nebulous meaning attached to terms such as knowledge or skill. They prefer observable, operational and tangible meaning for the term. Therefore, they define learning as change in observable behavior. The simplest definition psychologists have offered to the term is that *learning is relatively permanent change in behavior that occurs as a result of experience*. There are three components in this definition:

1. Learning is a change in behavior.
2. It is a change that results from experience; changes due to maturation, disease, fatigue, drugs or physical damage are not learning.

3. The change must be relatively permanent; it must last a fairly long time. Temporary changes resulting from drugs or fatigue do not qualify to be called 'learning'.

In short, learning can be defined as profiting from experience; the profit may be positive or negative as in the case of acquiring a good or bad habit respectively. We may learn things that hurt, as well as help.

There are several controversies about the process of learning. Psychologists have looked at learning from different perspectives. As a consequence, several theories of learning have emerged. Ernest Hilgard, an authority on learning theory, has discussed at least a dozen major theories of learning (Hilgard & Bower, 1975). It is beyond the scope of this chapter to review all of them. Instead, we examine three theories of learning that are popularly discussed in contemporary textbooks of psychology. These are classical conditioning, operant conditioning, and cognitive learning. Let us start with classical conditioning, which is a model of associative learning.

CLASSICAL CONDITIONING

Classical conditioning is often called Pavlovian conditioning after its founder the Russian physiologist Ivan Petrovich Pavlov (Fig. 5.1). When Pavlov was studying secretions such as saliva during digestion in dogs (he was awarded the Nobel Prize for his work on digestion), he observed dogs salivating not only when food was presented but also for some neutral stimulus such as the sound of a bell that was paired with food. He called the salivation for food an, unlearned response and later named it **unconditioned response (UCR)**. The food was called **unconditioned stimulus (UCS)**. The neutral stimulus, such as the sound of bell, that was paired with food, which also produced saliva, was called **conditioned stimulus (CS)** and the salivation to the neutral stimulus was called **conditioned response (CR)**. For a clear understanding of this phenomenon, we must examine in detail how the experiment was conducted by Pavlov.

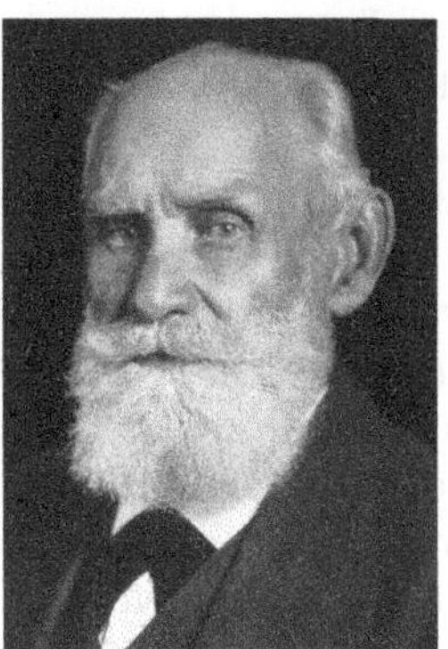

FIGURE 5.1: IP Pavlov

First, the dog was prepared for the experiment by performing a minor operation on its cheek, so that a part of its salivary gland is exposed. A graduated tube was attached to the cheek, so that the saliva secreted could be collected and measured. After the dog recovered from the operation, it was brought to the soundproof laboratory along with the fixtures and placed in a harness on a table. After the dog got itself acclimatized to the laboratory conditions, it was made to stand quietly on the table (Fig. 5.2). A cup was kept in front of the dog and it was so arranged that food could be delivered into the cup by remote control. The dog was completely isolated from extraneous

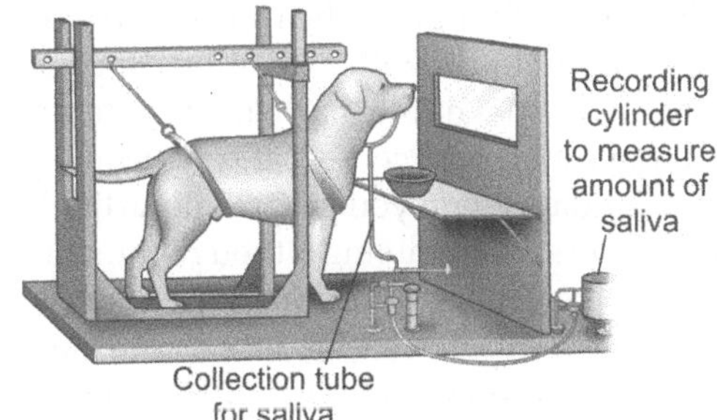

FIGURE 5.2: Pavlov's apparatus for studying conditioning

disturbances, but could be watched by the experimenter through a one-way glass panel. The salivation was recorded automatically.

Under these conditions, the sound of a bell (CS) is made. The dog may look up that way this way, but it does not salivate. After a few seconds, the food (UCS) is delivered into the cup. The dog eats the food and of course it salivates (UCR). A few more trials are given in such a way that when the bell is sounded it is always followed by food, which in turn produces salivation. The presentation of food (UCS) always after the sound of the bell (CS) is called **reinforcement**. After several reinforcements, the dog started salivating after hearing the sound of the bell even though food did not follow. When this happens, a CR (salivation to bell) has been established. The animal has come to associate the sound of the bell with the arrival food. Thus, a new type of learning has taken place. This is the process of conditioning and it is called classical conditioning to differentiate it from another kind of conditioning called **operant conditioning**.

Thus, classical conditioning is a process in which a neutral stimulus (CS) acquires the capacity to elicit a response (CR), which it did not do so earlier, by being paired with a natural stimulus (UCS), which always produced that response (UCS). We have several examples of such type of conditioning in our daily life: When you hear the word mango pickles, for example, you start salivating, although the hearing of the word has nothing to do with salivation. Suppose you saw a snake in a particular place and you have experienced fear; it is natural. But the next day, when you go to that particular place, you start trembling although the snake is not there. There are innumerable examples of such conditioned behaviors in our daily life. In all these situations a new learning has taken place. The basic processes involved in conditioning, which occur in three phases, are shown in **Box 5.1**.

Box 5.1: Three Phases of Classical Conditioning

1. Before conditioning	
Sound of bell (CS*)	No salivation
Food (UCS†)	Salivation
2. During conditioning	
Sound of bell + Food (CS + UCS)	Salivation (UCR‡)
3. After conditioning	
Sound of bell (CS)	Salivation (CR§)

*CS, conditioned stimulus; †UCS, unconditioned stimulus; ‡UCR, unconditioned response; §CR, conditioned response.

You have to remember one thing here. The salivation for food is called UCR and the salivation for bell is called CR. Are there no differences between these two? Yes, there are: one is that in the second case it is salivation to bell; the other is that the amount of salivation in the second case is slightly smaller.

Theories of Classical Conditioning

Although the discovery of CR as a form of learning revolutionized modern psychology, Pavlov never called himself a psychologist. He first called the phenomenon of the dog's salivating after hearing the sound of the bell *psychic secretion*. Since it looked mentalistic, he later named it conditioned response. Whatever that may be, the important issue here is: What are the psychological and physiological processes that occur when a conditioned response is acquired? There are differences of opinion in this regard. Two theories have been offered to explain the phenomenon of classical conditioning: one is the stimulus substitution theory proposed by Pavlov; the other is the information and expectation theory.

The stimulus substitution theory asserts that the CS, simply as a result of being paired with the UCS, acquires the capacity to be a substitute for the UCS in eliciting a response. That is, an associative bond or link between the UCS and CS is formed, so that the CS becomes an equivalent of UCS in evoking a response. Pavlov thought that such a linkage is established in the brain, and as a result of pairing of CS and UCS, the CS acquires the ability to excite the UCS area, thus leading to a reflex response.

The information and expectation theorists assert that the CS operates like a signal for the UCS and therefore, when the CS is presented, the UCS is expected and the learner responds in accordance with this expectation. The issue is not yet settled. Let us leave it to future research to decide the issue and proceed to examine the various other parameters of classical conditioning.

Factors Influencing Classical Conditioning

Acquisition of conditioned response is a gradual process and it depends on several factors. During the acquisition period, the CS-UCS pair must be presented a number of times. The CS is established quickly when it is reinforced copiously. When the UCS is intense and aversive (as in the case of sighting a snake, mentioned above), conditioning may occur with only one pairing. The sequence and time interval between the CS-UCS pairing are very important factors in conditioning. Under *forward short-delay pairing*, the CS (bell) appears first and is still present when UCS (food) is introduced; in this case, conditioning takes place quickly. In *forward trace pairing*, the CS (bell) is presented and stopped; a little later, UCS (food) is introduced. If the interval between the introduction of sound and food is more than 4 seconds (the so called **delayed conditioning)**, it is difficult to condition the animal. It is found that 2 to 3 seconds is the optimal interval for conditioning to occur. In *simultaneous pairing*, the CS and UCS are presented at the same time; in this case, acquisition of CR is less rapid. When the CS is presented after the UCS, the condition called **backward conditioning**, learning is the slowest. Once a conditioned response is established, generally it persists for a long time. In short, the acquisition of a conditioned response is easy, when the CS-UCS pairing is repeated several times, when the UCS is very strong, when there is forward pairing (CS appears first and is always followed by UCS) and when the time interval between the presentation of the CS and UCS is short (not more than 2 to 3 seconds).

Extinction and Spontaneous Recovery

What happens when the conditioned response is not reinforced? That is, what would be the result if ringing of the bell is not followed by food? During the first few trials, the dog salivates, but gradually the salivation decreases and finally stops. The frequency of conditioned response (such as salivation) gradually decreases and finally disappears. This process of weakening and finally disappearing of the CR in the absence of UCR is called **extinction**. Each occurrence of CS without UCS is called *extinction trial*. As the extinction trials are repeated, the CR weakens and finally disappears (the amount of saliva secreted by the dog diminishes and finally salivation stops). Therefore, it is necessary to reinforce the CS occasionally to retain the CR. One of the basic phenomena of conditioned learning is extinction—the decrease in frequency and eventual disappearance of conditioned response in the absence of reinforcement.

Two explanations are offered for the operation of extinction. One is that of Pavlov and the other offered by information-expectation theorists. According to Pavlov, two brain processes occur during conditioning: excitation and inhibition. During conditioning, the excitatory process is stronger and during extinction, the inhibitory tendency is stronger and hence the CR is suppressed. The information-expectation theory says that during extinction, the CS is not followed by UCS and therefore, the CS is no more the signal for the arrival of the UCS and the organism does not pay attention to it.

The disappearance of CR as a result of extinction is not permanent. After a few hours, if the animal is presented the CS, the CR appears suddenly. This phenomenon is called **spontaneous recovery**. In fact, the magnitude of CR in this case may be more than what it was earlier. It means that extinction does not completely erase the tendency to respond to the CS and some learning trace is still left there. This assumption is supported by the fact that reconditioning of the animal is easier and quicker than was the original conditioning.

Stimulus Generalization and Discrimination

During his experiments, Pavlov observed that the dog, which has learnt to salivate to the sound of a bell (CS), also salivates to other sounds that were similar to that of the bell. The greater the similarity among the stimuli, greater was the chance of the appearance of the CR. This phenomenon is called **stimulus generalization**—the tendency of any stimulus, similar to the original stimulus (CS), to elicit the CR. Generalization broadens the scope of classical conditioning in explaining several behavior patterns. A child who was threatened by a dog starts fearing all dogs and later all four legged animals and for that matter, the child may be scared even by a toy dog. Stimulus generalization plays an important role in the development of irrational fears and other maladaptive behaviors. For instance, one who has seen a snake in a green bush may develop a fear of all green bushes and later he/she may develop the fear of anything that is green. A girl went to take an examination and she did not do well that day. It so happened that on that day she was wearing a yellow saree. From then on, she never wore a yellow saree, while going to the examination. Later, she developed a dislike for yellow saree, and still later, all things that were yellow. Thus, many of our likes and dislikes as well as fears are the result of stimulus generalization.

On the other hand, people also have the ability to distinguish one stimulus from the other and respond to them differently. For example, we respond differently for red and green lights at traffic signal points. This process of learning to make one response to one stimulus and a different response or no response to another is called **stimulus discrimination**. Stimulus discrimination prevents stimulus generalization from running wild. It is necessary for us to discriminate between a good dog and a bad one; it should be possible for us to discriminate between a safe situation and a dangerous one although they look similar. In this way, stimulus discrimination works against the unnecessary hazards created by stimulus generalization.

Experimental Neurosis

Let us now examine an interesting phenomenon that Pavlov observed during his experiments. Suppose that showing the dog a circle is always followed by food and showing an ellipse is never followed by food. As we have seen, the circle will elicit salivation and the ellipse will inhibit salivation. Now, suppose the experimenter gradually changes the shape of the circle so that it appears more elliptical. What would happen? The animal cannot distinguish between the circle and the ellipse; that is, as Pavlov speculated the excitatory and inhibitory tendencies conflict and as a consequence, the animal's behavior breaks down. Since this behavioral breakdown occurs in a laboratory, it was called **experimental neurosis**.

An interesting fact in this connection was that different dogs exhibited different forms of "neurosis." Some dogs became highly irritable, tearing at the apparatus and barking violently. Others responded to the conflict by becoming depressed and timid. Based on these observations, Pavlov classified the animals into four categories; animals with:

1. High excitatory tendency.
2. Moderate excitatory tendency.
3. High inhibitory tendency.
4. Moderate inhibitory tendency.

Thus, Pavlov speculated that the way animals, including human beings, respond to conflicts depends on the nervous system they possess. He also said that much of human abnormal behavior is due to a breakdown of the inhibitory tendencies in the brain. Pavlov's views on conflict and the typology of the nervous system have influenced the subsequent researches in the areas of conflict, frustration, aggression and abnormal behavior.

Higher-order Conditioning

Suppose a dog is conditioned to salivate to the sound of a bell; that is, now the sound of the bell is the conditioned stimulus (CS) that produces salivation. Next, present a neutral stimulus, such as a green light, to which the dog does not salivate. Now, present the green light along with bell (but do not give food); still the dog salivates. If the green light and bell pair is presented several times, the green light acquires the capacity to produce saliva. This is called **higher-order conditioning** in which a neutral stimulus becomes a conditioned stimulus when it is paired with an already established conditioned stimulus. Generally, the conditioned response (CR) produced under higher-order conditioning is weaker and extinguishes more rapidly than the original CR. The dog salivates less to the green light than to sound of the bell and the salivation extinguishes sooner.

Applications of Classical Conditioning

The principles of conditioning discovered in the laboratory have been found to be useful in explaining several aspects of human as well as animal behavior. It has been shown that several of our aversions and attractions toward persons, objects or events are products of conditioning. Many of our subjective feelings of likes, dislikes, and several of our emotions are probably conditioned responses. The scent used by your spouse often triggers sexual arousal in you because the smell of the scent and your spouse have occurred together and have become associated. Similarly, the color of the dress your friend wears may be the source of attraction towards him/her. Several of our fears are conditioned. In fact, conditioning procedures may be used to get rid of several fears through deconditioning or unlearning. If fear is learned, it can be unlearned. Acquiring or eliminating fears has been a fascinating area of research in psychology.

In a classic experiment, Watson and Rayner (1920) demonstrated how children's fears are conditioned (see Chapter 10). In 1924, Mary Cover Jones successfully demonstrated how children's fears could be eliminated. Her approach to extinguish fear has become the basis for one of the current behavior therapies called **exposure therapy**. Recent laboratory experiments have convincingly shown that animals become afraid of neutral stimuli that were paired with electric shock. Today, behavior therapy techniques based on classical conditioning principles are among the most effective psychotherapies in treating phobias (refer Chapter 16).

Conditioning principles have been used to teach human body to learn to respond in ways that either promote or harm health. Classical conditioning explains why sometimes we develop physical symptoms that do not seem to have a medical cause. Suppose an individual is allergic to something, say a drug. If the drug is repeatedly paired with an odor, after some time, the individual exhibits allergic reactions to the odor itself. As you know, chemotherapy and radiation therapy, the popular treatments for cancer, produce nausea and vomiting among the patients. Many of these patients develop **anticipatory nausea and vomiting (ANV)**;

that is, they start vomiting hours before the commencement of the treatment. The sight of the hospital, the hypodermic needle, the doctor, the nurse, all neutral stimuli, by virtue of their being associated with treatment act as conditioned stimuli and trigger nausea and vomiting. Psychologist, Robert Ader (2001) demonstrated that the immune system among rats could be altered through classical conditioning. He administered an immune-suppressing drug to rats as they drank sweetened water. After several trials, the sweetened water itself became the immune suppressing agent. In another study, a German researcher administered a group of volunteer subjects sweet sherbet along with an injection of epinephrine (which increases the activity of the immune system). After a number of paired administrations, the subjects reacted to the sherbet alone with a stronger immune response. There are several other studies that have demonstrated that classical conditioning can be used to help fight disease.

Substance abuse, alcohol consumption and smoking can be eliminated using a conditioning technique called **aversion therapy**. People's attitudes, opinions and prejudices (racial discrimination, untouchability) can be modified, and several social evils can be eradicated using appropriate conditioning procedures. Advertising makes use of conditioning principles to make the products attractive to the consumer by pairing them with good-looking models. You have watched ads in which a pretty young woman standing by the side of a car. Looking at the woman elicits pleasant feelings in you. These feelings spread to the car by virtue of stimulus generalization and as a consequence, you develop a liking for the car and you may buy it. It has been shown that several allergic reactions and some of the disease symptoms are products of conditioning and they can be terminated by deconditioning.

OPERANT CONDITIONING

In spite of its importance and usefulness, classical conditioning cannot explain several other forms of learning we are familiar with. For example, it does not explain how we learn to drive a cycle, use a computer or make friends or fall in love. These are voluntary responses made by us, not reflexes (or responses) elicited by external stimuli. Pavlov's dog did not voluntarily salivate; it was elicited by a stimulus. The voluntary responses we make are *emitted*, not *elicited*. The learning of emitted responses is called **operant conditioning**. In learning of this type, we make (emit) a response and the response is either retained or dropped depending upon the consequences of making that response. If the consequence is desirable, the response is retained; if the consequence is undesirable, the response is not retained or dropped. For example, suppose you say "good morning" to a person in the street; if he reciprocates the response with a smile, the chances are that you will say "good morning" when you meet him next time. On the other hand, when you say "good morning," if the other person ignores your gesture, the chances are that you do not wish him good morning when you meet him again. So, in operant conditioning, the organism makes a deliberate attempt to produce a result; it operates on the environment to produce a result, hence the name operant conditioning or operant learning.

BF Skinner (Fig. 5.3), a renowned American psychologist, is generally recognized as the founding father of this form of learning. But, there was another great American psychologist, EL Thorndike (Fig. 5.4), whose pioneering work on learning has laid the foundation for the later work of Skinner, although Skinner claims that he was not aware of Thorndike's work when he first proposed his views. Whatever that may be, it is good to familiarize ourselves with the pioneering work of Thorndike before we

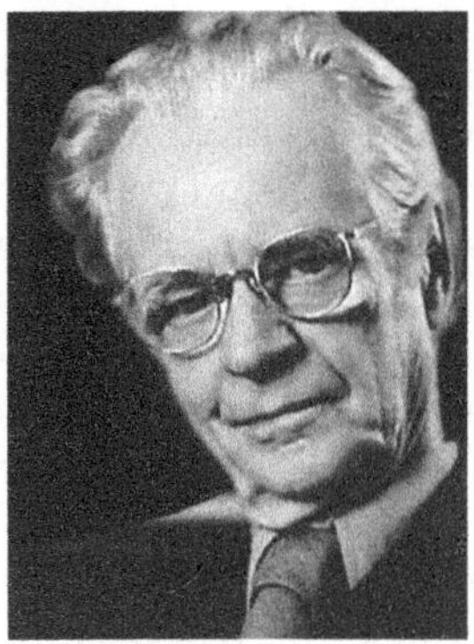

FIGURE 5.3: BF Skinner

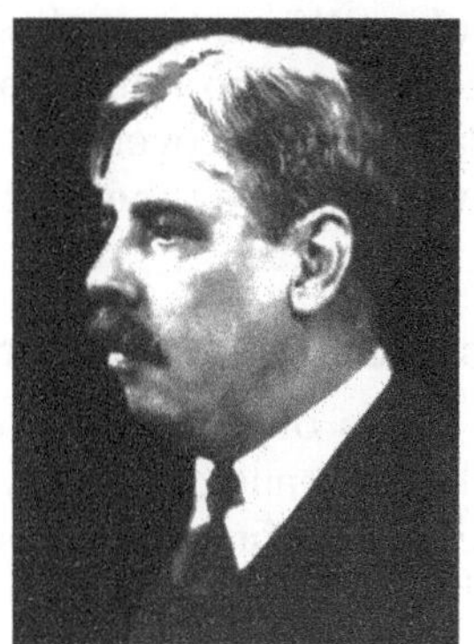

FIGURE 5.4: EL Thorndike

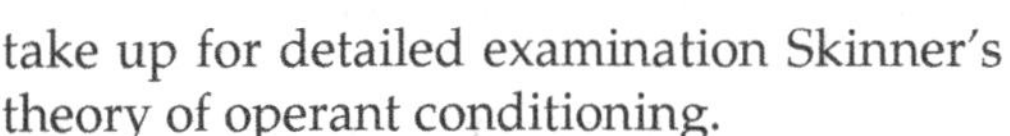

take up for detailed examination Skinner's theory of operant conditioning.

Thorndike's Connectionism

Thorndike's theory of learning is often called **connectionism** because it considers learning as establishing a connection (an association or relationship) between stimulus and response. He developed his theory, while exploring animal learning and problem solving. For the purpose of studying animals, he used a cage that has become famous in the history of psychology as Thorndike's *puzzle box* (Fig. 5.5).

Thorndike built the cage in such a way that its door could be opened from inside by pressing a lever. A dish containing some food was kept outside on the floor, which could be seen from inside. Under these conditions, when a hungry cat was put inside the cage, it actively moved around scratching the slats and the ground. Eventually by chance, the cat stepped on the lever, thus opening the door and reaching for the food. When the cat was put back in the cage for a second trial, the cat made random movements and again accidentally pressed the lever. After several such trials, it was seen that the escape time gradually decreased and finally the animal could escape as soon as it was put into the cage. The animal was gradually eliminating responses that failed and making responses that were successful. Thorndike called this type of learning **trial and error learning.** He explained this type of learning using a principle that came to be an important discovery in psychology, the **law of effect,** and the law has shaped the course of later theorizing on learning. The law states that responses followed by satisfying state of affairs are more likely to be repeated and responses followed by the annoying state of affairs are less likely to be repeated. In other words, a connection between stimulus and response (an associative bond) is strengthened, when the consequences are pleasant and weakened, when unpleasant. In addition to law of effect, Thorndike promulgated several other laws to explain the process of learning and later introduced

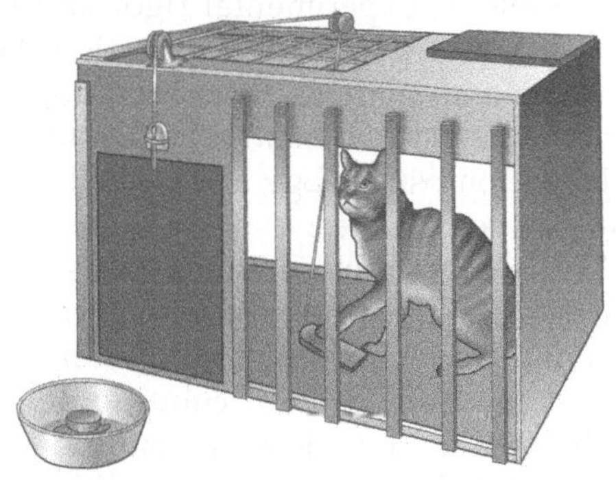

FIGURE 5.5: Thorndike's puzzle box

a number of modifications to these laws. In spite of the changes, Thorndike's law of effect remains a landmark discovery in psychology and the law has shaped the course of later theorizing on learning.

Principles of Operant Conditioning

Skinner's views on learning are elegant, economical, explicit and empirically anchored. He believed in the orderliness of behavior and said that an individual's behavior is as lawful as the movement of one billiard ball stuck by another ball. According to him, any behavioral law must apply to each subject, human or animal, observed under appropriate conditions. He asserted that the principle of determinism is as much applicable in the realm of human behavior as in the case of behavior of physical entities. One individual may commit a murder, another may save a life. Both varieties of behavior are the result of the interplay of identifiable variables that completely determine behavior. He believed that an individual's behavior is entirely a product of and can be understood purely in terms of the features of the objective world. Skinner believed that the same general principles will be uncovered regardless of what organism, stimulus, response and reinforcer that the experimenter chooses to study. Thus, Skinner was an ardent behaviorist, who was convinced of the importance of objective methodology, experimental rigor and the capacity of elegant experimentation. His concepts and methods have been applied in various areas of human behavior and his influence on psychology and related fields is highly perceptible.

We said in the beginning of this section that Skinner calls the form of learning he propounded as operant conditioning. He coined the term operant conditioning to distinguish it from classical conditioning, which he called respondent conditioning. Respondent learning is directly under the control of a stimulus as in the case of food producing saliva in the mouth. Because of its dependence on stimulus, Pavlovian conditioning was called Type-S conditioning. In the case of operant conditioning, the response often appears just simply to happen; it is *emitted*. That is, it is spontaneous rather than being a response to specific stimulus. Because of its emphasis on response, operant conditioning was called Type-R conditioning. The word "operant" is used because the response operates on the environment to produce a result. We can understand the principles of operant conditioning using an illustrative experiment such as the one conducted by Skinner. In most of his experiments, he used an apparatus called **Skinner box** (Fig. 5.6).

For all practical purposes, Skinner box can be viewed as an improved, modern version of Thorndike's puzzle box. The inside of the box is empty except for a protruding lever and a food tray beneath it. There is a small light bulb above the lever that can be lighted whenever the experimenter wants. The box is so built that when the lever is pressed a food pellet automatically drops into the food tray (sometimes instead of the lever a disk is used, which a bird has to peck to obtain food). When a hungry rat is left alone in the Skinner box, it makes some random movements and occasionally by chance, it presses the lever. The rate at which the rat first presses the lever defines

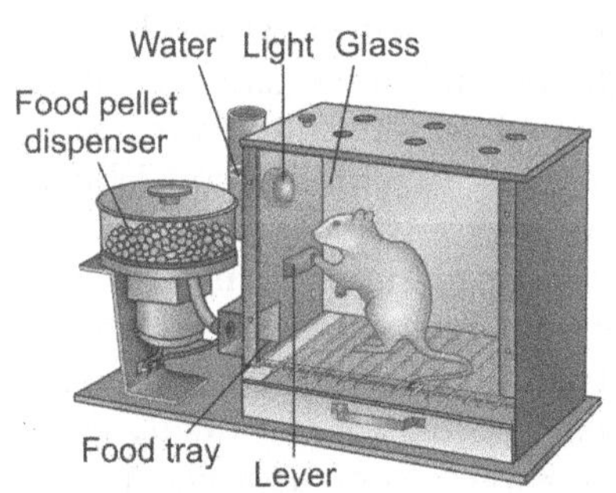

FIGURE 5.6: Skinner box

its preconditioned **operant level** of the lever-pressing behavior. After establishing the operant level, the experimenter attaches the food magazine so that every time the rat presses the lever, a food pellet falls into the cup. Initially the animal runs around exploring the box. After some time, it presses the lever accidentally and a food pellet is released. After eating the food, the rat again starts exploring the box and eventually presses the lever. Food arrives whenever the rat presses the lever. The food reinforces the lever-pressing behavior and the rate of pressing increases dramatically. That is, the rat has learnt to press the lever whenever it is put into the box. It operates on the environment to produce an effect. This in short is operant conditioning. If the food magazine is disconnected so that food is not delivered when the lever is pressed, the rate of lever-pressing gradually decreases and finally the lever-pressing behavior stops. That is, the response undergoes operant extinction because of non-reinforcement. The occurrence of extinction is similar to what happened in the case of classical conditioning.

The experimenter may introduce a new variable to the experiment; he presents food for lever pressing only when the light above the lever is on and not when it is off. Under this condition of selective reinforcement, the rat learns to press the lever only when the light is on. In this case, the light serves as a **discriminative stimulus**. Now, the discriminative stimulus controls the lever-pressing behavior of the animal.

The illustrative experiment above helps us to understand the process of operant conditioning and to distinguish it from classical conditioning. The lever pressing behavior (operant) "operates" on the environment to produce an effect—arrival of food pellets. In Pavlovian conditioning, the animal is passive; it does not do anything; simply it waits for the conditioned stimulus to arrive and is followed by the unconditioned stimulus. In operant conditioning, the animal is active; its behavior is not reinforced unless it does something (in this case, lever pressing). There is no unconditioned stimulus that connects the to-be-conditioned stimulus to the response. Although, classical conditioning and operant conditioning are different processes, it is *good* to note that many forms of learning involve both.

We may define operant conditioning as a form of learning in which the behavior is influenced by the consequence that follows. The consequence of making a response determines the fate in response; that is, the consequence decides whether the response is acquired or not. Skinner used the word reinforcement to refer to the consequence and the concept of reinforcement is central to his theory. In a nutshell, operant conditioning involves three steps:

1. An antecedent stimuli (the light above the lever is on).
2. A response (the animal presses the lever).
3. Reinforcement (arrival of food).

The relation between the response and reinforcement is called *contingency*. For the animal in the Skinner box, the receiving of food is contingent on pressing the lever. So the consequence that occurs after making response is crucial for the retaining or dropping out of the response. The effects of two important consequences have been extensively studied by Skinner and his associates in the laboratory. These are *reinforcement and punishment*. **Reinforcement** is the process in which the frequency of occurrence of a response is increased by an outcome that follows it. **Punishment** is the process in which the frequency of the occurrence of a response is decreased by an outcome that follows it. Let us examine the two concepts in some detail.

Reinforcement

Reinforcement is such an important construct in Skinner's system that, sometimes, his theory is called operant reinforcement theory (Skinner is averse to the word theory; often, it is said that his work is all facts and no theory; we use the term theory for purposes of easy communication). Skinner does not use any subjective mentalistic terms (terms such as consciousness that cannot be observed and manipulated objectively) in his theory. For all that we know Skinner's theory is similar to that of Thorndike's in several aspects. But Thorndike used terms such as satisfying affair and annoying affair in his theory; these are subjective, mentalistic concepts. Skinner asks: How to know whether the animal is satisfied or annoyed? Therefore, he completely avoided such terms and explained behavior in terms of objectively observable concepts. For instance, rewarding the animal (giving food) increases the frequency of response, while punishment (giving an electric shock) decreases the same. We can determine the number of times the animal is rewarded or punished. Skinner insisted that every concept used in his system is measurable. For example, '*operant strength*' was measured in terms of rate of response, that is, the more frequently the response occurs during a given interval of time, the stronger it is. Another measure of operant strength is the total number of responses the animal makes during extinction. Skinner used a *cumulative recorder* to measure the operant strength and obtained a *cumulative curve*. The lever in the Skinner box was attached to a recording pen that rests on a slowly moving paper. Each time the animal presses the lever, the pen moves upward, and then continues on its horizontal path. Because the paper moves at a fixed rate, the slope of the cumulative curve is a measure of response rate. A horizontal line indicates that the animal is not responding; a steep curve indicates a fast response rate.

There are two types of reinforcement that strengthen a response. These are **positive reinforcement** and **negative reinforcement**. A stimulus that increases the probability of occurrence of a response is called *reinforcer*. Similarly, there are two varieties of punishment that weaken the response; these are **positive punishment** and **negative punishment**. A stimulus that decreases the probability of occurrence of a response is called *punisher*. Therefore, we have positive reinforcers, negative reinforcers, positive punishers, and negative punishers.

Positive reinforcement: When the probability of occurrence of a response is increased by the subsequent presentation of a stimulus, it is called positive reinforcement. The stimulus that follows the response and strengthens it is called *positive reinforcer*. Food that follows lever-pressing is a positive reinforcer. Food when one is hungry, water when thirsty, rest when tired and a pay raise or some kind of special recognition (praise) for "good" work are examples of positive reinforcers. Uttering the word *good* when the child completes his homework is a positive reinforcer. A positive reinforcer is something given to the organism or introduced to the environment. There are two types of positive reinforcers: primary reinforcers and secondary reinforcers. A **primary reinforcer** is anything that acts directly and naturally to reinforce our behavior; for example, food and water are primary reinforces. On the other hand, a **secondary reinforcer** is something that becomes reinforcing because of its association with a primary reinforcer. It is a learned or conditioned reinforcer. Suppose a sound is made whenever the food pellet is delivered to the animal, the sound becomes the secondary reinforcer. A secondary reinforcer does not inherently satisfy a primary need; but by its presence every time the primary reinforcer is delivered, it becomes a reinforcer by its own right. The sound becomes the signal for food and at the same time, acquires the ability to act as a positive reinforcer. Secondary reinforcers play an important role in shaping behavior of children. Parents do not always use primary reinforcers to shape their children's behavior. Instead they use praise, encouragement, or show of affection, which are all learned reinforcers. Money is an important secondary reinforcer. We cannot eat or drink money, but we can purchase food or whatever we want using money. That is the reason why we are after money most of the time; money indirectly satisfies many of our needs. For a factory worker, recognition or promotion is a conditioned reinforcer and for a student, good marks in an examination.

Negative reinforcement: Not only is our behavior strengthened when we receive a positive reinforcer but also when some aversive condition or stimulus is withdrawn or removed. This process is called negative reinforcement. The stimulus that increases the probability of occurrence of a response when it is terminated is called *negative reinforcer*. Suppose you are in a warm room; you get up and put on the fan. This removes an unpleasant stimulus. When it starts drizzling, you open your umbrella; when you have a headache, you take Aspirin. These are instances of negative reinforcements. These operant behaviors are strengthened because they remove out of our way some unpleasant stimuli that were troubling us. Negative reinforcement should not be confused with punishment. Punishment is the introduction of an aversive stimulus that weakens a response. Negative reinforcement is terminating or removing an aversive stimulus which strengthens a response. Also, when you use the terms positive reinforcement and negative reinforcement, the terms positive and negative do not mean good and bad; they mean presenting and removing a stimulus. Remember, both positive and negative reinforcement increase the probability of occurrence of the preceding response. Negative reinforcement plays an important role in our learning of avoiding or escaping from unpleasant stimuli or situations. **Escape learning** and **avoidance learning** are two important examples of operant learning based on negative reinforcement.

Escape learning: Let us illustrate escape learning using a rat in the Skinner box. When the rat is in the Skinner box, a mild electric shock is applied to its feet. In response to the shock, the rat moves and runs about on the floor of the box and accidentally presses the lever. Pressing of the lever puts off the shock; thus the animal escapes the shock. After sometime, the rat is put into the box for a second trial under similar conditions. Even now, the animal makes random movements and eventually presses the lever terminating shock. After several trials, the animal learns to press the lever the moment it is put into the box, thus escaping from the shock. During the first few trials, the animal was slow to make the appropriate response (pressing the lever). But as more and more trials are given, the rat quickly presses the lever to escape the shock. The rat has learnt to make a response that terminates a noxious stimulus. This is escape learning based on negative reinforcement.

Avoidance learning: We can illustrate avoidance learning with slight modification in the experiment described above (for escape learning). In each trial as the animal is put into Skinner box, a buzzer sound is presented that continues for a few seconds (say 5 seconds) before the floor of the box is electrified to give a shock. If the animal presses the lever within the 5 second interval between the buzzer onset and the arrival of the shock, the buzzer is turned off and shock is avoided. In this case, the noxious shock is avoided by the response (lever-pressing). This is called avoidance learning (Box 5.2). The time the rat takes to make the response after it hears the buzzer sound is called the latency of response. If the latency on a trial is more than 5 seconds, the response is an escape response because the shock came on

Box 5.2: Avoidance Learning

Another Russian researcher, Vladimir Bekhterev, conducted experiments in conditioning using a slightly different procedure. He used a shock as an unconditioned stimulus (CS) and dog's withdrawal of its foot as an unconditioned response (UR). When a neutral stimulus such as bell (CS) was paired with shock several times, the dog learned to withdraw its foot (CR) after the bell, but before the shock. The dog has learned successfully to avoid the painful shock. This was an important extension of Pavlov's work, which became the basis of what is now called **avoidance learning**.

and the animal is escaping from it. But if the latency on a trial is less than 5 seconds, the response is an avoidance response because the rat pressed the lever before the shock appeared and thus the animal avoided it. Avoidance learning is a complicated phenomenon and a great deal of effort has gone into its explanation. We shall not go into those theoretical explanations.

Punishment

Punishment refers to the use of an unpleasant stimulus to decrease the likelihood of the occurrence of a preceding response. While reinforcement increases the probability of occurrence of a response, punishment suppresses or stops a response. It is not enough if we learn what to do; we must also learn what not to do. In a way, punishment promotes us to learn what we should not do. There are lots of things we should not do during our lifetime: we should not play with fire, we should not steal, cheat, lie, drive speedily, so on and so forth. These are taught by our parents and society by using punishment.

As in the case of reinforcement, there are two types of punishment: positive punishment and negative punishment. Positive punishment refers to the application of an aversive stimulus (*positive punisher*) such as spanking a child for misbehavior, cutting the salary of an inefficient employee, detaining a student for not performing well in the examination and giving an electric shock to a laboratory animal for making an unwanted response. Positive punishment is also called *aversive punishment* or *punishment by application*. In all the above instances, positive punishment reduces the probability of occurrence of the preceding response. On the other hand, negative punishment refers to the act of taking away something that one is already enjoying. Taking away the cell phone or the car key from your son or daughter is an example of negative punishment. Here, a privilege which one is already enjoying is withdrawn and as you can guess, the behavior preceding it will be weakened. Negative punishment is also called **response cost** or *punishment by removal*. So, negative punishment is the process of reducing the frequency of occurrence of a response by the subsequent removal of a stimulus (*negative punisher*). Negative punishment is often used in modifying behavior of children. You must have seen a mother saying often to her child "I shall not talk to you," or "Do not touch me," to bring about a change in the child's behavior. Since, the behavior really costs the child something, it will be weakened or discontinued. Different types of reinforcement and punishment are shown in Table 5.1.

Use of Punishment—Do's and Don'ts

Punishment is often the quickest and effective means of modifying undesirable

Table 5.1: Types of Reinforcement and Punishment

	Pleasant stimulus	*Unpleasant stimulus*
Presented	Positive reinforcement	Positive punishment
Removed	Negative punishment (response cost)	Negative reinforcement

behavior, but it must be used with discretion. In fact, using punishment to mold behavior is a tricky matter and many issues are involved in its use. Opinion is divided among psychologists and the public regarding the use of punishment. Let us discuss briefly why and when punishment is effective and the advantages and disadvantages of using punishment in changing behavior.

The following principles may be kept in mind while employing punishment as a means of modifying behavior:

1. It has been found that punishment is effective when it is sufficiently intense. Children engage in certain behaviors (running into a busy street, playing with fire, handling sharp instruments) that are dangerous. Strong punishment may be used to suppress such behavior. But it is important to see that punishment should be contingent on the behavior. Mild punishment suppresses the behavior temporarily. The punished behavior may return unless the punishment is rather intense. It is better that punishment is accompanied by simple explanation. Tell the child, why he should not do something he did and tell him also what he should do and praise him for doing so.
2. Punishment must be consistent. Once a behavior is punished, it must be punished consistently whenever it is exhibited. Punishing sometimes and not at other times gives a wrong signal. The child will be in conflict whether to do or not do. Inconsistent punishment does more harm than good.
3. Punishment must be closer in time and place to the behavior that is being punished. Punishing the child in the evening for what he did in the morning suppresses the behavior which he/she is currently engaged in. Delayed punishment is not effective. You recall what mothers do while punishing their children. When a mother notices the child's misbehavior, she often says "let your father come, I shall inform him what you have done." When the father comes home in the evening, the mother informs the child's misbehavior. The father spanks the child, while the child is engaged in doing homework. In this instance, the child develops a dislike for doing homework rather than to the misbehavior exhibited in the morning.
4. Even mild punishment can be effective if it is used to stop unwanted behavior, while at the same time, some desirable alternative behavior is positively reinforced. You may scold the child for doing something wrong, but at the same time, ask him to do something that is good and useful and praise him for doing it.
5. Often, humans and animals get used to punishment and this makes the punishment ineffective. When a child is punished for almost everything he does, he gets used to it and does not bother about it. Therefore, it is necessary that punishment is not used as a major means of controlling behavior. Punishment must be used sparingly.
6. One dangerous consequence of using punishment is that children may become fearful of their parents and even become hostile toward them. They may also develop a low opinion of themselves when most of what they do is disapproved.
7. There is a possibility that children who are over-punished often become resentful, rebellious, and antisocial.
8. There are disagreements regarding the type of punishments to be used. Should it be physical (spanking), verbal (scolding) or something else? Well, it depends on the person, situation, and the seriousness of misbehavior.

Extinction

As it happens in classical conditioning, in operant conditioning also, a response is gradually weakened and eventually disappears when it is not reinforced. This is called **operant extinction.** If lever pressing no longer produces food pellets, the rat finally stops pressing the lever. Operant extinction can sometimes be used as a substitute for punishment in reducing undesirable behavior. Often, a non-reinforced response may continue to occur several times or it may disappear soon. The degree to which a response, that is not reinforced, persists is called *resistance to extinction*. Resistance to extinction is influenced by the pattern of reinforcement that has previously maintained the response. This will become clear when you read the section on schedules of reinforcement.

Immediate and Delayed Reinforcement

The time interval between the occurrence of behavior and its consequence (reinforcement or punishment) affects operant learning. When the rat in the Skinner box receives food pellet immediately after pressing the bar, it is called **immediate reinforcement**. If the food pellet does not appear immediately and say it comes 30 seconds later, it is called **delayed reinforcement**. Generally, it is good to reinforce a response immediately after its occurrence. When training animals, immediate reinforcement helps the animal to associate the reinforcement with the desired response. If the reinforcement is delayed, the animal may associate it with some other subsequent, irrelevant behavior. For example, after pressing the bar, during the 30 second interval, the animal might have sniffed some part of the box, scratched its ear, or engaged in any number of other activities. It would be difficult for the animal to determine which of its behaviors had produced the food. But in the case of humans, the timing of reinforcement is not as important as in the case of subhuman organisms. Humans can imagine future consequences and wait for delayed rewards and gratifications. We work hard to get good marks in the examination, put extra effort to get a promotion in the workplace or please politicians to get an award. Often, the power of immediate reinforcement helps to explain why many people continue to engage in behaviors with maladaptive long-term consequences. Chronic drug users usually find it difficult to stop taking drugs because the immediate reinforcing consequences of the drug override the delayed benefits of not using the drug (improved health, living longer). With many drugs, such as cocaine, use is positively reinforced by feelings of pleasure, which appears to be the result of increased dopamine activity. Powerful negative reinforcers also play an important role in developing and retaining drug habits. For example, chronic cigarette smokers experience increased discomfort when the nicotine level in the blood drops as consequence of not smoking for some time. When they smoke again, the tension decreases. Thus, smoking is negatively reinforced by the removal of unpleasant tension.

Generalization and Discrimination

We have seen in classical conditioning that a response conditioned to a specific stimulus (CS) will also be elicited by other stimuli similar in some way to the original stimulus (CS). Similarly, an operant response will be made to a new stimulus that is similar to the original one. This is called **operant generalization**. For example, suppose a rat presses a lever that is rectangular in shape to obtain food pellets and this response has been well established and the rate of response is high, the animal will press the lever that is elliptical in shape. The degree to which the animal responds depends on the similarity between the original and the new stimulus. The amount of generalization is graded—it is more or less—depending on the similarity between the two stimuli. It is often called *gradient of generalization*.

We have also seen in classical conditioning that an animal learns to discriminate between two stimuli. That is, it learns to make one response to one stimulus and another response (or no response) to another stimulus. The same process occurs in operant conditioning also. An operant response will be made to one stimulus and not to the other. This is called **operant discrimination**. Operant discrimination is achieved by reinforcing a particular response to one stimulus and not reinforcing (or punishing) the same response to another stimulus. We learn a number of discriminations during our lifetime. We react in one way in one situation and in a different way in another; we respond in one way when we meet a friend and in another way in the presence of a foe; we learn to discriminate between red light and green light at a traffic intersection. The discrimination process in operant conditioning is often called *stimulus control of behavior*.

Schedules of Reinforcement

When every occurrence of a particular response is reinforced (every lever-pressing results in food pellets), it is called **continuous reinforcement**. In daily life, not all of our acts are reinforced always; sometimes we are reinforced and sometimes not. This is **partial reinforcement** or **intermittent reinforcement**. You will know later which type of reinforcement is good for effective learning. Reinforcements come in different times and in different frequencies. These patterns of reinforcement are called **schedules of reinforcement**. Skinner and his associates have made extensive study of schedules of reinforcement and have shown that specific schedules have a strong and predictable influence on the acquisition, extinction and performance of behavior patterns. Continuous reinforcement is generally used during initial operant learning. Once the response is established it is maintained by one or the other form of partial reinforcement. Skinner has proposed a number of schedules of reinforcement. We shall examine four of them that are being extensively used. These are fixed interval schedule, variable interval schedule, fixed ratio schedule and variable ratio schedule.

Fixed Interval Schedule

In a **fixed interval (FI) schedule**, the subject is reinforced only at known intervals of time. Suppose the experimenter has chosen a 100 second interval. The animal will not be reinforced (irrespective of the number of times the response is made) until 100 seconds have elapsed. The first response after 100 seconds is reinforced and then no more reinforcement is given until the first response after another 100 second interval has elapsed. In FI schedule, there will be a gradual acceleration of responding during the interval and a sudden decrease in responding immediately after the reinforcement, thus producing a pattern of response known as the **FI scallop** (Fig. 5.7) That is, the frequency of response comes down immediately after receiving reinforcement, and gradually increases as the time for the next reinforcement draws nearer. This pattern can be seen in the study schedule of students in our schools and colleges. Suppose there is a test every 3 months. Immediately after a test, students' study time suddenly decreases and as the next test is nearing the study time gradually increases.

Variable Interval Schedule

Under a **variable interval (VI) schedule**, the subject is reinforced for every first response after varying intervals of time. For example, if an animal is reinforced for its first response after 20 seconds, then after another response 40 seconds later, then 10 seconds later, then 30 seconds later, it would be on a variable interval schedule.

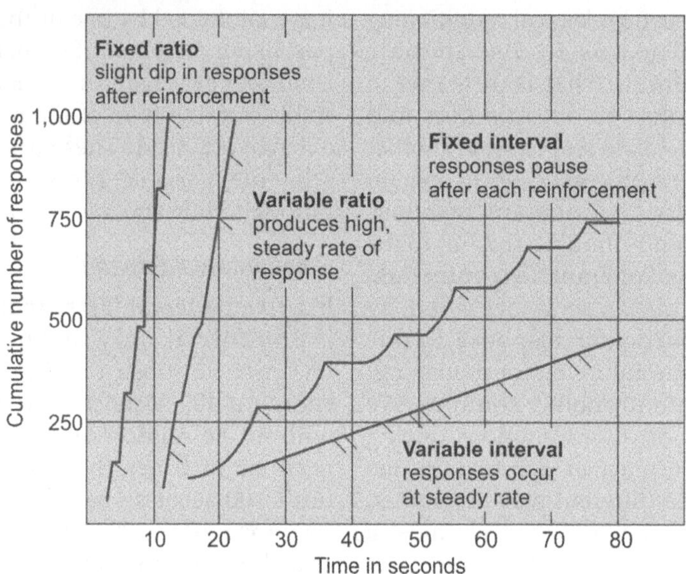

FIGURE 5.7: Schedules of reinforcement

Since, the occurrence of reinforcement is not predictable as in the case of FI schedule, the VI schedule results in relatively better performance. For instance in a workplace, if the supervisor visits at varying intervals of time to look up how people are working, they tend to perform better. If your teacher conducts the tests at random intervals, you will be always prepared to take the test. In laboratory animals VI schedule produces consistent, results although slow responding (refer Fig. 5.7).

Fixed Ratio Schedule

In a **fixed ratio (FR) schedule**, the reinforcement arrives after the subject makes a specific number of responses. For example, the animal may be reinforced after every 10th bar-pressing response regardless of how much time it takes to make those responses. It has been shown that FR schedule results in better performance. When the animal knows that every 10th response results in reinforcement, it tries to complete as many units of 10 responses as possible. Also, the animal may take a brief rest pause after reinforcement, because it knows for sure that the next response will not be reinforced. There is a high rate of response until reinforcement is given, then a lull, followed by a high rate of response until the next reinforcement and so on. FR schedule produces higher rate of responding than FI schedule.

Variable Ratio Schedule

In a **variable ratio (VR) schedule**, reinforcement is presented after a varying number of responses rather than after a fixed number of responses. For example, reinforcement may be given after 5, 18, 4 and 13 responses or it could be presented after 24, 1, 10 and 5 responses. The reinforcement occurs on average after every 10th response (5 + 18 + 4 + 13 = 40/4 = 10, or 24 + 1 + 10 + 5 = 40/4 = 10). The animal does not know when the reinforcement will come. The VR schedule leads to a higher rate of response and strong resistance to extinction. A good example of the effectiveness of the VR schedule can be seen in gambling behavior.

A card player wins sometimes and loses sometimes, but he cannot predict when he is going to win. He thinks he may win in the next game, so on, and continues to play. Because he wins sometimes (reinforced by variable schedule), he does not stop playing and ultimately he may become addicted to the card game. For this reason VR schedule is often called "gambling reinforcement schedule." Animals on this schedule tend to respond frequently, consistently and without long pauses. It is reported that one of Skinner's pigeons when shifted to VR schedule, continued to peck at a disk 150,000 times without reinforcement.

The four schedules of reinforcement mentioned above are the common ones used in the laboratory. There are several other more complex schedules, each with its own characteristics, used for special purposes. What we must remember in this connection is that, other things being the same, partial (intermittent) reinforcement schedules are better than continuous reinforcement schedules, and variable schedules are better than fixed ones.

Shaping

When a rat is left in the Skinner box, it takes lots of time to learn the lever-pressing behavior. The learning of this task can be hastened by using a technique called **shaping**. Shaping is the process of teaching an organism a complex skill by reinforcing responses that are closer and closer to the desired behavior. The final desired behavior is considered as a series of smaller behaviors, which become increasingly similar to the desired behavior; the smaller behaviors are called **successive approximations**. For example, the rat in the Skinner box has to become familiar with the apparatus, especially the food magazine. It is trained to associate the food tray with pressing the lever. To achieve this goal, the animal may be reinforced with food when it first looks at the lever, then when it moves closer to the lever, then when it touches the lever and finally when it presses the lever. This is shaping or teaching by the method of successive approximation. Using the shaping procedure, animals as well as humans can be taught to execute several complex skills. You must have seen the animals doing complex acts in the circus. They have been taught these skills by shaping. Skinner has taught pigeons to play table tennis, birds to deliver messages to spies working in foreign lands, so on and so forth. The essential feature in shaping behavior is teaching a series of simple responses leading to the final response; that is, the final response is learned because the steps leading to it were reinforced systematically.

Superstitious Behavior

Learning psychologists explain many of our ritualistic and superstitious behaviors in terms of learning and reinforcement. Suppose you went to an examination on the first day wearing green-colored dress and you did well in the examination; surprisingly, you will develop a tendency to wear similar dress, if not the same dress, the next day. A cricketer taps the ground three times with his bat before he hits the ball. Fortunately, he hits a boundary. Hereafter he begins to tap the ground three times every time before hitting every ball. This tendency occurs because his behavior is followed by a reinforcer the first time. If the behavior is followed by reinforcer, it is strengthened. Note that, the behavior which occurs prior to reinforcement is coincidental. Still a relationship is established between the behavior and the reinforcement and the behavior is continued. Several of our superstitious behaviors are thus products of accidental reinforcements.

Verbal Behavior

In Skinner's system, language related activities, such as listening, understanding, reading, writing, and speaking a language, are included under **verbal behavior**. He asserts that like all other forms of behavior, acquisition of language or verbal behavior can be explained within the context of operant reinforcement theory. We learn to talk and understand language just as we learn other types of behavior under the influence of reinforcement. Skinner classified verbal responses in terms of how they are related to reinforcement. Some of the classifications proposed by him are given below.

Mand: The word '**mand**' is coined by Skinner as a shortened form of ***demand***. When a demand, such as *look here, listen, run, stop, say yes* or *study*, is made on people and they obey them, they are reinforced. Thus, mands specify the responses or the behavior of the listener. They may also specify the reinforcement the individual requires. For example, one may say *water*, when he/she is thirsty. When the demand is met, the utterance (mand) is reinforced. When the need arises next time, the individual is likely to repeat the mand.

Tact: The term '**tact**' is coined by Skinner to refer to verbal behavior, which makes contact with some object in the external physical world. For example, when a child says *doll* in the presence of a doll, the child receives some sort of generalized reinforcement; the parents may smile, clap or hug the child. So, tact is a verbal operant elicited by an object, person or event, which is strengthened (reinforced) in a given verbal community. In simple terms, the tact involves naming objects or events in the environment appropriately and people reinforcing such verbal behavior.

Echoic behavior: When a child repeats someone else's verbal response verbatim, Skinner calls it **echoic behavior**. When such behavior is reinforced by people around, the child acquires such behavior, which later becomes a part of more complicated verbal behavior. Echoic behavior helps the speaker to learn more complex verbal relationships.

Autoclitic behavior: Skinner used the term autoclitic to suggest behavior that is based on or depends upon other verbal behavior. The function of **autoclitic behavior** is to qualify responses, express relations and provide a grammatical framework for verbal behavior. Autoclitics represent a class of utterances intended to suggest verbal behavior that is based upon the speaker's own role and dependent on other verbal behavior. *"I am inclined to add ..."* or *"I agree with..."* are good examples.

In short, we learn a language just as we learn all other behaviors. But several linguists, especially Noam Chomsky, do not accept Skinner's explanation of language learning. Chomsky asserts that language is too complex a phenomenon to be learned according to principles of operant conditioning. There must be certain other mechanisms that enable a 3-year-old child to make so many complicated verbal utterances. For example, according to GA Miller, there are about 10^{20} possible twenty-word sentences in the English language and it would take some thousand times the estimated age of earth just to listen to them all. Therefore, to say that we learn a language just by listening cannot be an acceptable explanation and operant conditioning does not explain the complexity of human language capacities. Chomsky believes that the human brain is structured to generate language. We are wired to produce grammatical utterances just as a computer can be wired to produce moves in a chess game. Chomsky's theory of language learning is based on heredity (nature) while, Skinner asserts that it is shaped by environment (nurture).

Applications of Operant Conditioning

Operant conditioning is not a game played by psychologists with rats and pigeons. Its author Skinner has proposed several uses of operant learning principles in human situations in his book, *Science and Human Behavior* (1953). He has described how parents, teachers, society and government are using operant learning principles to shape human behavior, without knowing they are doing so. These principles have been effectively used in education (programmed learning), certain forms of psychotherapy to treat mental disorders and a variety of business operations.

Programmed learning is an effective technique that uses a teaching machine to provide tutorial instruction to school and college students. Here, the subject matter to be learned is broken into smaller and easy units and are presented to students in frames. Each frame contains some new information and a question. The student enters the answer to the question and presses a button which tells him whether the answer is correct or not. Then, he moves to the next frame, which presents him with another piece of information and a question. Thus, a student proceeds stepwise through the entire subject matter. In programmed learning, there is no need for a teacher; the student learns at his own pace and is reinforced immediately (comes to know whether the answer is right or wrong). In fact, self-paced learning and immediate performance feedbacks are the important features of programmed learning. In business operations, application of operant learning principles has been found to be effective in increasing productivity and profit of the organization. You will learn about the application of operant learning principles in the treatment of psychological dysfunctions, when we discuss behavior therapy or behavior modification in Chapter 16.

Skinner's learning theory has attracted a number of enthusiastic followers and an equal number of critics and skeptics. The basic argument of Skinner is that all behavior is the product of operant learning and humans including animals can be trained to *"do whatever you want"* under controlled conditions. His ideas have been made public in his book, *Beyond Freedom and Dignity* (1971). But the most important question is: If you can make people learn to do whatever you want, *who should decide what is to be learned*? The question has dangerous implications because people may be trained to destroy the world including them! The philosophical basis of several of Skinner's ideas has been severely criticized by eminent intellectuals and the issue is still unsettled.

COGNITIVE THEORIES OF LEARNING

Classical conditioning and operant conditioning are often called stimulus-response (S-R) learning or associative learning. The focus here is on establishing a relationship (an association) between a stimulus and a response. According to S-R learning theorists, who are mostly behaviorists, the learner is an empty organism. There is no place for thinking, reasoning, problem solving or feeling. The organism is totally at the mercy of the environmental forces. External forces determine what the organism learns or what it does not. Is it as simple as that? No, say some psychologists. There is a large group of thinkers who emphasize the role of higher mental processes such as perception, memory, thinking and previously acquired knowledge on learning. These are called cognitive psychologists. The word **cognition** refers to the processes, such as thinking, conceiving, reasoning or simply knowing and processing of information about the world that is received through the senses.

Cognitive processes involve:

1. The selection of information.
2. The making of alterations in the selected information.
3. The relating of items of information with each other.

4. The elaboration of information in thought.
5. The storage of information in memory.
6. Retrieval of stored information when it is needed.

That is, there are several organismic processes occurring between stimulus and response; there is an organism (O) in between reception of the stimulus and responding to the stimulus. So, cognitive psychologists have challenged the S-R model and proposed the S-O-R model or cognitive model of learning. Today, cognitive psychology is playing a highly significant role in the understanding of processes involved in learning and other psychological activities. Here, we must remember one thing; the behaviorists did not deny the existence of higher mental processes such as thinking or reasoning. They only said that these concepts are not necessary to understand learning.

Insight Learning

Cognitive approaches to learning are not new; they have been in the air for a long time. For example, when Thorndike was proposing that learning was a matter of trial and error, the German Gestalt psychologist Wolfgang Kohler (1925) provided ample experimental evidence to show that animals learn by thinking and planning, a process he called insight. **Insight** refers to the sudden understanding of a meaningful relationship between environmental stimuli that leads to the solution of a problem. Kohler's studies of mentality of apes have become classics in psychology. In one of his experiments, Kohler (Fig. 5.8) left an ape (named Sultan) in an enclosure with a banana hanging from the roof beyond the reach of the animal. In the corner of the room, there were a few deal wood boxes (crates used for packing) lying helter-skelter. Sultan did not make any random movements as predicted by Thorndike, but looked around as though thinking about a plan to reach the banana and suddenly grabbed some crates, stacked them one above the other and obtained the banana and ate it (Fig. 5.9). This is a novel behavior reflecting insight. The animal saw a new relationship in using the crates to reach for the fruit. This is insightful learning.

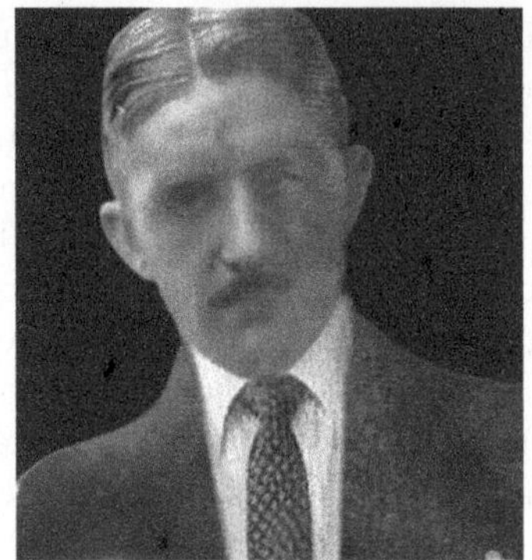

FIGURE 5.8: W Kohler

When we (humans) solve a difficult problem using insight, generally we experience a pleasant feeling and utter the sound *"a-ha."* Therefore, some prefer to call insight learning as **a-ha** learning. But how does insight learning occur? Cognitive psychologists say that insight emerges because of *perceptual reorganization* of elements in the environment, which in turn leads to sudden perception of new relationships among objects and events, which helps in the solution of the problem. Further, we make use of earlier learning in the solution of present problem. This carryover of learning is called *transfer of learning*. Some of the special features of insight learning are:

1. The solution occurs suddenly after a period of trying the various alternatives.
2. Perceptual reorganization helps in the emergence of insight.
3. The solution can be easily generalized to new situations.
4. Insightful learning is not easily forgotten.

Behaviorists argue that insight is one way of combining of previously acquired responses and there is nothing new in it.

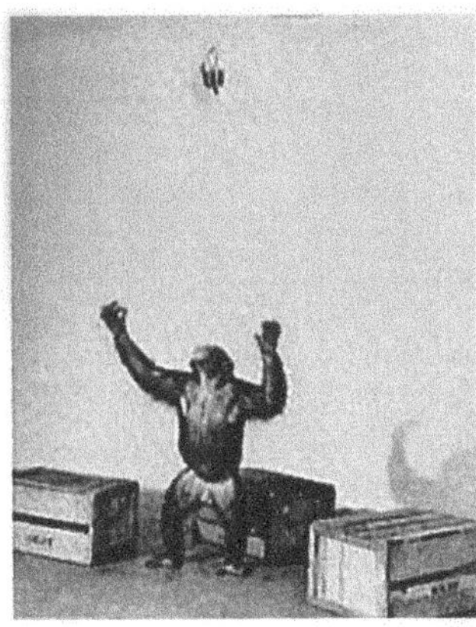
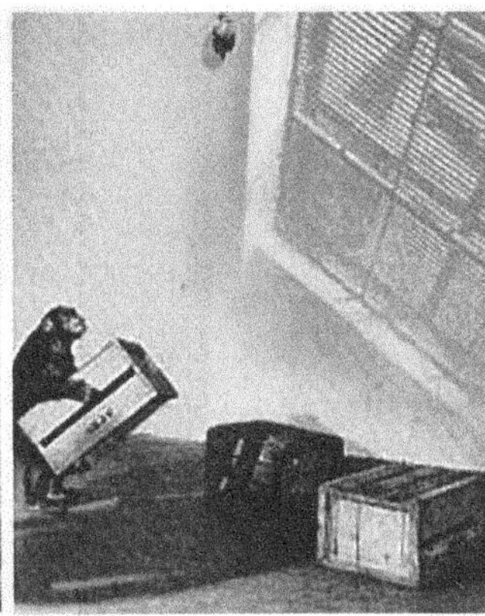
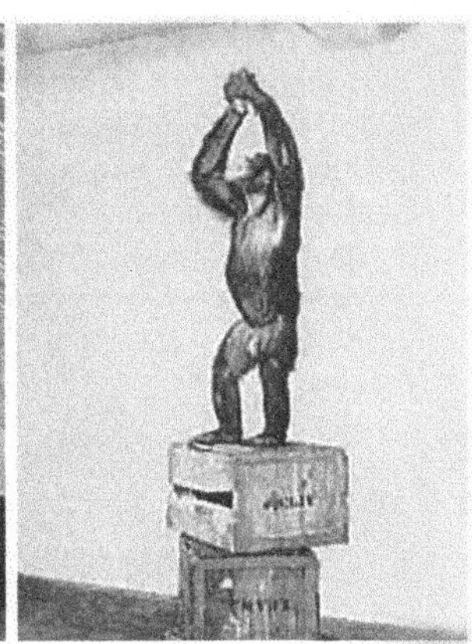

FIGURE 5.9: Insight learning

Well, the debate about the insight between S-R and cognitive psychologists continues even today. But the fact remains that Kohler's pioneering research helped the emergence of cognitive theories of learning.

Latent Learning

A second line of research that had a remarkable influence on the development of cognitive theories of learning came from American psychologist Edward Chase Tolman (Fig. 5.10). His experiments on latent learning, among others, demonstrated the role of cognitive processes. **Latent learning** refers to any learning that is not evidenced by behavior at the time of learning. As the word latent implies, it is hidden learning, learning that occurs but is not evident in behavior until later. Let us illustrate latent learning using one of Tolman's famous experiments. In this experiment three groups of rats (A, B, and C) were allowed daily to run in a maze (Fig. 5.11).

The rats in group A were given food (reinforced) when they reached the goal box at the end of the maze on each trial. The rats in group B were allowed to explore the maze, but were not given food when they reached the goal box; they were returned to the cage without any reinforcement. The procedure was continued once a day for 17 days for groups A and B. The rats in group C were treated just like the ones in the group B for the first 10 days and then given food, when they reached the goal during the remaining 7 days. The results were surprising. As you can see in Figure 5.11, all groups showed some learning as evidenced by the reduction in the number of errors. The reinforced group (A) learned more rapidly than the two non-reinforced groups. But, with the introduction of reinforcement on the 11th day, the rats in group C showed marked improvement in learning; their performance was as good as and even better than the ones in group A. The results clearly indicate that the rats were learning something about the spatial

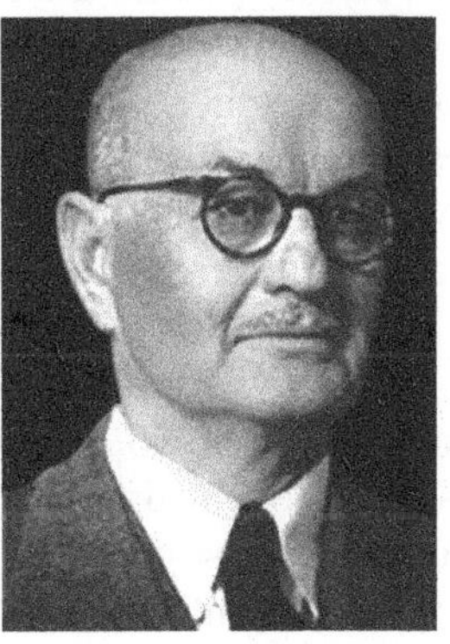

FIGURE 5.10: EC Tolman

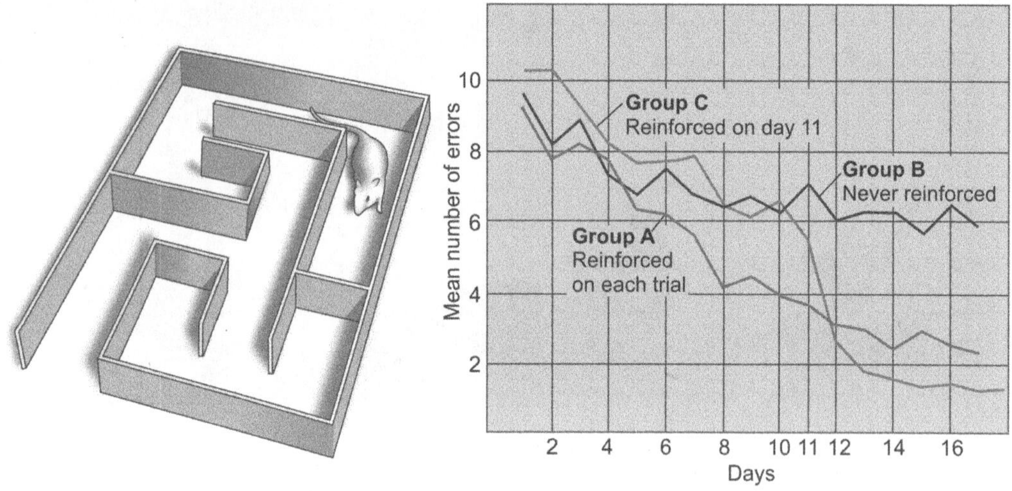

FIGURE 5.11: Tolman's maze and the learning curves

orientation of the maze prior to the time they were reinforced; probably, the rats were formulating a schematic representation (a **cognitive map**) of the maze, which was not evidenced in the performance until reward motivated the animal to perform. That is, the hidden or latent learning shows up when the animals are reinforced. These results have been replicated in several well-controlled experiments in later years.

Latent learning must have occurred on several occasions in your day-to-day life. Suppose you have been traveling between two cities regularly in a bus or car. If somebody asks you to name the towns and villages between the two cities, you can easily recite the same. Remember, you had not learnt these names voluntarily, but still you can give out the place names in the serial order. Is this not latent learning? You have learnt something, it was hidden in you; you did not display that knowledge until there was a need to demonstrate it. So, it is concluded that there is more to learning than forming simple stimulus-response connection; higher mental processes (cognitive activities) have an important role to play.

Cognition in Conditioning

Behaviorists assert that in classical conditioning there is nothing more than establishing a direct reflex-like connection between the conditioned stimulus (sound) and conditioned response (salivation). They do not postulate any other higher mental process other than a link between CS and UCS. Cognitive learning theorists also believe that there is a link between the CS and UCS, but they interpret the link as expectancy that the CS will be followed by the UCS. The expectancy model as proposed by Rescorla and Wagner (1972) states that the most important factor in classical conditioning is not how many times the CS and UCS occur together, but how well the CS predicts the appearance of UCS. Rescorla demonstrated how this phenomenon operates in a famous experiment. In one condition, rats received electric shocks (UCS), which was preceded by a tone. After a few trials, the tone became a (CS) that triggered fear reaction when presented alone. In the second condition, rats received the same number of tone-shock pairings as the first group, but they also received as many shocks that were not preceded by the tone.

According to the classical conditioning model, the tone should have produced a fear reaction in the second group of rats, because they received the same number of tone-shock pairings as in the first group. But the second group of rats did not develop fear reactions because, as predicted by the expectancy model, the tone did not reliably signal the appearance of shock. Thus, Rescorla's hypothesis that conditioning only occurs when a particular CS is a good predictor of the UCS was supported. Incidentally, the theory answers the question "Why did not Pavlov's dog salivate to Pavlov since he was the one who administered the food?" It is because Pavlov was also there when the food was not delivered. Unlike the bell, he was not a reliable predictor of the arrival of food. The moral of the story is: *When a neutral stimulus does not consistently predict the arrival of the UCS, it is less likely to become a CS.*

Similarly, S-O-R theorists assert that cognitive processes play a crucial role in operant conditioning also. They emphasize that organisms develop an awareness or expectancy of the relations (contingency) between their responses and probable consequences. According to them, the best predictor of behavior is the perceived contingency, not the actual one. Often the two are identical, but sometimes people perceive contingencies that do not exist. An example for this can be seen in superstitious behavior, which we discussed earlier. Here people misperceive that a specific behavior produces favorable consequences and engage in superstitious behavior to gain a sense of control over environmental events. You go to a temple every time before you make a journey, because you think that will guarantee a safe journey. This behavior of yours is reinforced each time by safe arrival. Thus, it is your perception of the relationship (between temple going and safe journey), not the actual relationship, which determines your behavior.

Observational Learning

Another form of cognitive learning is **observational learning** or learning by **imitation**. This is learning that occurs as a result of watching and imitating the behavior of others. You must have observed young children playing the 'mummy-daddy game' in your backyard. Who taught them this game? What was the reinforcement? They simply are imitating their parents. So, we learn great many things in life just by observing others. Since this observation takes place in the social setting, it is often called *social learning*. We learn by watching the behavior of our parents, teachers, friends and several others. The person whose behavior we are imitating is called the model and therefore observational learning is also called **modeling**. Observational learning has high adaptive value. We learn what we should do and what not to do at certain situations, which behavior is desirable and which is not, and what behavior will be rewarded and what will be punished by observing other's behaviors. Often we learn our fears, prejudices, likes and dislikes by watching others. Even animals are found to learn several forms of behavior by observing other animals' behavior. For example, monkeys are found to learn the fear of snakes by observing the reactions of other monkeys' reaction when the latter see a snake.

Albert Bandura (Fig. 5.12) has done extensive research and theorizing in the area of observational learning. His theory is called *social-cognitive theory* or simply **social learning theory** and it asserts that people learn by observing the behavior of models and acquire the belief that they can produce behaviors to influence events in their lives. He has challenged the behaviorist's S-R theory of learning and helped the development of S-O-R model. Social learning involves four cognitive processes:

1. We must watch carefully the behavior of the model; pay attention to what the model is doing.

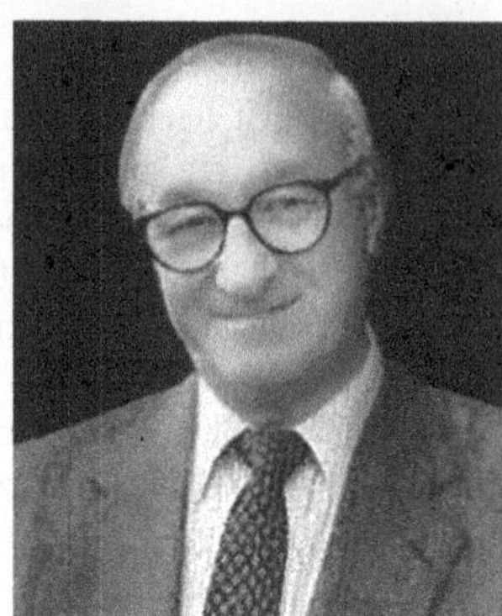

FIGURE 5.12: Albert Bandura

2. We must remember what we have watched.
3. We must be capable (physically and mentally) of reproducing the model's behavior or something similar to it.
4. We must be motivated to display the model's behavior; there must be the desire and opportunity to reproduce the model's behavior.

According to Bandura, a large part of human behavior is a product of observational learning. One of his experiments that demonstrated how modeling operates has become a classic in psychology. Young children were shown a film in which an adult was wildly hitting an inflatable doll (called Bobo doll). Later, when the children were given an opportunity to play with the Bobo doll, most of them displayed the same kind of behavior (hitting the doll), often imitating model's aggressive behavior identically. This experiment has led to serious research to determine the effect of media watching (watching violence on TV and movie) on the development of aggressive behavior. Later researchers have found that watching live aggressive behavior has more of an impact than watching a video of a person exhibiting the same behavior. Do not think that only negative behavior is acquired through observational learning. Even desirable altruistic behavior has been found to be learned by observing a model. Modeling has been used in the treatment of certain types of psychological disorders.

Of course, not all behaviors we watch are learned or executed. Whether we imitate the model's behavior depends on a number of factors. An important factor that facilitates imitation is the consequences of model's behavior. If the model is rewarded for what he/she does, we are more likely to imitate that behavior than when the model is punished. Often, the status of the model plays a crucial role. We generally imitate movie stars, sports persons, political leaders and glamorous models. That is why advertisers make extensive use of these people to promote their products and services. Observational learning plays a very important role in the acquisition of skills that cannot be shaped by conditioning. For example, performing brain surgery cannot be learned by trial and error procedure. We may have to watch experts engaged in this and several other skilled acts for learning them. Bandura's demonstration that we learn by observing others and such learning occurs with or without imitation, and with or without reinforcement is a significant contribution to learning theory.

Constraints on Learning

The principles of learning discussed so far have neglected certain important factors. The learning theories have been successful in explaining how certain forms of learning occur. But they have not taken into account the characteristics of the learner and the response being learned. Learning theorists were interested in establishing general laws that would apply to human beings and animals. They did not consider the response being made and the animal that is making the response as important. Now we know that both the learner characteristics and the nature of response are important in explaining how learning takes place. We know that some animals are biologically prepared to learn certain types of responses more easily than others and some responses are very difficult, if not impossible, to learn for certain animals. You cannot teach a rat to fly and an ape to speak a language. Not all behaviors can be taught to all species of organisms equally well. There are built-in limitations in the ability of animals to learn certain types of behaviors. In several cases, the organism's brain is wired in such a way that it can learn certain responses easily and quickly, but not others. There are biological, cultural and psychological constraints on learning.

As a result of evolution, certain species of animals have developed suitable brain structures that helped them to adapt to the environment they live in. Certain species of animals are thus biologically predisposed to learn some response more easily than others and such responses are often called **prepared behaviors**. It is almost impossible for some animals to learn some responses. These are known as **contraprepared behaviors**. There is a third class of responses, which can be learned when special learning procedures are applied; these are known as **unprepared behaviors**. The phenomenon of learned food aversion is an example of prepared behavior. Humans and animals develop food aversions quickly even with a single exposure. These aversions are quite resistant to extinction. Food aversion must have developed during the course of evolution as a way of avoiding poisonous substances and it must have become a biological tendency to avoid foods that are tainted. John Garcia conducted numerous experiments on the development of taste aversion that have challenged several assumptions of classical conditioning. It is sometimes said that humans are prepared to learn a language while subhuman animals are not. Similarly, humans are prone to develop certain phobias easily; for example, fear of snakes or cockroaches. While unprepared behaviors can be learned with some effort, it is almost impossible to teach animals some contraprepared behaviors. The idea of biological constraints on learning has been very well demonstrated by two students of Skinner.

Keller & Marian Breland (husband and wife), students of Skinner, became famous animal trainers (Marian Breland later became Marian Bailey). They were successful in training thousands of animals for commercial purposes (advertisements, circuses, TV serials, movies and the like), using operant conditioning procedures. On one occasion, they tried to train a pig to place a wooden disk (a token) into a piggy bank (a box). Brelands thought it would be an easy task to teach the animal to do it. But what happened is interesting. Every time they tried to make the animal put the disk into the bank, they failed. When the animal saw the disk, it was willing to do nothing but to root the wooden disk along the ground. Probably, the pigs were biologically programmed only to push stimuli in the shape of disks along the ground. Later, the Brelands substituted raccoons in the place of pigs and repeated the procedure to make the raccoons to drop the disk into the box. The raccoon treated the disk as a tidbit of food, rubbed it against the side of the box, pulled it out, held it tightly, and rubbed it again and so on. At last, the animal dropped the disk into the box and it was reinforced. But when the second disk was added, the problem started. Now, the raccoon had two bits to play with and started rubbing the disks together endlessly for such a long time, the Brelands had to abandon the project of training the raccoons. Similar difficulties were encountered when they tried to train chickens to play baseball. These and other experiments suggested that the animals are biologically prepared to learn only some types of responses more readily than others. Certain responses (like the raccoons rubbing the disk as though it was food) were so deeply rooted that they overrode the conditioning procedure. Brelands called this behavior **instinctive drift**—a tendency for conditioned response to drift back toward instinctive behavior. Based on their experience of training animals, they wrote an article titled '*Misbehavior of Organisms*' (1961) as a takeoff on the title of an influential book by Skinner, *The Behavior of Organisms* (1938), in which Skinner had proposed the general laws of operant conditioning. Later researches have provided additional evidence to the phenomenon of instinctive drift, suggesting that there are limitations to conditionability of animals.

Nowadays, several researchers doubt the contention that conditioning occurs automatically if any CS is paired with a UCS or if a freely emitted response is followed by a reinforcer. There is a growing recognition that the genetic endowment of an organism must be taken into consideration when we talk about learning. For example, Robert Bolles has proposed an evolutionary theory of learning, which emphasizes innate predispositions that limit the associations that an organism can learn. William Timberlake has extended and elaborated Bolles' ideas. Seligman (1970) maintains that some species learn associations more easily than other species because they are biologically prepared to do so. Similarly for some species, it is difficult to learn some associations because they are not biologically prepared to learn them. Therefore, where an association falls, on the *preparedness continuum*, determines how easily it is learned.

LEARNING AND BRAIN

All along, the learning theorists focused on overt behavior and ignored the role of the brain in learning. Pavlov had tried to explain conditioning in terms of excitation and inhibition, which governed all central nervous system activity forming what he called *cortical mosaic*. His views did not find favor with modern neuroscientists. Recently, researchers have shown that certain other brain functions play an important role in learning. According to them, the action of neurotransmitter dopamine lies at the core of forming associations between stimuli, responses and the consequences of making responses. These are complex theories that are still at the stage of their infancy and no final words have been said about them. Today, it is generally held that ability to learn depends not only on brain structure and nerve circuits, but also on the brain's ability to modify its structure and function in response to experience. No single part of the brain is involved in all learning. Hypothalamus is involved in the regulation of our ability to experience the pleasures of being rewarded. Hippocampus plays an important role in allowing an individual to learn the cues that signal the appropriate context for a behavior. Several parts of the frontal lobes are involved in operant learning; some parts store representations of goals and expectations, other parts are involved in representing the emotion associated with an event and still other parts monitor the relationship between how one expects to perform and his/her actual performance, signaling when one has made an error or is in danger of making an error. The cerebellum plays a major role in classical conditioning and the amygdala is important in the acquisition of conditioned fears. Learning is an exceedingly complex process that relies on interactions among many brain areas and activity of different neurotransmitters that affect these areas in subtle ways. Biology influences learning, but do not forget that learning can also affect biology. Several studies have shown how certain forms of learning change the structure of the brain. For example, in an individual who continuously engages in complex movements (as in the case of a musician who plays on violin), it has been seen that the somatosensory strip (at the right hemisphere) associated with movement is enlarged.

Learning represents an individual's continuous process of adapting to changing circumstances and its effects on the brain occur throughout the life cycle. Researchers compared the brains of rats raised in standard cages with rats raised in enriched environments—with toys and greater opportunities for learning—and found that rats raised in enriched environment having heavier brains with more dendrites and synapses and greater concentrations of neurotransmitters. These rats performed better on subsequent learning tasks. Human beings, who had been exposed to stimulating environments with ample learning opportunities early in life, were found to exhibit a slower decline in brain functioning during late adulthood. So remember, everyday during your life your brain adapts and continues its own evolution. The brain's structure and functions are affected not only by your genetic endowment but by your learning experiences as well. In addition, your cultural and psychological conditions may also affect what you learn and what you do not.

Chapter Summary

Learning is the key psychological process that has made you what you are today. You know who you are, what you are and where you are; know a thousand and more things. You have learnt to speak a language, to read and write, to respect certain things and to dislike certain others, to appreciate the good and the beautiful and detest the bad and ugly. You have learnt to fear some things, fight against certain other things, to love some people and hate some others, and about your culture, festivals and rituals. You have acquired specific attitudes toward certain objects and events; you have acquired certain stereotypes, and certain prejudices. The list is endless. All these are products of learning. But what is learning? This chapter has attempted to give a broad idea of the concept of learning and the factors associated with it.

Although, defining learning in such a way acceptable to everyone has not been possible, psychologists have given a simple, but non-controversial, definition to the term. They have defined learning as a relatively permanent change in behavior brought about by experience. For one thing, the change is not temporary; secondly, it is not the result of maturation, disease, accident or drugs. There is no agreement on types of learning; some propose two types, some three and some others eight types of learning. Generally three types of learning are considered important. These are: classical conditioning, operant conditioning and cognitive learning.

Classical conditioning was propounded by the Russian physiologist Pavlov. Classical conditioning is the process of learning by which a previously neutral stimulus (CS) comes to elicit an identical or similar response to the one originally elicited by another stimulus (unconditioned stimulus) as the result of pairing of the two stimuli. The response elicited by the CS is CR. When the CS is not followed by UCS, the CR gradually weakens and ultimately stops. This is extinction. After sometime, when the CS is presented, suddenly the organism may respond with CR. This is called spontaneous recovery. The tendency to produce CR to stimuli that are similar to the CS is called stimulus generalization. Organisms can also learn to differentiate among stimuli that are related to the conditioned stimulus, but not identical to it. This is stimulus discrimination. If a new stimulus acquires the ability to elicit a CR when it is paired with an established CS (that already produces a CR), the process is called higher order conditioning. Examples of CR in real life are many. Several of our fears, positive and negative attitudes including sexual attraction, are conditioned. We also develop certain food aversions due to conditioning. Techniques based on classical conditioning have been developed to treat irrational fears.

The author of operant conditioning was Skinner. The basis for operant learning had already been laid by Thorndike through his law of effect. The law of effect states that responses that have satisfying effects will be strengthened, while those that are annoying will be weakened. In a way, Skinner's work can be seen as a systematic elaboration of the principles enunciated by Thorndike, although Skinner states that he was unaware of Thorndike's contribution for several years of his career. Operant conditioning is a form of learning in which the consequences of behavior determine the likelihood that the behavior will be

Contd...

Contd...

repeated. That is, what happens when a response is made determines whether that response will occur again. Two important consequences studied by Skinner were reinforcement (reward) and punishment.

Reinforcement is the process by which a stimulus increases the probability that a preceding response will be repeated. A reinforcer is any stimulus that increases the probability that a preceding behavior will occur again. There are several kinds of reinforcers. Stimuli such as food and water that are naturally reinforcing (satisfying basic needs) are called primary reinforcers. Stimuli such as money, social approval or praise that acquire reinforcing value because of their association with primary reinforcers are called secondary reinforcers. Those stimuli, whose presentation following a response strengthens the response, are known as positive reinforcers. Those stimuli (generally aversive ones), whose removal following a response strengthens the response, are known as negative reinforcers.

Schedules of reinforcement are predetermined plans for the delivery of reinforcers. In continuous reinforcement schedule, every correct response is reinforced. In the partial reinforcement schedule, only some of the responses are reinforced. In a fixed ratio schedule, reinforcers are given after a specified number of correct responses. In a variable ratio schedule, the number of correct responses needed before a reinforcer is given varies around some average. In a fixed interval schedule, a specified period of time must pass before a correct response can be reinforced. In a variable interval schedule, the period of time that must elapse before a response can be reinforced varies around an average interval.

Reinforcement and punishment operate in opposite ways in learning. Reinforcement strengthens the response it follows; punishment weakens or suppresses the preceding response. When an unpleasant stimulus is used to remove a response, it is called aversive or positive punishment. When a positive reinforcer is removed, it is called negative punishment or response cost. In general, reinforcement is more effective than punishment. It is clear that punishment if used with discretion may be effective. The processes of stimulus generalization, stimulus discrimination, extinction and spontaneous recovery are applicable in the case of operant learning also. Principles of operant conditioning are used in behavior therapy, biofeedback training, programmed learning and training animals.

Cognitive psychologists believe that we need to go beyond conditioning in understanding learning. They assert that certain types of learning depend on higher mental processes such as thinking, information processing, planning, problem solving, and imaging. Among cognitive psychologists, Kohler worked on insight learning, Tolman on latent learning and Bandura on observational learning. Insight learning is a mental process in which the restructuring of a problem into its component parts leads to the sudden emergence of a solution to the problem. Latent learning is a kind of hidden learning that occurs without apparent reinforcement and is not displayed until reinforcement is provided. In observational learning, behaviors are acquired by observing and imitating the behaviors of a model. Bandura, a social cognitive theorist, states that modeling involves four steps: attention, retention, reproduction and motivation. Children are found to learn aggressive or prosocial behavior by watching models.

An organism's evolutionary history determines what it can learn and what it cannot, implying that there are certain biological constraints to learning. Certain associations are easily acquired than others. It is difficult to operationally condition animals to perform behaviors that are contrary to their evolved natural tendencies. Organisms abandon conditioned behavior in favor of a more natural response, a phenomenon that has come to be called instinctive drift. The brain's ability to adapt and modify itself in relation to experience underlies the ability to learn. No single part of the brain is involved in all learning. Studies have shown that learning alters the brain.

6 CHAPTER Memory: Remembering and Forgetting

PREVIEW

In the previous chapter, we discussed some of the fundamental ways in which learning takes place. Here we shall try to find out what happens to what we have learned. Suppose yesterday you learnt how to ride bicycle. If you want to use this learning, this information must be stored somewhere within you and you must be able to get it back (remember) today, so that it can be used. This is the process of memorization. Learning is acquisition of skills and knowledge. But learning is of no use without memory. Memory is the system by which we retain information and bring it to consciousness. Without memory, experience would leave no mark on our behavior, we would be unable to retain the information and skills we acquire through experience. In this chapter, we shall see in some detail how the learned information is processed by human mind. Perception, learning and memory are the three processes that are intricately connected. One cannot exist without the other. You have to remember what you perceive or learn if it were to be of any consequence. If you do not remember, not only you cannot use the information, but further learning will not be possible. What you are learning today depends on the memory of what you learned yesterday. Unless you know what you have learned, you cannot proceed with further learning. Psychologists conceptualize human memory as a type of information processing that involves three basic psychological activities: encoding, storage and retrieval. Encoding is the process of converting information into a form usable in memory; storing is retaining information in memory and retrieval is bringing back to mind information stored in memory. In short, memory consists of three processes: registration (learning), retention and recall.

As you read through the chapter, you will come across some surprising facts about memory. Suppose you utter the following five digits 8-3-5-4-2 and ask your friend to repeat them after you. She will do it without any difficulty. Next, you ask her to repeat the following digits, 6-2-8-9-2-1-7-1. In all probability she will fail. In the next trial, you present the same digits in the following order: 26-12-1978; she will repeat them easily. Find out why. Very often, it so happens that you know the person in front of you very well, you can recognize the face, but you cannot remember her name. You feel that you know her name as well as yours; but still you cannot recall it. Why? You can easily recall your childhood memories; but it is difficult to remember what you ate for breakfast yesterday morning. This is especially so with the elderly people. Remote memories are intact while recent memories are fragile. Why? Some people have poor memory for numbers, but their memory for names or faces is good. How do you explain this phenomenon? Does it mean there are several kinds of memory, such as memory for names, memory for faces and memory for numbers? Finally, why do people forget? Or, do they forget at all? These are questions that psychologists are trying to answer. You will have a glimpse of what psychologists are saying about these issues in this chapter.

As usual, psychologists accept that there are several gaps in their knowledge about memory; but they have learned a good deal about memory during the last century. Psychologists, like all other scientists, are skeptics; they do not believe in anything blindly. They want accurate answers with evidence. That is not always easy. Scientists move toward perfection; they never reach it. However research on memory has enabled psychologists to make some practical suggestions about improving your memory. They have demonstrated the extent to which human memories could be trusted and especially the extent to which the report of the so-called eyewitness to a crime can be trusted. Read the chapter carefully; you will be a great deal wiser about the accuracy of others' and often your own memories.

Chapter Outline

In the previous chapter, we discussed how learning occurs. Learning helps us to adapt to the environment that is ever changing; learning has survival value. We search for food, plan our actions, think about the consequences of our actions, so on and so forth. That is, we use what we have learned for successful living. Learning, to be useful, must be stored in mind. But what do we mean when we say "store it in mind?" What happens to the materials we have learned? Where and how are the learned materials stored? How do we get them back when we want? These are important questions pertaining to the process called memory. In this chapter, we try to understand the phenomenon of memory. But then, what is memory? Memory is the process involving registration (encoding), retention (storing) and recall (retrieval) of information that has been learned and stored in the mind. When memorizing, mind acts as a processing system that encodes, stores and retrieves information. **Encoding** refers to the process of receiving and organizing the information and converting it into neural code that the brain can understand. **Storage** refers to the process of retaining the information in memory over time. Finally, **retrieval** is the process of accessing the stored information in memory.

MEMORY AS INFORMATION PROCESSING

The computer analogy is often employed to explain the processes involved in memory. When you type some information on your computer keyboard, the keystrokes are converted into electrical code that a computer can understand and process; this is encoding. The next step is filing and saving the information in the computer; this is storing. The information may be stored temporarily in random access memory (RAM) or it may be stored permanently by sending it into the hard drive. When you give a command to the computer such as "open file," the information you have stored (saved) appears on the screen for you to examine; this is retrieval. But you must not stretch the analogy too far. Memory is a highly dynamic human process and its complexity cannot be captured by the information processing model used in the context of a computer. Human beings more often forget what they have learned or distort what they have stored in the memory; sometimes they remember events that never occurred. However crude it is, the **information processing model** is still useful in explaining memory. But before proceeding with the information processing model of memory involving encoding, storing and retrieval, we have to learn certain other aspects of memory.

THREE STAGE MODEL OF MEMORY

Many psychologists studying memory suggest that any information acquired has to pass through three different stages before it is remembered. A highly influential model of this variety was offered by Waugh & Norman (1965), and Richard Atkinson & Richard Shiffrin in 1968 (modified in 1971). According to these researchers, there are three kinds of memory storage systems, each of which differing in its function and the length of time it holds the information. These are **sensory memory**, which refers to the initial momentary storage of information in memory lasting only for a brief interval of time (typically a fraction of a second or a little more); **short-term memory (STM)**, which holds relatively small amount of information (typically five to nine items) for only a few seconds (15 to 30); and **long-term memory (LTM)** in which huge amounts of information are stored relatively permanently for longer duration, from hours to years (Fig. 6.1). Let us examine briefly the nature and functions of these three storage systems of memory.

Sensory Memory

Sensory memory system holds the incoming sensory input for a very brief interval of time. Sensory memories occur automatically without effort. These memories arise as a result of temporary activation of sensory-perceptual areas in the brain by the stimulus. There are different subsystems of sensory memory called **sensory registers**, which are the initial processors of information. We can think of several types of sensory memories depending on the sense modality from which the information emanates. When the information comes from visual system, it is called **iconic memory**. The message from auditory system is called **echoic memory**. Whatever the source, sensory memory does not last long. The iconic memory lasts less than a second and the echoic memory fades within 2 or 3 seconds. Whatever the type, the sensory memory can retain information only for very brief interval of time. Unless it is transferred to STM, the information fades away. But in spite of its short duration, the precision of sensory memory is found to be of high order. Experiments have demonstrated that sensory memory can store the exact replica of stimulus to which it was exposed. Sensory memory should not be confused with eidetic memory. Description of eidetic memory is given in Box 6.1.

Box 6.1: Eidetic Memory

There are some people who can recall a visual image in such vivid detail as if still they are looking at it. This form of visual memory is called **eidetic memory** or photographic memory. The critical features of those with eidetic imagery are:

1. They continue to see a representation of a visual stimulus some time after it has been removed.
2. That they are seeing a true visual image and not merely the memory of the stimulus. Eidetic memory is rare in adults (one in 1,000 or even one in a million), but it occurs in about 5% of young children. It typically disappears before the age of 10.

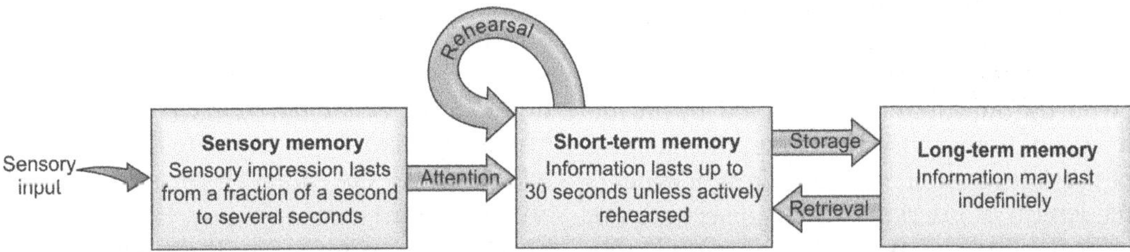

FIGURE 6.1: Three stage model of memory

If the storage capacity of sensory memory is so limited and the information stored is so fleeting, how do we know whether such a memory system exists at all? It would not have been known but for a series of novel experiments conducted by George Sperling (1960), which is regarded as a classic in psychology. Sperling exposed on a screen a series of 12 letters in three rows and four columns (as shown below) for $\frac{1}{20}$ of a second, and asked the participants to report what they saw.

MTLQ
RYNS
DKBF

The participants could report only four or five of the letters flashed although they knew they saw more. It is possible that the information was accurately registered in the sensory memory, but during the time the subjects took to verbalize the first four or five letters, the memory of the remaining letters faded. To test this possibility, Sperling conducted another experiment. This time, he presented a high, medium, or low tone immediately after the array of letters were flashed, and the participants were instructed to report the first row of letters if they hear the loud tone, the second row of letters if they hear the medium tone, and the last row if they hear the low tone. Surprisingly, the participants reported the letters accurately regardless of whether they were at the top, middle, or the bottom row, based on the type of tone they heard. The results demonstrated that the information stored in sensory memory was an accurate representation of what the subjects had seen. Sperling has also shown that the ability to recall the information depended upon the length of time elapsed between the flashing of the information and sounding of tone. If the length of interval exceeds a second, the information fades away, and the participants cannot recall the letters in any row. In short, the experiments demonstrated that there is a sensory memory store, the information stored in it is an accurate representation of the sensory input, but the information stays in it only for a brief period because it is displaced by other stimuli entering into it, and unless it is transferred to STM store it will be lost forever.

Short-term Memory

As you know, the input into the sensory memory fades away soon because it is displaced by other incoming stimulus information. But when it is selectively attended to, it will be transferred to the second memory store, (STM), which can hold a limited amount of information for a short period of time (about 15 to 20 seconds and with effort up to 30 seconds). There are differing theories suggesting how information in sensory memory is transferred to STM. According to one theory, the information is transformed into mental images, and according to another, it is converted into meaningful words. That is, when information leaves sensory store, it must be converted into some type of code if it were to be retained in STM. These are called **memory codes**, which are mental representations of some stimulus or information. Mental codes take several forms; mental images of seen stimuli become *visual codes*, auditory stimuli take the form of *phonological codes*, and meaningful materials are retained as *semantic codes*.

The storage capacity and duration of STM are limited. STM can hold about "seven plus or minus two" independent units of information at any given time; it could be letters or digits or other units (A paper titled *The magical number seven plus or minus two: Some limits on our capacity for processing information* by GA Miller [1956] is considered an important event in psychology). But how do we remember long sentences? This is possible because of a process called

chunking. Chunking is grouping of stimuli into meaningful units so that they can be remembered easily. Examine the following array of letters:

'TSAPSIHOTNIEESTONDLUOCOHWNAMEHT'

Can you remember these letters by looking at them once? It is difficult. Now, look at them from the other end; it is a sentence, "The man who could not see into his past." The entire array can be easily remembered because the 31 letters are chunked into nine meaningful units (words) constituting a sentence. Sometimes, a complete sentence may become a unit and you may retain five or six sentences in your STM. Chunks can vary from a single digit or letter to complex groups of digits or letters, such as a telephone number, letters forming a word (*complementary*) or words forming a sentence (Ram is planning to go to Delhi to attend an international conference on solar energy). How chunks are formed depends on your knowledge and past experience.

Although you can hold in your STM 5 to 9 units of information, their stay there will be short lived. Suppose you want to telephone a person whose number you do not know, but it is there in the telephone directory. You look into the directory, notice his number, give him a ring, talk to him for a while, and put down the phone. Now you try to recall his phone number! You have forgotten it. The number has disappeared from your STM. Psychologists are of the opinion that information cannot be held in STM for more than 15 to 25 seconds, unless it is transferred to LTM. Transferring information from STM to LTM occurs largely through a process called rehearsal.

Rehearsal

Rehearsal is the process of keeping the items of information in the center of attention by repeating them silently or aloud. In the example above, suppose the phone number you noticed is important and you may have to use it again, then, you try to repeat the number several times till you learn it "by heart". Rehearsal serves two purposes: firstly, it retains the information in the STM and secondly, transfers the information into LTM. The more an item is rehearsed, the more likely it will become part of LTM. There are two types of rehearsal namely, maintenance rehearsal and elaborative rehearsal. **Maintenance rehearsal**, as the name suggests, is the act of keeping the material in the focus of attention; it may not help the material to be consolidated in the LTM. On the other hand, **elaborative rehearsal** is an active process; it gives the material organization and meaning as it is being rehearsed, so that it fits into the material that already exists in the LTM. We shall learn more about elaborative rehearsal when we discuss levels of processing later in the chapter.

Working Memory

According to the three stage model of memory, STM is a temporary holding station along the route from sensory memory to LTM. Rehearsal is the only process that is operating in STM. The notion that information in STM can be used in several ways led researchers to expand the conception of how this kind of memory works, which in turn led to the theory of **working memory**. The theory of working memory is an improved version of STM. Here, working memory is considered as a mental workspace that retrieves and stores information, actively manipulates it, and helps other cognitive functions, such as planning and problem solving; it finely characterizes how information is stored in STM. It has distinct stores, which retain different kinds of information. According to British psychologist Alan Baddeley (1992), there are several components of working memory, four of which are important; these are phonological loop (or articulatory loop), visuospatial sketchpad, episodic buffer and the central executive.

Components of working memory: The **phonological loop** is the speech-based component of working memory. It stores mental representations of auditory stimuli; it is active when you hear a sound or word or when you utter a word to yourself while reading something. Rehearsing silently what you hear will refresh the acoustic codes stored in the phonological loop. In the absence of rehearsal, the acoustic traces may fade away. The mental image of spatial information, such as the face of a person or a scene you see is stored for a brief period in the **visuospatial sketchpad**. The visuospatial sketchpad is like a notepad with patterns drawn in fading ink; it briefly retains mental images. The phonological loop and visuospatial sketchpad may work simultaneously. For example, when you are introduced to a person, you may utter his name silently to yourself while holding the mental image of his/her face. The third component of working memory, **episodic buffer**, carries out an integrative function. Information from LTM, phonological loop and/or visuospatial sketchpad are manipulated, coordinated, integrated and made available to conscious awareness. Suppose your teacher asks you a question such as: What is the area of a rectangle? The phonological loop maintains the acoustic codes for the sound 'rectangle' in the working memory; visuospatial sketchpad maintains the mental image of a rectangle; the formula for the area of a rectangle is retrieved from LTM.

All these bits of information are stored temporarily in the episodic buffer, where they are integrated to provide you with the conscious awareness that the area of a rectangle is: length multiplied by width. Baddeley maintains that episodic buffer plays an important role in chunking groups of words into phrases and sentences, thus enabling us to retain at a time 15 to 16 words. The fourth component of working memory is the **central executive**. As the name suggests, it supervises the entire set of activities of the working memory; it plans and controls the sequence of activities to be performed (mentioned above in determining the area of a rectangle) and allocates attention to other subsystems and integrates information within the episodic buffer. It is believed that the functioning of central executive is controlled by certain areas of frontal lobe. Some researchers speculate that the breakdown in the central executive processor may lead to serious memory disturbances such as those found in **Alzheimer's disease (AD)**. The components of working memory are shown in Figure 6.2.

Long-term Memory

When we use the term memory, we generally refer to **LTM**. All that we have learned about the world and ourselves is stored more or less permanently in LTM. It contains words, sentences, ideas and the experiences we had. Our memories of the past, our sense of continuity as individuals, the names of individuals we know, our relationships with them and a whole host of other things, essential for our survival, are all stored in LTM. We are not sure how much information can be stored in LTM and for how long. The storage capacity of LTM is infinite. LTM may last for days, weeks, months, years or even a lifetime. In one study, an investigator showed participants more than 600 pictures; then some other pictures (not seen by participants) were mixed with them, and after 2 hours, the participants were asked to pick out those they had

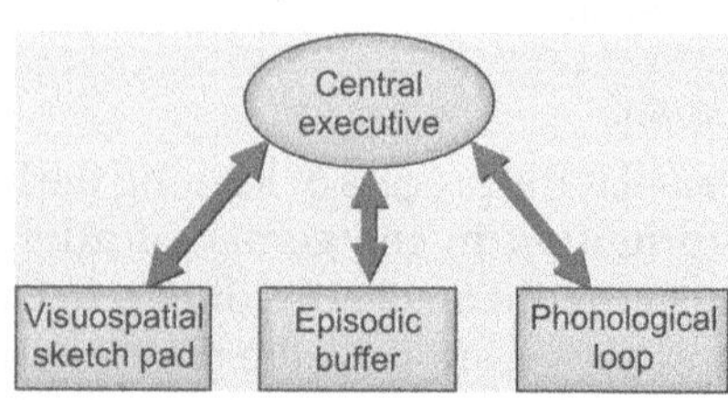

FIGURE 6.2: Components of working memory

seen earlier. Surprisingly, the participants could recognize 99 percent of the pictures correctly; they recognized 87 percent after a week (Shepard, 1967). This remarkable degree of retention occurred even though the participants had seen the pictures only for about 5 to 6 seconds.

Some psychologists assert that memories are never lost. Once information is stored in LTM, it is there forever. Only, sometimes, we have difficulty in accessing them, which may be because we have not stored them in organized fashion or because we are not searching for them at the proper place. LTM is our vast library of stored information. Like a library, LTM must be organized if information is to be retrieved. We must know where to search for a book in the library; a misplaced book in the library cannot be accessed easily. The same principles hold good for LTM. Memory store must be well-organized and be in order; that is, there must be proper encoding. Memory, especially LTM, is essential for our survival. It is one of the basic cognitive processes that play an important role determining our behavior and experience.

We have said that information is passed on to LTM from STM for being stored. But often information may move from LTM to STM. In fact, contents of working memory are generally drawn from LTM, not from STM. For example, when you look up a telephone number, you must first access LTM in order to know how to pronounce the numbers and then keep them in STM as you prepare to make the call. Thus, LTM plays an important role in perception; you recognize and identify something only after the appropriate information is activated in LTM.

Information stored in the LTM must be properly organized. Only then, it can be retrieved easily. Organization of information depends on how the information is encoded. When the information is encoded more effectively into LTM, the likelihood of its retrieval is better. There are two basic types of encoding: effortful processing and automatic processing. In your day-to-day life, you are bombarded with innumerable items of information—names of people and places, your work schedule, social activities, familial commitments, so on and so forth. When you are remembering all of them, you are engaged in effortful processing. Encoding of this type is intentional and requires conscious attention. You rehearse the items, take notes and make lists of them when you are engaged in effortful processing. On the other hand, certain information is encoded into your LTM without intention or with minimum of attention. For example, on your way to college, you must have watched several landmarks (houses, shops, medical clinics, trees, etc.), which are stored in your LTM without your being aware of it. When someone asks you about the medical clinic, you can remember its exact location and inform the person about it. This information got into your LTM through automatic processing.

Levels of Processing Theory

The three stage model of memory, which we discussed above, is only one of the explanations of how we remember information. There are other explanations that are equally valid and influential. One such exposition is called the **levels of processing theory** (LOP theory). This theory holds that the capacity to remember depends upon the degree to which the input is processed. The deeper the processing, the more likely it will be stored in memory for later recall. If we do not focus our attention closely to the material that is presented, it is processed scantily and hence the memory will be poor. On the other hand, if the material is critically analyzed and deeply processed, it will be stored well and easily remembered. For example, let us say you are exposed to the word 'chair'. If you merely perceive the structural properties of the word (such as whether the word is in upper case or lower case, italics or bold letters), your processing is shallow. If you utter the word for yourself, hearing its sound, you are phonetically coding the word; this is slightly better and you are processing at the intermediate level. On the other hand, if you pay close attention to the word, understand its meaning and implication, you are engaged in the deepest level of processing called *semantic coding*. When the material is processed at the deepest level, it is stored well and remembered better.

Rehearsal plays a very important role in deep processing of information as it does in the case of three stage memory theory. As we know, rehearsal is the process of retaining information by repeating it often. According to the level of processing model, mere repetition (maintenance rehearsal) is not sufficient for effective memorization. **Maintenance rehearsal** keeps input active in short-term (working) memory and the information may not enter long-term store. For consolidation of information to take place, one must engage in elaborative rehearsal. **Elaborative rehearsal** takes into consideration the meaning of the material presented and expands on it. If the meaning is understood, the material will be remembered better. Thus, the idea of elaboration has been added to the level of processing theory. Elaboration involves the active search for meaning and integrating the information with the existing memories. So, elaborative rehearsal is more effective in transferring information to LTM; that is, the greater the elaboration, better the memory. The LOP theory has important practical implications. For example, when you study a passage, the theory suggests that:

1. You must understand the material and organize it instead of simply memorizing it.
2. You must think about the ways in which it can be applied to your own life.
3. You must try to relate the material you are learning to what is already known to you.

   In short, it is advised that you engage in elaborative rehearsal if your memory has to be long-lasting.

Organization of Long-term Memory

Human memory is not an untidy collection of bits of information. It is well classified and organized. As mentioned earlier, our LTM is like a well-organized library. Information in LTM is classified and grouped in some logical manner; it is arranged in some way to make sense. There are several organizational schemes that enhance LTM.

Hierarchies and Chunking

One effective way to memorize information is to arrange the material into a hierarchy. A logical hierarchy enhances our understanding of the items because of the intrinsic relationship among the individual items. Let us illustrate the value of hierarchical arrangement of items with a simple experiment. Try to learn the two lists of words given in Table 6.1 one list at a time. Find out the number of trials you need to master each list. You may need several trials to learn the list-A, while one or two trials may be enough to learn and remember list-B. It is because list-A contains unrelated discrete words, while list-B

Table 6.1: Effect of Hierarchical Arrangement of Items on Memory

List-A	*List-B*
Spiral	Boy
Bench	School
Water	College
Profession	Study
Window	Examination
Bottle	Degree
Green	Employment
Telephone	Money
Carbon	Love
Harbor	Marriage
Literate	Family
Receiver	Children

contains words that are arranged logically to form a hierarchy. In list-B, as you proceed from top to bottom, each word operates as a cue for the word below it and hence you can learn and remember the words with ease.

Chunking is another factor that helps remembering. As we have seen earlier, chunking is grouping of items into meaningful units. Chunk is a unit of information, such as a digit, letter or word. Chunks are easier to rehearse, keep alive in working memory (STM) and transfer into LTM.

Role of Imagery

According to Allan Paivio (1969), information is stored in LTM in two forms: verbal codes and visual codes. A code is simply a kind of internal mental representation of a stimulus or event. In his **dual coding theory**, Paivio states that it is advantageous to encode information both in visual codes (imagery) and verbal codes, because the chances are that at least one of them will come to our help when we want to recall the information. Paivio and his colleagues have shown that pictures are generally remembered better than words because pictures are stored using dual codes using visual and verbal codes; that is, you can describe what you see (the picture) in words as well as store it visually. That is why textbooks are illustrated copiously to improve remembering. The one difficulty in Paivio's theory is that visual imagery cannot be produced in several cases. For concrete objects like chair or table, it is easy to form visual imagery, and definitely, visual imagery aids recall. But, how can we form images of abstract concepts such as justice, love or jealousy?

CONSTRUCTIVE PROCESSES IN MEMORY

When we encode certain complex events of life or something we have read, there is a possibility that these materials are modified. With passage of time, some details may be added, some may be deleted and others may be changed in such ways that the remembered material is not an exact copy of what we have experienced or read. These modifications are called constructive processes. We may encode only the gist or the meaning of what we read in a book or a newspaper. Long ago in 1932, the British psychologist Sir Frederick Bartlett conducted some classical experiments to demonstrate the role of constructive processes in memorizing. He asked his subjects to read a story and obtained from them successive recalls of the story after 1 day, 3 days, a week and a month. He found that the subjects have shortened or simplified the story, adding or omitting several details. Mostly the participants remembered the gist of the story. He also found that the subjects were using inferences in their encoding of the story. Recent experiments have shown that we remember what we inferred at the time of encoding.

Inferences are made on the basis of the memory organizations called schemas. A **schema** is a mental picture about some aspect of the world— an organized pattern of thinking stored in our memory, which influences how we interpret, store, and recall new information. For example, when we see a young man and a woman walking together, we tend to see them as lovers; in fact, they may be siblings! Schemas often distort our memories by leading us to encode or retrieve information in ways that make sense. The information is changed so that it fits in with our pre-existing notions about the objects and events in the world. When we rely on schema, it means that our memories are general reconstructions of our previous experience. Bartlett has shown that schemas are based on specific information to which people are exposed, their understanding of the situation, their expectations about the situation and their awareness of the motivation underlying the behavior of others. Therefore beware, your memories may not be reliable and your imperfect recollections may have dangerous implications. Let us examine one instance (eyewitness testimony in courts) where imperfect memories can play havoc.

Mistaken Eyewitness Testimony

The fact that an individual's knowledge, expectations and emotional state can distort recall resulting in unfortunate consequences has been well-documented in experiments as well as real life situations. One such instance is in the courtroom where some people are called on to give evidence as witnesses to an accident, crime, rape, murder or robbery. Because the events that are witnessed are almost always totally unexpected, of brief duration and stressful, even an honest, intelligent and well-meaning person may be inaccurate when asked to recall the details of a past event or to identify a suspect. Because of this, several innocents have been convicted and sent to jail. Feldman (2002) reports of a victim who was sentenced to serve 14 to 50 years in jail because two people picked him out of lineup of several others by mistake. Five years later, the actual criminal was determined and the innocent victim was released. But the unfortunate fellow had lost precious 5 years of his life. Several such instances have occurred all over the world. It is generally believed that if memories are constructed, then information that occurs after an event may shape that construction process. The distortion of memory by misleading post-event information is called *misinformation effect.*

Researchers have found several factors that affect the accuracy of recall during testifying in a court. For example, when a person witnesses an event and then he is exposed to misleading, suggestive statements about it, the person will be confused and his/her report tends to be inaccurate. Those who are exposed to media (TV, radio, newspaper) reports about the event have a tendency to be influenced by the report rather than what actually happened. What witnesses have heard from others about the event may also enter into the constructive process. If there is a weapon in the hands of the alleged criminal, accuracy of testimony generally decreases. Witnesses who are under the effect of alcohol tend to be less accurate than when they are sober. During identification parade, the suspects change their appearance, which often leads to inaccurate identification. Often an innocent wearing the dress similar to that of suspect has been identified as the criminal. Sometimes, the personal bias may lead to wrong identification. For example, if the witness and the suspect belong to different races or ethnic groups, the person belonging to the other groups are picked up as the offender.

Nowadays, brain-imaging techniques are being introduced to study the neural activity that occurs when false memories are created by misinformation, but the fact whether misinformation can permanently change the original memory is far from being established. But overall, the researches indicate that misinformation can distort eyewitness reports. In the light of available information, doubts have been raised about the reliability of eyewitness testimony. There is a popular belief that children's report is more reliable than those of adults. But research has shown that like adults, children also experience misinformation effects. Vulnerability is found to be more among young children when suggestive questions are asked repeatedly. It has not been possible to determine when children are reporting accurate memories or when they sincerely believe in false memories.

Storage of Information

People store an incredible wealth of information in their LTM. But how and where is the information stored? As of now, we do not have the correct picture, but several theories have been proposed to explain how information is retained in memory. Most of these theories view memory as a network. One group of theories holds that memory can be represented as an **associative network** of ideas or concepts. We have seen that memory is improved by forming associations between new information and other items we already have in our memory. So, we can assume that we have in our memory store a huge network of associated ideas and concepts. Each idea or concept exists as a node or unit. When we think of one idea (a node) it activates another. For example, when we think about a concept such as crime, it activates related concepts in the network; thus, crime may activate related concepts such as law, court, trial, judgment, punishment, fine, jail, and a number of others. Some of them are closely related to crime and some remotely. The activation of one concept by another is called **priming**. The concept "crime" primes punishment. We have well-knit associative networks for several categories such as flowers, fruits, animals and so on and so forth. When you think of one item in a category, it activates other nodes in the same category.

Another group of theories assumes that there are neural networks underlying memory. The neural network model attempts to explain the spreading of activation and priming in a different way. In the associative network model, each concept resides in a node. It is not so in neural network model. Here each node does not contain an individual unit of information. There is no single node for crime or rose. Instead, each node operates like a small information processing unit. Each memory is represented by a unique pattern of interconnected and simultaneously activated nodes. Various nodes distributed throughout the network fire in parallel at each instant and simultaneously spread their activation to other nodes. Thus, certain nodes prime other nodes, and concepts and information are retrieved. For this reason, often the neural network models are called **parallel distributed processing models**.

Retrieval of Information

If information coded and stored in LTM were to be used, it must be accessed or retrieved. How do we retrieve (recall) or read out the required information from the LTM library? Several retrieval cues that help us in finding the information have been identified. The retrieval cue may be a word, a sound, a scene or an emotional experience. It operates as a reminder and leads the memory search to the appropriate location in LTM. Several experiments have shown that it is important to have the retrieval cues encoded along with information as it is put into LTM. The cues may be objective or subjective; objective cues are stimuli that coexist with the information and the subjective cues are self-generated. Suppose you met a person on a beach during sunset. The beach and sunset are objective cues. A friend of mine has a poor memory for numbers. It is difficult for him to remember even his date of birth. He was born on 15-4-1911. Can you guess the strategy he uses for remembering his date of birth? Look what he does; 15 + 4 = 19 and 15 – 4 = 11 and combining them he arrives at his date of birth 15-4-1911. This is self-generated internal cue. Of course, the cue appears to be more complicated than the information to be remembered. Still he remembers it easily because it has undergone elaborate processing. We have seen earlier how deep and elaborate processing aids memory; that is what is happening in this case.

Having multiple cues is beneficial in retrieving information. If one of them fails, the others may help. Remember the friend you met on the beach. Remembering him is aided by the beauty of the beach, the sound of the water waves, and the sight of the setting sun and so on. The distinctness of the material often works like a cue in remembering. Distinctive events such as date of births, deaths, wedding and accidents are remembered better. We often say that such and such a thing happened 4 days after the birth of a child or 10 days after the death of somebody. Similarly, emotion-arousing events (pleasurable ones or even painful ones) are distinctly remembered.

Often, memory is enhanced when the conditions present during retrieval match those that were present during encoding. This is said to be due to the operation of the **encoding specificity principle**. Suppose a person met with an accident and he does not remember anything about it. When he is brought back to the place of the accident, he may remember all about it. That is, when certain stimuli associated with an event become encoded as part of the memory, they may later serve as retrieval cues. The encoding specificity principle has two parts. When it is applied to environmental cues it is called **context-dependent memory** and when applied to an internal state of the learner while encoding, it is called **state-dependent memory**. Context-dependent memory states that it is easier to remember something in the same environment in which it was originally encoded. You must have heard about the police people taking a witness of a crime to the site of crime with the hope that he/she will remember the events accurately. State-dependent memory proposes that the ability to retrieve information is greater when our internal state at the time of retrieval matches our original state during learning. Suppose you encoded something when you were in a state of arousal; it is easier to recall the same thing when you are in a similar state. Similarly, there is a condition called **mood-congruent memory**, which states that there is a tendency to recall information that is congruent with our current mood. That is, we tend to remember positive events when we are happy and negative events when sad.

LONG-TERM MEMORY MODULES

We have seen earlier how STM is accorded the status of working memory. Similarly, modern cognitive psychologists view LTM as a complex process consisting of several components or modules. One theory has identified two components called declarative memory and procedural memory; another theory has called the same memory systems as explicit memory and implicit memory. It is speculated that each of these modules is controlled by separate area in the brain.

Declarative and Procedural Memory

Declarative memory (sometimes called **explicit memory**) is involved in remembering factual information such as names, faces, dates and facts. Verbal and visual memories that one carries with are explicit memories. These memories are stored after cognitive learning. Declarative memory is further divided into semantic memory and episodic memory. **Semantic memory** refers to memory for general knowledge and facts about the world, especially the meaning and use of words and concepts in the language we speak and the rules of logic we use to deduce other facts. Semantic memory is very well organized and considered to be very stable; there is little forgetting of the meaning of words, the ways they are related to one another and about the rules for using them in communication and thinking. Information is stored logically in hierarchies that go from general to specific categories. Words are organized in clusters with related meanings, which can be seen in what is called **tip-of-the-tongue** (**TOT**) phenomenon. **Episodic memory** refers to long-term memories of our personal experiences and biographical details; it consists of memories of specific things that happened to us at various times and places. It is the memory of episodes in our life: when, where and what happened to us in the past. In other words, remembrances of past constitute episodic memory. Episodic memory can be surprisingly detailed. You may remember what you did on a specific day, in a specific place, at a specific time accurately. Suppose, I ask you to tell me where you were 10 years ago on this day; with some difficulty, you can recollect the information and give the correct answer. This is made possible because of your episodic memory. Episodic memory is less well-organized and is not as stable as semantic memory; hence it is liable to be forgotten sooner than semantic memory.

Procedural memory (also called non-declarative or implicit memory) consists of memories of motor and cognitive skills and habitual activities. You are guided by procedural memory when you ride a cycle, drive a car or type a letter. You are not aware of these memories; they simply dispose you to behave in particular ways. Information *about things* is stored in declarative memory; information about *how to do things* is stored in procedural memory. Five major types of procedural (implicit) memories are generally recognized; these are classically conditioned responses, memories formed through non-associative learning, habits, skills and priming. Suppose you had burnt your hand while touching a hot iron rod, you avoid going near it; you may not even be aware why you are doing it. You do it simply because you are conditioned to do so. Implicit memories are formed through non-associative learning; for example, non-associative learning occurs when repeated exposure to a stimulus alters an organism's responsiveness. The learning that occurs when repeated exposure to a stimulus decreases an organism's responsiveness to the stimulus is called *habituation*. For example, if you are walking in a city and hear a car horn you may be startled the first time. But after several days of stay there you may not be startled by car horns. You get used (habituated) to the sound of horns.

The third type of procedural memory is habit. A habit is a well-learned response that is carried out automatically, without conscious thought. A car driver automatically lifts his foot from the accelerator and presses the break at the sight of a red light without being aware of what he is doing. The behavior has become habit and it is stored in the implicit memory store. A skill is like a habit, but more flexible. Learning to ride a cycle is a skill. Once you learn it, you pedal, balance and steer the cycle automatically. When you first begin to learn cycling, you rely on controlled processing; you pay attention to each step and coordinate the steps using working memory. When you have learned cycling, you rely on automatic processing, which allows you to carry out a sequence of steps without having to pay attention to each step. Researches have shown that controlled processing relies heavily on the frontal lobes and to some extent, on anterior cingulate gyrus, while automatic processing relies partly on the basal ganglia and cerebellum. The fifth type of implicit memory is priming, which refers to the effect that occurs when exposure to a stimulus influences how an individual responds to that same or another stimulus (the activation of one concept by another). Priming that makes the same information more easily accessed in the future is known as repetitive priming. You can recognize a word or picture more quickly if you have seen it before than if it is novel. Such priming can be very long-lasting. A way of classifying memory is given in Figure 6.3.

Tip-of-the-tongue Phenomenon

The fragmentary nature of memory is revealed in the tip of the tongue phenomenon. Suppose you are trying to recall a piece of information (a word, a concept, a name or an event), which you are sure you know but cannot recall it. This experience is called **tip-of-the-tongue (TOT)** phenomenon. The word seems to be on the tip of your tongue, but you have difficulty in accessing it immediately. You search for it frantically; you get words that sound similar but not the 'target word.' Investigation of people having

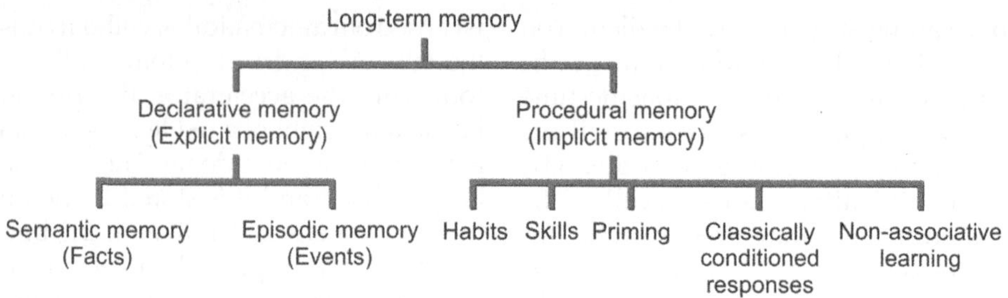

FIGURE 6.3: Types of memories

TOT experience has shown that they can recall accurately several characteristics of the target word—the number of syllables in the word and its initial letter. TOT phenomenon demonstrates how words are clustered in semantic memory; it also indicates that retrieval is not an all-or-none process; we can forget certain characteristic of the word while retaining other relevant information. In short, semantic memory can be thought of as the mental almanac of facts.

Flashbulb Memories

There are some long-term memories of certain life-events, which are so clear and vivid that it becomes virtually difficult to forget them; they become part and parcel of our lives. For example, it may be the scene of an accident, the assassination of an important person (like JF Kennedy, Indira Gandhi or Rajiv Gandhi) or a traumatic event (jetliners crashing into the World Trade Center on September 11th 2001). The pictures of these events stand out like sharp snapshots and these are often called **flashbulb memories**. These memories are formed when we experience an important life-event that is of immense consequence to us. The existence of these hard to forget sharp memories cannot be denied, but their accuracy is disputed by several researchers. On closer examination, it seems that flashbulb memories are not necessarily accurate and these are most probably products of an individual's later elaborations and constructions.

FORGETTING

Forgetting is a normal, natural phenomenon, which refers to the apparent loss of information that has been encoded and stored in LTM. Several people complain about their poor memory and are even worried about their forgetfulness. What would happen if you do not forget? Life would be miserable. So, thank god you forget. That apart, what actually is forgetting? Why do we forget? What happens to the material we encoded? Do we forget at all? These and several other questions concerning memory have bothered psychologists for ages. Some researchers assert that there is nothing like forgetting; once you learn something, it is there for good; only sometimes, you cannot access it. Others believe that there is decaying of memory; the memory traces are obliterated with time. Still others think that you forget because you want to forget what has happened to you. Historically, the study of memory and forgetting can be traced back to the pioneering work of the German psychologist Hermann Ebbinghaus (Fig. 6.4).

Psychologists are indebted to Ebbinghaus for his groundbreaking studies of memory. He developed a novel method of studying memory, used nonsense syllables as the material for memorizing and conducted experiments on himself. The results of his experiments and the conclusions he derived are classics in psychology. Ebbinghaus developed, for the first time in psychology, a set of over 2,300 **nonsense syllables**

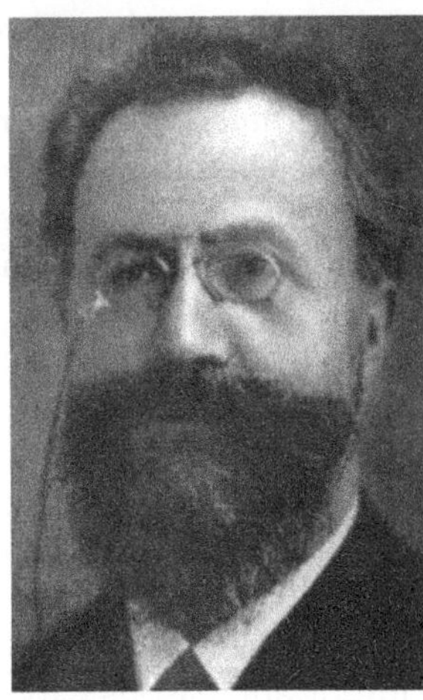

FIGURE 6.4: H Ebbinghaus

(meaningless three-letter combinations such as BEK, CEZ, MEB, etc. the material that is being used all over the world for studying memory); proposed a novel method of studying memory, called the **relearning method** or **savings method**; used only one participant that was himself and came out with a curve of forgetting that has become a landmark in psychology as Ebbinghaus 'curve of forgetting'. The curve (Fig. 6.5) indicates that memory loss is very rapid at first and then it is gradual, and finally the curve becomes an asymptote to X-axis indicating that loss of memory is never complete.

In spite of its primitive nature, Ebbinghaus' work had tremendous influence on subsequent research in the field of memory and some of his basic findings remain valid even today. Today, we use nonsense syllables for studying memory, employ his method of relearning to assess forgetting and his conclusion, that memory loss is rapid during the initial period (during the first 9 hours) and it proceeds gradually later with passage of time, has stood the test of time.

Theories of Forgetting

Why do we forget? The question is simple but like several simple questions, we do not have a definite answer. There are several theories of forgetting. Each of them is partially true, but none of them explain the phenomenon adequately. Let us discuss some of the major theories of forgetting.

Decay Theory

One of the oldest views, the **decay theory**, assumes that the loss of information is a function of time and non-use. As time passes, what you have learned just decays

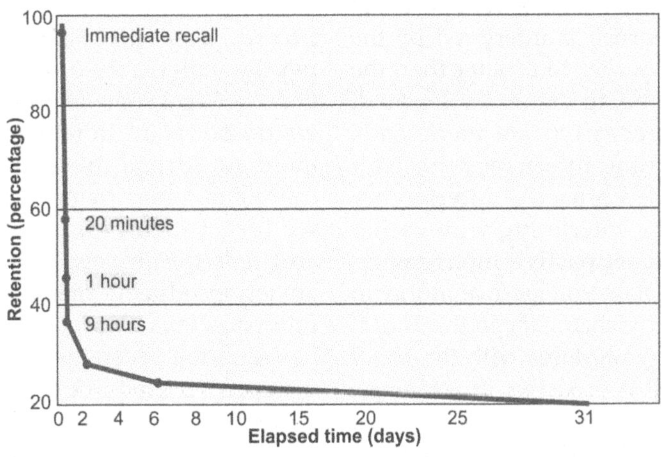

FIGURE 6.5: Ebbinghaus curve of forgetting

and becomes weaker and weaker until it finally fades away. In other words, the *memory trace* in the brain (often called the '**engram**') undergoes a physical change (decay) with the passage of time. Although there is some decay in memory traces, it is not an acceptable explanation for forgetting. If the decay theory were to be true, we would not be able to remember several pieces of information, which we learned a long time ago. Some of our remote memories are vivid and intact while we find it difficult to recall some of the recent events. Therefore, the assertion that the passage of time alone causes memory loss is not tenable. The experiments on a phenomenon called reminiscence bump contradict decay theory. *Reminiscence bump* refers to a sudden increase in the items recalled with the passage of time. For instance, when subjects learning a list of words were tested after two different intervals of time, it was found that in the second testing they recalled more words than they did during the first testing. Therefore, memory researchers have proposed alternatives to decay theory to explain the causes of forgetting. One such view is called interference theory.

Interference Theory

Interference theory assumes that recall of what we have learned is interfered by the material learned earlier to or later than the material that is being currently learned. Therefore, there are two types of interference. When prior learning interferes with later learning, it is called **proactive interference** and later learning interfering with earlier learning is called **retroactive interference**. Suppose in your class you learn anatomy in the 1st hour and biochemistry in the 2nd; if learning anatomy interferes with the recall of biochemistry it is proactive interference; if learning biochemistry interferes with remembering anatomy, it is retroactive interference.

Although interferences have been found to be important causes of forgetting, how they operate on memory is still not clear. One view assumes that the brain takes time to convert STM into LTM and the entry of new information disrupts the conversion process (retroactive interference). Another view holds that the competition among the retrieval cues causes interference. When different memories are associated with similar retrieval cues, confusion can occur and a cue may access wrong memory.

Encoding Failure

One of the important reasons why we forget is that we did not learn things carefully; that is, we did not attend to the material, organize the information properly or processing was not deep enough. In short, we did not encode the information, so that it is well-stored in LTM. Suppose you are watching a TV news channel while you are eating your dinner; can you remember all the news items? Probably not; you may remember an item because of its relevance to you and since you showed interest in (attended to) it. All other items are forgotten because you just heard them but did not process deeply enough to commit to memory.

Motivated Forgetting

Some psychologists, especially psychoanalytically-oriented ones, believe that we forget some information just because we do not want to remember them. True, there are several things that are shocking, humiliating and painful to remember. So, we forget them; this is called repression and it is the process of blocking certain anxiety-producing memories from coming into conscious awareness. Sigmund Freud has reported several instances of repressed memories buried in the unconscious of his patients. For example, during the funeral of her sister, a young woman thought, "*My brother-in-law is now free to marry me.*" The idea was so shocking that it was repressed and Freud unearthed the memory during one of his treatment sessions. There are several instances illustrating motivated forgetting in our daily life; you may forget the names of people you do not like, forget to bring a vegetable your wife has asked because you hate it, etc. In short, we forget several pieces of information just because we want to forget and do not want to remember them.

Failure of Prospective Memories

Very often we forget to do things; we forget to post a letter, to put off the light, to meet a friend, so on and so forth. These are prospective memory failures. **Prospective memory** refers to remembering to do something in future in contrast ***to retrospective memory***—the memory for past events. Prospective memory—to do things in the future—has little content in LTM and hence the failure. To be successful, prospective memory has to draw from other cognitive abilities, such as planning and allocating attention to the things to be done. Laboratory experiments have shown that adults and the elderly have poor memory for things to do. Outside the laboratory, it is found that the elderly fare better in prospective memory, not because their memory is good, but because they are highly motivated to do things (such as taking a medicine) or because they engage in them as a matter of habit.

Amnesia

Partial or total loss of memory for life experiences is referred to as **amnesia**. You must have seen instances of amnesia in movies: somebody forgetting his past after a psychological shock or an accident and later he/she remembering everything when a similar situation that produced amnesia is recreated. However badly it is portrayed, the movie is telling you one important thing: the memories lost in amnesia are not completely destroyed and the forgotten events can be retrieved without relearning.

Amnesia is a clinical condition that refers to one kind of memory disorder. It is caused by special conditions such as illness, brain injury or psychological trauma. If the memory loss is for events that occurred prior to a shock, injury or illness, it is called **retrograde amnesia**. If the memory loss is for life events that occurred after the shock or injury, it is called **anterograde amnesia**. Based on whether the amnesias are due to functional or organic disturbances, they are called **psychological amnesia** or **biological amnesia** respectively. The distinction between these two types of amnesia is blurred; there may be psychological factors in biological amnesia and biological impairments in psychological amnesia.

Psychological Amnesia: Psychological amnesia results from major disturbances in the process of encoding, storing, and retrieval of information. There will not be any known biological disturbances such as brain injury or inflammation of organic tissues. One type of functional (psychological) amnesia that all of us encounter is **infantile amnesia** (also called childhood amnesia)—the inability to remember the experiences of the first 3 or 4 years of our life. Why our memory for childhood events is poor? According to Freud, childhood memories involve forbidden, anxiety-producing, sexual and aggressive urges and therefore these are repressed and cannot be retrieved. In recent times, several alternative hypotheses of infantile amnesia are proposed. One view suggests that most of our memory is coded verbally and tied to language; language development and richness of memory go hand in hand; the childhood memories are encoded non-verbally and are in the form of images or feelings; our language-dominated memory organization does not have retrieval cues appropriate to access childhood memories stored in the form of images and feelings. Another view suggests that the child's brain is evolving and still immature to code information in LTM. Still another view proposes that children do not have clear self-concept and hence lack a personal frame of reference around which memories could be organized.

Biological Amnesia: In biological amnesia, there is an organic involvement, especially some disturbance or impairment in the brain. The major causes of biological amnesia are brain diseases or/and use of certain drugs. Among the diseases of the brain that produce memory dysfunctions are strokes, brain tumor, concussion in the brain, disorders of brain metabolism, stoppage of blood supply to the brain, syphilis of the brain, multiple sclerosis, senile dementia, primary degenerative dementia, various conditions caused by drugs and toxic chemicals, and other brain infections. We discuss a few of them here.

Impairment of mental functions such of memory, reasoning, planning, etc. associated with degeneration of the brain is called **dementia**. There are several kinds of dementia. Dementia may occur at any point of time in life, but it is most prevalent among the elderly. Dementia occurring during old age is called **senile dementia**; it is generally caused by lack of sufficient blood supply to the brain due to hardening of blood vessels (cerebral arteriosclerosis). The condition is marked by disorientation and deficits in memory, attention, judgment and abstract thinking.

Alzheimer's disease (**AD**) is a form of primary degenerative dementia and is the most common cause of amnesia among people over the age of 65. It is estimated that 2 to 4 percent of the elderly suffer from this condition. The symptoms of AD include forgetfulness, confusion, faulty judgment, disorganized thinking and disorientation; these symptoms worsen gradually with advancing age. Initially, there is memory loss for recent events, but later spreads to both recent and remote past. The precise cause of AD is not known, but there is some evidence that it is related to deficiency of neurotransmitter acetylcholine in the brain.

Normal aging may also produce some amount of memory loss, but it is not as severe as is in the case of senile dementia. Older people generally suffer memory loss for recent events, but they compensate for the loss by writing down things to be done, engaging in less number of activities, and organizing their lives into routines, thus reducing the burden on their information processing activities.

Drug abuse, especially alcohol abuse, may produce amnesia. Heavy drinking over a period of years may produce some irreversible damage to the brain, which results in a condition called **Korsakoff syndrome**. A prominent symptom of Korsakoff syndrome is the inability to form new associations (anterograde amnesia), but later it spreads to remote items. Drugs such as marijuana also produce some temporary disturbances in encoding, storing and encoding of information, but this condition is not called amnesia.

MEMORY AND BRAIN

A great deal of research, reasoning and speculation has gone on to answer questions such as: Where are the memories stored in the brain and how are memories formed? For example, several years ago, a group of researchers (Babich, Jacobson, Bubash & Jacobson, 1965) conducted a fascinating experiment. Assuming that memory is stored in ribonucleic acid (RNA) in the brain, they trained a group of eight rats to reach the food cup in the Skinner box every time a click was sounded. After the animals learned the response, RNA was extracted from each of their brains. Similarly, RNA was also extracted from nine untrained rats. Eight hours after extraction, the RNA from each of the rats, trained and untrained, was injected into two groups of live untrained rats. Both groups were tested in the Skinner box by presenting the sound of click 25 times and the number of times they approached the food cup was determined. Surprisingly, the experimental group (rats that received RNA from trained group) performed better than the control group (those that received RNA from untrained rats) on the experimental task (approaching food cup in the Skinner box after hearing the sound of click). Some researchers replicated these findings and others could not. Still the results are inconclusive. In spite of dead ends, scientists have thrown some light on the memory processes in the brain. Today, it is suggested that memory involves a number of interacting brain areas.

The following suggestions emerge from contemporary research: sensory memories are processed in the sensory area of the cortex; working memory involves a network of several regions; the frontal lobes play important role in performing the executive functions of working memory; the cerebral cortex and hippocampus are implicated in storing and consolidation of long-term declarative memory; amygdala is believed to process emotional aspects of events, and cerebellum in the procedural memory; damage to thalamus produces amnesia. These observations are tentative and we may have to wait for several years to hear some substantive statements about brain functions in memory.

IMPROVING MEMORY

After having read the chapter, you may be wondering whether the knowledge derived from memory research could be applied to improve your memory. Yes, some of them can be used in your day-to-day activities, especially in school and college (academic) learning. There are no magical or effortless ways of enhancing memory. You may have to work hard and adopt some of these principles. Psychologists suggest the following techniques that you can use to your advantage, especially in academic learning and memorization.

Organize the material: When you organize the information, you are making it meaningful. When you are reading, try to understand the outline of the subject and how the material is logically developed. Try to recognize how the major theme is logically connected to the subordinate items in a hierarchical fashion. Then, you will have multiple retrieval cues, which make recall easy.

Link the new information to what you already know: This is a well-known principle, which states that fitting the unknown with the known facilitates learning and remembering. This way, you are making the material personally relevant and meaningful. Try to concentrate on the illustrations and examples; and see if you have had similar experiences in your life.

Use imagery: Try to have images of the material you are studying. Visual, auditory and other sensory images provide additional cues. Try to use multiple imageries; if one fails others may come to your help as predicted in dual coding theory. When you are reading, try to recall the image of the classroom, the face and the voice of your teacher. When you do so, recalling may become easy.

Avoid interference: When you have to take examination on several papers, set up time schedule for each paper. Do not study for two papers on the same day; this will avoid the occurrence of proactive or retroactive interference. Do not study mathematics and history on the same day one after the other;

one may interfere with the other. You may study history and geography; the similarity of contents allows for transfer. Plan a study schedule and stick to it. During the time set out for study, do not entertain friends or watch TV.

Overlearn the material: This refers to reading of the material even after mastering the same. There is experimental evidence to show that overlearning improves performance on memory tests.

Rehearsal: It refers to going through the material mentally, reviewing silently within you, repeating subjectively, trying to remember the material after reading and correcting the mistakes, if any. This is active, ego-involved learning. Elaborative rehearsal helps you to understand the meaning; it is processing material at a deeper level. Rote learning, i.e. learning by-heart without grasping the meaning of the subject, does not facilitate retention.

Distributed learning: Experiments have shown that **distributed practice** is better than **massed practice**; that is, instead of reading a lesson five times continuously, read it three times with rest pauses between the practice sessions. You may rehearse during the rest passes. A good sleep after studying some information avoids interference and helps consolidation of the material.

Mnemonics: This is a method for remembering discrete concepts, which uses a set of symbols (letter, numbers, words, images, etc.) as substitutes for the materials to be learned. Suppose you want to remember the names of cities such as Tirupati, Agra, Bengaluru, Lucknow and Ellora. You can recall all of them by associating each town with the letters in the word TABLE. The letters are called pegs and the names of the cities are hung on the pegs. Another example is VIBGYOR, in which each letter refers to the colors of the rainbow—violet, indigo, blue, green, yellow, orange and red.

There are several **mnemonic devices** such as the **method of loci**, number and letter peg systems, making a story and chunking. In the method of loci (the word loci means places), you imagine a scene, a building, your house or anything you like. For example, imagine your house; remember the several rooms (hall, bedroom, kitchen and guest room) and the furniture in each room and several other items located at appropriate locations. Rehearse this picture so that it is very well fixed in your memory. Now you try to associate the materials you wish to remember with the rooms and objects therein. For instance, suppose you have to remember a list of vegetables, grocery items, a list of words or anything. Associate each item with a room and with the items there in. For example, you may associate the bedroom with milk, kitchen with a knife, guest room with pillows, so on and forth. In the number and letter peg systems, you establish the items in the list to be remembered either with a letter or a number. Similarly, you may create a story out of the materials to be remembered. In chunking, we may combine several items into chunks. Suppose you want to remember an eight digit phone number such as 35198067; the first six digits can be remembered as a date, 3-5-1980 and 67 as the age of somebody you know.

Whatever the information you want to remember, if you make use of the processes such as planning, rehearsal, organization, feedback and review, the matter will be well fixed in the LTM and it will be easy to retrieve the same.

Chapter Summary

Memory permits us to retain and recall what we have learned through experience. Without memory, experiences would leave no mark on our behavior. Learning is useless when it cannot be used. To be used, the experience (information) must be encoded, stored and remembered. Where and how acquired information is stored and recalled has been the subject matter of this chapter. You have learnt that memory involves three main processes: encoding, storage and retrieval. Encoding is the process of organizing and transforming incoming information, so that it can be stored in memory; storage is the retaining of information in memory; and retrieval is the process of accessing stored information. There are three types of memory stores: sensory memory (momentary storage of sensory information), STM (working memory in which information is held in awareness for up to about 30 seconds) and LTM (permanent storage of information). Some information reaches working memory to be acted upon immediately; some information goes to LTM where it is represented by visual, phonological, semantic or motor codes. Working memory consists of four components:

1. The speech-based phonological loop.
2. The visuospatial sketch pad for holding visual or spatial information.
3. Episodic buffer.
4. The central executive, which coordinates the other subsystems, processes material held in working memory and filters out distracting thoughts.

LTM stores large amounts of information, which may last a lifetime.

Effortful processing involves intentional encoding with conscious attention. Automatic processing occurs without intention and requires minimal effort. Deep processing enhances memory. Elaborative rehearsal provides deeper processing than maintenance rehearsal. Hierarchies, chunking, dual coding that includes visual imagery and other mnemonic devices facilitate deeper encoding. Schemas are mental frameworks that shape how we encode information. According to one view, memory is a representation or reconstruction of past events or experiences and may be distorted under the influence of expectations, emotions and other psychological factors such as schema. Eyewitness testimony in law court may be distorted.

Retrieval cues activate information stored in LTM. Retrieval is easy when there are multiple cues. Encoding specificity principle states that memory is enhanced when cues present during retrieval match cues that were present during encoding. Typically, it is easier to remember a stimulus when we are in the same environment in which it was originally encoded (context-dependent memory) or we have the same internal (psychological) state as when the stimulus was originally encoded. In general, people tend to recall stimuli that are congruent with their current mood.

There are two major types of LTM: declarative and procedural memory. Declarative memories involve factual knowledge and include episodic memories (knowledge of personal experiences) and semantic memories (facts about the world and language). Procedural memory is reflected in skills and actions. Declarative memories are explicit memories in that they involve conscious or intentional retrieval. Procedural memories are implicit memories in that they influence our behavior without conscious awareness. Flashbulb memories are vivid, highly detailed and long-lasting memories of emotionally charged personal or historical events.

Forgetting tends to occur most rapidly soon after initial learning, but the time frame and degree of forgetting can vary widely depending on many factors. Information that was never coded properly cannot be retrieved. Decay theory holds that memory traces in LTM deteriorate with disuse over time. Interference theory holds that forgetting is caused by the material one has learned before or after what one is currently learning. Proactive interference occurs when materials learned in the past impairs recall of newer material. Retroactive interference occurs when newly acquired material impairs the ability to recall information learned at an earlier time. Psychodynamic theory proposes that we forget painful, anxiety-producing material through the unconscious process of repression.

Retrospective memory refers to memory of past events and prospective memory refers to the things to be done in future. Amnesia is partial or total loss of memory. Retrograde amnesia is memory loss for events that occurred before the onset of amnesia. Anterograde amnesia refers to memory loss that occurs after the initial onset of amnesia. Alzheimer's disease produces both types of amnesia and is the leading cause of dementia among the elderly.

The search for the brain areas involved in memory has not yielded conclusive results. It is suggested that numerous interacting brain regions are involved in memorization. Sensory memory depends on input from sense organs and sensory areas of the brain. Working memory involves a network of brain regions. The frontal lobes are involved in performing the executive functions of working memory. Several areas of cerebral cortex are involved in declarative memory and hippocampus helps consolidate declarative memories. Amygdala is implicated in processing emotionally charged memories. Cerebellum helps in procedural memory and damage to thalamus produces severe amnesia. Based on the available evidence, psychologists have proposed several techniques (mnemonic devices) of improving memory.

7 CHAPTER Thinking and Language

PREVIEW

It may look strange why thinking and language are clubbed together in one chapter. The two are intimately related and you will know how, later in the chapter. Thinking, problem solving and acquisition, comprehension and production of language are cognitive processes that are central to the branch of psychology called *cognitive psychology*. Cognition refers to the psychological processes underlying all forms of thinking, perceiving, remembering, planning and problem solving. Cognitive psychology along with diverse fields, such as experimental psychology, psycholinguistics, computer science, mathematics, neuroscience and engineering, constitute an emerging scientific discipline called *cognitive science*. Cognitive psychologists investigate among others, how we think and process information, use language and solve problems. As you can guess, your ability to think, reason and communicate with others is what sets you apart from other living beings. Therefore, it is not surprising that psychologists are deeply engaged in the investigation of these higher mental activities.

Human beings may be smaller and weaker than several other animals. They may not be able to run like a cheetah or fly like a bird. But still they dominate the world because they can think better and communicate more effectively than all other living beings. Humans have the marvelous capacity to create mental representations of the world and manipulate them. Mental representations include images, ideas, concepts and principles. Remember, the entire process of education is all about transferring ideas and skills from one mind to another. In this chapter, you will be introduced to two important themes of cognitive psychology namely, thinking and language. The former half of the chapter deals with the various forms of thinking, the important tools used in thinking and the impediments to correct thinking.

Early psychologists were not enthusiastic about studying thinking. During the first half of the 20th century American psychologists, under the influence of dominant behaviorists like Watson & Skinner, believed that it was a waste of time and energy to study about thinking. Behaviorists discouraged the study of subjective mental phenomenon such as thinking that is not available for direct observation and manipulation. Studying mind was not considered respectable within experimental psychology. Such a line of thinking changed during the 1960s with the emergence of cognitive psychology. Many experimental psychologists, who were engaged in studying animal behavior for understanding human behavior, shifted their interest toward studying higher mental processes among human beings. By 1970, this movement became so widespread that it came to be recognized as 'cognitive revolution'. As you know, scientific psychology started its career in Wundt's laboratory as the study of 'immediate experience' using introspection. Such a psychology was opposed by several psychologists and as a consequence, several schools such as functionalism, behaviorism and Gestalt psychology sprang up. All these were protestations toward Wundt's psychology. But with the rise of cognitive psychology, it appears that psychology has traveled the full circle and came back to the starting point, the study of mental experience.

In the second half of the chapter, we will examine the nature and functions of language. Language and thinking are so intimately related that some people believe that all thinking is determined by language. You will come to know that although language influences the way we think, it does not determine all thinking; thinking is more than language. It is now known that we share certain fundamental cognitive abilities, which remain intact regardless of language particulars or environmental influences. This chapter may appear a bit abstract; but it is essential that you should know what you do when you think and communicate using a language.

Chapter Outline

Most of the time, humans are thinking about something or the other. When we get up in the morning, our day starts with thinking about a hot cup of coffee, a warm bath, a good breakfast, going to school or college, about paying the fees, or preparing for the examination; you may think about your mother's health, father's business, you may even think of your lover; the idea of getting married and there is no end to thinking. Even when you are asleep and dreaming, you are thinking. Dreaming is a form of primitive thinking. In fact, it is difficult not to be thinking. You are always thinking. If thinking is such an all-encompassing or pervasive activity, actually, what is it that you do when you are thinking? The first part of this chapter attempts to apprise you with some elementary ideas about thinking. Loosely, it is said that we are mentally processing or manipulating information when we are engaged in thinking. Some of the information may be coming from the environment through sensory-perceptual processes and some of it may be emerging from within in the form of memories, images and symbols. That is, thinking may involve remembered, absent or imagined objects and events, as well as those currently impinging on the sensory systems. Psychologists consider this process of manipulating symbols as a higher mental activity called *cognition*. Thinking is the major area of interest for cognitive psychologists. Basically, thinking is symbolic; it consists of rearrangement or manipulation of symbols. A symbol represents or stands for some object or event, other than itself. The most often used symbols in thinking are images, words (language) and concepts. Images are mental representations of objects and events. Concepts are mental categories or classes of objects, events, or persons that share some common features. Most of the concepts are language symbols. Almost all words, except those that are proper nouns are concepts. So, we can tentatively define thinking as the process of mentally representing and manipulating information that is in the form of language (words), mental images and concepts. Thinking and language are intimately related because the most often used symbols in thinking are words. Let us briefly try to examine the role of language, images, and concepts, which are the most common tools used in thinking.

TOOLS OF THINKING

Thinking and Language

Many people say they think with words. At the first glance, it seems plausible. Language provides us with thousands of symbols and gives us rules for using them. It is the use of language symbols that has made human thinking so much more sophisticated than the thinking of subhuman beings. For many of us, thinking means use of language symbols (words) grammatically. The words, their meanings and the rules for joining words into phrases and sentences are stored in our semantic memory. When we use language as a tool of thinking, we draw information from this long-term memory store. Watson, the founder of behaviorism, claimed that thinking was subvocal speech; "you are talking to yourself, when you are thinking." But there are certain flaws in this argument. If thoughts were already formed in language, expressing them would be very easy. But you have difficulty in putting some thoughts into words. You must have sometimes said "I don't know how to put it in words." So, all thoughts cannot be translated into words. Secondly, words are often ambiguous, but thoughts are not. For example, when you are thinking about the word "port," you do not wonder whether you are thinking about a "wine" or a "harbor." You are sure about what you are thinking. Thirdly, psychologists have shown that several animals can think and can even solve problems although they do not use a language.

Some theorists have exaggerated the role of language in thinking. An amateur linguist, Benjamin Lee Whorf (1956), asserted that language not only influences but also determines what and how we think, a view that has come to be known as **linguistic relativity hypothesis**. Research has shown that this is an overstatement. For example, the Dani of New Guinea have only two color words in their language, one for bright warm colors, and the other for dark cool colors. Still the Dani could discriminate among and remember a wide range of colors in much the same way as can speakers of the English language, which contains many color names. The truth is that language influences how we think, and how well we think, but it does not entirely shape and determine thought. Thought is more than language.

Thinking and Images

Philosophers like Plato, Aristotle, and later John Locke, described thought as a stream of mental images. A mental image is a representation of a stimulus that originates inside the brain (mind), rather than from external sensory stimulus. Image is a revived percept. The picture of your mother in your mind, when you are looking at her, is a percept. The picture you have of her in your mind in her absence is a mental image. Images arise from information stored in your long-term memory. They are perceptions without sensations. Images may pertain to any of the senses, but visual images are the most predominant. You may form mental images of different objects—faces of known people, the picture of your classroom, the layout of your dining hall, a recently held religious ceremony, a political party meeting, the smell of a favorite dish, the hand shake from a friend or the melodious song you heard in a movie.

People differ with regard to the use of images in their thinking. Some people use images extensively in their thinking. There are some who almost never use images; they think mostly verbally, using words. Usually, images are vague and incomplete. Some people can have vivid images. There are some rare people who can have extremely vivid, lifelike images called eidetic images. Investigators have reported some gender differences in imagery. Women are reported to have more vivid images of past experiences than men. Women can form better still images of objects. That is the reason why husbands ask their wives where they have put the keys or their glasses. Men use images more often in solving problems. The ability to hold and manipulate images help people to perform many cognitive tasks, such as remembering directions to reach a destination in a big city. It is said that Einstein used imagery extensively in developing his theory of relativity. He commented that words did not play any significant role in his creative thought; they came only after he was able to reproduce mental images of the new ideas he had formulated (Nevid, 2007).

Images have some limitations as tools of thought. They cannot represent abstract ideas such as justice or liberty. You may imagine the statue of a blindfolded lady holding a balance, but that is not what you have in mind when you think of justice. Further, not all of us are good in forming images. There are vast individual differences among people in their ability to have images. There can be thought without images. One German student of Wundt, Oswald Kulpe of Würzburg University, became famous for demonstrating *imageless thought*. Therefore, like language, imagery can contribute to our thought processes, but it cannot be the only means by which we think.

Thinking and Concepts

Concepts are the next most important tools in thinking. Concepts are mental categories we use to group objects, events and ideas according to their common features. We use innumerable concepts in thinking and communication. As said earlier, almost all words of a language, except those referring to proper nouns, are concepts. Car, tree, man, woman, boy, girl, beauty, justice, circle, table, snake, so on and so forth, are all concepts. When you use the word 'car,' you are not referring to a particular car. It is a term referring to a group of vehicles with certain common features. Concepts help us to respond quickly to objects and events by reducing the need for new learning each time we come across a familiar object. Having acquired the concept of snake we immediately know how to respond when we encounter one.

Based on how clearly they are defined, concepts are classified as logical concepts and natural concepts. Concepts with clearly defined rules for determining membership are called logical concepts. For example, you do not have difficulty in saying that any three-sided figure is a triangle. It is a clearly defined concept. When you see a three-sided form you decide that it must be a triangle. But many of the concepts we use in our day-to-day life are poorly defined or ambiguous natural concepts, such as furniture, fruit, animal, freedom, justice, respect, sports, work, etc. For example, we do not have a precise idea of what makes an 'animal.' When we come across ambiguous concepts, we usually think in terms of examples called prototypes. A **prototype** is a typical, highly representative example of a concept. We decide which category something belongs to by its resemblance to the prototype. We decide quickly that dove is a typical 'bird' prototype. When I ask you to name a vegetable, if you come up with 'potato,' then, 'potato' is a good prototype of a vegetable. The use of prototype is an elementary method of forming concepts. We note similarity among objects or events and put them together. All flying animals are birds. Thus, we have the concept of bird. This way of forming concepts is arbitrary and sometimes may lead us into difficulty. For example, what you call a 'terrorist' may be for me a 'freedom fighter'.

Psychologists order concepts into categories such as broad, superordinate concepts, middle or basic level concepts and narrow subordinate concepts. For example, 'furniture' is a superordinate concept, 'chair' is basic level concept and 'cane chair' is a subordinate concept. People are more likely to use basic level concepts than superordinate or subordinate concepts when identifying objects. We recognize a chair as a 'chair' more often than as a furniture or cane chair. When you see an apple, you are more likely to say that it is an 'apple' rather than a 'fruit' or 'Simla apple.'

Thinking and Reasoning

Most of our thinking is goal directed. We think in order to solve problems, make decisions and draw conclusions. Logical, intelligent, goal-directed thinking is often called reasoning. Thus, reasoning helps us to acquire knowledge, make sound decisions and solve problems. It saves our time and effort by avoiding haphazard, time-consuming trial and error efforts. We solve problems by developing solutions mentally and then translate them into action. When you want to build a house, first you will develop a mental picture of the finished product to direct your actions. You will prepare a plan; decide how much money you can spend on the project, what materials you need to construct and where will you purchase them. In this type of thinking, you consider what follows from what and decide what to do next. In decision making, we evaluate the possible outcomes and choose one alternative or course of action over others. Two types of reasoning underlie many of our attempts to make decisions and solve problems. These are deductive reasoning and inductive reasoning.

Deductive Reasoning

In **deductive reasoning**, you start with a set of assumptions or general principles and reach a conclusion about a specific case. In logic, this is called *syllogistic reasoning* and logicians use the following well-known example to explain the same:

All men are mortal.
Socrates is a man.
Therefore, Socrates is mortal.

The first statement is called major premise, the second one minor premise, and the third one the conclusion. Because the first two premises are true, logically we come to an accurate conclusion. We can also write the above syllogism as follows:

All A's are B.
C is an A.
Therefore, C is a B.

Sometimes, even when the first two premises are right, we may apply logic incorrectly. Examine the following example:

All A's are B.
C is an A.
Therefore, all A's are C.

Although not immediately apparent, this conclusion is illogical. You can see that when we make the syllogism more concrete:

All men are mortal.
Socrates is a man.
Therefore, all men are Socrates.

Often an individual's beliefs and emotions come in the way of reasoning. Examine the following syllogism:

All things that are smoked are good for one's health.
Cigarettes are smoked.
Therefore, cigarettes are good for one's health.

Will you agree with the conclusion? Probably you do not. But the conclusion is logically correct. Because of the *belief bias*, you do not accept the conclusion. Belief bias is the tendency to reject logically correct conclusion because of your personal beliefs. This is also called retentive bias. Similarly, emotional bias about the concepts used may lead you to reject the conclusion. For example, look at the following syllogism:

Pressure groups are dangerous to democracy.
The opposition party X is a pressure group.
Therefore, the opposition party X is dangerous.

Many people judge this syllogism as false even though it is logically correct. Simply, people do not believe that the opposition party is dangerous. Here their emotional bias distorts their capacity to reason logically. What we are implying here is that man must adapt to reality. If he allows his beliefs, motives and emotions to bias his reasoning, he may be tempted to make wrong conclusions that may lead to undesirable consequences.

In deductive reasoning, the rules of logic are applied to a set of assumptions, stated as premises, to discover what conclusions inevitably follow from those assumptions. The *content*, the actual meaning of the premises, is irrelevant to logic; only the *form*, the sequence of what-implies-what, counts in logic. If you accept the premises, then the rules of the logic dictate that you must accept the conclusion. Deductive reasoning is the basis of formal mathematics and logic. It is said to be the strongest and the most valid form of reasoning. If the premises are true, the conclusion cannot be false. Deductive reasoning involves what researchers call top-down form of reasoning.

Inductive Reasoning

Inductive reasoning is bottom-up form of reasoning. Here, we start with specific facts and based on them we try to derive a general principle. This is the form of reasoning extensively used by scientists. They observe a number of specific instances of a phenomenon and discover general principles or laws. Suppose you observe that several people who smoke develop lung cancer, you come to the conclusion that smoking causes cancer, or at least, smoking is associated with cancer. Inductive reasoning uses individual examples to figure out a rule that governs them.

There is an important difference between deductive and inductive reasoning. You can be sure of the accuracy of deductive conclusions, if the premises are true. You cannot be sure of your conclusion when you follow inductive reasoning. You might have seen several smokers developing cancer. But there may be one who smoked all his life, still did not develop the illness. The possibility of error is always there in inductive conclusions. One new observation may disprove your conclusion. The belief that inductive reasoning works may not be acceptable, but often it works. Much scientific discovery relies on just this kind of reasoning. In reality, much of our reasoning involves a combination of deductive and inductive reasoning. Flawless reasoning is the key factor in drawing conclusions and solving problems. However much we may try, there are certain factors that prevent us from drawing sound conclusions. You will know them a little later in this section.

PROBLEM SOLVING

Life is full of problems; successful living consists of effective problem solving. When you come out of your home to go to work, your vehicle does not start, now, you have a problem. You have gone to a hotel for breakfast, then you realize that you have forgotten your purse; here also you have a problem. These are simple problems. But problems may be more complex, severe and serious. Whatever the problem, fortunately, human beings are endowed with capacity to solve problems. Problem solving is a cognitive activity in which you employ mental strategies to find out an answer to the problem. In solving problems, people generally go through four steps: Understanding or framing the problem is the first step, second is generating the possible or potential solutions; third is testing the solutions and finally, evaluating the results.

Our initial understanding of a problem is a key step toward a successful solution. When a problem is poorly framed, we will enter into a maze of blind alleys and be confused about the solutions. Optimal framing can generate effective solutions. A knack in framing problems in effective ways is a prized skill in many academic and work settings. A clearly stated problem helps you to formulate potential solutions. Then you test the solutions in the light of the data and finally evaluate them to determine the best one among them.

Problem-solving Schemas

A **schema** is a mental framework, an organized pattern of thinking or organized knowledge structure that guides our interpretation of the world. While solving problems, people learn to use certain shortcut strategies called *problem-solving schemas*. These are a set of rules found to be useful in solving problems. The two strategies often used in problem solving are **algorithms** and **heuristics**. Algorithms are formulas that automatically generate correct solutions. They are step-by-step set of rules for solving problems. Most of mathematical formulas are algorithms. For example, there are sets of rules for carrying out addition, subtraction and multiplication. There are formulas for finding out area of a triangle, circle, and rectangle. If you apply them correctly, you will always get right answers. Heuristics are general problem-solving strategies that are applied to certain classes of situations. Heuristic is a rule of thumb that does not guarantee a solution, but may help in arriving at one. One heuristic is **means ends analysis**, in which we determine the difference between the present situation and the desired situation and then try to make changes to reduce the difference. Another is **subgoal analysis**, which involves breaking down the problem into smaller, more manageable parts.

Although heuristics help in problem solving and in decision making, they sometimes steer us toward wrong decisions. Take for example, the **representativeness heuristic**. The representativeness heuristic assumes that the more similar something is to a prototype stored in memory, the more likely it is that the thing belongs to the category of the prototype. That is, often we assume that a given sample is representative of a larger population and make a wrong judgment. We overhear someone saying that, some brand of TV is good and we purchase it. This way we might end up having a bad set. Another source of error is the **availability heuristic**, which is the tendency to base decisions on information that readily comes to mind (Kahneman and Tversky, 1973). We tend to remember events that are important or glaring. We judge that more people die because of airplane accidents than automobile accidents although the deaths due to the latter are several times more than the former. It is because we remember air accidents easily than the road accidents. Daniel Kahneman and Amos Tversky performed groundbreaking studies of such errors and received a Nobel Prize for their contribution in 2002 (only Kahneman received the prize; Tversky did not live to see his work honored).

Another impediment to right thinking is **confirmation bias**, which refers to a tendency to look for evidence that confirms our current opinion or belief. The best thing we can do to test our belief is to search for evidence that will disconfirm it. But that is not easy, because we are unwilling to challenge our cherished beliefs. When we have a strong belief, we select and expose to such information that confirms our belief. We mix with like-minded people; we read newspapers and watch TV channels that support our line of thinking. We tend to avoid and forget evidence that is not in line with our cherished ideas. The fact that we find it difficult, and even upsetting, to challenge our beliefs will be a major obstacle in getting the evidence needed to take the correct decision. Sometimes, confirmation bias gives rise to a distorted sense of overconfidence in which we feel we are generally infallible and capable of taking correct decisions almost always. Overconfidence and confirmation bias are formidable adversaries in our accurate decision making, we will be blind toward truth because of them.

Habit and Mental Set in Problem Solving

Practice in solving problems in specific ways creates **mental set** in us. When we followed a procedure and solved a problem, next time we face a similar problem, we tend to follow the same procedure. It is natural and quite useful. But sometimes mental sets hinder problem solving and often we may fall into a trap. Suppose we are shown the following words: MacDonald, MacIntosh, MacAndrew, MacHinery; how will you pronounce the last word? Will you really pronounce it as *machinery*?

Abraham Luchins conducted a series of interesting experiments to demonstrate the operation of mental sets in problem solving. One of the problems Luchins used is given in Table 7.1. The problem is to use the jars in each row to measure out the required amount of water. Try it yourself before reading further to realize the power of mental set in problem solving.

If you have tried to solve the problem, you realize that the first five problems are all solved the same way. Fill B; take out using A once from B; and finally take out from B using C twice. You are left with required amount of water in B. Simply apply the formula B – A – 2C. But when you come to problem 6, you fall into a trap. Watch carefully, the sixth problem (6th test) can be solved directly by subtracting C from A once (A – C). If you were given the sixth problem first, you would have solved it without any difficulty. Because you solved the first five problems using a particular procedure, you have developed a mental set and you apply the same formula here also, which is not necessary. The mental set hinders your problem-solving ability. In Luchins' study, nearly 75 percent of a group of college students were blinded by the mental set at the level of the sixth problem. They were blind to the easy method after having practiced the long method for five trials.

The hindering effect can be reduced by:

1. Warning the subject, "do not be blind now," or "Look sharp, now," before the sixth problem.
2. Reducing the number of practice trials.
3. Separating practice and test trials by days or weeks.

There is another kind of mental set called functional fixedness, which can create difficulties in solving problems. We shall examine it now.

Functional fixedness is a mental set to use objects in the same way we are accustomed to use them, even if a different use might solve a problem. The phenomenon was demonstrated by Adamson (1952) in one of his famous experiments. The problem was to mount a candle on a vertical screen. All of the subjects were given candles, cardboard boxes, tacks (small broad-headed nails) and matches (Fig. 7.1).

Adamson used two groups: an experimental group and a control group. The participants of the experimental group were provided with the material as shown in the first figure at left. The control group participants were given the

Table 7.1: Luchins Jar Problem

Problem number	Given the following empty jars			Obtain the required amount of water
	A	B	C	
1 Practice	21	127	3	100
2 Practice	14	163	25	99
3 Practice	18	43	10	5
4 Practice	9	42	6	21
5 Practice	20	59	4	31
6 Test	23	49	3	20

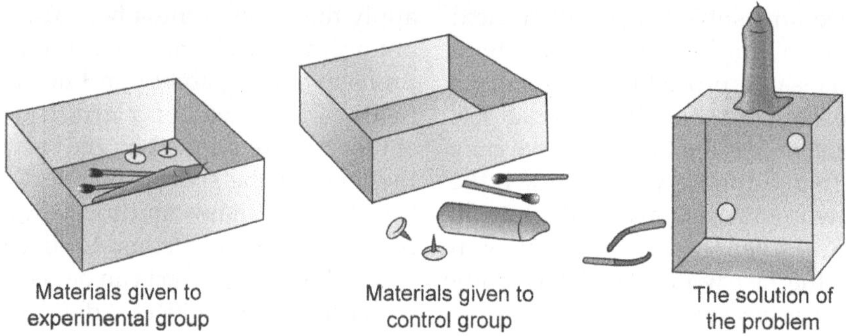

FIGURE 7.1: Functional fixedness (the arrangement of materials as provided to the two groups and the solution to the problem)

materials as shown in the middle figure. The solution to the problem is shown in the last Figure at the right. The problem was simple; it consisted of sticking the candle on the box with melted wax and then attaching the box to the screen using the tacks. Experimental subjects found it difficult to solve the problem. They thought of the box only as a container for the materials, it never occurred to them that it could be *used* as a platform to mount the candle and be fixed on the screen. Such a fixation on the *function* of the box was created in their minds by placing the materials (candle, tacks and matches) as shown in the left figure. No attempt was made to establish such functional fixedness in the subjects of the control group; the empty box, together with other materials was simply placed on the table, as shown in the middle figure. The results provided strong evidence for the operation of functional fixedness as a set that hinders problem solving; only 12 of the 29 (41%) subjects of the experimental group solved the problem within the allotted time (20 minutes). On the other hand, 24 out of 28 (86%) members of the control group solved the problem.

Several researchers obtained similar results with other problems providing strong evidence that functional fixedness operates as a kind of set hindering problem solving. In some studies, the participants were asked to stop trying to solve the problem temporarily and were asked to solve the problem after some rest. Surprisingly, for several of them the functional fixedness had disappeared and they were able to solve the problem with a fresh approach. So, when you are stuck up with a problem, it is better to take some time off and come back to solve the problem; you may get the solution.

CREATIVE THINKING

Creative thinking is a special type of thinking, which involves the combining of ideas or responses in novel ways. A creative thinker creates something original, new and useful. He may be an artist, a poet or a scientist. Creative thinkers think in unusual ways, produce objects that are unique, come out with solutions that others have not thought of before. The emphasis of creative thinking is on novelty. It is believed that creative thinking involves considerable amount of unconscious rearrangement of symbols. Creative thinkers struggle in the beginning, but then after some time, a new idea or a solution appears suddenly like a bolt from the blue. The sudden appearance of the idea, as you know, is called **insight**. The following famous story attributed to Archimedes, illustrates the role of insight in creative thinking.

Hiero, king of Syracuse got a gold crown made to be presented to a temple. The weight of the crown was equal to the weight of the gold the king had given to the goldsmith. But the king doubted that the goldsmith had cheated him by removing some gold and replacing it with an equal amount of silver in making the crown. Archimedes was asked to find out whether the crown was made of only gold or some silver was mixed in it. While he was struggling to solve the problem, one day Archimedes happened to get into his bath and noticed that when he got into the bathtub, exactly the same amount of water flowed over the side, as the volume of his body that was under water. Realizing that he got the solution, he ran home naked shouting "Eureka", "Eureka" ... (I have found it, I have found it). Archimedes established that the goldsmith had indeed cheated the king. The silver in the crown, having a larger volume than an equal weight of gold, made the crown displace more water than it would have, had it been made of gold alone.

Archimedes could not solve the problem until an environmental circumstance triggered his creative solution. A number of creative people have reported that after conscious thought has failed them, insight suddenly appears when they are doing something completely unrelated to the problem. Remember the story of Newton getting the idea of gravity, when he watched an apple falling to the ground. Similarly, Valmiki got the idea of an appropriate rhyme to use in writing The Ramayana, when he watched one of the two mating birds being killed by a hunter. However, insights do not really spring from nowhere; they emerge in prepared minds that have studied the problem from various angles.

Graham Wallas, after studying some outstanding creative thinkers, proposed that such thinking occurs according to a recurring pattern in five stages: *preparation, incubation, illumination, evaluation*, and *revision*. In the first stage (preparation), the thinker formulates the problem and collects the necessary information to solve the problem. Often, he finds that the problem cannot be solved. Having failed, he turns away from the problem. Thus, the thinker enters into the second stage (incubation), in which he is probably working at the subconscious level. If he is lucky, the third stage (illumination) occurs; the solution suddenly dawns in his conscious mind. He has insightful experience of "aha". In the fourth stage, the solution is evaluated to see whether it is satisfactory. In the last stage, if the solution is not a good fit, necessary modification is made.

This is a general picture of creative thinking; there may be individual differences in reaching the solutions.

Guilford (1967) made an elaborate study of creative thinking using a battery of carefully constructed tests. He proposed two varieties of thinking: convergent and divergent. **Convergent thinking** is concerned with the search for a specific solution. An individual collects required information and goes step by step following the problem-solving procedure to reach the right answer. He reaches an answer that has been established by others. This is not the type of thinking engaged by creative thinkers. Creativity involves **divergent thinking**; it is a type of thinking in which novel ideas, which are unusual, are generated. Creative people are intellectual rebels. They are not bound by traditional constraints and they do not follow the off-beaten path.

Convergent and divergent thinking can be illustrated with an example. Suppose you asked a question: "What do you do with a newspaper? If you say "I read it," it is convergent thinking. On the other hand, if you say that it can be used as a 'dustbin,' it is divergent answer. In one study, a

10-year-old boy gave the following answer to the question: "How many uses can you think of for a newspaper?"

> *You can read it, write on it, lay it down and paint a picture on it. You could put it in your door for decoration, put it in the garbage can, and put it on a chair if the chair is messy. If you have a puppy, you put newspaper in its box or put it in your backyard for the dog to play with. When you build something and you do not want anyone to see it, put newspaper around it. Put newspaper on the floor if you have no mattress, use it to pick up something hot, use it to stop bleeding, or to catch the drips from drying clothes. You can use a newspaper for curtains, put it in your shoe to cover what is hurting your foot, make a kite out of it and shade a light that is too bright. You can wrap fish in it, wipe windows, or wrap money in it. You put washed shoes in newspaper, wipe eyeglasses with it, put it under a dripping sink, put a plant on it, make a paper bowl out of it, use it for a hat if it is raining, tie it on your feet for slippers. You can put it on the sand if you had no towel, use it for bases in baseball, make paper airplanes with it, use it as dustpan when you sweep, ball it up for the cat to play with, wrap your hands in it if it is cold (Ward, Kogan and Pankove, 1972).*

The boy must have been extraordinarily creative. An important aspect of creativity is cognitive complexity—the preference for elaborate, intricate, and complex stimuli and thinking styles. Surprisingly, one factor that is not related to creativity is intelligence. Most of the traditional tests of intelligence rely on convergent thinking. They require you to give one correct answer. Researches have consistently shown that creativity is only slightly related to school marks and intelligence as measured by contemporary intelligence tests. In fact, some of the creative thinkers may fail in these tests.

Creative thinkers appear to share certain personality characteristics. They prefer complexity; they are more independent in their judgment; they are more self-assertive and dominant, also they are slightly low in impulse control. A researcher in the field of creativity, psychologist Welsh (1975), has identified a personality dimension called *origence* that is related to creativity. According to him a person high on this dimension resists conventional approaches that are used by others. He/She would rather do his (or her) own thing, even if it is unpopular or seems to be a bit rebellious or non-conforming. Such a person is more interested in artistic, literary and aesthetic activities that do not have a correct answer agreed upon by consensus and that allow a more individualized interpretation and expression.

Improving Creative Thinking

Contemporary cognitive psychologists are of the view that most of us have the potential to be creative; of course, some of us are more creative and some less. They believe that abstract rules of logic and reasoning can be taught, and such training can improve our reasoning about the underlying causes of everyday events in our lives. They assert that critical and creative thinkers are made, not born. They suggest the following hints to improve our critical and creative thinking.

Redefine the problem: Rephrase the problem, modify the assumptions; when you state your problem clearly, it is half solved. Many of us cannot solve the problem because we do not know what the problem is.

Use fractionation: Break the problem into parts and examine each part for new possibilities. Remember what we said under subgoal analysis. Solving a subgoal may become a step toward the ultimate solution.

Adopt a critical perspective: Do not accept the assumptions or arguments passively, critically evaluate the material, consider its implications and think about the possible exceptions and contradictions.

Consider the opposite: It is possible that you understand the issue better when you think of its opposite. For example, you will appreciate mental health better when you think about mental illness.

Use metaphors and analogies: Often, use of metaphors and analogies lead us to creative solutions. A metaphor is a figure of speech for likening one object or concept to another. You may liken love to honey or moonlight. Analogy is comparison between two things based on their similar features. Bell developed telephone using the analogy of ear. Radar was designed after studying the bat.

Engage in divergent thinking: Think of the multiple uses of a common object. For example, think of the multiple uses of a pencil or a brick.

Take the perspective of another person: Look at the problem from another person's point of view. You may gain fresh insights.

Use heuristics: We have seen how cognitive shortcuts can be used in solving problems, especially, when there is a single solution to the problem.

Experiment with various solutions: Take different routes to find solutions, think of different solutions and evaluate them. You may stumble upon an original idea.

Conceptual expansion: Adapt the available material for new use. Expand the concepts into new ones. Remember how humans have created the images of gods after their own form, by increasing the number of hands or heads.

Conceptual combinations: You may combine two are more concepts into one concept resulting in the creation of a new idea or application. Examples are cell-phone, home-page and facebook.

Concluding Words about Thinking

The status of theory and research in thinking is difficult to evaluate, especially, after the emergence of cognitive psychology. An American cognitive psychologist (G Oden) has summarized the position of thinking in contemporary psychology succinctly in one sentence: "Thinking, broadly defined, is nearly all of psychology, and when narrowly defined, it seems to be none of it." The term thinking generally denotes any covert, cognitive or mental manipulation of ideas, images, symbols, words, propositions, memories, concepts, percepts, beliefs or intentions. In short, it encompasses all of the psychological processes associated with concept formation, problem solving, intellectual functioning, creativity, complex learning, memory, symbolic processing and imagery, among others. No other word in psychology casts such a broad net and few encompass such a rich array of connotations. However, all are agreed on three points:

1. Thinking is a symbolic process; it does not refer to observable behavioral activities that can be explained otherwise.
2. Thinking is a covert, implicit process that cannot be directly observed; it has to be inferred either from the reports of one who is thinking or by observing certain behavioral activities that suggest thinking is taking place (such as producing a solution to a problem).
3. Thinking is generally assumed to involve the manipulation of certain theoretically proposed elements. But there is no agreement on the nature and number of these elements. Different theorists have proposed dissimilar elements, such as muscular movements (Watson), words or language (Whorf), ideas (Locke), images (Titchener), propositions (Anderson), operations and concepts (Piaget), scripts

(linguist Schank) and so on and so forth. Interestingly, all these elements have at least some evidence to support their involvement in thinking. Because of the breadth of the concept, often qualifying terms are used to distinguish various forms of thinking, such as convergent thinking, divergent thinking, logical thinking, critical thinking, creative thinking and autistic thinking.

LANGUAGE

An important cognitive activity that has put humans at the pinnacle of evolution is their capacity to think and communicate with others using language. Noam Chomsky (1972) called language the *human essence.* Others have referred to it as *the jewel in the crown of cognition*. A good deal of human thinking, reasoning and problem solving involves the use of language. Our knowledge, wisdom and expertise are all stored in the long-term memory in the form of language. Our history, culture and civilization have been transferred from generation to generation through the use of language. What are we without a language? Language underlies so much of what we do, that it is impossible to imagine life without it. If you find two or more people together anywhere on earth, the chances are they are talking to each other. When there is no one to talk, you may talk to yourself, to a pet or even to a plant. Not only is language the central tool for communication, it is also said to be a major determinant of our thinking. Therefore, it is not surprising that psychologists have devoted considerable amount of time and energy to study the topic of language. They have studied the structure and functions of language and its adaptive value. They have shed light on the neuropsychological mechanisms involved in the acquisition, understanding and production of language. The area of psychology that is concerned with the study of language has come to be known as '**psycholinguistics**'.

During the course of evolution, people realized that, it is advantageous to live in groups; a socially oriented lifestyle helped them to survive and reproduce. But living in groups created new demands such as cooperative living, division of labor, development of social customs, passing on of knowledge and wisdom to the next generation and communication of thoughts. Development of language thus became adaptive necessity and people developed some 5,000 to 6,000 languages around the world. Humans gradually evolved into highly social creatures for whom the need to communicate with one another became essential; for this purpose, they had to develop physical structures that allow them to communicate in the most flexible way; the result is the evolution of language.

Properties of Language

People speak different languages. The interesting characteristic of languages is not their differences, but the underlying features they have in common. Language is generally defined as system of symbols that can generate an infinite number of messages and meanings. This definition encompasses four properties of language: *symbols, structure, meaning* and *generativity*; some will also include a fifth property: *displacement*. All languages use sounds, written characteristics or some other symbols (hand signs) to represent objects, events, ideas, feelings, and actions. The symbols used in any given language are arbitrary. For example, examine the words used to represent the animal 'dog' in different languages. It is called 'dog' in English, 'chien' in French, 'hund' in German, 'cane' in Italian, 'perro' in Spanish, 'kutha' in Hindi, 'naayi' in Kannada and Tamil, 'kukka' in Telugu, so on and so forth. None of these words or the sounds we use to refer to them has anything to do with the animal 'dog.' In fact, we could have used any other word to refer to the animal; but we do not. The word "dog" has an agreed upon meaning to people who speak English.

Language has a structure governed by a set of rules. The set of rules that dictate, how symbols can be combined to create meaningful units of communication is called *grammar*. A portion of grammar, known as *syntax*, dictates the rules for ordering words in a sentence. The grammars of all languages have rules for changing present tense into past tense, declarative statement into interrogative statement, active voice to passive voice and so on. In English, an adjective is placed before the noun (*big* river). In French, it is placed after the noun (*Rio Grande*). Language conveys meaning, an aspect determined by semantics. The meaning may be denotative or connotative. Denotative meaning denotes an object. For example, the word 'table' denotes an identifiable object; it is the accepted meaning of an object. Connotative meaning refers to the emotional and evaluative meaning of words. For example, words such as justice, beauty or conservative connote something. Psychologist Osgood and his associates have developed a technique called *semantic differential* to measure the connotative meanings of words in the English language.

Language is generative and permits displacement. Generativity means that the symbols of language can be combined to generate an infinite number of messages that have novel meaning. For example, the 26 letters in English can be combined into over half a million words. The words can be combined into an infinite number of sentences. Displacement refers to the fact that language allows us to communicate about events and objects that are not physically present. We can discuss the past and the future, as well as people, objects, and events that ordinarily exist or are taking place elsewhere. We can even discuss completely imaginary situations. We shall examine some of these properties in some detail.

Structure of Language

So far, we have learnt that language is a system of communication composed of symbols (mainly words) arranged according to a set of rules (grammar) that govern the proper use of words, phrases and sentences to express meaning. Psycholinguists study language under four heads: phonology, syntax, semantics and pragmatics.

Phonology is the scientific study of the organization of the speech sounds. The sounds of any language are built up from sets of **phonemes**. A phoneme is the smallest unit of sound that is recognized as separate. The word 'players' has three phonemes: 'pley,' 'ər,' and 'z'. Humans can produce about 100 phonemes, but no single language uses all 100. Some languages use as few as 15 phonemes and others more than 80. English has about 40 to 45 phonemes to sound out about 500,000 words found in a standard dictionary. Phonemes have no inherent meaning, but they change meaning when combine, with other elements. Changing one phoneme in a word can change the meaning of the word. When you change the 'r' sound in 'reach' to a 't' sound, it becomes 'teach.' The same letter can make different sounds in different words. The 'o' in 'two' is a different phoneme from the one in the word 'one.' Similarly, the words 'boy' and 'toy' differ in one phoneme. The ability to produce phonemes depends on your having heard others say them. Different languages have different phonemes.

Phonemes are combined into **morphemes**, which are the smallest units of meaning in a language. Simple words like *boy*, *girl*, *tree*, *time* are morphemes. But there are other units of language, such as un-, sub-, -ed and -ing, which also convey meaning. These suffixes and prefixes that convey meaning are also morphemes. The prefix 'un-' conveys the meaning 'not.' The suffix '–ing' conveys continuing action; '-ed' implies that the act occurred in the past. A word like 'pretested' has three morphemes—'pre,' 'test,' and 'ed.' Morphemes are not always syllables. For example, the letter 's' in English is not a syllable. But when it is added to noun, the noun becomes plural. Thus, the word 'fans' has one syllable, but two morphemes. The word "players" has two syllables, but three morphemes. In every language, there are rules that determine how phonemes can be combined into morphemes. There are specific rules that dictate the use of morphemes. For example, we cannot add *-'ing'* at the front of a word or *'mis'* (another morpheme) at the end. The 40 phonemes in English can be combined into more than 100,000 morphemes.

Language is a system of symbols. It has a structure. Morphemes are the stuff with which words are made. Words are combined into phrases and phrases into sentences. **Grammar** and **syntax** dictate how words and phrases are combined to create meaningful sentences. Grammar tells us how symbols are combined to create meaningful units for communication and syntax tells the rules that govern the order of words in phrases and sentences. The sentence "drink water I" sounds odd because it violates the basic rule of English syntax—the subject 'I' must precede the verb 'drink'. People follow rules of syntax even if they are not aware of them or cannot verbalize them. An analysis of the syntactic structure of a sentence (Cultured people speak good language) is shown in the Figure 7.2.

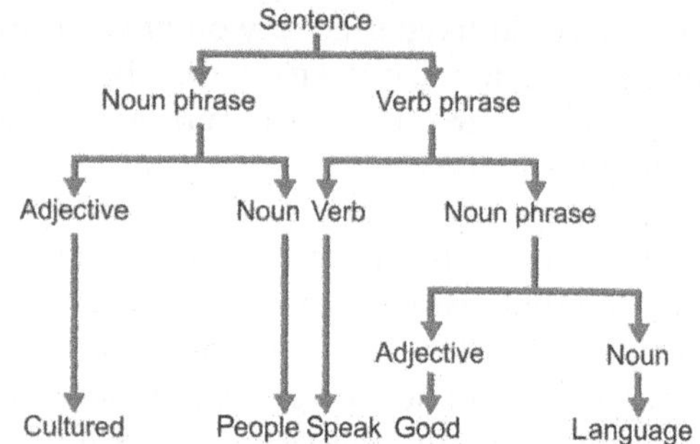

FIGURE 7.2: Syntactic structure

Language is more than a matter of sound and structure. We have said earlier that it must convey meaning. **Semantics** is the third component of language that is concerned with the rules that govern the meaning of words and sentences. Semantics is a tricky affair. The meaning of a sentence (semantics) and its syntax are to a large extent distinct. A syntactically correct sentence need not be meaningful. Chomsky pointed out that the sentence "Colorless green ideas sleep furiously" has an acceptable syntax, but it is meaningless. The same word may convey very different meanings depending on the context. The word *park* means differently in the following sentences: "*Park* the car." "We shall go to the *park* tomorrow." The same set of words can express different propositions depending on how they are organized. Look at the following illustration: An English teacher wrote a sentence on the blackboard and asked his students (men and women) to punctuate it. See how it was punctuated by boys and girls:

> The sentence given as: *Woman without her man is a brute.*
>
> As punctuated by men: *Woman, without her man, is a brute.*
>
> As punctuated by women: *Woman, without her, man is a brute.*

The fourth component of language is **pragmatics**. Speaking in such a way as to have an impact on others is pragmatics. Language researchers use the word pragmatics to refer to the practical knowledge used to understand the intentions of the speaker and to provide an effective answer. Suppose someone makes an indirect request such as: "Could you close the door?" If you process the information literally, you might say: "Yes, I have enough energy to go to the door and close it." Here, you are violating the pragmatic rule. In fact, the other person may think that you are making a sarcastic statement. Suppose a stranger asks you: "Where will this road go?" Your literal answer should be "It will not go anywhere; it only stays where it is." Again you are violating the pragmatic rule.

Pragmatic rules dictate how you speak depending on whom you are speaking to and his/her social status and the social context in which you are speaking. If your father happens to be the teacher in your class, you do not address him as 'father' there. You simply address him as 'Sir' only. You may use some slang words when you are with your friends, but you do not utter them in your home. Psycholinguists have identified social rules that guide communication between people. Depending on whether you are speaking to an adult, a child or a foreigner, you adjust your rate of speech, choice of words, and the complexity of your sentences. Speech is social and interpersonal. We speak to communicate information to another person, to influence the behavior of another or to obtain a favor. In all these, we make use of pragmatic rules.

Surface Structure and Deep Structure

Psycholinguists think of language as having a surface structure and a deep structure. According to Chomsky (1957), the **surface structure** refers to the symbols (words) used and the order in which they are used (the expressed sentence). Syntax provides the rules for proper ordering of words. In contrast, the **deep structure** refers to the underlying meaning of the combined words (the mental representation of what a person intends to say). This is the semantic aspect of the language. Sentences may have different surface structures, but the same deep structure. Examine the following examples:

1. Rama ate the apple.
2. The apple was eaten by Rama.
3. Eaten by Rama the apple was.

Each sentence conveys the underlying meaning that the apple ended up in Rama's stomach. The syntax in the third sentence is incorrect; still its meaning is clear enough.

Sometimes, a single surface structure can give rise to two deep structures. It happens, when we speak in ambiguous sentences. Examine the following sentences:

1. The police must stop drinking after midnight.
2. Visiting relatives can be a nuisance.

The first sentence may mean either: "The police must prevent people from drinking alcohol after midnight," or "The police people must not drink after midnight." Similarly, the second sentence may mean either: "Relatives visiting you may be a nuisance," or "Your visiting the relatives may be a nuisance."

Generally, we move from the surface structure to deep structure. We infer the meaning based on the way the sentence is spoken or written. Even when all the words are not used (as in telegraphic language), we understand the meaning. But when we express our thoughts to others, we transform the deep structure into a surface structure that others can understand. According to Chomsky, language production requires the transformation of deep structure into an acceptable surface structure using *transformation rules*; to explain how it is done, he has proposed the theory of **transformational grammar**. The rules can also be used to change the surface structure into deep structure.

Language Development

Children all over the world acquire language basically in the same way, more or less according to a time table. Until about 6 months of age infants communicate through non-language symbols such as crying and cooing (these sounds are known as *prelinguistic speech*). Around the same time they start babbling—speech-like, but meaningless sounds. By the time children are approximately 1-year-old, they produce short words that start with consonants such as b, d, m, p or t. They may produce words such as *papa*, *mama* or *dada*. Later, they produce two word combinations. By the age of 2 years, the average child may have a vocabulary of about 50 words. At about the same age, children use telegraphic speech, where unimportant words are left out as is done in sending a telegram. By age 3, children learn to make plurals by adding 's' to nouns, and to form past tense by adding 'ed.' In doing so, they make errors such as 'mouses' instead of 'mice', 'runned' instead of 'ran,' 'eated' instead of 'ate.' This phenomenon is called overgeneralization. Children apply the rules rigidly, not knowing that some rules have exceptions. Most children acquire the basic rules of language by about 5 years. However, the subtle rules of grammar are not attained until later. Table 7.2 shows major milestones in language development during the first 3 years (there will be individual differences).

Table 7.2: Major Milestones in Language Development (During the First 3 Years)

Age in months	Development
Birth	Can cry, make some response to sound; can perceive speech
1–3	Coos and laughs
3	Plays with speech sounds
5–6	Makes consonant sounds
6–10	Babbles
9	Uses gestures to communicate
9–10	Begins to understand words, usually own name and words like "no"
10–12	Uses social gestures; does not discriminate words not in own language
10–14	Utters first word, usually a label for something
10–18	Says single words
13	Understands symbolic function of naming; uses elaborate gestures
14	Uses symbolic gesturing
16–24	Learns new words; increase in vocabulary, uses verbs, adjectives
18–24	Says first sentence; two-word sentences
20	Names things
20–22	Spurt in comprehension
24	Uses many two-word sentences; wants to talk; no more babbling
30	Learns new words almost every day, speaks in three-word sentences; understands very well; still makes grammatical mistakes
36	May say up to 1,000 words, 80% intelligible; makes some mistakes

Theories of Language Development

How do children learn the secrets of verbal communication? Is linguistic ability learned or inborn? No simple and straightforward answer can be given to the question. There has long been a debate about how language is acquired. At least three camps are actively discussing this issue.

Behaviorist Theories

According to behaviorists, especially Skinner, language is entirely a product of learning. Why do people of China speak Chinese, people of France speak French and those born in Japan speak Japanese? The answer is simple. They have learnt their languages from their parents, teachers and friends. We teach our children language, they learn it. Children acquire words and sentences by watching and imitating others. When a child utters the word 'mama', he/she is hugged and praised by the mother; when the child says 'dog' at the sight of a pup, his/her father smiles and says 'good.' This way the child is reinforced to utter the word 'mama' at the sight of the mother and 'dog' the next time he/she sees a canine. So, the behaviorists assert that language is learned according to the same principles of learning that apply to all other forms of learning. This line of thinking is rooted in a philosophical theory called '**empiricism**' according to which all our knowledge, including language, comes to us through experience (learning), especially sensory experience. The theory, although partially true, does not explain all aspects of language learning. For one thing, parents praise their children even when they speak ungrammatically, but the children learn to speak grammatically. When a child says "I have two foots", generally we do not correct them; we are not worried about the syntax. But ultimately children learn to speak correctly and grammatically. Adults do not teach grammatical rules to children or even systematically correct grammatical errors, but even 4-year-old children acquire rules of grammar. One researcher showed that most children at the 4th year generalize grammatical rules. This is true even when sentences contain nonsense words. For example, a child is given the following problem:

There is a kud. Now there is another one. Now there are two _______.

When asked for the missing word, most 4-year-olds have no trouble saying *kuds*. How does this occur? Further, children produce novel words, phrases and sentences, which you have never taught them. Cognitive psychologist GA Miller (1965) points out that there are 10^{20} possible 20-word sentences in the English language and it would take one thousand times the estimated age of the Earth just to listen to them all, let alone teaching or learning them. American psychologist Steven Pinker estimates that we would need at least 100 trillion years to memorize all the sentences any one of us can possibly produce. Obviously, Skinner's operant conditioning cannot explain the complexity of our language capabilities. Therefore, many psychologists have come out with alternatives to behaviorist theory of language learning.

Nativist Theories

The nativists firmly hold that the crucial aspects of language acquisition are innate (inborn), not learned. This theory is rooted in the philosophical viewpoint called '**nativism**', which asserts that people are born with some knowledge, including the capacity to learn language. The similar course of language development across various cultures and the ease with which children naturally acquire language suggest that language depends on an innate mechanism that might be built into the brain. American linguist Chomsky has championed the nativist approach to language acquisition. He is the most severe critic of Skinner's theory of verbal behavior, which states that language is acquired according to the principles of operant learning principles. According to Chomsky, humans are born linguists; people inherit a biological readiness to recognize and eventually produce the sounds and structure of whatever language they are exposed to. According to him our brain is simply structured to generate language. The underlying grammatical structure of all human languages reflects an underlying brain structure. People are 'wired' to produce grammatical utterances just as a computer can be wired to produce moves in a chess game. Chomsky says that all the world's languages share a similar underlying structure called *universal grammar*; we are all born with an internal **language acquisition device (LAD)**, which both permits understanding the structure of language and provides strategies and techniques for learning the unique characteristics of a given native language. That is, the LAD contains a set of grammatical rules common to all languages; we do not actually *learn* the grammar of language, rather, we *discover* which particular language is being spoken around us and our LAD 'tunes' in our built-in set of rules, so that we can speak that language. Chomsky argues that language is uniquely a human phenomenon made possible by the presence of the LAD. This theory allows us to understand how children acquire language even when the input stimuli are not sufficient to specify all the rules. We acquire the ability to speak, much as we do the ability to walk and jump, because we have an inborn propensity to develop it. We do not teach our children to sit, stand, and walk; they do it anyway. Children learn to use the rules of grammar without any formal instruction. Children in English-speaking societies begin to place subject before the verb even before they know what the terms *subject* and *verb* mean. Children are able to learn grammatical structures as rapidly and easily as they do because the human brain contains the basic blueprint or neural circuitry for using grammar.

Chomsky's theory is not without critics. The critics of this theory assert that LAD is not an actual physical structure in the brain; it is only a hypothesis, an abstract concept of how language centers in the brain work. It does not explain the mechanisms by which language is produced.

Regardless of the exact mechanisms involved in language production, there is little doubt that both *nature* and *nurture* are necessary for the language to develop. Chomsky & Skinner seem to be continuing the age-old nature-nurture controversy launched by Plato & Aristotle. Chomsky's deep-brain structures theory of language acquisition represents the nature or Platonic side & Skinner's view that verbal behavior is shaped by the environment represents the nurture or Aristotelian side.

Interactionist Theories

Interactionist theories draw materials from both behaviorist and nativist theories to explain language acquisition; and in addition they add the social factor. They hold that language acquisition depends partly on social environment and partly on our genetic heritage. Social learning is a crucial contributor to language acquisition and the interplay between biological and environmental is a basic postulate for most modern theorists. American psychologist Jerome Bruner proposed the term **language acquisition support system (LASS)** to represent factors in the social environment that facilitate learning of a language. One could say that when LAD and LASS interact in a mutually supportive fashion, normal language development occurs. There are many interactionist theories, which vary in the relative emphasis placed on general language-specific innate abilities. An important feature of these theories is that they have formulated testable propositions, which in turn have brought to light several diverse facts about language acquisition. However, no general consensus on a final form of such a theory has yet emerged.

Biological Bases of Language

Studies of people suffering from aphasia have revealed some of the brain mechanisms underlying speech comprehension and speech production. **Aphasia** is a general term referring to any of a variety of language impairments caused by brain damage. Aphasia may be partial or complete; there are literally dozens of varieties of aphasia. The discovery of neurological basis for aphasia has an interesting history. In 1861, a French neuroanatomist Paul Broca described how damage to the left frontal lobe disrupts speech production. This is a significant discovery in the history of neurophysiology. It happened as follows: In 1831, a patient was admitted at the Bicêtre hospital for insane. His sole defect was that he could not talk; otherwise he was normal. He was capable of communicating intelligently by signs. He remained in the Bicêtre hospital for 30 years. On April 12, 1861, he was put under the care of Broca, the surgeon, because of a gangrenous infection. Broca examined the patient thoroughly for 5 days and found that everything was normal. On April 17, unfortunately (or fortunately for science) the patient died. Within a day, Broca performed an autopsy, and discovered a lesion in the third frontal convolution of the left cerebral hemisphere. Broca concluded that this area is responsible for speech production. Since then, the area has come to be known as **Broca's area** and the speech disorder caused by damage to this area is called **Broca's aphasia**. This kind of aphasia disrupts production of speech much more than comprehension. Today, a patient is diagnosed as suffering from Broca's aphasia if he/she produces little speech, the production tends to be slow and very poorly articulated and speech is generated with considerable effort. The condition is often called *motor aphasia* and *expressive aphasia*. Interestingly, these patients can comprehend spoken and written language fairly well.

About a decade after Broca's discovery, a German neurologist Carl Wernicke reported that damage to the posterior part of the left temporal lobe disrupts language comprehension. This area was later named **Wernicke area** and the speech disorder caused by damage to this area is called *Wernicke aphasia*. The patient with this type of aphasia articulates normally, even fluently, but the speech tends to be empty without coherency. Comprehension of both written and spoken language is impaired. The condition is also known as *receptive aphasia* and *sensory aphasia*. Traditionally, Broca's area has been identified with speech production and Wernicke's area with speech comprehension, but now it is known that Broca's area is involved in the use of syntax in both production and comprehension. The Broca's & Wernicke's areas are shown in the Figure 7.3.

There are other forms of aphasia. An aphasia presumed to be due to lesions of *angular gyrus* is known as *anomic aphasia*. The dominant symptom here is severe loss of the ability to name objects. *Conduction aphasia* is believed to be caused by lesions in the *arcuate fasciculus*, which connects Broca's area with Wernicke's area. Patients suffering from this form of aphasia find it difficult to repeat a sentence just heard. When there are lesions in both Broca's & Wernicke's area, the condition is called *global aphasia* in which language is impaired on a global scale. Aphasia caused by a lesion that is outside of Broca's & Wernicke's area is called *transcortical aphasia*.

Although it is now known that production and comprehension of language are complex phenomena that rely on different mechanisms, the effects of brain damage demonstrate that both these functions rely on at least some of the same processes. Damage to Broca's area and related brain areas can produce difficulties

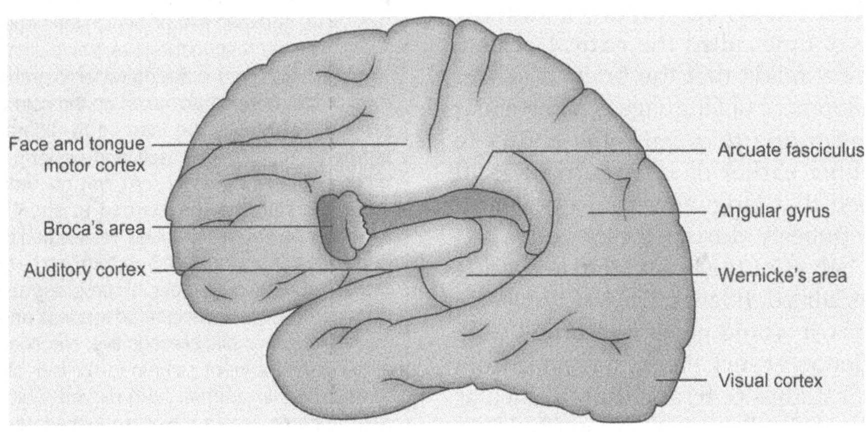

FIGURE 7.3: Language areas

not only in forming sentences with correct syntax, but also in understanding syntactic relations. Thus, the Broca's area is involved in the use of syntax in both production and comprehension. Comprehension however, being more completely tied to the meanings of words, may be less disrupted than production when the interpretation of syntax is impaired. For all that, we know there may be several other areas in the brain that are involved in language production and comprehension. For example, scientists have reported that men who suffered a left hemisphere stroke are more likely than women to show severe aphasic symptoms. In females, who suffered from left hemisphere damage, the language functions are more likely to be spared, suggesting that more of their language function is shared with the right hemisphere. It is reported that when males process phonemes, the left cerebral hemisphere is primarily activated, but when females process, both hemispheres are strongly activated. May be this is one reason why females tend to be better with language than males. Neural systems involved in several aspects of language may be organized differently in women than in men.

Critical Period Theory

There is a theory suggesting that language can only be learned during a narrow window of time called the **critical period.** This theory holds that the brain is set for the development of language at a particular point and trying to acquire the ability to speak either earlier or later is fruitless. It is claimed that language has to be learnt prior to puberty during the period when the two halves of the brain were becoming fully specialized. If language was not learnt before this, it would never be learned well. The evidence for such theory has come from anecdotal studies of **feral children**, such as Victor, the Wild Boy of Aveyron (Box 7.1). Victor was found naked and filthy in the woods near Paris, in 1799. He was behaving like a wild animal. A physician named Itard tried to educate him, but without much success. It was very difficult to teach Victor the language skills. Some people thought that Victor was probably a mentally retarded child; that may be the reason why he was abandoned by his parents and that is why he could not learn a language.

Recently, another case has been reported that throws light on language learning. A girl named Genie, the daughter of deranged parents, was locked up in a back room from the age of 20 months until she was 13-year-old. Genie was intelligent and had no difficulty to talk as toddler. Only later she was isolated from human company and was punished when she attempted to make any sound, and nobody was allowed to talk

Box 7.1: Wild Boy of Aveyron

In 1799, three hunters found a child living in the forests of Aveyron, France. Probably abandoned by parents at an early age, the child grew up without human contact in the wild forest and lived like animal. Aged 12 when found, he climbed trees, ate nuts and roots, bit people who interfered with him and made few sounds. He walked on all fours, although he could stand upright. People regarded him as half human, half beast and they called him Wild Boy of Aveyron. The boy was later placed under the care of a physician, Jean Marc Gaspard Itard, who named him Victor and tried to train him. In the beginning, Victor was not responsive to aversive stimuli; he would put his hand to boiling water to grab some food or roll around half naked on the cold winter ground. Eventually, he learned to differentiate temperature, dress himself and perform some other self-care behaviors. At first his emotions were flat, but later he learned to show some affection toward his caregiver. He learned to read and write some words and perform some simple tasks. But as he grew older, his progress declined considerably. He never learned to speak and after 5 years of education, his cognitive, emotional and social development remained limited. Unable to improve him further, Itard moved Victor to a nearby home where a woman looked after him for the rest of his life.

to her. After she was discovered, the girl was given intensive training in language with mixed success. She was able to learn many words; she had reasonably good language comprehension. Therefore, no evidence was found to support the critical period hypothesis. But Genie was never able to grasp the rules of grammar fully, and thus there does seem to be a critical period for acquiring grammar. The existence of a critical period for grammar explains why brain damage has much greater long-term effects on language when it occurs in adults than in children.

Research has shown that if parts of the brain that are assumed to be devoted to language functions are damaged in young children, other parts can take over these functions. In fact, even when the entire left half of a young child's cortex, including the areas normally used in language, has to be removed because of injury or disease, the child will nevertheless learn the language. On the other hand, it is very difficult for an adult to recover language abilities following brain damage that produces of aphasia.

Genetic Basis of Language

Some researchers have claimed that human beings have special genes for language. The evidence for such a view has come from the studies of a speech disorder called *specific language impairment*. People suffering from this disorder have trouble understanding grammar and complex words made up of many morphemes, such as *predisposing*. These people belong to certain families and the disorder is not caused by cognitive difficulties or lack of intelligence. The disorder is more likely to occur in both twins in identical sets than in both twins of fraternal sets. So, it is argued that there is a genetic basis for language. In fact, some researchers have identified a gene that is associated with specific language impairment. These claims have yet to be confirmed. It is also reported that the communication disorders run in families and are about 80 percent heritable. Stuttering in part is genetic. These observations cannot be accepted as final. Language is a highly complex phenomenon and it is unlikely that it is controlled by one gene. It involves many factors, any of which may be affected by a different gene or a set of genes.

SOME SPECIAL ISSUES

Apart from what we discussed here, psychologists are interested in certain special issues relating to language, such as bilingualism, non-language communication among humans and animals. They have tried to teach a language to certain higher mammals. These issues are briefly mentioned below.

Bilingualism

All people learn a language (mother tongue) and most of the people in the world learn a second language at some point in life. It has become a necessity in several countries. The use of two languages (**bilingualism**) in daily life is common throughout the world. Many Europeans speak two or more languages. Canada officially is a bilingual country. People there speak both English and French. English is the official language in the United States, but some 50 million people who speak their mother tongue at home also speak English fluently. In India, which is a multilingual country, a person must know at least three languages. Therefore learning a second language is a necessity for most people today and psychologists are interested in the issues associated with the learning of more than one language. Specifically, psychologists are interested in three issues:

1. What are the problems associated with learning of a second or a third language, and is learning a second language the same as learning a first one?

2. Does bilingualism affect other cognitive abilities?
3. Are the neural processes involved in learning a second language the same as in learning a native language (or different)?

These are important issues and have been fairly well studied by psychologists. Without going through the voluminous literature in the area, let us examine the major conclusions arrived from the researches:

1. Children can learn languages better during early years. It appears therefore that a second language would be learned best and spoken most fluently when acquired early in life.
2. Some linguists believe that there is a critical period for learning a second language that ends in childhood or possibly in the early teens. However, the critical period hypothesis is not fully supported.
3. The data suggests that there may be a *sensitive period* (rather than a critical period) for learning a second language that extends through mid-adolescence. Sensitive period is a window of time when learning a language is the easiest, but is not the only time when learning can occur.
4. Studies suggest that bilingualism is at least correlated with greater thinking flexibility and higher performance on non-verbal intelligence. Bilingual children also perform better than monolingual children on certain perceptual tasks in which selective attention is crucial. Learning a second language helps children to perceive the unique grammatical features of their mother tongue.
5. In general, it appears that when people acquire a second language early in life or learn it to a high degree of proficiency later in life, both languages use a common neural network. Yet, some brain regions become more active when fluent bilinguals use the language to which they have been less extensively exposed. This suggests that they are exerting more conscious effort to process the less dominant (second) language.

People vary widely in their ability to learn and communicate a second language. It is reported that Albert Einstein was so poor in language skills that his parents were worried that he might be mentally retarded. He could not speak fluently and grammatically, English and French both of which he learned later in life. But he spoke both of them with a native German accent. There have been several polyglots. MD Berlitz, who invented a system for teaching foreign languages, spoke 58 of them. Sir John Bowring, a former British Governor of Hong Kong, could speak 100 languages and read 100 more. The Jesuit missionary Benjamin Schulze (1699–1760) is reported to have recited the Lord's Prayer in 215 languages (Passer & Smith, 2007).

Non-verbal Communication

Although language is the best and the most powerful medium of communication, it is not the only medium used by humans and non-human beings. People are remarkably proficient in using non-verbal communications such as gestures, postures, and other forms of body language to convey their thoughts to others. Social psychologists have shown how body language helps us in understanding (social perception) the current moods of people with whom we are interacting (See Chapter 13 for more of this). It is found that women generally are better than men in decoding non-verbal communication. But men can decipher unspoken signs of anger better than women. Men and women are found to differ in their non-verbal behavior. Studies of non-verbal behavior have shown that men are generally more restless and more expansive than women, but women are more expressive than men in front of emotional events. However efficient these expressions are, they do not qualify to be called language. Non-verbal communications do not have units like phonemes, which can be combined to form new units. There is no syntax. The physical signs and gestures cannot be combined to form new meaningful expressions. Still, these rudimentary forms of communication are used by some non-human species.

Communication Among Animals

Chimpanzees grunt, bark, scream and make gestures to communicate with other chimps. Dolphins make clicking sounds and high-pitched vocalizations. Many animals use special calls to warn about impending dangers from approaching predators and to attract mates. Insects demonstrate highly specialized forms of communication. Honey bees use a special form of body movements (waggle dance) to indicate the availability of nectar and its location. Communication patterns among certain bird species show interesting parallels to human language. It is reported that each songbird species has its own songs just as humans have different languages. Some songbirds have even local dialects. Bird watchers can recognize from their songs the area from which they have come. Some experts say that certain species of animals have critical periods for acquisition of songs. Although animals use diverse forms of communication, the capacity to use a language is beyond their reach. Several attempts have been made to teach human language to chimps but with little success.

Can Animals Learn Human Language?

In terms of Darwinism, chimpanzees are our nearest ancestors. It is estimated that, we share with them about 99 percent of our genes. Therefore, several researchers have made heroic attempts to teach human language to chimps. Several years ago, two researchers (Kellogg and Kellogg, 1933) raised a chimp named Gua along with their son, Donald. Gua & Donald were exposed to the same experiences and careful attention was paid to rewarding the appropriate vocalizations. But in the end, the Kelloggs had merely produced a fine speaking son and an effectively mute chimp. Later efforts to teach chimps to speak yielded the same discouraging results. Since chimps lack the vocal system that is necessary to produce human-like speech, the researchers failed in their attempts. It is something like a bird trying to teach a boy to fly by raising him in a nest. Without wings how can the boy learn to fly?

Taking advantage of chimps' hand and finger dexterity, some investigators tried to teach these animals sign languages (Box 7.2). Allen Gardner & Beatrice Gardner tried to teach American Sign Language to a 10-month-old female chimpanzee named Washoe. The researchers raised Washoe at home and treated her like a human child. By the age 5, Washoe had learned 160 signs. The striking thing was that Washoe could combine signs (e.g. 'more fruit') in novel ways. Another researcher trained a gorilla named Koko to use 600 signs.

In California, psychologist David Premack taught a chimp named Sarah to manipulate plastic shapes that symbolized words (for example, a plastic triangle stood for the word *banana*). Sarah was able to respond to simple symbol-based sentences (such as insert banana into pail). In Georgia State University, one researcher worked with a special species of chimpanzees. One chimp named Kanzi, at the age of one and half years, learned to use plastic geometric symbols that were associated with words. By the age of 4, with only informal training during social interactions, Kanzi has learned more than 80 symbols and produced a number of two- and three-word communications. Kanzi learned to respond to English commands. It is reported that Kanzi correctly responded to 74 percent of the novel requests compared with the researcher's daughter who complied with

Box 7.2: Sign Language

It is a language based on gestural communication. The term refers to the rich elaborate grammatical manual system used by deaf children and adults. Deaf children, raised by speaking parents who do not use signs to communicate, will spontaneously invent their own sign languages. Sign languages are not like the movements one might make when playing charades. Here the gestures refer to the manual equivalents of phonemes, small units that are combined to make appropriate perceptual signals. Symbols for individual words are combined according to syntactic, semantic, and pragmatic rules. Just as there are different spoken languages, there are different sign languages. American Sign Language (ASL) is different from British Sign Language (BSL). One who understands ASL cannot understand BSL. The two are simply two different languages.

Sign language is a true language. Brain damage disrupts it in ways that parallel the impairments of spoken language. Brain damage in the same area results in similar defects in normal people (who can speak) as well as deaf people (who use sign language). For example, damage to Broca's area can cause in both the groups trouble in using grammar and producing and comprehending sentences. In addition, just as in the case of spoken language there is a critical period for acquiring a sign language. In fact, the right cerebral hemisphere only is activated when one uses ASL before puberty; in some who learned ASL after puberty, the right hemisphere is not activated when signing is used.

The gestures made by normal people while talking are not sign language. But they do enhance communication, partly because they lighten the cognitive load on the speaker. Such gesturing is learned. Even people who are born blind make gestures as they talk and these are similar to gestures made by people who can see. The blind people make gesture even when they know they are talking to another blind person. Gestures can supplement information conveyed in speech, but they are not in themselves a distinct language.

65 percent when both of them were between the ages of two and two and a half. It can be seen that Kanzi comprehended human speech at the level of a human toddler.

These are very impressive demonstrations and are quite convincing when you see them in a circus or a movie. But have chimps like Kanzi really acquired a language? Some psychologists assert that the chimps' behaviors simply reflect reinforced learning rather than true language ability. Remember that human language is symbolic, structured, generative, conveys meaning and permits displacement. The extent to which these properties of language are found in apes' communication remains controversial.

Chapter Summary

Thinking and other higher mental processes were not favorite subjects of study within psychology until 1960. With the advent of cognitive psychology, things changed. Contemporary psychologists are starting to look into the minds of people to see what they are doing while thinking, solving problems and communicating with others. Psychologists define thinking as the process of mentally representing and manipulating information. When people think, they represent information in their minds in the form of words, images and concepts. Sometimes, thinking can occur without these elements, but most of human thinking involves words, concepts and images. Images are mental pictures or representations of objects or events. Concepts are mental categories for classifying objects, events and ideas on the basis of their common features or properties. Prototypes are representative examples of concepts. Almost all noun words (except proper nouns) in any language are crystallized concepts. Therefore, one has to concede that language plays an important role in thinking. Watson thought thinking is subvocal speech; that is, when we think, we are talking to ourselves. Whorf asserted that language completely determines our thinking. Now we know that language influences the way we think, but does not determine thought completely. People can think without language and without images (imageless thought). Thought is more than language and imaging.

When we are engaged in decision making, we employ one of the two types of reasoning: deductive or inductive reasoning. In deductive reasoning, we reason from general principles to a conclusion about a specific case. Inductive reasoning involves reasoning from a set of specific facts or observations to a general principle. Deduction is the most valid form of reasoning

Contd...

Contd...

because the conclusion cannot be false if the premises are true. Inductive reasoning cannot yield certainty. Still that is the type of thinking employed in science.

Problem solving proceeds through several steps: understanding the nature of the problem; formulating an initial hypothesis; testing the solutions in the light of the existing evidence and evaluating the results of these tests. People use several schemas when solving problems. Algorithms are formulas that guarantee correct solutions. Heuristics are general strategies that may or may not provide correct solutions. Means-end analysis is a common heuristic. The representativeness heuristic is the tendency to judge evidence according to whether it is consistent with an existing schema. The availability heuristic is the tendency to base conclusions and probability judgments on what is readily available in memory. People exhibit confirmation bias, a tendency to look for facts that support hypothesis rather than those that disprove it. They also suffer from overconfidence, a tendency to overestimate their knowledge, beliefs and capacity to make accurate decisions. Functional fixedness is a mental block that can blind us to new ways of using an object or procedure thereby interfering with problem solving.

In creative thinking, something new is sought. Some novel ideas seem to come suddenly after little progress has been made over a long period of time; this sudden appearance of new ideas is called insight. Creative thinking is said to proceed in five stages: preparation, incubation, illumination, evaluation and revision. Divergent thinking is conducive to creativity. Creative people seem to have some personality feature in common; they are believed to possess a personality trait called origence.

The use of language as a tool of thought and a medium of communication distinguishes humans from all other living beings. Thousands of languages spoken all over the globe share some common features. Language is symbolic and structured, conveys meaning, is generative and permits displacement. Comprehension and production of language relies on certain aspects such as phonology, syntax, semantics and pragmatics.

Language elements are hierarchically arranged: from phonemes to morphemes to words, phrases and sentences. The surface structure of a language refers to how symbols are combined; the deep structure refers to the underlying meaning of the symbols. The set of rules used for changing the deep structure into surface structure and vice versa are dictated by transformation rules. Chomsky has offered a theory of transformational grammar.

Language is acquired gradually by children without explicit instruction. In infancy, babies emit all the phonemes that exist in all the languages of the world. At about 6 months of age, babbling sounds narrow down to include only the sounds specific to their native language. By age 4 to 5, most children develop mastery over the basic grammatical rules for combining words into meaningful sentences. There is probably a critical period for learning grammar. Language development also depends on exposure to the speech of others. Thus, both nature and nurture are necessary for the development of language.

Three groups of theories have been proposed to explain language development. According to behaviorist theories, language is learned like learning of all other things. Nativistic theories hold that language development depends heavily on innate mechanisms. Interactionist theories explain acquisition of language in terms innate mechanisms blossoming in a social environment. Language acquisition and production are controlled by specific brain centers. Broca's area in the left frontal lobe is believed to control primarily (not exclusively) language production and Wernicke's area primarily (not exclusively) language comprehension. With minor modifications these assumptions are found valid. Some researchers have gone so far as to invoke the presence of a specific gene that controls language, but the evidence is not sufficient to accept such a view. Researchers have proposed a critical period for proper development of language, especially for understanding grammatical rules.

The pros and cons of bilingualism and difficulties involved in learning a second language, other than the native tongue, are examined by scientists. It appears that a second language is most easily mastered and spoken well if it is learned during a sensitive period that ranges from early childhood possibly through mid-adolescence. Bilingual children are found to perform better than monolingual children on some of the cognitive functions. In general, it appears that when people acquire a second language early in life or learn it to a high degree of proficiency later in life, both the mother tongue and the second language share a common neural network.

Although language is the major tool of communication, other non-verbal means of conveying information are extensively used by both humans and animals. Gestures, postures, facial expressions and movement of hands add to the effectiveness of communication through language. Several species of animals such as birds and bees have specialized systems of non-verbal communication. The songs of birds and the dance of bees communicate specific messages to other members of their species. Several psychologists and other researchers have made heroic attempts to teach chimpanzees human language, but with little success. Apes are not equipped with the necessary anatomical structures to produce language sounds. As an alternative, researchers have tried, with some success, to teach a sign language to apes. Several apes were found to understand what has been said to them and respond back successfully using sign language. Although they do not understand key aspects of language, some apes have exhibited remarkable abilities to form novel utterances, which reveal the use of rudiments of grammar.

8 CHAPTER Intelligence

PREVIEW

You are familiar with the word intelligence; you may even be quite sure what the word means. But you will be surprised to learn that psychologists are not agreed upon what actually intelligence is. The word *intelligence* is used in several contexts to mean several things. We say one is an intelligent student, another is an intelligent driver, a third is an intelligent cook and fourth is an intelligent businessman and so on and so forth; the list will be endless. Is the ability behind each of the above activities the same? Difficult to answer! Then, what is intelligence? If there is something called intelligence, can we measure it? Intelligence testing is big business today; there are hundreds of tests that are supposed to measure intelligence. To what extent can we trust the intelligence tests that are designed to measure it? Is intelligence inherited or is it acquired? Were you born intelligent or became intelligent? Why and how do people differ with regard to their level of intelligence? Can intelligence of an individual be boosted? As a consumer of psychology, you need answers to these questions. Finally, is it necessary for you to be highly intelligent to succeed in life? Many extremely intelligent people were failures in life. The power of a car is separate from the way the car is driven! This chapter tries to discuss with you several issues pertaining to the concept of intelligence. An attempt is made to answer some of the questions raised above. These may not be satisfactory answers; they are only sincere attempts to answer. There are no final answers to any question anywhere in science; so it is with psychology.

Intelligence is a complex phenomenon. It encompasses most of the psychological activities we discussed in the earlier chapters. It underlies accurate perception, effective learning, memorization and problem solving. See the contradiction: You cannot perceive, learn, memorize and solve problem if you are not intelligent. At the same time, perception, learning, memory and thinking constitute what we call intelligence. Which of the following assumption is true: You learn well because you are intelligent or you are intelligent because you learn well? It is difficult to say which is the cause and which the effect. Examine a definition of intelligence, which accommodates most of the contemporary viewpoints: *Intelligence is the ability to acquire knowledge, to think effectively and deal adaptively with the environment.* Can you say which is the cause and which the effect? That is the reason why intelligence is considered the most controversial concept in psychology. Parents, educators, policy makers and psychologists are struggling to understand the exact meaning of intelligence.

We may bring in some clarity to the idea of intelligence by adopting the following line of thinking: We know that people differ in their capacity to learn, remember, think and act. We assume that there is something that makes them differ in doing these things. Shall we say that it is this "something" which makes people differ is intelligence? If our assumption is correct, should we not measure that something called intelligence so that we can predict people's success or failure in real life. This assumption has made intelligence testing a huge enterprise all over the world. Generally, when psychologists talk about intelligence, they are normally referring to the differences people show in their ability to perform tasks. People clearly differ in ability and the measurement of this difference is used to infer the capacity called intelligence. Think about it, if everyone in your class gets the same grade, the term intelligence would lose its meaning. Just because they get different grades, we assume they differ in their intelligence. Psychologists who study intelligence attempt to measure the differences among people and then determine how and why those differences occur. One of the important goals of such venture is to use individual differences to predict things like success in school or performance in an occupation. In this chapter, you will learn about the different attempts psychologists have made to understand, explain and measure intelligence.

Chapter Outline

INTRODUCTION

Intelligence is a word most of you are familiar with. You must have used the word often with reference to people in utterances such as "She is very intelligent," or "He is not intelligent". What exactly do you mean when you use the word intelligence? You may find it difficult to say precisely what you mean, but do not feel bad about it. You are not the only person in that group. Not many people know the exact meaning of the word intelligence, including experts. Long ago in the 1950s, when in an introductory course in psychology, one might have read a sentence which appeared somewhat as follows: "*Teachers try to cultivate intelligence, psychologists try to measure intelligence and several others talk about intelligence, but none of them know precisely what intelligence is.*" The position remains very much the same even today. However, intelligence is a focal construct for psychologists who are interested in understanding how people adapt their behavior to the changing environment in which they live and work. Intelligence is also the key concept in explaining how people differ from one another in the way in which they learn about and understand the world around them. It is composed of almost all other psychological processes that we discussed in earlier chapters, such as sensation, perception, learning, thinking, reasoning and problem solving among other cognitive activities. In this chapter, we discuss the nature of intelligence, determiners of intelligence and the difficulties involved in defining and measuring intelligence. We ponder over the different conceptions of intelligence developed by psychologists and their attempts to develop standardized tests as means of measuring intelligence.

WHAT EXACTLY IS INTELLIGENCE?

Intelligence is not a concrete material substance that can be observed, studied and measured objectively; it is a concept. Like many other important human characteristics such as attitude, interest, aptitude, motivation and personality studied by psychologists, intelligence has to be inferred from certain behavioral manifestations. As a consequence, there is considerable amount of disagreement among psychologists with regard to the definitions offered to intelligence. But what most of them mean when they refer to intelligence is pretty close to the standard dictionary meaning. One of the Oxford dictionaries defines intelligence as "the ability to gain and apply knowledge and skills." Accordingly, a student who performs well in school or college is intelligent; a merchant who sells his goods well and earns more money is intelligent; so is a tribal person who can hunt better than others. Thus, intelligence is the mental ability to learn complex skills and use them effectively; it is the ability to profit from experience and adapt to the environment; also the ability to think, reason, and solve problems. In fact, all tests of intelligence rely on the assumption that intelligent people can acquire knowledge, think and reason effectively, solve problems and deal adaptively with the environment. Psychologists and educators first tried to measure intelligence and then started thinking about the nature of intelligence. Therefore, it would be necessary to learn about the early attempts to measure intelligence and how scientists have gone about theorizing about it.

HISTORY OF INTELLIGENCE TESTING

Historically, it was a British gentleman-scientist Sir Francis Galton (a cousin of Charles Darwin), who initiated the study and measurement of mental skills. Galton (Fig. 8.1) was influenced by Darwin's theory of evolution and believed that eminent people inherited certain psychophysical constitutions that made them more fit to think and act effectively than their less successful counterparts. He started an anthropometric laboratory in 1884 to measure several bodily characteristics such as the keenness of sight, hearing and touch, speed of respiration, reaction time, muscular strength, height, weight and related characteristics, which he believed constituted the building blocks of an important human trait, called intelligence.

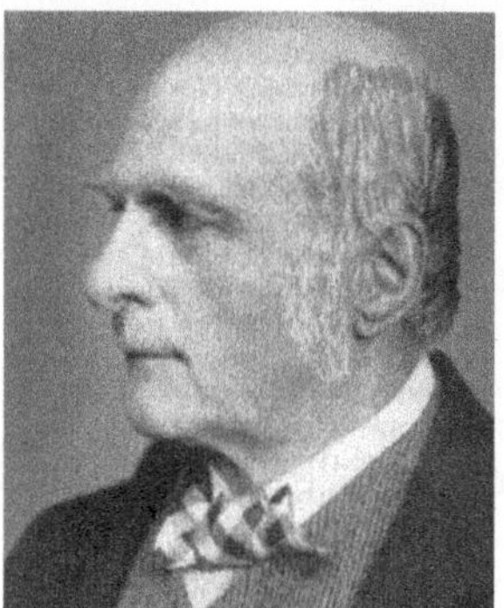

FIGURE 8.1: Francis Galton

This belief of Galton might have partly grown out of his observation of mentally retarded people, who exhibited poor sensory discrimination and inability to perceive pain. He reasoned that these disabilities hamper people's ability to profit from experience (intelligence). Thus, he came to the conclusion that sensory and physiological measures might yield a means of measuring intelligence. Unfortunately, later researches demonstrated that Galton was wrong; scores on sensory and motor tests did not correlate well with teachers' ratings of intelligence, with students' scholastic achievement or even with one another. Naturally Galton's tests were not good measures of intelligence.

The second initiative to study and measure intelligence came from the well-known French psychologist Alfred Binet (Fig. 8.2). In 1904, French Ministry of Public Education asked Binet and his colleague Theodore Simon to develop a test to identify children who did not profit from formal education and needed some sort of special instruction. The tool the two pioneers developed, the *Binet-Simon Scale of Intelligence* (1905), became the forerunner of all modern intelligence tests. The test was revised in 1908 and again in 1911.

In developing this test, Binet asked experienced teachers what sort of skills children should have at each age for successful learning. Thus, he developed

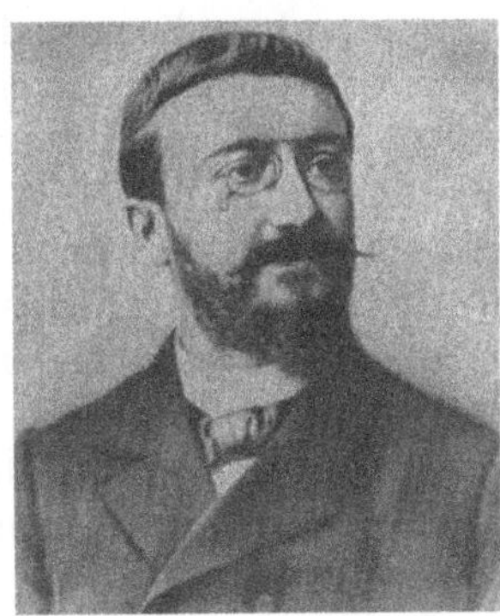

FIGURE 8.2: Alfred Binet

test items suitable for ages 3, 4, 5 and so on. Using these items, he could determine whether a 5-year-old child was as good as a standard group of 5-year-olds; if it was so, Binet concluded that the child had normal intelligence, and developed a score to indicate the level of intelligence, which came to be known as **mental age (MA)**. That is, if a 5-year-old (**chronological age** or **CA**) child could answer all questions meant for the average 5-year-old, his mental age is 5; if he could solve the problems meant for 10-year-olds, his MA is 10. The French school system thought that a 10-year-old (chronological age) with an MA of 6 or less could not profit from normal instruction.

Binet's views of intelligence are noteworthy. He believed that intelligence was not a single ability, but composed of several abilities. He did not accept the view that intelligence was inherited, but thought that heredity may set an upper limit on intellectual potential. He asserted that almost everyone functions below their potential and everyone could improve a great deal intellectually if properly stimulated. He also believed that some kind of mental orthopedics (exercises that would improve a child's will, attention and discipline) could prepare disadvantaged children for school and help them to learn how to learn. It is unfortunate that Binet died young, at the age of 54, when he was at the height of his career.

A few years later, the German psychologist William Stern introduced a concept that is now well-known as the **IQ** or **intelligence quotient**. Stern defined IQ as the ratio of mental age to chronological age multiplied by 100; that is

$$IQ = \frac{MA}{CA} \times 100$$

Here MA divided by CA and multiplied by 100. Thus, a child whose CA is 5 and MA is also 5 has an IQ of 100.

$$\left(\frac{5}{5} \times 100\right)$$

If MA is 10 and CA is 5, the IQ will be 200.

$$\left(\frac{10}{5} \times 100\right)$$

Nowadays, psychologists do not use the concept of MA or IQ in intelligence testing. The concepts of MA and IQ worked well with children, but not with adults. For example, if a 25-year-old performed at the level of a 75-year-old, he would be taken as having an IQ of 300! Because of these difficulties, today intelligence tests provide an IQ score that is not a quotient at all. Instead a **deviation IQ** score is calculated. The deviation IQ is a type of *standard score* (an IQ expressed in standard deviation units). For this purpose, the average test score for a specific age group is determined and this average score is assigned an IQ of 100. Then, using a statistical technique that calculates the differences (deviations) between each score and the average, IQ scores are assigned.

In later years, Binet's test was revised by several people in other parts of the world to suit their own local conditions. One of the most well-known of these revisions, undertaken by Lewis Terman of Stanford University in the United States, is known as the *Stanford-Binet*. Terman and Merrill (1972) have made the test a household name in the

Americas. The test, now in its fourth edition, is called Stanford-Binet IV (Thorndike et al, 1986), and consists of a series of items that vary in nature according to the age of the person being tested (refer Table 8.1 for sample items of Stanford-Binet III revision).

The intelligence tests that are most popularly used in the United States today were devised by David Wechsler (1975). There are three forms of Wechsler test, one for adults, one for children and the third one for preschool children. The adult's version called *Wechsler Adult Intelligence Scale (WAIS)* appeared in 1939 and its third revision (WAIS III) is currently in use (refer Table 8.2 for some sample items). The children's version called *Wechsler Intelligence Scale for Children (WISC)* was published in 1955 and it is in its fourth edition (WISC IV). The third test called the *Wechsler Preschool and Primary Scale of intelligence (WPPSI)* was put out in 1967.

The Stanford-Binet and Wechsler tests are individual tests; they can be administered to one person at a time and it is difficult and time consuming to administer and score them on a large scale basis. Therefore, a number of group tests have been developed. During World War I, a verbally oriented group test called the *Army Alpha* was developed to screen large numbers of US Army recruits for intellectual fitness. In order to test people who could not read and write, a non-verbal tool-consisting of mazes, picture-completion problems and symbol substitution problems called the *Army Beta* was developed. During Second World War, the *Army General Classification Test* was developed. Later, new group tests such as *Lorge-Thorndike Intelligence Test, Otis-Lennon School Ability Test* and several other tests were developed to be used in schools. These are paper-pencil tests in which subjects read the questions and write down their answers. The main advantage of group tests is that they can be administered to large groups of people and can be scored quickly. However, there are some disadvantages in group testing. For instance, they contain fewer items than individual tests. Further, it is possible that people work better on individual tests. Another disadvantage of group tests is that they cannot be used with children and people with low IQ. We shall learn more about intelligence testing later in the chapter. For now, let us examine the nature of intelligence.

NATURE OF INTELLIGENCE

Intelligence has been a major area of research in psychology for the past several years. Psychologists have been trying to find out answers to questions such as: Is intelligence one single entity, or is it made up of several specific abilities? Is intelligence inherited or is it a product of upbringing? What are the biological bases of intelligence? Are there many kinds of intelligence? It is not easy to answer these questions satisfactorily even after one century of research. But, while scientists were attempting to answer these questions, many important discoveries were made and several theories of intelligence promulgated. In general, there have been two approaches to the studies of the nature of intelligence: the factor-theory (psychometric) approach and the cognitive process (information processing) approach. We shall discuss briefly these two approaches.

Factor Theories of Intelligence

Is intelligence one single characteristic or is it a collection of specific abilities? One group of theories that tried to answer this question is called *factor theories*. Factor theorists make use of a psychometric procedure called **factor analysis** for this purpose. Factor analysis is a statistical technique used to determine the basic components of a complex phenomenon. It is something like a physicist's analysis of sunlight into seven colors; only the method is different. In factor analyzing intelligence, a researcher collects as many different kinds of intelligence tests that are available, administers them to as many people as possible, determines the correlation of each one of the tests with every other and analyzes the intercorrelations using one of the methods of factor analysis (there are several methods) to determine the factors that constitute intelligence. It is a complex procedure that you do not have to bother about. It is enough if you understand that factor analyses are complex statistical procedures to determine the basic components that constitute intelligence.

One difficulty with factor analysis is that there are different methods of analysis and each of them produces different factors of intelligence. But, because factor analytical procedures have enriched our understanding of intelligence and have provided us with different theories of intelligence, it is necessary that we have some knowledge about them.

Spearman's Two-factor Theory

One of the earliest to use factor analysis to analyze intelligence was the British psychologist Charles Edward Spearman (Fig. 8.3), who was working in this field at the same time when Binet was developing his test. Spearman (1927) found that performance on any intelligence test could be explained by postulating two factors: a **general factor (g)** and a **specific factor (s)**. All the tests share the same general factor to varying degrees, but each test has its own specific factor. For example, suppose there are three tests each measuring competence in mathematics, language and music. The common factor among all the three is g; in addition, each test also has a specific ability such as mathematical, verbal and musical abilities. He equated his general factor with general intelligence. Spearman's theory is well known in psychology as **two-factor theory of intelligence**. Spearman's views about intelligence are important in psychology for four reasons:

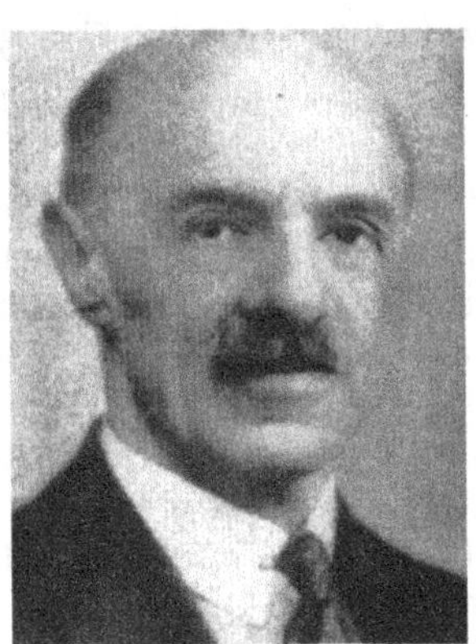

FIGURE 8.3: CE Spearman

1. He emphasized the unitary nature of intelligence, whereas Binet emphasized its diversity.
2. He asserted that intelligence was largely inherited; whereas Binet thought that it was modifiable by experience.
3. It was largely Spearman's conception of intelligence that was adopted by the testing movement all over the world and not Binet's. That is, most of modern tests of intelligence measure Spearman's g rather than Binet's multifarious intellectual abilities.
4. For introducing the concept of factor analysis as a research method in psychology; in fact, Spearman is called father of factor analysis.

Modern intelligence tests, notably Wechsler's tests, include subtests such as picture completion, vocabulary, block design and arithmetic subtests. Recent researches have shown that people who do well on one subtest tend to do well on others indicating that these tests are positively correlated. This led researchers to conclude that there is a single form of intelligence that cuts across the various subtests, thus supporting the central intellectual factor "*g*" postulated by Spearman.

Thurstone's Multiple Factor Theory

The second important factor theory of intelligence, *multiple factor theory*, was proposed by one of the most outstanding American psychometricians Louis L. Thurstone (Fig. 8.4) of Chicago University. Thurstone did not agree with Spearman's concept of 'g' and instead felt that intelligence could be broken down into a number of primary abilities. He administered to large groups of people a number of intelligence tests containing many different types of items and determined the intercorrelations among them. He analyzed the intercorrelations using a different method of factor analysis called **centroid technique**. This procedure yielded seven factors, namely, verbal comprehension, word fluency, number ability, spatial relations, memory, reasoning and perceptual speed. He called these factors **primary mental abilities** (Thurstone, 1938). He and his wife, Thelma Thurstone developed a battery of tests to measure each of these abilities called the *Primary Mental Abilities Test* (*PMA*). The test is being widely used all over the world. Later, researches have shown that Thurstone's primary abilities are not completely independent and there are significant correlations among them, thus providing some support to Spearman's concept of "g". However, we must remember that Thurstone denied the existence of "*g*", and argued that a single score does not hold much value in assessing intelligence.

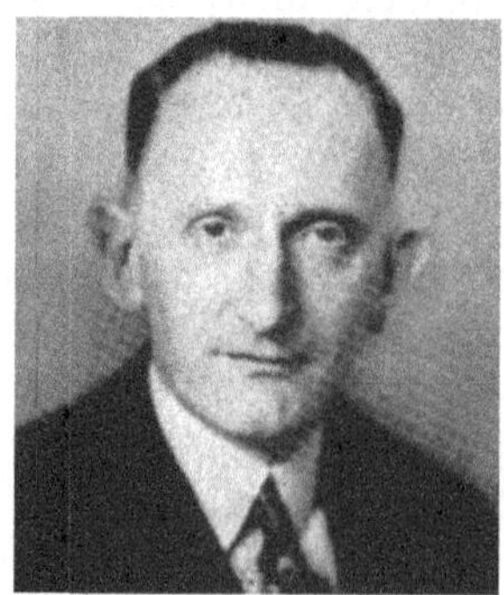

FIGURE 8.4: LL Thurstone

Cattell's Theory of Crystallized and Fluid Intelligence

Raymond B Cattell (Fig. 8.5) in 1971 proposed an influential alternative to Thurstone's model of intelligence, which was further elaborated by his student John Horn. According to this model, there are two distinct, but related subtypes of general intelligence (*g*), namely, crystallized intelligence and fluid intelligence. **Crystallized intelligence** refers to the ability to apply previously acquired information and procedures to solve current problems. This is the kind of intelligence that develops as one becomes an expert in an area. For example, a college professor has an accumulated store of crystallized intelligence; it has become crystallized by being practiced over time. It depends on the ability to retrieve previously learned knowledge such as problem-solving strategies from long-term memory and apply them to day-to-day issues. Most of the language usage skills stem from crystallized intelligence.

On the other hand, **fluid intelligence** refers to the ability to deal with current problems for which previous knowledge and experience does not provide a solution. It is the ability to solve new problems here and now. It is used to invent novel solutions to problems "on the spot." Fluid intelligence relies on inductive reasoning and creative problem solving. People with

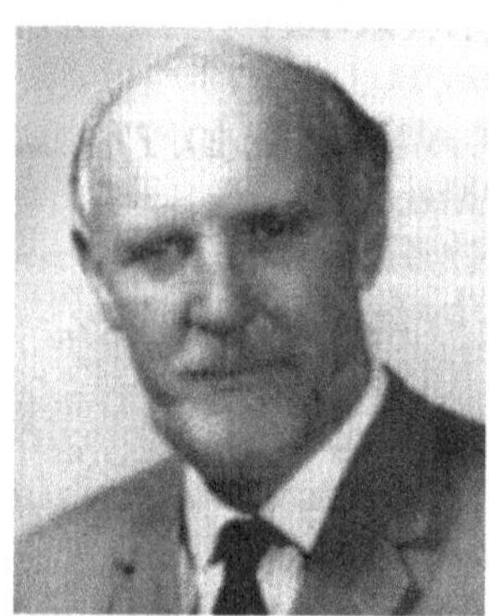

FIGURE 8.5: RB Cattell

high fluid intelligence can perceive new relations among stimulus patterns and draw inferences from relationships; they are capable of abstract reasoning and logical thinking. They rely on short-term (working) memory more than on long-term memory store (Horn and Cattell, 1966).

Both Cattell & Horn argue that over a life-time people progress from fluid intelligence to crystallized intelligence. With advancing age, there will be a decline in fluid intelligence, while crystallized intelligence does not suffer much. The two forms of intelligence develop at different rates during childhood and it is speculated that these are controlled by different brain areas; the two are not equally heritable; also, different facets of academic achievement are controlled by the two forms of intelligence. This line of thinking has tempted researchers to assert that these are actually two kinds of intelligence that are distinct.

Guilford's Structure of Intellect Model

American psychologist JP Guilford rejected both Spearman's general intelligence factor (g) and Thurstone's broad primary abilities and proposed a multifactor model (**structure of intellect model**) composed of 120 factors of intelligence. After a massive analysis of a vast number of available intelligence tests, Guilford (1959) came out with a three-dimensional theory. The three dimensions proposed by him are *operations, products* and *contents.* There are five kinds of operations, namely, *evaluation, convergent production, divergent production, memory* and *cognition;* six kinds of products, namely, *units, classes, relations, systems, transformations* and *implications;* and four kinds of contents such as *figural, symbolic, semantic* and *behavioral,* giving rise to 120 factors (5 × 6 × 4 = 120). The cubical model of Guilford's theory is given in Figure 8.6 wherein, each factor is represented by a cell and is some combination of the three dimensions (refer Fig. 8.6).

Hierarchical Theories of Intelligence

Vernon's Hierarchical Model

A perusal of the factor theories does not appear to give us a clear picture of the number and nature of intellectual abilities.

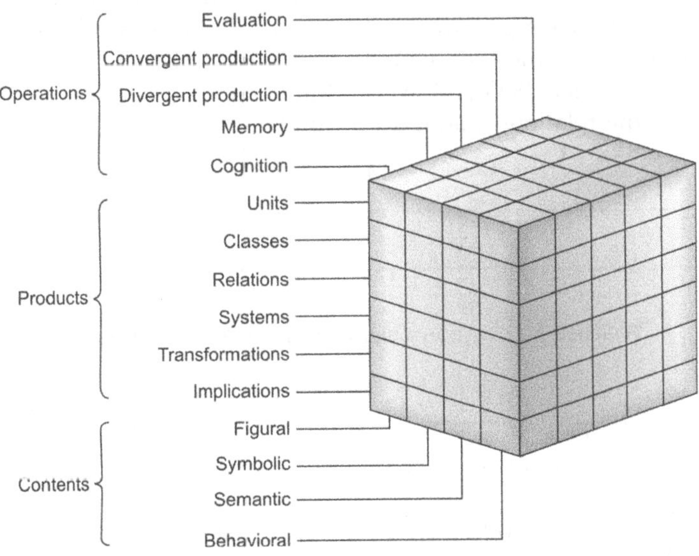

FIGURE 8.6: Guilford's structure of intelligence model

However, there is some truth in each of the theories presented above. Psychologists have identified some ability factors that are relatively independent of one another. But on closer examination these factors appear to be significantly correlated, indicating an underlying *g*-factor. As a compromise between the conflicting views, the British psychologist PE Vernon (1950) proposed a *hierarchical theory of intelligence*, which combines both *g*-factor and multiple factor theories. Such a view is presented in Figure 8.7.

We see at the top of the hierarchy the general factor, which shows up in all kinds of intellectual activities. Underneath it are several moderately specific broad factors like those of Thurstone's primary mental abilities. At the bottom are a large number of highly specific abilities like those of Spearman's specific factors that may come into play at one particular task and not in others. The hierarchical theory, as you can see, borrows from several factor theories to form a multilayered view of intelligence—a view that may turn out to be more reasonable.

Carroll's Three-stratum Theory

John B Carroll (1993), after a reanalysis (factor analysis) of test data from a large number of (over 450) high-quality studies conducted all over the world between 1935 and 1980, demonstrated that the relations among the test scores could be neatly arranged into a three-stratum hierarchy that very much resembled the one proposed by Vernon. Carroll's three-stratum theory of cognitive abilities contains elements of Spearman's, Thurstone's, & Cattell & Horn's models. The theory establishes three levels of mental abilities—*general, broad* and *narrow*—arranged in a hierarchical model. The hierarchy is shown in Figure 8.8. The general intelligence factor (*g*) at the top underlies most of the intellectual activities. Below g, at the second level, are eight broad factors arranged from left to right according to the extent to which they are correlated with *g*.

For instance, fluid intelligence is strongly related to *g* and crystallized intelligence is next, indicating Cattell-Horn factors. The other six factors of the second stratum represent basic cognitive activities such as learning and memory, perceptual functions, speed of functioning, and some of these resemble Thurstone's primary abilities. Finally, at the bottom are 69 specific abilities that contribute to the broad factors. These specific ability measures tend to correlate around 0.30 with one another, reflecting the common *g* factor at the top of the model. Thus, Carroll has given us a comprehensive model encompassing virtually all known cognitive abilities that attempt to sketch the most complete and detailed picture of human intellect.

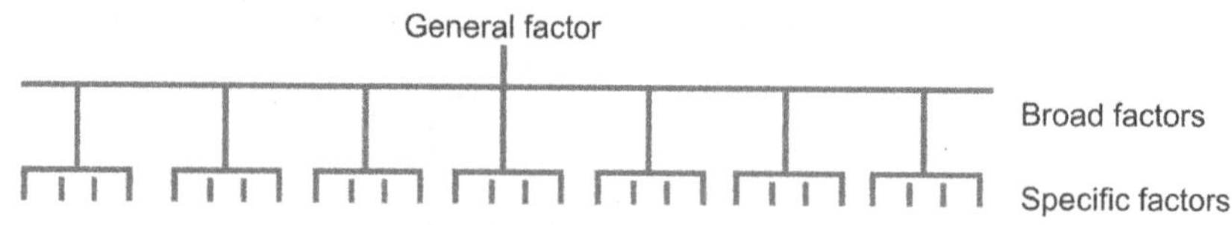

FIGURE 8.7: Vernon's hierarchical model of intelligence

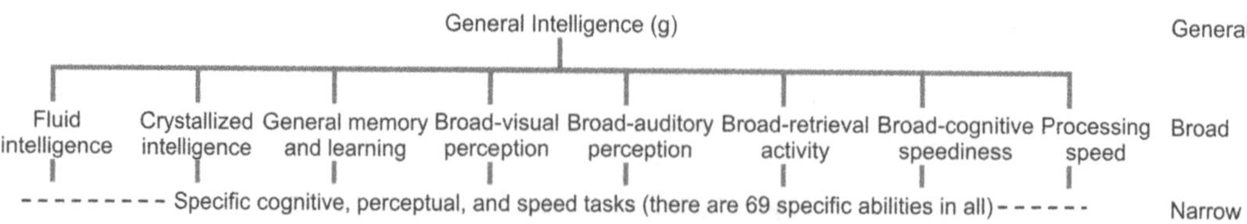

FIGURE 8.8: Carroll's model of intelligence

Cognitive Process Approaches

The theories of intelligence discussed above describe the components of intelligence and how those components (factors) fit together. These are statistically sophisticated ways of describing how people differ from one another. But they do not tell us why people differ in their intellectual activities. An alternative approach, called the cognitive process approach, focuses on intellectual processes—the patterns of thinking and reasoning that people use when they are engaged in intelligent behavior and solving problems. The vocabulary used by these theorists is different; for example, they speak of cognitive processes rather than intelligence. They are more interested in *how* people go about solving problems rather than *how many* problems they have solved. They are thus more process-oriented rather than product-oriented; they are interested in the development of intellectual processes—how the processes change as the individual matures. Cognitive theorists consider intelligence from the information-processing perspective. According to them, the way people store information in long-term memory, retrieve information from long-term memory and use the information in working memory for solving problems, give a better picture of intelligence. Rather than emphasizing the structural components of intelligence, they focus on the processes involved in intelligent behavior. One of the most important theories of this variety, especially concerning cognitive development, was proposed by the eminent Swiss psychologist, Jean Piaget. Piaget's theory is discussed in Chapter 12. Here, we examine a modern theory of intelligence built around cognitive processes.

Sternberg's Triarchic Theory of Intelligence

The most influential cognitive process theory, which is currently making news, is the **Triarchic theory of intelligence** proposed by Robert Sternberg (2004). The theory is concerned both with the psychological processes involved in intelligent behavior and the diverse forms in which intelligence manifests. Sternberg has identified three cognitive processes underlying intelligence and has called them as cognitive components—the steps an individual go through when solving a problem. These are *metacomponents, performance components* and *knowledge acquisition components*. The metacomponents are the higher mental processes that are put to use in planning and executing an intellectual function. These include processes such as identifying the problem, formulating possible solutions (hypotheses) and ways of testing them. According to Sternberg, metacomponents are at the root of fluid intelligence; people who think more before they act are the ones who possess this component to a large degree.

Performance components are the processes that are used to perform the task. These include perceptual processing, retrieving information and schemas from long-term memory store and generating suitable responses. The knowledge acquisition components help us to learn from past experience, store information in memory and develop new insights. As you have probably guessed, this component is similar to crystallized intelligence.

Sternberg assumes that there is more than one form of intelligence. This is explained in his triarchic theory. According to Sternberg, there are three types of intelligence: *analytical intelligence, practical intelligence* and *creative intelligences*. Analytical intelligence is the ability to learn to read and write well, do arithmetic problems and understand and appreciate literature. This is what is generally called 'scholastic ability'. Practical intelligence is the ability to engage in skilled activities such as driving automobiles, tailoring, or repairing machines. These and such other activities depend upon implicit memories, learned responses and skills that guide people to engage in them even without their being aware of the steps involved. Creative intelligence, on the other hand, resembles Cattell & Horn's fluid intelligence. This is the ability to solve problems in novel ways.

In short, our IQ tests measure analytical intelligence. Practical intelligence is what our vocational tests measure, and creative intelligence is difficult to measure; but attempts are on to develop tests of creativity. Although Sternberg claims that there are three different forms of intelligence, opinion is divided on this issue. For example, can one be creative without having some sort of scholastic and occupational skills? The answer is probably not. There are others who forcefully plead that there is more than one type of intelligence; one of the strongest proponents of such a view is the Harvard psychology professor Howard Gardner who has proposed a theory of multiple intelligences.

Gardner's Multiple Intelligences Model

Howard Gardner (2000) proposed a theory of intelligence, in which there are nine types of intelligences; Gardner is sure of eight of them, but is tentative about the ninth variety. The following is the list of his multiple intelligences.

Linguistic intelligence: The ability to produce and use language efficiently; writers, journalists and lawyers possess this ability markedly.

Visuospatial intelligence: The ability to deal with spatial relations effectively as is done by artists, architects and surgeons.

Logical-mathematical intelligence: The ability to manipulate abstract symbols logically as is done by scientists, mathematicians and computer specialists.

Musical intelligence: The ability to understand and produce music.

Bodily-kinesthetic intelligence: The ability to plan and execute bodily movements in a controlled manner as is done by actors, dancers, and athletes.

Interpersonal intelligence: The ability to understand people (their intentions, emotions, moods) and interact with them as is done by politicians, teachers and corporate executives.

Intrapersonal intelligence: The ability to understand internal aspects of oneself, such as one's own feelings and emotions as found among clergy, saints and philosophers.

Naturalistic intelligence: The ability to analyze and understand the natural environment, which is found among biologists, forest officers and meteorologists.

Existential intelligence: The ability to think about the meaning of life and existence as is done by the existentialists. Gardner is only tentative and not sure of the existence of this type of intelligence.

The first three types of intelligence in Gardner's list are measured by contemporary IQ tests; for others, there are no proper and suitable assessing tools. In fact, some critics observe that the other six are not aspects of intelligence at all as the concept is traditionally understood and at best they can be considered as some special talents. Gardner's theory of multiple intelligences is quite provocative, but it is also highly controversial because it goes beyond the traditionally defined concept of intelligence as a complex manifestation of cognitive skills.

Practical and Emotional Intelligence

In recent times, several psychologists have started talking about two types of intelligence: **practical intelligence** and **emotional intelligence**. Practical intelligence is intelligence related to the overall success in living. Traditional tests relate to academic success; they do not relate to career success.

For example, although successful business executives usually score moderately well on intelligence tests, the rate at which they advance and their ultimate achievements are only minimally associated with their test scores. Sternberg, a proponent of this view, argues that career success requires a very different type of intelligence apart from academic success. Academic success comes from reading, listening, and acquiring information. Practical intelligence, on the other hand, is learned mainly through observation of others' behavior. People who have high practical intelligence learn general norms and principles and apply them appropriately. Practical intelligence involves the ability to employ broad principles in solving everyday problems.

Some psychologists have broadened the concept of practical intelligence even further beyond the intellectual realm and consider intelligence from an emotional point of view. According to a group of researchers in this area (Mayer et al, 2004), we are given to understand that emotional intelligence (EI) is the ability to read other's emotions accurately, to respond to them appropriately and also to be aware of one's own emotions and control and regulate them effectively. EI helps us to get along with others, to understand what others are feeling and experiencing and to respond to others' needs appropriately. EI is at the root of social skills, empathy and self-awareness.

Emotional intelligence has two major components. One of them involves intelligence as it is traditionally understood. It is a composite of four complex processes, namely,

1. Perceiving emotions: Ability to identify emotions on the basis of perceptual cues.
2. Facilitating thought with emotion: Ability to harness emotional information to enhance thinking.
3. Understanding emotion: Ability to comprehend emotional information about relationships, changing emotional states and verbal information about emotion.
4. Managing emotion: Ability to manage emotions and emotional relationships.

A psychological tool called emotional intelligence test has been devised by Mayer, Salovey & Caruso to measure the four processes of EI. The second component involves subjective experience and inclination. It can be assessed by asking test-takers to rate themselves subjectively regarding relevant characteristics, such as their degree of assertiveness, empathy, stress tolerance and optimism. Objective measures of EI are found to be correlated with general intelligence (g), while subjective measures appear to be well correlated with scores on personality tests.

In recent years, the concept of EI has become a fertile area of research and a number of suggestive findings have been making the rounds. For example, it has been found that women tend to score higher than men on some dimensions of EI, especially those that pertain to social skills; men believe that they have better EI than women, which is not true; in the US, minority groups score better than Whites on tests of EI; older people score better than college students on EI tests, and people who can read variations in other people's moods tend to exhibit better social adjustment. It is claimed that EI tests explain and predict certain behaviors that were not explained by tests of personality and intelligence. Well, it is too early to accept these findings as final; the utility and limitations of EI measures have yet to be established.

Now that we have acquired some elementary knowledge about the nature and types of intelligence, we shall proceed to review some of the important intelligence tests that are in use today. But before that we have to learn about the general characteristics of psychological tests.

GENERAL CHARACTERISTICS OF PSYCHOLOGICAL TESTS

As it is, today we know more about intelligence tests than intelligence. It is true; intelligence tests came first, and then attempts to understand and explain the concept of intelligence. Psychological testing, especially intelligence testing, is a big industry today. Tests are being used for various purposes by different groups of people all over the world. There are several varieties of tests and it may take an entire volume to describe all the published tests. In this section, we shall discuss some of the very important tests and the general characteristics of these tests and how these are constructed and used.

Intelligence tests are one kind of psychological tests. Some of the essential characteristics of humans cannot be seen by a casual observer. For example, abilities, aptitudes, attitudes and personality characteristics cannot be observed directly. However, we can systematically observe people's behavior and make inferences about the underlying attributes that are believed to stimulate that behavior. Psychological tests help us in this endeavor.

What is a Psychological Test?

A psychological test is a standardized procedure designed to measure individual differences pertaining to some psychological construct based on a sample of relevant behavior. There are many kinds of psychological tests and they come in different forms. The special value of these tests lies in three characteristics:

1. There are specific, uniform procedures so that whosoever uses the test will follow the same steps in administering and scoring it. This enables us to compare the performance of different individuals on the test.
2. The scoring is objective; whosoever scores the test gets the same result. There is no scope for the tester's subjective bias to influence the score.
3. The test scores are interpretable meaningfully. We can infer from the test scores what characteristics are believed to be associated with high or low scores.

Types of Psychological Tests

There are different types of tests to measure different human characteristics. For example, there are achievement tests, ability tests and personality tests. Achievement tests are designed to measure what people have learned so far in their schools, colleges, occupations and in short, while living. Ability tests are designed to measure capacity or potential to achieve rather than actual achievement. Ability tests come in two forms; intelligence tests and aptitude tests. As we have seen, intelligence is made up of many abilities and the term refers to overall capacity for learning and problem solving. Aptitude tests usually are designed to measure the potential ability of people to learn certain skills, provided they are given necessary training; these tests go beyond prior learning and are believed to measure a person's potential for future learning and performance. They may measure a person's capacity to become a mechanic, a pilot or a salesman. Personality tests are designed to assess an individual's characteristic ways of thinking, feeling and behavior. They may also measure an individual's attitudes, interests, emotional states, sociability, interpersonal skills and level of adjustment.

PSYCHOMETRIC CHARACTERISTICS OF A GOOD TEST

In order to design a test, we must first decide, which specific behaviors serve as indicators of the psychological construct we plan to measure. Then, we have to devise test items that allow us to measure individual differences in those behaviors. Item selection to construct a test is a specialized process involving complex statistical procedures. Items must be relevant and representative of the behavior that is being measured.

One has to estimate the item's capacity to discriminate and its difficulty level. For example, if all persons pass an item, it is useless; similarly if all fail the item, even that is useless. We shall not go into the details of test construction and standardization here. But it is necessary to know the characteristics that a test should possess if it were to be really trustworthy and informative. Three of the most important characteristics of psychological tests are reliability, validity and norms.

Reliability

Reliability refers to the consistency of measurement; that is, the extent to which a test would yield the same result if repeated again. It is the most basic requirement of a test and a correlation coefficient is its typical index. Reliability may be estimated by correlating the scores obtained from a sample of participants at two different points in time. It is called **test-retest reliability**. It may be estimated by correlating the scores on one-half of the test with scores on the other half; then it is referred to as **split-half reliability**. The third way of determining reliability is to develop two sets of similar items (parallel forms) and administering the two sets to a group of people and correlating the scores on the two forms; this is called **alternate forms reliability**. Actually these are three forms of reliability: test-retest reliability measures stability of test scores, split-half reliability is an estimate of consistency, and parallel forms reliability indicates equivalence. There are also several more complex procedures of estimating reliability of a test about which we may not worry. It is enough to know that when the index of reliability (correlation coefficient) is high, the test is consistently measuring what it is measuring. If it is low, it means the test in question has a high probability of error and any prediction we make based on the test score is not trustworthy.

Validity

Validity of a test refers to the extent to which the test measures what it has been designed to measure. Assessment of validity is a special problem in psychology. It is only in psychology that we have to prove what we are measuring is actually what we want to measure. In other sciences, this problem does not arise. For example, when a physicist measures length using a meter stick, he does not have to prove that he is measuring length. In psychology, when we measure intelligence, we have to prove that what we have measured is intelligence only. As in the case of reliability, there are several ways of estimating the validity of a test. Some important types of validity are content validity, criterion-related validity and construct validity.

Content validity refers to the representativeness or the sampling adequacy of the content of the test; that is, it refers to whether the items of a test measure all the knowledge or skills that are assumed to underlie the attribute that is being assessed. For example, we must be sure that a numerical ability test we want to develop includes all operations pertaining to numbers such as addition, subtraction, multiplication, division, fractions, and equations and so on. **Criterion-related validity** refers to the extent to which the test scores correlate with some meaningful *criterion measure*. **Criterion** is some behavior or characteristic that reflects the attribute the test is designed to measure. For example, if an intelligence test is valid, its score must predict some behavior that is assumed to be influenced by intelligence, such as school marks. In this case, school marks are the criterion measure. Since criterion-related validity is based on the ability of the test scores in predicting a criterion, it is often called **predictive validity**. The third type of validity, called **construct validity**, is a more complex concept. It is determined by finding the relationship between the test scores and other behavior variables with which the construct being measured is supposed to be related. One of the easiest ways of validating a test is by determining its correlation with an already validated test. This type of validity is called '**concurrent validity**'.

Norms

The third important characteristic of a test is its norms. **Norms** are sets of scores obtained from a sufficiently large sample of people for whom the test is intended. Based on the norms, an individual's raw score can be compared with similar person's score and interpreted. A test without norms is useless. Suppose you score 80 on a test. What does that mean? Unless you compare your score with a standard (say 100), you do not know whether your score is a good score or not. One important point here is that the sample from which normative scores are obtained must be representative of the population with which the test will be used. Further, the norms must be revised with the passage of time. Otherwise they become outmoded. Psychological test construction, item selection, establishing reliability and validity, suggesting uniform procedures of administering and scoring the test and development of norms, all these activities are subsumed under the term standardization of a test and of course, it involves a lot of time, effort and resources.

ASSESSING INTELLIGENCE

We have seen that intelligence testing was started by Binet & Simon in France. Henry Goddard (1865–1957) an American, who was working with mentally retarded children, brought the Binet-Simon test to the United States and translated it into English for use with American children. Later, the Binet-Simon test was revised by psychologists in several countries to suit their local population. You will be surprised to know that the test was revised in India by Kamath to test children of Karnataka. However, the most popular of these revisions was the English version of the test called the *Stanford-Binet Intelligence Scale* published in 1916 by Lewis Terman (1877–1956). The test includes items that tap a wide range of abilities including abstract reasoning and problem solving (Table 8.1). This was an age scale, individually administered that yielded an MA score. Later, the concept of IQ was derived from the MA. Since IQ as conceived by William Stern had several problems, another score, called **deviation IQ**, was developed, which is the most preferred concept now-a-days.

Two decades after Terman introduced the American version of the Binet test, David Wechsler developed a family of tests for people at various age levels. Today, Wechsler tests (WAIS-III, WISC-IV and WPPSI) are the most extensively used tests in the United States of America and other English-speaking countries. Wechsler believed that Stanford-Binet relied too much on verbal skills. He thought that intelligence tests should include both verbal and non-verbal abilities and included in his tests some performance (non-verbal) items. The types of abilities measured by the WAIS-III are shown in the Table 8.2. The test yields three types of scores: a verbal IQ based on the sum of the scores on the verbal subtests; a performance IQ based on the scores on the performance subtests and a full-scale IQ based on both the performance and verbal subtests. The IQ scores on WAIS-III are adjusted so that the mean is 100 and standard deviation is 15 points. As shown in Figure 8.9, about two thirds of all people have IQs of 85 to 115 points; that is, one standard deviation above or below the mean. A little more than a quarter have IQs either between 70 and 85 or between 115 and 130 (within the second standard deviation above or below the mean). Only 4.54 percent of IQ scores

Table 8.1: Sample Items from Stanford-Binet Intelligence Scale

Age	*Test items*	*Description*
2	3-hole form board Block building: Tower	Inserts forms (circle, triangle, square) in correct holes after watching a demonstration Builds a four-block tower from model after demonstration
3	Block building: Bridge Pure vocabulary	Builds a bridge consisting of two side blocks and one top block from model after demonstration Names 10 of 18 line drawings
4	Naming objects from memory Picture identification	One of three objects (such as car, dog or shoe) is covered after child has seen them; child then names objects from memory Points to correct pictures of objects on a card in response to: "Show me what we cook on?" or "What do we carry, when it is raining?"
7	Similarities Copying a diamond	Answers questions such as "In what way coal and wood are alike?" or "Ship and automobile are alike?" Draws three diamonds following a printed example
8	Vocabulary Memory for stories	Defines eight words from a list Listens to a story, then answers questions about it
9	Verbal absurdities Digit reversal	Says what is foolish about stories similar to: "I saw a well-dressed young man who was walking down the street with his hands in his pockets and twirling a brand new cane" Repeats four digits backward
Average adult	Vocabulary Proverbs	Defines 20 words from a list (same list as at age 8 above) Explains in own words meaning of two or more proverbs
	Orientation	Answers questions similar to: which direction would you have to face so your left hand would be toward the south?"

Table 8.2: Subtests in Wechsler Adult Intelligence Scale (WAIS-III)

Verbal subtests	*Description*
Information	Items pertain to factual knowledge about historical events, geography, nature, etc. (e.g. on which continent the river Nile flows)
Comprehension	Understanding of social conventions, rules (e.g. "People living in glass houses should not throw stones at each other")
Arithmetic	Arithmetical reasoning and computation through verbal problems (e.g. Suppose you buy a shirt that was Rs. 200, but is now marked "20% off," how much should you pay?)
Similarities	Determining ways in which objects are similar (for example, How are a tree and a blade of grass are alike?)
Letter number sequencing	Tests of attention and ability to retain and manipulate information in memory; a set of alternating numbers and letters are presented orally and the participant is required to repeat first the numbers and then the letters in order of magnitude and alphabetical order (e.g. 8-K-6-B-3-T to be converted into 3-6-8-B-K-T)
Vocabulary	The subject is required to define increasingly difficult words (e.g.: what does 'plausible' mean?)
Performance Subtests	
Digit symbol	The task is to learn a coding system in which symbols represent numbers (e.g., if the symbols # ^ * @ ~ represent 1 2 3 4 5 respectively, fill in the numbers for * # ~ * @ ~ #)
Picture completion	The test consists of finding missing parts of pictures that are otherwise complete
Picture arrangement	Putting a set of pictures in the right sequence, so that they make a meaningful story
Block design	Arranging colored blocks into a design that matches the one given on a card; tests the ability to perceive and analyze patterns
Object assembly	Putting pieces of a jigsaw-like puzzle together correctly; measures the ability to deal with part-whole relationship

Note: The examples given in the brackets are not from original test.

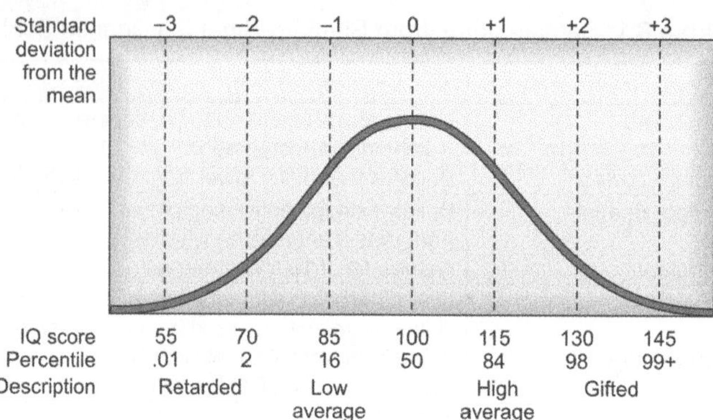

FIGURE 8.9: The distribution of intelligence

are above 130 or below 70. The bell-shaped curve is called **normal probability curve.**

Varieties of Intelligence Tests

There are several other types of intelligence tests. The Stanford-Binet & Wechsler tests are individual tests. These can be administered to one person at a time. Psychologists have devised a number of group tests that can be administered to groups of people at a time; for example, Thurstone's Primary Mental Abilities (PMA), Differential Aptitude Test (DAT) and Army General Classification Test (AGCT). Thurstone's test measures factorially derived abilities such as *verbal comprehension, word fluency, perceptual speed, memory, numerical ability, spatial ability* and *reasoning*. DAT includes eight subtests such as *verbal reasoning, numerical ability, abstract reasoning, space relations, mechanical reasoning, clerical speed and accuracy, language usage: spelling* and *language usage: grammar*. DAT is specifically designed for counseling high school and college students. AGCT is an omnibus test including verbal, numerical and non-verbal (paper-pencil) items. Tests that make use of language are called verbal tests. There are non-verbal paper pencil tests such as Raven's Progressive Matrices Tests. Raven's test is designed to measure Spearman's "g." There are three scales; standard, children's and advanced scales. In performance tests, the subject is required to do something manually. A large number of performance tests, such as Alexander's battery (consisting of the well-known *block-design, pass along* and *cube construction* tests) and Pintner-Paterson Scale of Performance, are being used all over the world.

In addition, there are achievement and aptitude tests. **Achievement tests** measure how much a student has learned so far in school or college in one or the other subjects. **Aptitude tests** measure a person's potential for future learning. Achievement tests are good predictors of future performance in similar situations. The aptitude tests depend less on prior knowledge than on an individual's ability to react to the problems presented on the test. Both achievements and aptitude tests are being extensively used in educational and industrial institutions. The best known test of this type is the Scholastic Aptitude Test (SAT) routinely administered to students who want to enter liberal arts colleges in the United States. Graduate Record Examination (GRE) is another well-known test that is administered to students who plan to do advance (doctoral) work in a number of areas in the arts and sciences. Similar tests are used for selecting students to schools of medicine, dentistry, nursing, law and other professions. In fact, most modern tests of intelligence measure a combination of aptitude and achievement, thus emphasizing the importance of both native ability and previous learning.

Several tests of intelligence are theory based. Thurstone's test of PMA was devised to measure the factorially established intellectual dimensions. Raven's Progressive Matrices tests are measures of Spearman's general factor of intelligence. Recently, attempts have been made to develop some other theory-based tests. For example, the Kaufman Adolescent and Adult Intelligence Test and the Woodcock-Johnson Psycho-Educational Battery have been constructed to measure Cattell-Horn's crystallized and fluid intelligence separately. The Kaufman test has three subtests for each of fluid and crystallized ability and separate IQs can be calculated for them. Sternberg Triarchic Ability Test (STAT) measures the three forms of intelligence analytic, practical and creative, identified by Sternberg in his model.

There are good books describing the available tests of intelligence, aptitude and achievement; for example, Anastasi A (1982). *Psychological testing* (5th Ed.), Kaplan RM & Saccuzzo DP: *Psychological Testing—principles, applications and issues.*

INDIVIDUAL DIFFERENCES IN INTELLIGENCE

As seen in the Figure 8.9 showing the distribution of IQs, intelligence is distributed in the general population in such a way that most people possess average intelligence (about 100 IQ points), some people possess superior or poor intelligence and a few have very high (the mentally gifted) or very low ability (mentally retarded). The intellectual level of individuals determine their ability to cope with the demands of living in contemporary society that is characterized by technological sophistication, high level of competition, mobility, and to adjust to fast changing circumstances around them. While high intelligence may not guarantee success in life, low intelligence definitely creates barriers preventing active participation in the achieving society.

Mental Retardation

Generally, people who score below 70 IQ points are considered mentally retarded. Their adaptive skills are inadequate to cope with ordinary problems of day-to-day life. During childhood, their psychomotor developments such as walking and talking were delayed; in school, their reading, writing and arithmetic skills were very poor; they may not be able to tell the time of the day, date and month correctly; they cannot count money properly; as adults their vocational performance and social adjustment are inadequate. It has been estimated that about 2 to 5 percent of people in the general population are mentally retarded. On the basis of IQ scores, mental retardation has been classified into four categories such as mild (50–75 IQ), moderate (35–50 IQ), severe (20–35 IQ) and profound (below 20 IQ).

Mildly disabled children constitute about 85 percent of the mentally retarded group; they can attend school, but exhibit difficulty in acquiring skills in reading, writing and arithmetic. Moderately disabled children constitute about 10 percent; they are slow in everything and with some difficulty, they can be trained to look after themselves. The third group (about 4 percent) exhibit marked delay in walking and speech and cannot profit from formal education. The last group (about 1 percent) exhibits gross difficulties in all walks of life and they do not survive if not nursed properly.

The psychomotor disabilities exhibited by retarded children are due to several causes; some genetic, some due to other biological factors and some are due to environmental factors. About 25 percent of all mental retardation has been reported to be due to genetic factors and it is said that there are about 100 genetic causes. For example, a condition called **Down syndrome** (mongolism), which is characterized by mild to severe mental retardation, is usually caused by an abnormal division of the 21st chromosome pair. Down syndrome is more likely to occur in births to older women whose eggs have been dormant for many years. The second genetic cause is referred to as **fragile X syndrome**. Children suffering from this condition inherit a peculiar genetic defect; a small bit of deoxyribonucleic acid (DNA) on the X chromosome repeats itself many times. This defect makes the chromosome prone to breaking up and hence the name fragile X syndrome. Mental retardation can be caused by accidents at birth, such as severe oxygen deprivation (anoxia); it may result if the mother is suffering from rubella (German measles), scarlet fever or syphilis; it may also be the result of the pregnant mother taking certain drugs (antibiotics and analgesics) and/or alcohol. If the pregnant mother drinks heavily, especially during the first few weeks without being aware that she is pregnant, her child can be born with a condition called **fetal alcohol syndrome** part of which is mental retardation. A pregnant woman who is malnourished, diabetic, human immunodeficiency virus (HIV) positive, or exposed to high doses of X-rays, may also give birth to a mentally retarded child. It is believed that mental retardation may be due to certain still undetected brain anomalies, extreme environmental deprivation, or a combination of the two.

As of now, there is no known cure for mental retardation. However, special training can sometimes produce modest improvements in psychosocial activities. In advanced countries, such as the US, there are special provisions to look after cognitively disabled children. This has resulted in the practice called '**mainstreaming**' or 'inclusion program' which allows mentally and behaviorally challenged children to attend school in regular classrooms and experience a more normal environment. There are provisions to give such children special attention and individualized instruction.

Gifted Children

At the other (right) end of the normal probability curve showing the distribution of IQ scores (refer Fig. 8.9) are the people who are intellectually gifted. Generally, these are people with superior ability who have IQs beyond 135 (it is common to include in this group people in the 150–180 range). It is estimated that about 2 to 3 percent of the people in the general population are gifted. There is a misconception that the gifted people are generally awkward, shy and social misfits who cannot get along well with others. This is a wrong stereotype. Because of their superior intellect, they may be deeply absorbed in certain cognitive tasks and hence appear to be not very social. But research has shown that they are mostly outgoing, well-adjusted and can do things better than others. The longitudinal studies of the gifted children undertaken by Lewis Terman have shown that these people are mentally, physically, academically, socially and personally better than others. They are stronger, healthier, taller and heavier than their non-gifted peers. They receive many awards in school, distinctions in life and earn more money in their occupation. But, not everyone of the group Terman studied was successful in all walks of life. Superior intelligence does not mean that success is guaranteed. Gifted people may not be good at everything. As can be expected from theories of multiple intelligences, one individual may be enormously talented in some special area of mental competence, but is average in other fields. There are some mathematical prodigies who are just mediocre in other areas. One researcher has found that 95 percent of the gifted children had sharply different mathematical and verbal skills.

Researches indicate that success is a product of three interacting factors. The first is of course high intelligence; the second is creative problem-solving capacity and the third is high level of motivation. Studies of eminent scientists, artists, musicians, writers, actors and athletes revealed that they were highly devoted to their profession and worked harder than their less eminent counterparts. Albert Einstein, Sigmund Freud, Charles Darwin and several others were not exceptionally gifted as children, but their motivation, single-minded devotion and hard work helped them to achieve eminence in their chosen field. According to one researcher, gifted children do the same kinds of processing as average children but simply do it more effectively. They are driven by an extraordinary passion to excel in their chosen field. In fact, it is not clear what contributes to giftedness, whether it is heredity or environment. There are some research hints that gifted boys tend to have lower testosterone levels than non-gifted ones, whereas gifted girls may actually have higher amounts of testosterone than non-gifted girls. Such research findings indicate that there might be some biological basis for giftedness.

Before closing this section, mention must be made of a lacuna in social science research: although there are several programs to improve the performance of mentally retarded children, not many attempts have been made to study the gifted children, identify the area of giftedness and encourage the special ability in them. Without special attention, a gifted child may become bored and frustrated in a class full of mediocre peers. There is an urgent need to organize special programs designed to enrich the environment in which the gifted ones live and learn. There must be attempts to nourish their talents, so that they may flourish. There are indications that many eminent people had the help of efficient teachers, mentors or guides at crucial periods of their lives. Having an apprentice relationship with an appropriate role model can be of great help in nourishing giftedness. It is something like having a good supervisor when one is pursuing a doctoral degree.

GROUP DIFFERENCES IN INTELLIGENCE

Contemporary researchers on intelligence have been interested in determining whether there are group differences in IQ scores among various racial groups such as African Americans, White Americans, Asians, Chinese and Jews. Another area of interest is gender differences in intelligence. Let us see what psychologists have to say about race difference and gender difference in intellectual abilities.

Race Differences

In contemporary world, it is not easy to identify persons as belonging to specific race because several races blend seamlessly into one another. In fact, several researchers assert that the concept of race is a social invention and not a biological fact. They doubt the idea that several races exist. Nevertheless, people have been grouped into several races based on certain (doubtful?) assumptions and their intelligence assessed. Studies of race differences in the USA have repeatedly shown that Asian Americans tend to score better on IQ tests than White Americans, and White Americans tend to score better than African Americans. National comparisons show that Japanese children have the highest mean IQ in the world. Asian Americans score better than White Americans on tests of spatial and mechanical reasoning, but score slightly lower on verbal skills. African Americans score, on the average, about 12 to 15 IQ points below White Americans. The fact that the Blacks tend to score lower than Whites has led some researchers to the controversial conclusion that the latter's inferior scores are rooted in their genes.

There are heated discussions and bitter debates concerning the racial and national differences in intelligence and their political, social and educational implications. An article by Arthur Jenson in the "*Harvard Educational Review* (1969)" sparked a bitter debate in the US. Jenson concluded that intelligence is inherited and that there are genetic differences among the various ethnic groups. Some 25 years later, Richard Herrnstein & Charles Murray in their book: "*The Bell curve: Intelligence and Class Structure in American Life* (1994)," painted a similar picture. Of course, as we have seen in the previous paragraph, there are differences in the average intelligence test scores. But the unanswered question is: Where do these differences come from? Do they emanate from genes, sociocultural differences or the built-in bias of the intelligence tests themselves? These questions are highly complex and simple answers are not available; the debate is unlikely to be resolved soon.

Gender Differences

Men and women are biologically different. Every cell in the female body is different from those in the male. There are differences in the structure and functions of the brains of men and women. It is reported that the cerebral hemispheres are not as sharply specialized in women as in men. There are hormonal differences between them. Fortunately, there are no significant differences between them in the overall intelligence test scores. But, there appears to be slight, but consistent differences in certain cognitive skills that constitute intelligence. For example, men perform better than women in certain spatial tasks; that is, they do well in tests that involve mentally rotating or manipulating objects in space. Men are also more accurate in target-directed skills, such as throwing and catching objects and they perform slightly better on tests of mechanical and mathematical reasoning. Women, at the other hand, perform better on tests of verbal fluency, perceptual speed, and arithmetical calculation; they are also good at precise manual tasks involving fine motor coordination. The interesting thing is that these differences between men and women are small, but appear consistently.

Psychologists have attempted to explain these gender differences both in terms of biological and environmental factors. The environmental explanations focus on the differential forms of socialization that men and women have undergone during their development. For example, boys are encouraged to engage in the so called 'masculine tasks', such as climbing trees and sports involving throwing, catching and hitting the targets. That may be the reason why they score better than girls in tests involving these skills. Girls are encouraged to undertake 'feminine tasks,' such as nursing, child-rearing, knitting and cooking, which favor the development of verbal skills. Biological explanations focus on hormonal differences between men and women. The effects of hormones go beyond reproductive activities; they influence the brain organization and the consequent behavioral tendencies such as aggressiveness and problem-solving strategies. But, the extent to which hormones produce gender differences in intelligence has not yet been clearly established and hence no definite conclusions can be drawn in this regard.

HEREDITY, ENVIRONMENT AND INTELLIGENCE

Is intelligence determined by heredity or by environment? This question has long been a source of controversy and bitter debate among social scientists. The issue has not yet been resolved. The simplest answer could be that both nature and nurture influence the development of intelligence. There is no doubt that heredity plays an important role in determining intelligence, but the precise nature of that role is difficult to establish among humans. Let us see the roles of these two factors in some detail.

Genetic Influence on Intelligence

The best way to determine the genetic influence on intelligence is to mate individuals selectively and study the offspring. This cannot be done on humans and therefore psychologists have resorted to animal experiments. Long ago in 1940, Tryon undertook a classical experiment to study the inheritance of ability in rats. He trained rats in maze learning; selected the brightest among them and bred them to produce a superior race of rats. He bred the dull ones to produce a dull race of rats. He continued the process of selective breeding for seven generations and produced two strains of rats: the bright and dull ones. At this point Tryon found that virtually 100 percent of bright rats learned faster than any rat in the dull group. The conclusion is unambiguous; intelligence can be determined to a high degree by heredity. Rigorous selective breeding can sort out intelligent genes so that one family line is superior and another inferior in intelligence.

Unfortunately, we cannot conduct such a controlled breeding experiment on human beings. As an alternative, psychologists have chosen the easy route of analyzing intelligence as it unfolds naturally over the course of people's development. For this purpose, they began comparing intelligence of individuals who differ in their degrees of genetic resemblance. For example, they compared intelligence quotients (IQs) of fraternal twins with those of identical twins. Fraternal twins, on the average, have 50 percent of their genes identical, and identical twins have 100 percent identical genes. If genes determine intelligence, the identical twins must have more similar IQs than the fraternal twins. In fact, this is what has happened. Studies conducted in several countries all support the contention that intelligence is genetically determined.

Other researchers studied the problem from a different angle. They studied the similarity of IQs among identical twins who were separated early in life and were reared apart. These children, as you can easily infer have same heredity, but different environments and thus give us an idea of the relative influence of heredity and environment. Studies of this type have found correlations of IQs between separated identical twins in the range of 0.67 and 0.78. These are significantly high correlations and suggest that genetic similarity leads to intellectual similarity.

Environmental Influence

Although there is overwhelming evidence to suggest the influence of genes on intelligence, the role of environment should not be underestimated. Researchers have studied the similarity in intelligence between the biological parents and their children on one hand, and the similarity between parents and their adopted children on the other. The first group has similar heredity and similar environment; in the case of second, heredity is different and environment same. The correlations between scores of parents and their natural children were, on the average, higher than those found in the case of parents and their adopted children. This again suggests that it is heredity, not environment, which leads to similarity of intelligence between parents and children. This does not mean that environment has no role to play in the development of intellectual skills. Some studies have compared the scores of identical twins who were reared together (both heredity and environment same) with those that were reared apart (heredity same, but environment different). These studies have found lesser resemblance in the second group than in the first. That is, although the heredity is same, the rearing conditions have a role to play in determining the intellectual status. Several studies have shown that the shared home environment, enriched environment and educational experience do have significant influence in shaping intellectual skills. Siblings who are reared together (shared home) appear to be more similar to one another than those reared apart. Children who are removed from deprived environment and placed in middle class or rich homes have shown improvement in their intelligence. Also, good education can have significant influence in increasing IQ scores. All these findings lead to the conclusion: genes may set limits on what one can achieve, but environmental conditions determine the extent to which the potentiality is actualized. The relative influence of heredity and environment is summarized in the Table 8.3.

In short, the conclusion can be that heredity and environment both influence intelligence, but they rarely operate independently. The environmental conditions such as good food can influence how genes express themselves. Similarly, genetic factors can influence the effects produced by the environment; for instance genetic factors influence which environment people choose for themselves and how they respond to the environment. Therefore, the question is not the extent to which heredity or environment determines intelligence; it should be: How does heredity and environment interact to affect intelligence? As of today, we do not have unambiguous answers to questions pertaining to the role of heredity and environment as determiners of intelligence.

BRAIN AND INTELLIGENCE

Some researchers have claimed that people with larger brains perform better on intelligence tests. Larger brains, of course, contain more neurons. But it is not clear whether larger brains cause more intelligence or more intelligence causes larger brains. Also, the relation between the brain size and intelligence is not that simple. For instance, women have smaller brains than men, but they have about the same average intelligence as men. The Neanderthals (the human subspecies who lived 75,000 years ago) had larger brains than we have, but there is no evidence that they were more intelligent. The observed correlation between brain size and intelligence is small and correlation does not mean causation. However, some neuroscientists claim that the key variable is not the overall brain size, but the crucial areas in the brain. For example, it is reported that Einstein's brain had an unusually large number of glial cells (these cells help in the care and nourishing of neurons, influence the communication

Table 8.3: The Correlations in Intelligence Among People Who Differ in Genetic Similarity

Relationship	*Percent of shared genes*	*Correlation of IQ scores*
Identical twins reared together	100	0.86
Identical twins reared apart	100	0.75
Fraternal twins reared together	50	0.57
Siblings reared together	50	0.45
Siblings reared apart	50	0.21
Biological parent-children reared by parent	50	0.36
Biological parent-children not reared by parent	50	0.20
Cousins	25	0.25
Adopted child-adoptive parent	0	0.19
Adopted children reared together	0	0.32

among neurons, and are involved in information processing), especially in the bottom portion of the left parietal lobe. This portion of the brain is believed to play an important role in mathematical reasoning and spatial visualization. As you know, Einstein was a genius and made extensive use of these abilities. The extra glial cells may have helped this portion of the brain to function efficiently. Einstein's brain had more neurons in this key area and his parietal lobes were about 15 percent wider than normal, but the overall size of his brain was only average. Thus, the meaning of correlation between the brain size and intelligence is complicated and not clear.

Studies of the brain have also demonstrated a relationship between working memory and intelligence, especially fluid intelligence. Researches have shown that frontal lobes are involved in working memory and fluid intelligence (damage to frontal lobes impairs fluid intelligence). Cognitive scientist John Duncan and colleagues have observed activation in the lateral prefrontal cortex when subjects were taking certain IQ tests such as Raven's Progressive Matrices (a good test of *g* or fluid intelligence involving visual-spatial reasoning). In general, these findings suggest that there is a global workspace in the brain that organizes and coordinates information, helping to transfer material to other parts of the brain. The functioning of the workspace represents general intelligence.

CAN INTELLIGENCE BE BOOSTED?

In spite of the general assumption that intelligence is genetically determined, one cannot rule out altogether the importance of environmental influence in shaping cognitive activities. Varying the environment can boost intelligence as measured by the IQ tests. In several advanced countries, attempts have been made to raise the level of intelligence of school-going children coming from disadvantaged families by enriching the environment through some special educational and social programs. One such program, called the Project Head Start, was initiated in the US during the 1960s. Under the program, additional intellectual stimulation was provided to socioeconomically disadvantaged children. Unfortunately, the outcome was not encouraging; there were some short-term gains in IQ points that evaporated with time.

Flynn Effect

Still, modern psychologists look upon intelligence as more flexible and modifiable than originally envisioned. James Flynn (1999), a researcher from New Zealand, has reported that much of the world's population today is scoring progressively higher on intelligence tests. There has been an IQ increase of 28 points in the US since 1910 and a similar increase in Britain since 1942. On average, there has been an increase of about three points per decade. It means that current average IQ would be about 115 if the tests were scored according to the norms used in 1955. The increase is occurring to the same degree for both men and woman and for different ethnic groups. This tendency of rising IQ is often called the '*Flynn effect*', named after the researcher who reported the phenomenon. The suggested causes of Flynn effect are effective child rearing practices, better nutrition, improved health conditions (contributing to increased brain functioning), richer and more complex learning environment in schools requiring more coping skills, improved social environment, and the technological advances that may have helped shape the kinds of analytical and abstract reasoning skills involved in intelligence tests. Whatever the cause, the increase in IQ scores is not due to genetic factors!

Rosenthal Effect

Two American psychologists, Rosenthal and Jacobson (1967), have reported another interesting phenomenon. They studied the way in which student-teacher interactions affect intelligence of children. In one of their studies, they have demonstrated that if teachers thought the children in their classes were going to become smarter, those expectations led the teachers to behave in such a way that the children actually did become smarter. This is called the **self-fulfilling prophecy**; what the teachers expected to happen, they made happen. In a large-scale study in the US, the researchers administered a non-verbal test of intelligence to elementary school children; then selected 20 percent of them at random and they told their teachers that these children have scored exceptionally well in the test and they would bloom in intelligence in the next 8 months. Actually, there was no difference in intelligence between these children and other children in the class, and the teachers did not know this fact. At the end of the year, all the children in the class were again tested. Surprisingly, those whom the teachers thought were going to bloom intellectually did score higher than others. How could this happen? Rosenthal and his associates explain that this was the result of the treatment meted to the students by their teachers. The teachers treated the students they thought had greater potential for growth in intelligence differently. They behaved more warmly toward them, put more effort to teach them, gave them more information, gave more time for them to answer the questions and corrected them when they went wrong. So, what the teacher thought would happen did happen. This self-fulfilling prophecy, which is also called *Rosenthal effect*, has been repeatedly found by other researchers, especially if the teachers did not know the children well.

Chapter Summary

Although intelligence is defined differently by different theorists, most people agree that intelligence is the capacity to learn and acquire knowledge, think rationally, act effectively and adapt to the changing environmental conditions encountered in life. Historically, it was Sir Francis Galton of Britain who thought of measuring intelligence using anthropometric indices. But the real intelligence testing started in France by Alfred Binet and his associate Theodore Simon who developed the first intelligence test. The two measured intelligence in terms of a score called mental age (MA). Later, William Stern, a German psychologist, introduced the concept of intelligence quotient (IQ) as an index of intellectual level. Today, the term IQ is known all over the world. The Binet-Simon test became such an important measure of intelligence that it was revised and adapted by researchers all over the world. The most famous revision of the test was undertaken by Lewis Terman in the USA. The test became well-known as Stanford-Binet. During World War I, group tests such as Army Alpha and Army Beta were developed to screen army recruits. During World War II, another group test, Army General Classification Test (AGCT), was developed. Later, David Wechsler in 1939 developed Wechsler Adult Intelligence Scale (WAIS), in 1955, Wechsler Intelligence Scale for Children (WISC), and in 1967, Wechsler Preschool and Primary Scale of Intelligence (WPPSI). Wechsler tests have been revised several times. Today, Wechsler tests (WAIS-III and WISC-IV) are the widely used individual tests of intelligence in the USA and other English-speaking nations.

Early psychologists spoke more about intelligence tests than about intelligence. Understanding of the nature of intelligence came later, especially from factor theorists. One of the earliest factor theories of intelligence was proposed by Charles Edward Spearman of London University. His two-factor theory stated that intelligence was made up of one general factor (g) that partakes in all the tests and a specific factor (s) that was specific to each test. Later, g was found to be made up of several factors. Thurstone proposed a set of seven primary mental abilities (verbal comprehension, word fluency, numerical ability, memory, reasoning, spatial relations, and perceptual speed). Cattell introduced the concepts of fluid and crystallized

Contd...

Contd...

intelligence and Guilford came out with a model of intellect consisting of 120 factors. After reanalyzing the available test data, Carroll proposed a three-stratum model of intellect in which there was 'g' at the top, several broad abilities at the second level and a number of specific cognitive, perceptual, speed tasks at the third level.

Cognitive theorists like Robert Sternberg suggested a triarchic theory of intelligence that focused on the cognitive processes that underlie intelligence. Sternberg believes that there are three types of intelligence: analytical intelligence involving academically oriented problem-solving skills, practical intelligence that deals with day-to-day problems and creative intelligence that aims at finding novel ways of adapting to life. Recently, Harvard psychologist Howard Gardner suggested that there may be more than one type of intelligence. His multiple intelligences include linguistic intelligence (ability to use language), logical-mathematical intelligence (ability to think logically), visuospatial intelligence (ability to deal with spatial problems as in architecture), musical intelligence (ability to understand and produce music), bodily-kinesthetic intelligence (ability to make skillful body movements as in dance or surgery), interpersonal intelligence (ability to understand and relate with people), intrapersonal intelligence (ability to understand oneself), naturalistic intelligence (ability to understand the natural world) and existential intelligence (ability to deal with philosophical problems dealing with life and death). In recent times, researchers have introduced the concept of emotional intelligence as the ability to read and respond appropriately to other's emotions, and to be aware of and control one's own emotions.

Psychologists are extremely careful in developing tests to measure any human attribute including intelligence. Three important standards for psychological tests that psychologists emphasize are reliability (consistency of measurement over time, within tests and across scorers), validity (the extent to which the test measures the intended attribute) and standardization (development of standard procedures of administration, scoring, and norms). There are innumerable varieties of psychological tests that are in use today. In addition to assessing intelligence, psychologists have developed tests to measure aptitudes, achievement, attitudes, interests and personality among others. Psychological testing has become a billion dollar industry in the United States and among other developed and developing countries. Today, there are thousands of tests to measure all conceivable forms of human attributes.

Intelligence is distributed normally in the general population. Some people are brilliant (gifted), some are dull (mentally retarded) and most are average. The top one to two percent of people in the general population having an IQ of 130 or more is classed as gifted. The bottom 2 to 5 percent of people are branded as mentally retarded. All gifted children may not attain eminence. Only those who have had special educational opportunities make a mark in life. Unless given special social and educational support, the intellectually disadvantaged children may not survive in the competitive society. Intervention introduced early in life will have positive effects. They have little effect when applied later in life.

Although the differences are not large, men as a group tend to score higher than women in certain spatial and mathematical reasoning tasks. Women perform better in verbal fluency, arithmetic calculations and fine motor coordination. Group differences in intelligence have been well documented. Consistent differences between whites and nonwhites and between white Americans and Asian Americans have been reported. Whether these differences are due to biological factors or environmental influences is being debated. Differences in intelligence among individuals may arise due to genetics or due to upbringing. Recent evidence suggests that the brains of intelligent people function more efficiently. Researchers attribute about 50 percent variability in IQ test scores to genetics. But it has not been possible to sort out accurately the relative contributions of nature and nurture to differences in intelligence. In all probability, heredity establishes a reaction range with upper and lower limits for intellectual potential and environment affects the point within that range that will be reached. Intensive, early training may increase IQ scores but not very much. Intelligence test scores generally have been increasing with passage of time (Flynn effect), probably because of the challenges posed by complex issues in contemporary society. People today are taught new strategies of decision-making, problem solving and remembering information, all of which may have contributed to the apparent increase in the ability. The operation of Rosenthal effect may not be ruled out in assessing intellectual functions.

9 CHAPTER

Motivation

PREVIEW

All living beings, including humans, are always active, doing something or the other. Sheela is busy preparing for an entrance examination to get a seat in a medical college. Gowri feels lonely and searching for a companion. Krishna is working hard to get elected to a post in his college union. Mary is planning to get married. Ram is doing all that is possible to get relief from the severe headache. Your friend may be working hard to get a promotion in his organization. Another person may be going to a restaurant to eat his favorite dish. There may be a person planning to burgle a house, to snatch a chain from a pedestrian or even to murder someone, whom he does not like. The list can be endless. All these people are engaged in doing something and trying to reach a goal; in short, they are behaving. These examples show that behavior is driven by some needs, wishes and desires. People are being pulled toward certain goals. We need a term to refer to these driving or pulling forces. The term is motivation. Why do people engage in activities (or behave) like these? Where do the organisms get the energy to engage in these activities? Both the questions are answered by psychologists using the term motivation. Then, what is motivation?

It is difficult to deal with the subject matter of psychology without understanding the concept of motivation. Motivation is an internal psychological state that alerts and energizes organisms to do something, or directs them toward a goal. The motivated organism is in a state of readiness to act and its behavior is focused toward an end or goal. The organism desires to do something and often it is actually driven to do so. Without this central concept of motivation, the study of psychology becomes meaningless. Motivation tells us why an organism behaves the way it does. Take your own example. Why are you studying? Why did you choose to become a nurse? Why do you earn money? Why do you eat? Why do you get married? Why do you raise children? In short, why do you behave the way you do? Psychologists assume that you do all these because you are motivated to do so. As you can see, there are several kinds of motives. Some of them are triggered by internal conditions such as hunger, thirst, sex, avoidance of pain, etc. Organisms are driven or pushed by them and these are biologically based motives that are common to all living beings. These are often called "push motivations". On the other hand, there are certain motives that are unique to humans, such as the need to achieve, the need to affiliate, the need for power, etc. These occur in the psychosocial context and hence are called social motives or psychological motives. Sometimes certain properties of external stimuli pull us toward them. The color of a garment in the showcase of a shop or the aroma of the dish in a sweet meat stall may pull you toward them; if you had not noticed them you would not have bothered about them. When you see them, they pull you toward them; you develop a desire to possess them, have them. These are called the "pull motivations". Motives are internal states; they are not directly observed; they are inferred from behavior. They are inferred from what people say and do. Living organisms are always engaged in some activity or the other. The energy for doing these things is assumed to come from motives. Can there be activity in the absence of energy? Can there be any behavior that is devoid of a purpose? That is why motives are called energizers of behavior, dynamics of behavior, the causes of behavior or simply, "the why of behavior."

In this chapter, we discuss the issues concerning the topic of motivation. We shall learn about the factors that energize and direct behavior of humans and animals. The study of motivation consists of identifying why people work to do the things they do. All of us are interested in questions such as Why do people choose particular goals for which they strive? Can individual differences in motivation account for behavior variability? Can we motivate people to behave in certain ways, such as stopping bad habits and cultivating good habits? Can we motivate people to do more work and produce more? A careful reading of the chapter will give you an idea why people behave the way they do, and more specifically, why you behave the way you do? Why do you work? Why you prefer some kind of food? Why you seek the company of some people, but not others? Why you choose to dress in certain ways? Read on; you may get an answer.

Chapter Outline

MEANING OF MOTIVATION

The term motivation, as it is generally used, refers to the causes of behavior. If psychology is the study of behavior, motivation is used to explain why we behave; that is the reason why motivation is often referred to as the "Why of behavior." Behavior is all that living organisms are engaged in doing during their lifetime. For example, we eat, we drink, we make love, we fight, we think, we help somebody who is in difficulty, we work, and we do innumerable other things; why do we do all these things? In short, why we act as we do? Psychologists try to answer these questions in terms of the concept of motivation. Used in this sense, motivation runs through the entire gamut of psychology, but there are also certain other aspects of behavior that are not governed by motivation; e.g. maturation. Therefore, psychologists have somewhat narrowed the scope of the term motivation to refer to those internal or external conditions that alert the individual, energize his/her behavior, direct it toward a goal and maintain the energy supply till the goal is reached. A motivated organism is active, focused toward a goal and acts more efficiently than the unmotivated one. The term motivation is derived from the Latin root *motivus*, which means a 'moving cause'. So, we can say that motives are the moving causes of behavior (the terms motivation and motive are used interchangeably). Motives direct living organisms to behave in a particular way, in a specific situation, at a particular time.

When we talk about motivation, it should be remembered that we are talking about a psychological construct developed to explain behavior; no one can directly observe a motive; the existence of a motive is inferred from what living beings do. In other words, motives are inferred from behavior. For example, think of a student who attends classes regularly, visits the library often, discusses what he has studied with teachers, peers, and at home, he/she studies day and night. When we observe these patterns of behavior, we infer that the student is motivated to achieve a good grade in the coming examination. For that matter, all most all of our day-to-day behaviors are explained in terms of motivation. That is why psychologists who study personality give so much importance to the concept of motivation. Understanding of motivation helps us to predict behavior. If we can infer correctly why a person is doing what he is doing, it is possible to say what he/she will do in the future under a set of given conditions. An individual, who works hard to achieve success in his chosen field (in school, in business, in play and in many other situations) is driven by the **achievement motive**. One who is interested in people (friendship, companionship, etc.) is under the grip of **affiliation motive**. A politician, who strives hard to seek position and power, is driven by **power motive**. These three motives, **need for achievement (nAch), need for affiliation (nAff), and need for power (nPow)** have been extensively studied by an American psychologist David McClelland. In short, motives help us to predict what an individual will do in different situations.

Although the above description of the term motivation appears quite reasonable, the status of the concept is not at all that clear; several psychologists do not agree with this description. Some researchers assert that the term motivation could be used to account for the energizing aspects of behavior. But determiners of the direction of behavior, they aver, are cognitive factors. Some even argue that the concept of motivation is unnecessary and could be dispensed with altogether. In fact, as of today, there is no single widely accepted theory of motivation that can explain all behavior. There are biological motives, such as hunger, thirst and sex; there are learned motives such as earning money, seeking a promotion and aspiring for name and fame. Motives may be triggered by internal forces (hunger) or challenges from the external world (climbing the Everest); they may be determined by the current state of affairs or by future expectations. In order to understand and clarify some of these controversies about motivation, it is necessary to examine the various approaches to the study of the concept of motivation that have emerged over the years.

THEORIES OF MOTIVATION

The term motivation was not in use within psychology until the beginning of the 20th century. Philosophers, especially rationalists among them, thought that humans are rational beings; they are endowed with intellect and a free will; they are free to choose their course of action, and hence the concept of motivation has no place in the determination of human behavior. Reasoning for them was the important determinant of human action. Whether man's actions are good or bad depends on his intellect and training, and the person alone is responsible for his/her behavior. As opposed to rationalism, there was the mechanistic viewpoint. According to this view, some of the actions of individuals are impelled by internal or external forces over which the individual has no control. For example, most of our behavior is directed by our desire to seek pleasure and avoid pain, a view called *hedonism*. Whatever the explanations given for behavior, ultimately, pleasure seeking and pain avoidance are the two basic tendencies that are at the root of most of behavior. The hedonistic view is still prevalent in several of the contemporary theories of motivation. One of the most prominent theories holding this mechanistic viewpoint is the instinct theory.

Instinct Theories

Instinct (often called *fixed action pattern*) is an inherited biological tendency that predisposes organisms to behave in certain ways that are unalterable. Some birds and fish migrate to certain places only at certain times to lay eggs; birds and wasps build their nests in specific ways, and spiders weave fixed kinds of web only. These are instinctive behaviors. Instinctive behaviors are inherited, biologically determined and not products of learning. Instincts cannot be modified. According to instinct theorists, humans and animals are genetically programmed to behave in certain ways, which are essential for their survival. Instincts energize and direct behavior to run in appropriate channels. Early philosophers thought that animals have no souls and hence their behavior was governed by instincts, but humans have souls, they are rational and capable of reasoning. They can decide and choose what they want because they have free will. But with the advent of Darwin's theory of evolution, which suggested that there was no big gap between humans and animals, people started explaining human behavior in terms of instincts.

The most vociferous proponent of the instinct theory was the British psychologist William McDougall. He asserted that instincts are the prime movers of human behavior and believed that human nature never changes. McDougall (1908) maintained that all our behaviors and thoughts are guided by instincts and postulated a list of about 18 instincts, which included food seeking, reproduction, pugnacity, flight, gregariousness, self-assertion, self-submission and curiosity. McDougall's theory fell into disrepute because of several difficulties. There was a huge controversy over the nature and number of instincts. One sociologist, Bernard, claimed that there were about 5,759 instincts. It is possible that a significant portion of animal behavior is instinctive, but human behavior is remarkably flexible and a good deal of it is acquired. Because of these and other shortcomings, instinct theories were replaced by newer conceptions of motivation. However, the concept of instinct has not completely disappeared from psychology. In modern times, ethologists (such as Konrad Lorenz & Nikolaas Tinbergen who studied animal behavior in their natural habitat, and were recipients of the Nobel Prize for their work), sociobiologists and evolutionary psychologists have revived interest in instincts.

Drive Theories

Some psychologists, who were dissatisfied with instincts, proposed that behavior was directed by certain drives. A **drive** is an aroused state of an organism resulting from certain bodily needs such as the need for food, water, sex, oxygen and avoidance of pain. The aroused condition drives an organism to engage in appropriate behaviors that satisfy the need. For example, lack of food produces certain chemical changes in the body, indicating a need for food, which in turn creates a drive state of arousal and tension. Now the organism seeks to reduce this drive by engaging in certain activities that reduces the need. An important drive theory of motivation was proposed by Clark Hull in 1943, which is well known in psychology as **drive-reduction theory**.

Before we proceed further, it is necessary to clarify the difference between the terms *"drive"* and *"need."* The need refers to the physiological state of tissue deprivation whereas drive refers to its psychological representation in the consciousness. Thus, a drive is the consequence of the need. Drives and needs are parallel, but not identical. An increase in the need may not necessarily produce an increase in the drive. For example, after prolonged starvation, an organism may be so weakened that its drive-strength is reduced. When one is fasting for long duration, the feeling of hunger comes and goes, but the need for food persists.

The drive, like instinct, is a hypothetical construct. We do not see a drive; we infer it from the behavior. Although drive is an inferred construct, it is amenable to manipulation in the laboratory. An animal that has been deprived of food behaves differently from those that are fed regularly. For example, a food-deprived rat runs rapidly in a maze to obtain food than a non-deprived one. We can infer from its behavior that the animal's drive-state (hunger) has been activated. Needs could be defined objectively and conditions could be specified for creating or eliminating them. As a result, the drive has turned out to be a more useful concept in psychological research than instinct. During the second quarter of the 20th century, innumerable studies were conducted by Hull & his associates to determine the relationship between drive-reduction and learning.

Homeostasis and Drive Theory

An important principle that is basic to drive concept is homeostasis. **Homeostasis** refers to the tendency of the body of a living organism to maintain an internal steady state; that is, the body strives to maintain a state of internal equilibrium. For example, your body temperature remains more or less constant irrespective of the changes in the environmental temperature. When it is hot outside, your body starts perspiring and the peripheral blood vessels dilate to let the heat escape, thus keeping your body temperature constant. When it is cold, the blood vessels on the body surface constrict in order to retain the warmth of the body and your body generates warmth by shivering. These are automatic mechanisms designed to keep body temperature within normal limits. There are several such mechanisms that help retain steady states in blood sugar concentration, the level of oxygen and carbon dioxide in the blood, water level in the cellular environment, etc. Probably, there are certain sensors in the body that detect these discrepancies and activate mechanisms to correct the imbalances. The concept of homeostasis, which was introduced by the American physiologist, Walter B Cannon in 1932 to explain the maintenance of physiological study states, turned out to be a very useful construct within psychology to explain several aspects of behavior. Today, researchers talk not only of maintenance of bodily steady states, but also of psychological steady states as well as sociological steady states. They have proposed several learned drives (learned drives are called **secondary drives** to distinguish them from biological, physiological or **primary drives**) such as anxiety, achievement, affiliation, power, etc., which are acquired and motivate people. When the physiological imbalance is corrected, drive reduction occurs and the motivated activities come to a halt. Many physiological imbalances are corrected automatically. But, often the automatic mechanisms are not enough to set right the imbalance in the organism and then the organism becomes aroused, and a drive is activated. Now, the organism itself has to do something to set right the situation; that is, it is motivated to restore the imbalance and reduce the drive. For example, an individual goes in search of food when the blood sugar level falls, which is experienced as hunger; he goes in search of water when there is dehydration. Similarly, psychological states of fear, anger, discomfort or anxiety can create a drive state and the person will be motivated to do something to reduce the tension. In short, drive theorists assert that physiological or psychological imbalance will motivate behavior designed to restore equilibrium.

Incentive Theory of Motivation

Drive theories may be called "push theories of motivation." During 1950s psychologists became disenchanted with the push theories and began showing interest in the "pull theories of motivation." Drive theories have completely overlooked the environmental instigators of behavior. Pull theorists argue that behavior is not only pushed by internal drives, but also pulled by external factors called incentives. An **incentive** is a valued object or goal that draws the individual toward it even in the absence of an internal drive. For example, look at an individual, who has had a full stomach after a satisfying dinner, moving toward delicious ice cream!

He is not hungry, but still he consumes the ice cream. Some animals that are well fed start eating when they see other animals eating. In a work-a-day world, motivation appears to be a matter of expected incentives, such as wages, bonuses, vacations and the like, rather than the drives and their reduction.

People generally approach positive incentives and avoid negative ones. Thus, an incentive may arouse the organism and direct behavior either toward or away from the goal object. Incentive theories suggest that motivation stems from the desire to obtain valued external objects and the need to strive to reach desirable goals and avoid undesirable goals or objects. But, incentive theory does not provide a complete explanation of motivation; there are instances where organisms try to fulfill needs even when incentives are not apparent. Therefore, it is fair to say that drives work in tandem with incentives. Drives and incentives do not contradict each other; they work together in motivating behavior. Motivation could be better understood as an interaction between attractive stimulus objects in the external environment and an inner physiological state of the organism.

Approach and Avoidance Motivation

Generally, we move toward certain things and away from others; we seek to maximize pleasure and minimize pain and we move toward rewards and avoid punishment. It is hypothesized that these two seemingly universal tendencies are mediated by two distinct neural systems in the brain. According to one neuroscientist (Jeffrey Gray, 1991), there is a **behavioral activation system (BAS)**, which is aroused by signals from rewarding objects and a **behavioral inhibition system (BIS)**, which responds to signals from potentially painful objects. Activation of BAS causes a person to move toward positive goals in anticipation of pleasure. The BAS also produces the emotions of hope, elation and happiness. The BIS causes the person to move away from potentially non-reinforcing, threatening stimuli in anticipation of pain and BIS is associated with the emotion of fear. Neuroscientists have been searching for specific brain sites underlying the pleasure-seeking and pain-avoiding behaviors. They believe that these mechanisms involve different brain regions and different neurotransmitter systems. Studies suggest that prefrontal area in the left hemisphere controls BAS and several structures in the limbic system and the right frontal lobe are involved in the functioning of BIS. These findings have to be confirmed before the neural underpinnings of the BAS and BIS are firmly established. The researches on BAS and BIS are important because they address the important distinction between approach and avoidance motivation and also because they help in the organization of the physiological, cognitive, and behavioral processes that underlie seeking pleasure and avoiding pain. BAS and BIS also show how motivation and emotion are tied together because the former is closely associated with seeking desired rewards and positive emotions and the latter with avoiding undesirable objects and negative emotions.

Arousal Theory of Motivation

Arousal is a common component of all motivational states. Psychologists like Berlyne have developed a theory of motivation around the concept of arousal. Just like homeostasis approach, which states that there is an optimal physiological condition, which the organism strives to maintain, the arousal theory asserts that the organism is motivated to behave in such a way as to maintain an optimal level of arousal. According to arousal theory of motivation, people try to maintain or increase a certain level of stimulation or activity. If the stimulation level is too high, we try to reduce it as suggested by the drive reduction model. But, when the stimulation level is too low, we try to increase it by seeking stimulation. So, it is postulated that there is a need to maintain an optimal level of arousal. People vary widely with regard to the level of arousal they seek out. There are some who are prone to search for exciting stimuli and situations. They are called "sensation seekers" by Zuckerman (1978), who has developed a test called the **Sensation-Seeking Scale** to assess the preferred level of arousal of people. According to Berlyne (1967), stimuli from the environment arouse all of us, and each of us has an optimal level of arousal, which we seek. Being at or near the optimal level of arousal is pleasurable; too high or too low level of arousal produces feelings of discomfort. Moderately novel and complex stimuli are good at producing an optimal, pleasurable level. These findings conform to what is now known as the **Yerkes-Dodson Law**, named after the two researchers who first described a similar principle. This law states that people perform best when they are at an intermediate level of arousal. Under-aroused conditions make people sluggish; over-aroused people cannot stay focused and attentive. When we are under-aroused, we become bored and seek additional stimulation. One difficulty with this theory is that there is no precise definition of levels of arousal and how they vary.

Cognitive Theory of Motivation

Cognitive theories of motivation suggest that motivation is a product of people's thoughts, expectation and goals, in short, cognitions. According to one cognitive theory of motivation, goal-directed behavior is jointly determined by the strength of the person's expectation that particular behaviors will lead to a goal and by the incentive value the individual attaches to that goal. The theory is represented in the form of an equation: *Motivation = Expectancy × Incentive value*. Cognitive theorists also distinguish between intrinsic motivation and extrinsic motivation. **Intrinsic motivation** implies that we engage in an activity for its own sake; we perform an activity because it is enjoyable in itself and not because we gain any concrete, tangible reward by doing so. On the other hand, **extrinsic motivation** implies that we do something for money, recognition, grade or some other concrete, tangible reward. For example, if you play tennis for pleasure, it is because intrinsic motivation; when you play for money, it is extrinsic motivation. Let us learn a bit more about the concept of intrinsic motivation.

Intrinsic Motivation

Psychologists use the term **intrinsic motivation** to describe behaviors that appear to be entirely self-motivated or self-determined. Behavior does not always have to be triggered by either external pulls or internal pushes. Often, our activities may be self-determined. We go for a long walk, hum a tune or engage in solving a crossword puzzle just for the fun of it. A child may spend lots of time coloring a picture. There is no biological urge to do so, nor is there an obvious external reward for such behaviors. Nobody pays you for solving the crossword puzzle nor are you biologically pushed from inside to do so. You do it just because you enjoy doing it. A surprising feature in this context is that when people are engaged in an intrinsically motivating act, providing them an external reward can actually lower their interest in the task. In one experiment (Lepper et al, 1973), preschool children who were naturally interested in drawing were asked to draw either for its own sake or for a reward. The children in the rewarded condition evinced less liking for drawing a week later. The reward apparently reduced the children's interest in drawing. Why? Probably people come to think that external rewards in a way are controlling their behavior. The children in the experiment may have felt that they are drawing for the sake of someone else and not because it was pleasing to do so. There is some truth in this argument. We play football, cricket or tennis for pleasure. When we start receiving huge amounts of money for playing, the game suffers! That is what is happening to certain games nowadays. But not all psychologists agree with this point of view. They argue that when you expect a reward for doing something, then the performance may not suffer. The negative effect of reward on intrinsic motivation may be related to expectation or promise of reward rather than the reward itself (Cameron and Pierce, 1994). The debate is still continuing.

Self-determination Theory of Motivation

While working on the concept of intrinsic motivation Edward Deci & Richard Ryan have proposed a theory called self-determination theory of motivation (Deci, 1975; Deci and Ryan, 1985; Ryan and Deci, 2000). This theory focuses on three fundamental psychological needs such as *Competence, autonomy* and *relatedness*. Competence refers to the need to master new challenges and to develop skills; this need encourages exploratory and growth-inducing behavior in such a way that the behavior becomes its own reward, that is, the behavior becomes intrinsically motivating. Autonomy represents the need for freedom and self-regulation rather than regulation by external factors; it leads to self-integration, feelings of personal control and self-actualization. Relatedness refers to the desire to develop meaningful bonds with others. It is proposed that people experience self-fulfillment when these three needs are satisfied. The importance of these three needs in human life has been well supported by research. The three needs appear to have independent and additive effects in producing positive consequences such as psychological health, happiness and satisfaction in occupation. In a way, self-determination theory of motivation attempts to provide support for the humanistic concept of self-actualization.

Psychoanalytic Theory of Motivation

Sigmund Freud in the context of his personality theory proposed two groups of instincts, life instincts (Eros) and death instincts (Thanatos), which he believed were the mainsprings of most of actions among humans. Although, there is little research to support Freud's dual-instinct model, the fact remains that sex (a derivative of life instinct) and aggression (a derivative death instinct) are the two major forces that drive most of human behavior. Another important aspect of Freud's theory is its emphasis on unconscious nature of motivation. He asserted that many of us are not aware of the origins of our motives. More than anything else, Freud's model of motivation stimulated a great deal of thinking and theorizing in this area.

Maslow's Hierarchical Theory

Abraham Maslow (1954) tried to provide a comprehensive model of motivation, which organized the human needs in the form of a hierarchy. The model can be conceptualized as a pyramid (Fig. 9.1) in which basic needs are at the bottom and the higher-order needs at the top.

The most basic needs are physiological needs, such as the need for food, water, sex, avoidance of pain and the like. When these needs are satisfied, the safety or security needs are awakened. These are needs for a safe and secure environment for the individual to live, a safe home, protection from hazards and crime. When these two sets of needs are satisfied, people start experiencing the need for love and belongingness. It is not enough if we eat, sleep, have sex and have a secure environment to live. We want to love people and belong to a group such as family and feel that we are wanted by people

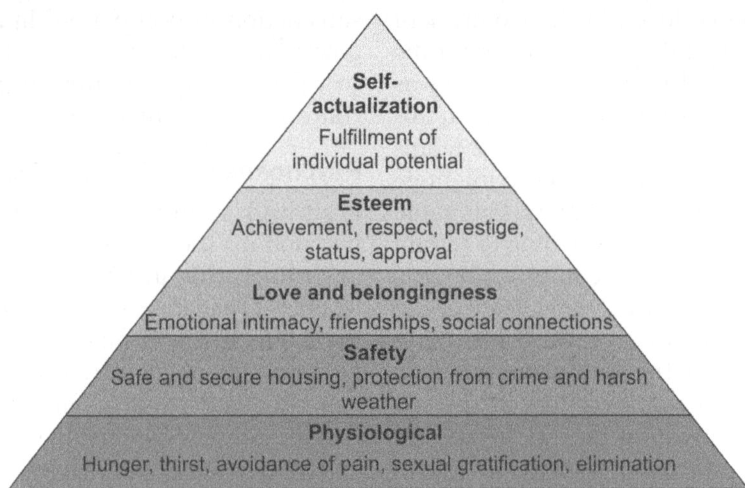

FIGURE 9.1: Maslow's hierarchy of needs

around us. When the need for love and belongingness are satisfied, the needs in the fourth level of hierarchy become operational. It is not enough if we love somebody and be loved in turn; we want to be recognized, admired and valued as worthy persons by others around us. These are called esteem needs. The third and fourth level needs in the hierarchy are called social needs. When all the four sets of needs are fulfilled, the individual begins to experience the highest need, the need for **self-actualization**. Self-actualization is a superior order need that is distinctly human; it refers to an urge to fulfill one's potentiality—a desire to become what one could become; it is the ultimate human motive. It motivates people to be emotionally mature, socially helpful and artistically creative and to live a meaningful life that is dedicated to the betterment of all people, not just themselves.

One of the characteristics of Maslow's hierarchy is that unless the lower order needs are satisfied, the higher ones will not become operative. Only when physiological needs are satisfied, the security needs are aroused; when security needs are satisfied, social needs emerge, so on and so forth. The final need to emerge in the hierarchy is the need for self-actualization. Maslow believed that people are so very much engaged in satisfying the lower-order needs (called deficiency needs) and they find little time to realize the higher-order needs (also called growth needs). He once said that deficiency needs *shout* and growth needs only *whisper*! Only rarely people approach self-actualization. People like Mahatma Gandhi, Abraham Lincoln, Albert Einstein & Mother Teresa, who made an enormous contributions to the betterment of humanity, qualify to be called self-actualized. Maslow belonged to a group of psychologists called humanistic theorists and made an extensive study of the personality characteristics of self-actualizers, which will be discussed in Chapter 12.

The validity of Maslow's theory of hierarchy of needs has been questioned by several critics. They have argued that the hierarchy breaks down in several occasions. For example, how do you explain the behavior of people who go on hunger strike to defend some valued principles? Why do some soldiers risk their lives to save a buddy? Does the need to know wait till the lower needs are satisfied? Has self-actualization any adaptive value? Critics say that the concept of self-actualization is vague and hard to measure. For some of them, the ordering of needs seems intuitive and arbitrary. Despite the criticisms, Maslow's theory has appealed to several researchers and has influenced thinkers in the fields of psychology, philosophy, education and business (Zinovieva, 2001).

MAJOR MOTIVES

The review of the different approaches to the study of motivation discussed above indicates the complexities of the concept. No one approach gives us a comprehensive view of motivation. The picture becomes still more complicated when we study the major motives, their origin and development. In the following section, we discuss some of the important motivational forces that have been the subject of extensive research both in physiology and psychology. Motives are generally grouped into two major categories such as biological motives and psychological motives. Biological or physiological needs such as hunger, thirst and sex are common to all living beings. Psychological needs such as need for achievement, affiliation, and power are secondary or learned needs and these are found among humans.

Biological Motives

The biological motives are largely rooted in the physiological state of the body. There are a number of biological needs such as hunger, thirst, sex, sleep, avoidance of pain, regulation of body temperature, and need for oxygen. As we have seen, most of these biological motives are triggered partly by the departures from the steady states of the body and the body automatically tends to maintain the steady states (homeostasis). Generally, the automatic physiological mechanisms that maintain homeostasis are supplemented by motivated behavior. For example, when the body does not get nutrients from food or fluid in the blood, the physiological processes may start conserving the substances that are lacking (such as seen in the **antidiuretic hormone** acting on the kidneys to reabsorb water when one is thirsty). This is not enough; sooner or later food and water must be obtained from outside. Thus, the biological motives are aroused largely by departure from the homeostatic equilibrium; the motivated behavior driven by the imbalances restores the equilibrium. Let us see how these mechanisms operate in three of the most important motives, namely, hunger, thirst and sex.

Hunger Motivation

Hunger is a universal motive. It is a primary, basic motive necessary for survival. The biochemical processes, which sustain life, get their energy and chemicals from food. Thus eating is a necessity; for many, it is also one of the cardinal pleasures of life. But, what is hunger? What triggers hunger motivation? What stops hunger? How is food intake regulated? In spite of advances in physiology, these simple questions have not yet been answered satisfactorily. Our eating behavior is not as simple as it appears; it is influenced by a number of factors. Numerous physiological, psychological and environmental factors regulate our food intake. Let us briefly examine some of these factors.

Physiology of hunger: Life is sustained by body's metabolism, the set of chemical events in each of our cells, events that convert food molecules into energy that enables the cells to function. Eating food is necessary to maintain our metabolism. Then, what are the factors that determine what and when we eat and when we stop eating? The mechanisms, which help us to know whether we require food or should stop eating, are complex. It is not just a matter of the empty stomach causing hunger pangs or a full one relieving hunger. Filling the stomach with salt water does not remove the feelings of hunger as much as filling it with milk. The stomach contains a mechanism that can detect the food value of its content and this information is fed into the brain. Even people whose stomachs have been surgically removed for medical reasons report hunger. One of the important factors which cause hunger is the change in the glucose level of blood. The glucose levels are monitored by the hypothalamus in the brain. Several years ago, researchers thought that they have discovered the "start" and "stop" eating centers in the **lateral hypothalamus (LH)** and the **ventromedial hypothalamus (VMH)** respectively. They reported that a very small lesion in the LH caused an animal to stop eating even when it is dying out of starvation. When the same structure was electrically stimulated, the animal ate 400 times more and worked hard to obtain food. In contrast, when VMH was stimulated, the animal thought its stomach was full and stopped eating. But recent researchers have found several difficulties in interpreting these findings. Lesions in the LH not only suppressed the animal's interest in eating, but also in drinking, sex and caring for the young; animals generally became sluggish. The lesions were disrupting neurons in the hypothalamus as well as the connections between other brain areas. Similarly, when VMH was damaged, the animals just did not stop eating; they became picky eaters and consumed more carbohydrates. Improved methods have suggested that hypothalamus works in coordination with several other brain centers in regulating hunger. When chemicals were used to destroy only neurons in the LH and none of the connections that go through it, hunger is reduced more than most other drives. When VMH is damaged, the animals keep on eating because the VMH appears to affect other brain centers that allow stored food molecules to be released. However, we have to go a long way before we fully understand the neural basis of hunger.

Psychosocial factors in hunger: Our habits, attitudes and psychological states also regulate eating behavior. You must have seen people in parties not consuming much even when there is a desire to eat more. Here, the feeling that "What others think of me when I eat more" is affecting the food consumption. Similarly, you have seen people moving toward ice cream or fruit salad even after consuming a full meal. Most of us are instructed in our homes not to leave food on the plate; therefore, we eat all that has been served even when it is nauseating to do so. While watching a television serial, we go on eating snacks without knowing what we are doing. When we are alone we eat less; we think about what and how much we ate during the last meal and adjust our food intake. When we are in a group we may eat "more" or "less" depending on the nature of the group, and what and how much other group members eat. When the group is large, meal takes longer to complete and there is enough time to eat more; sometimes, we eat less because we do not want to be considered gluttons. The figure-conscious women do not eat (some may even starve) well because of the fear of becoming fat; they want to remain slim and retain their curves. Dieting has become a fashion in several societies. There are countless other psychosocial pressures that either restrict or relax the desire to eat.

The taste and variety of food also regulate eating behavior. When the food is tasty we consume more of it. When there is no variety, when we eat the same stuff for lunch and dinner (as it happens in several of our hostels), we become bored and reduce food consumption. Remember, you are tempted to eat more at a buffet! Because of classical conditioning, we associate the smell and sight of food with taste; these sensory inputs trigger hunger. Eating may be the last thing in your mind until your nose detects the inviting aroma of hot *pakoda* or *bajji* in a fast food center!

Set point: Living beings, including humans settle on a particular body weight that is the easiest to maintain; this weight is referred to as the **set point**. For many years, researchers thought that the set point remains constant because of homeostatic mechanism. But nowadays, it is argued that the body does not maintain the set point automatically; it can change with the changes in an individual's environment, his/her activities and the emotional state. For example, when you are transferred to West Bengal, you may start eating rasgulla, which is the popular dish there and your body weight may increase. Often, the set point changes when you are engaged in hard work or exercise regularly, and when you are elated or depressed.

Obesity: We humans like tasty food and we eat more than what our body needs; the result is obesity. An obese person is defined as one who is more than 20 percent heavier than the medically recognized ideal weight for that person's age, sex and height. According to this definition, around 30 percent of people in developed countries are obese. But why do we eat more? It is argued that the cognitive system in the brain, which has connections with the hypothalamus, overpowers the latter (the hypothalamic system that regulates hunger) in influencing eating behavior. Thus, we eat more, not because we are hungry, but because we are lonely or bored or simply because it is time to eat. So, if one eats when the body does not need, he/she is overeating. When overeating is continued for a prolonged time, the number of fat cells in the body increases to store the additional fat and the person gains weight. On the other hand, when a person tries to lose weight, the fat cells decrease in size, but not in number. Therefore, remember, it is easy to gain weight, but not to lose it.

Several researchers implicate that some personality traits are associated with obesity. According to one view, obese people eat more when they are under stress and when they are aroused positively or negatively. But the results about this issue are not conclusive. The majority view holds that there are no personality differences between obese and non-obese people. Overeating is not the same as an eating disorder; people do not overeat because of psychological problems. Researchers believe that at least some forms of obesity have genetic basis. Over 200 genes have been identified as contributing to obesity. Some genes are hypothesized to affect appetite, some satiety, and some others metabolic rate. Among identical twins, if one is obese, chances are more that the other one also will be obese; the heritability has been estimated to be 70 percent. A gene called *"ob"* is believed to play a role in regulating eating behavior and weight control and this particular gene is assumed to be defective among the obese people. Yet another gene has been discovered that is hypothesized to determine whether the excess fat is converted into body fat or is turned into surplus body heat. It may take quite some time before these conjectures are verified and confirmed or even rejected. However, as genetics play an important role in obesity, so does the environment. Genes have not changed in recent times, but the number of obese people is increasing. This may be due to increased economic affluence, availability of inexpensive food items that are tasty and rich in fat and carbohydrates. Technological advances have made our lifestyle inactive, devoid of physical activity; so, we are becoming fat.

Dieting and losing weight: Dieting has become a fashion in modern society, especially among women. It often stems from social pressure to conform to cultural standards of beauty. There has been a trend to remain thin from 1950s to 1990s under the misconceived belief that *thin equals attractive*. Mass media messages, fashion modeling and beauty contests have all been emphasizing an unrealistic ideal female body shape. Surveys in Australia, China, America and other parts of the globe indicate that women of healthy body weight consider themselves as overweight. Compared with men, women are increasingly becoming dissatisfied with their body image. In general, women want to be thin; men who are overweight want to be thinner, but those who are thin want to be heavier. It is believed that what begins as diet may unfortunately evolve into a health-threatening eating disorder.

Does it mean that we should remain overweight? Definitely not. For millions of people who are overweight, being fat primes them to stay fat, in part by altering body chemistry and energy expenditure. Obese people have higher levels of insulin than do people of normal weight. Increased weight makes it harder to exercise vigorously. Therefore, dieting is necessary, although some say it is a losing battle. Diet experts suggest the following points to keep in mind when trying to lose weight:

1. *Exercise:* One medical expert has said that if exercise could be prescribed as a capsule, it would be the most sought after drug in the world. Exercise burns the fat stored in the body, which may help lose weight; it might lower the set point. It is recommended that people should engage in at least 30 minutes of moderate exercise 3 times a week. Walk briskly, climb the stairs or engage in some vigorous work. If nothing else, the endorphins released during exercise makes you feel better even if you do not lose weight.
2. *Beware of the calories:* Some foodstuff is loaded with calories. Try to avoid them. Instead of a fruit drink, eat the actual fruit itself or dilute the fruit juice with water.
3. *Develop good eating habits:* Limit (if not avoid) excessive fat foods; fatty foods can be dangerous to your health. Eat small quantities slowly; do not be tempted by desserts; do not eat in between meals. Eat at regular times and if possible in the same place. Do not yield to persuasive serving of food items.
4. *Set reasonable goals:* Decide how much weight you want to lose and proceed toward the goal gradually; do not try to lose too much weight too soon; you will be doomed to fail.
5. *Eat slowly:* It takes around 15 minutes for the brain to register that your stomach feels full; give it a chance to catch up with your stomach.
6. *Do not feel guilty:* If you do not succeed in losing weight, do not feel guilty. There are several people who have failed like you. Remember, you may be genetically predisposed to be obese.
7. *Remember, it is not easy to lose weight:* You may have to make permanent changes in your food habits, which may be difficult. Cut down the quantity of food gradually but have an eye on the nutrition value of your intake.

Eating disorders: There are two types of eating disorders, i.e. anorexia nervosa and bulimia nervosa. **Anorexia nervosa** is a severe eating disorder characterized by refusal to eat because of an intense fear of becoming fat. It is more prevalent among women who are overly concerned about their body weight. Many people become skeleton-like, but do not think that their appearance and behavior are unusual. Anorexia causes disturbances in the menstrual cycle (it may even stop menstruation) in women, constipation, gastrointestinal problems, bone loss, stress on the heart and even death. **Bulimia nervosa** is a peculiar disorder; it is characterized by *binge eating* (uncontrolled overeating) followed by purging of the food. About 90 percent of people suffering from these two disorders are women and the conditions are more prevalent among affluent, industrialized, and advanced countries, where thinness is equated with beauty. Eating disorders are far less common in non-Western countries. One reason may be that there is not enough food to eat or the emphasis on slimness is lacking. The complete explanation of anorexia and bulimia is still elusive. The disorders probably are caused by a combination of biological, psychological and sociocultural factors.

Thirst Motivation

Food and water are essential for our survival. We can go without food for several weeks, but we cannot survive without water for a few days. Maintenance of water level in the body is essential for survival. All organisms replenish water deficit in two ways, i.e. by recovering water from the kidneys before it is excreted as urine and by drinking water. The first is executed by the homeostatic mechanism and the second by motivating the organism to drink water. In the first case, water deficit sets off a homeostatic mechanism by stimulating the release of the **antidiuretic hormone (ADH)** from the pituitary gland. The ADH acts on the kidneys so that water is reabsorbed into the blood leaving concentrated urine. That is why urine appears colored after a long sleep, especially during summer. This process can maintain the body water level only up to a point. When the water deficit is too great, a need is created and the organism is driven to search for water.

Thirst motivation and drinking water are not as simple as they appear. A number of complicated activities are involved in water-intake behavior of which two are very important. Among others, water consumption is triggered by two conditions in the body such as loss of water from cells (cellular dehydration) and reduction in blood volume (hypovolemia). When there is water loss in the body, water is released from the cells leaving them dehydrated. Under such conditions, certain nerve cells in the anterior hypothalamus, called osmoreceptors, generate nerve impulses, which act as signals for thirst and drinking. Thirst triggered by osmoreceptors is called **cellular-dehydration thirst**. Drop in the blood volume is monitored by volumetric receptors. Loss of blood volume produces thirst even in the absence of cellular dehydration. When blood volume comes down (hypovolemia), blood pressure also drops. The drop in the blood pressure stimulates the kidneys to release an enzyme called *renin*. Renin is involved in the production of a substance called *angiotensin II* that circulates in the blood and this hormone is hypothesized to trigger the thirst (there is no unanimity of opinion about the role of this hormone in drinking). The idea that cellular dehydration and hypovolemia cause thirst is often called **double depletion hypothesis**.

Thirst or drinking water is more complicated than what is said above and appears to be under the control of several other mechanisms. Experiments with animals have demonstrated that receptors in the mouth and throat also play a role in the regulation of water consumption. For example, in an experiment, dogs were fitted surgically with a plastic tube in such a way that the water consumed is drained out of the body. The dogs could drink water normally, but the water does not get into the stomach; it is simply drained out. Under such conditions, the dogs drank their usual amount of water and then stopped as though satisfied by the fluid that never entered their stomach. After about 10 minutes, the dogs began drinking the same amount of water. This cycle continued with dogs gradually increasing their water intake as the water deficit builds up. This shows that there are some receptors in the mouth and throat that measure the water intake, because the animals stopped drinking after swallowing its usual amount. After a few minutes, however, the body realizes that it has been duped and starts sending other signals (from osmoreceptors and volumetric receptors) that motivate the animals to consume water. In another experiment, water was directly placed in the stomach using a tube through the mouth and throat. In spite of the presence of enough fluid in the body, the animals drank water. After 5-, 10- or 15-minute delay, the water intake gradually decreased and after 20 minutes water consumption stopped. These experiments indicate that a certain amount of water must be absorbed through the stomach wall into the blood stream before the mechanism that responds to water intake is activated.

Sexual Motivation

Why do people crave for sex? You may think that the answer is obvious. But, science asserts that sexual behavior is not that simple. Generally, it is believed that people engage in sex to have babies and for obtaining sensual pleasure. The description of sex as a biological reproductive motive does not explain why people masturbate or why couples in their 70s and 80s have sex. Even when the sexual motivation is considered from a biological angle, it has certain characteristics that differentiate it from other biological drives. First, sex is not necessary for survival of an individual. Sex deprivation does not cause death; sex is not necessary for self-survival, although it is necessary for the survival of the species. Second, sexual drive is not triggered by a lack of any substance in the body as in the case of hunger or thirst; there is no demonstrable tissue need. Third, in higher animals at least, sexual drive is perhaps more under the control of sensory information (mostly visual) from the environment than are other biological drives.

If you think that sex is only for pleasure, you are correct only partially. A vast majority of people (about 98%) have sex for pleasure, as opposed to procreation. Sex leads us to one of the most pleasurable experiences. Evolution has shaped our body in such a way that having sex feels good; we can have sensual pleasure and also children to carry our genes and perpetuate our species. But, consider the following findings:

- In one study, when teenagers were asked why they have sex, both boys and girls reported that they have sex because of peer pressure rather than for pleasure (Stark, 1989)
- In the 1920s, one British sex researcher Helena Wright found that most women she surveyed, viering sex as an unenjoyable marital duty (Kelly, 2001)
- According to Laumann et al (1994), 10 percent of American men and 20 percent of American women consider sex as not at all pleasurable.

So, people have sex for different reasons; for reproductive purposes, for obtaining and giving sensual pleasure, for expressing love and affection, for fostering intimacy, for fulfilling a duty, because of peer pressure and for a host of other reasons.

Research on sexual behavior: Although sex is an important aspect of human life, it is unfortunate that authentic information about sexual behavior based on scientific research is few and far between. Naturally conducting research on sex is not easy. As you know, nobody permits a behavior scientist into his/her bedroom to conduct research on sex. In spite of the difficulties, it is noteworthy some groundbreaking researches on sex were undertaken in the 20th century. The most frequently used research method in this area is survey. Survey is not a reliable method for collection of information for several reasons. For one thing, not many people volunteer to participate in such surveys; secondly, those who participate may not answer questions posed truthfully. *Sampling bias* and *response bias* make survey data about sex suspect. Still survey method is a popular tool for obtaining information about human sexual behavior.

The first major attempt to survey sexual behavior was launched in the USA by a biologist, Alfred Kinsey, during the late 1930s. The result was the publication of two monumental volumes, highlighting the sexual practices of American men and women, namely; *Sexual Behavior in the Human Male* (1948) and *Sexual Behavior in the Human Female* (1953). Kinsey & his coworkers interviewed thousands of individuals and elicited sensitive information about their sex lives without causing embarrassment. The researchers found that people engage in a variety of sexual activities (apart from heterosexual ones), which were generally considered rare or even abnormal. It was reported that people masturbate, daydream about sex and even have sexual contact with animals. There was a public furore when Kinsey published his work. He was branded as an immoral pervert. A congressional committee charged him with undermining the nation's moral fiber. Scientists criticized him for several procedural shortcomings (such as biased sampling). Despite the criticisms, the fact remains that Kinsey's work set the stage for later surveys. One of the most comprehensive surveys, based on a representative sample conducted by a group of researchers (Michael et al, 1994), sheds light on the sexual behavior of contemporary Americans. This and other surveys have reported reliable information about the frequency of sex acts, prevalence of premarital sex and deviant forms of sexual behavior. In one survey, 41 percent of boys and 29 percent of girls said that they had sex by the first year in American high school. The incidence of premarital sex among 19-year-old girls was 19 percent in 1960; it rose to 72 percent by 1995. The frequency of premarital sex has been increasing in several other countries during the second half of the 20th century. Changing social values and the tendency to delay marriage are the reasons given for this trend. However, some recent surveys indicate a decline in the unbridled sex practices probably because of the fear of acquired immune deficiency syndrome (AIDS) and an increasing social emphasis on depth of relationship.

Physiology of sex: In 1953, William Masters and Virginia Johnson made a landmark study of the actual sexual behavior of men and women under laboratory conditions. They monitored several thousands of sexual episodes and measured what goes on in the body during sexual intercourse. The outcome was a description in detail of the happenings within the human body, which has now become famous as the **sexual response cycle** (Masters and Johnson, 1966). According to these researchers, most people, when engaged in intercourse, go through a four-stage sexual response cycle, which includes *excitement*, *plateau*, *orgasm* and *resolution*. These stages merge into one another with no sharp dividing lines. There are obvious gender differences in how the human body responds to sexual stimulation during these phases. During the excitement phase, there is penile erection in men and vaginal lubrication in women, which are caused by vasocongestion (pooling of blood in bodily tissues). In the plateau phase which precedes orgasm, sexual arousal "plateaus" at a fairly high, but stable level. Orgasm is a reflex action. During orgasm phase, rhythmic contractions in the pelvic muscles occur resulting in a release of sexual tension and feelings of intense pleasure. The resolution phase follows orgasm. The body now returns to its prearousal state. The resolution phase is characterized by an important gender difference. Unlike women, men enter a *refractory period* during which they are incapable of another ejaculation or orgasm. The refractory period may last a few minutes among adolescent males, but it may last a few minutes to a day among men aged fifty and above. Women do not experience a refractory period. With continued stimulation they are capable of becoming quickly re-aroused to the point of multiple orgasms. The huge amount of research conducted by Masters & Johnson led them to the following conclusions:

- The bodily reactions of men and women are mostly similar during sex
- Women generally respond more slowly than men, but remain aroused for longer duration
- Women can have multiple orgasms, whereas men cannot engage in sex immediately after orgasm; they go through a period of sexual inactivity, called the refractory period, during which they cannot be sexually aroused
- The size of the male sexual organ has no relation to sexual performance (as reported by women), unless the man is worried about it.

The role of hormones on sexual behavior: Sex hormones play an important role in sexual motivation. They not only activate sexual desire and behavior during adulthood, but also influence development of sexual characteristics during the prenatal period. Hypothalamus plays a significant role in the secretion of sex hormones. It controls the pituitary gland, which regulates the secretion gonadotropins. Gonadotropins are hormones that regulate the rate at which **gonads** secrete sex hormones. Testes in the males and the ovaries in the females are called gonads. Testes secrete **androgens**, the male sex hormones such as testosterone and ovaries secrete **estrogens** such as *estradiol* (one of the most important estrogens). It must be remembered that both men and women produce both androgens and estrogens, but to different degrees.

In a genetically male embryo, testes are formed around the 8th week after conception. The sex hormones produced by the testes during this critical period are sufficient to produce a male pattern of development (genital and reproductive organs as well as the brain). When the male reaches puberty, the hypothalamus stimulates an increased release of sex hormones from the testes, which determines male sexual characteristics and activities. In the genetically female embryo, the absence of sufficient androgen activity during the prenatal period causes the female pattern of development. At puberty, the hypothalamus stimulates the release of sex hormones from the ovaries in a cyclical manner that regulates the female menstrual cycle. The secondary sex characteristics in men such as growth of body hair, pitch of voice and shape and structure of the body are determined by androgens. Similarly, feminine sex characteristics such as growth of breasts and voice are controlled by estrogens. These processes are often called organizational effects of sex hormones.

Stimulation of sexual desire and behavior by the sex hormones is called activational effect. Among mature non-human males, the secretion of sex hormones remains relatively constant and their sexual readiness largely depends upon the external stimuli such as a receptive female. But in females, hormonal secretion follows an *estrus cycle*, and they are receptive to sex only during ovulation—the period during which there is an increased estrogen production (that is, when they are in heat). Humans are different in this aspect; normal short-term hormonal fluctuations have relatively little effect on human sexual behavior. Females can be receptive to sex throughout their cycles depending on the external stimuli and men are ready most of the time. Although biological factors are important, it takes more than hormones to motivate sexual behavior among human beings. Humans are very versatile; not only a receptive partner, but nearly any object, sight, smell, sound, or other stimuli can lead to sexual excitement among humans. Hormonally-ready humans are aroused by the "look" of the other sex people, their voice, style, dress and odor or simply what they say. In short, much of sexual behavior is turned on by external stimuli. Learning plays an important role in sexual arousal and expression among humans. The arousing stimuli may be different for different people.

Sexual stimuli: Although hormones play a dominant role in sexual arousal, they do not tell the whole story. Human sexuality is a very complex phenomenon. Sensory stimulation, especially touch, vision and smell trigger and sustain sexual motivation. Freud once said that the skin is the erotic organ par excellence. Do not be surprised if you are told that the "major human sex organ is the *brain*" and the resulting conscious experience. Much of what is considered sexually arousing for humans has little or nothing to do with their genitalia, but instead is related to external stimuli, which through a process of learning have come to be recognized as erotic or sexually arousing. The cognitive process and the interpretation given to the stimulus are important. For example, although touching is a very important component of sex, its arousing value depends on who is touching and when. When a physician touches the breasts or the genitalia of a female patient, there will be no arousal; but when her lover or husband touches the same spot, she will be sexually aroused. In both instances, the information sent to the brain is the same. It is the interpretation the brain gives to the nerve impulses reaching it that makes it either sexual or otherwise.

Vision is the most important sense modality among human beings. About half of the cerebral cortex is engaged in processing visual stimuli. These stimuli play a dominant role in arousing sexual motivation, especially among men. When men and women were shown sexually stimulating video pictures, they were found to respond differently. Brain scanning studies have shown that erotic visual stimuli activated the hypothalamus only in men and not in women. The degree of arousal (the desire for sex) was directly proportional to the intensity of hypothalamic arousal. When visual stimuli did arouse women, they did so differently than in men. Women were found to be aroused by both male and female sexual stimuli. In contrast, men were aroused by female sexual stimuli only. A recent report says that the male brain is wired in such a way that men cannot help looking at attractive women; it may not mean that they will go after them; just they cannot help looking at them. Biologically men are predisposed to look at women. It is reported that when men look at women, more than 40 percent of them look at the breast of women. The tendency for visual stimuli to be less important in sexual arousal among women is reported to be more due to cultural factors rather than their lack of interest in male figure.

Psychosocial factors influencing sexual behavior: By now it must be clear that sexual arousal involves more than physiology. Psychological factors play a dominant role in the arousal and initiation of sexual behavior. Sex begins with a desire and an attractive stimulus. The stimuli may be real or imaginary. Sexual fantasy is an important component of sexual arousal, especially among men than women. Fantasy illustrates how psychological factors influence physiology of sex. Studies have shown that half of American men and a fifth of women fantasize about sex at least once a day. Sexual fantasy alone can trigger sexual arousal and even orgasm in some individuals. People are found to engage in fantasizing not only during masturbation, but also during intercourse. The kind of fantasies that men and women have (among American college students) during coitus are found to be more or less similar. Interestingly, such fantasies often include having sex with someone other than one's partner of the moment. However, it is important to note that having a particular fantasy may not mean that one has an inclination to fulfill it in the real world.

Psychological factors may also inhibit sexual behavior. A person engaged in sexual activity may terminate it when the partner says or does something silly. You may be surprised when told that there are several people who are just not interested in sex, but it is true. Some people desire sex, but are afraid of engaging in it. Others have difficulty in becoming or staying aroused. Arousal difficulty may emerge from performance anxiety or it may be a psychological consequence of sexual abuse during childhood or sexual assault in later life. Disease, injury, stress, fatigue, drugs and anger at one's partner may turn off the sexual desire at least temporarily.

Social and cultural factors determine sexual motivation in several ways; sometimes what appear to be erotic stimuli are dictated by sociocultural norms. For example, in many societies breast size is often the standard by which males estimate female appeal, but in several other cultures breast size is irrelevant. In some societies, women are found to poke a finger into their partners' ear during sex, or bite off and then spit out hairs from their partner's eyebrow; in some other societies kissing is unknown. In fact, the psychological meaning of sex itself is dictated by culture. In several religious societies, premarital sex is forbidden; sex for anything other than procreation is frowned upon. In many societies clotting that are sexually revealing are not permitted. In contrast, there are some societies where women dress scantily. Some societies openly encourage premarital sex. Clearly, what is regarded as sexually right, desirable and moral varies from one culture to other.

Complexity of sexual behavior: Human sexual behaviors—what triggers sex, the choice of partners, varieties of sexual practices, and sociocultural determinants of sexual drive—are so complex that several books have been written about the subject. The major factors that affect human sexual activity are many and varied. The most important ones are anatomy and physiology of the participants, their age, race, culture and religion, the law of the land, which they inhabit and their educational and socioeconomic status. People also vary with regard to their *sexual orientation*; they may be heterosexuals, homosexuals or **bisexuals**. Heterosexuality refers to sexual gratification with members of opposite sex; homosexuals prefer members of the same sex; and bisexuals are attracted toward members of both sexes. You may probably know that homosexuality was considered abnormal till recently. But, nowadays *gay marriage* (between two men) and *lesbian marriage* (between two women) are tolerated in several societies. There are several theories about sexual orientation. One theory proposes that male homosexuals come from families in which mother is dominant and father ineffectual. Another theory hypothesizes that male homosexuals and heterosexuals differ in their adult levels of sex hormones. Some researchers report that there are anatomical differences in the brains of homosexuals and heterosexuals. Many of these theories have taken a scientific beating. But there is growing evidence that heredity influences sexual orientation. It appears that biological predisposition combines with socialization processes in determining sexual orientation.

Atypical sexual behaviors: Several people derive sexual gratification through deviant means. These are called **paraphilias**. **Masturbation** (solitary sex) was once considered a mental disorder; it is now known that a majority of people engage in this form of sexual outlet and it is considered normal. Oral sex, which was once considered obscene, is being practiced today as a preferred mode of sexual practice. Several atypical sexual behaviors such as **pedophilia** (having sex with children), **exhibitionism** (exposing one's genitals), **fetishism** (deriving sexual arousal and gratification with some object that is generally not considered erotic), **transvestism** (deriving sexual satisfaction by cross-dressing), **voyeurism** (sexual arousal by clandestine observing of others when they are undressing, nude or engaged in intercourse) and **bestiality** (sexual contact with animals) are prevalent in contemporary society.

Attitudes toward sex have been changing rapidly all over the world in recent times. Sexual liberation and availability of effective birth control measures have increased premarital sex and led to the so-called "free sex" movement during the 1960s in the US. It is reported that over one half of women between the ages 15 and 19 have had premarital sexual experience. The trend recently has been toward more women engaging in premarital sex. Males are also having premarital sex, but the increase has not been as dramatic as for females because it is already high among males. But, with the spread of AIDS and the resurgence of fundamentalist religious attitudes, sexual behavior is changing. People are becoming more careful; it is a good sign. Cultural influence on sexual behavior appears to be very strong; it clearly determines how, when and where one should indulge in sex.

Psychological Motives

Several powerful motivational states that are not rooted in biology operate as wellsprings of human behavior; these are called psychological motives, learned motives, secondary motives or social motives. These are called social motives because they are acquired in the social context, especially in the family as children grow up and also because they generally involve other people. A long list of social motives (also called needs) was proposed by Henry Murray long ago in 1938. He has distinguished between primary (viscerogenic) needs and secondary (psychogenic) needs. Some of Murray's major needs are shown in the Table 9.1.

Social motives are generally inferred from observing people's behavior, answers to questionnaires and projective tests such

Table 9.1: A Brief Description of Some of Murray's Needs

Motives	*Characteristics*
Abasement	Submitting passively to external force; accepting criticism, blame, punishment.
Achievement	Accomplishing something difficult; desire to master, manipulate or organize.
Affiliation	Trying to please others, winning their affection, enjoying their company.
Aggression	Overcoming opposition forcefully, wanting to attack, to fight and to punish.
Autonomy	Trying to be free, independent; removing restraints, resisting coercion and restriction.
Defendence	Defending oneself from attack, blame and criticism; justifying and vindicating oneself.
Deference	Admiring, praising, honoring, emulating, eulogizing and supporting superiors.
Dominance	Controlling and influencing the behavior of others; commanding and persuading.
Exhibition	Making an impression on others; wanting to be seen and heard.
Nurturance	Helping and taking care of those in distress such as infants, disabled and sick.
Order	Arranging things in order; keeping things clean, neat and tidy.
Play	Engaging in sports; enjoying leisure; acting for fun without further purpose.
Succorance	Desire to be nursed, supported, loved, protected, consoled and guided.
Understanding	Asking and answering general questions; theorizing and speculating.

as the Thematic Apperception Test (TAT). Researchers have proposed several other psychological motives such as the need for competency (Robert White), autonomy and self-esteem. David McClelland made in depth study of some of the major social needs, especially the need for achievement (nAch), the need for affiliation (nAff), and the need for power (nPow). Let us learn some information about the three McClelland's needs.

Achievement motivation: David McClelland, John Atkinson & their coworkers have studied **need for achievement (nAch)** in detail and their work is continuing even today by others. McClelland defined nAch as a positive desire to accomplish something in life and to compete with some standard of excellence. Achievement behavior may emerge from the positively oriented *need for success* and the negatively oriented need to avoid failure (or fear of failure). McClelland et al, (1953) inferred nAch from stories written by participants to TAT-like pictures. The stories were analyzed for achievement-relevant themes using a standardized procedure. For example, a person who writes a story in which the hero is seen as studying hard to get good grades in college, trying to beat an opponent in sports or working studiously to get a promotion in his office shows clear signs of achievement need. The fear of failure (avoidance motive) was assessed by psychological tests that asked participants to report how much anxiety they experienced when they were engaged in achievement tasks. The researchers found that nAch and fear of failure were independent (uncorrelated) dimensions and hence a person could be high in both, low in both or higher in one and low in the other.

People with high nAch strive to become accomplished in their chosen area and try to improve their task performance. They prefer to work on tasks that are challenging and on which their performance can be evaluated in some way against a standard. It may be in achieving high grades in college, earning more money in business, or achieving glory in sports. They tend to avoid situations that are easy (unchallenging) and also those in which success is unlikely; they are realistic and choose tasks of intermediate difficulty. They like tasks in which their performance can be compared with those of others. They like feedback on how they are progressing. They enjoy the thrill of victory. On the other hand, those motivated by fear of failure seek to avoid the pain of defeat. They choke under pressure. The anxiety associated with failure may negate the impact of need for achievement and can impair performance. They prefer tasks that are easy (where success is assured). People who exhibit high nAch and low fear of failure are often called *high need achievers*. When tasks are challenging and importance of good work is stressed, high-need achievers outshine *low need achievers*. Their performance is of high order; when they encounter obstacles in their path to success, they exhibit extraordinary skills in overcoming them.

Why people differ with regard to nAch? This need, as we know, is a social need and the answer may have to be sought in the developmental history of the person in the familial and social environment. Social needs—including nAch—are acquired (learned) by imitating the behavior of parents and other significant models. According to Albert Bandura, this is an instance of observational learning (modeling); children take on or adopt many characteristics of the model, including the nAch if the model possesses this motive to a marked degree. Parental expectations from their children can also influence the development of need for achievement. A cognitively stimulating family environment in which parents encourage and reward achievement, but do not punish failure, is the fertile ground for the growth of nAch. On the other hand, fear of failure seems to develop when parents take successful achievement for granted but punish failure, thereby inculcating in the child a dread of failing. Providing a mastery motivational climate in the home, the school and the sport field encourages the development of need for achievement.

Culture also shapes achievement need. In North America and much of Europe, individual achievement is given more importance. In countries like India, Japan and China collectivism is nurtured; in these countries, children care more about meeting parental expectations. In Japan, workers are encouraged to work for organizational improvement; the company looks after the employees welfare, promote them and retain them for life. Naturally, the workers are devoted to the organization and remain loyal to their managers.

Apart from all these factors, there appears to be an intrinsic human desire to achieve, which expresses itself in intriguing ways. Throughout history, we have seen people migrating to other countries seeking greener pastures. Studies have shown that people who expressed a desire to emigrate to other countries seeking better life had higher average achievement motivation scores than those who wanted to remain in their homeland. On the whole, studies suggest that achievement motivation is an important predictor of success in school, business and several other professions.

Need for affiliation: The second well-researched social motive is the need for affiliation (nAff). According to McClelland, those who are eager to establish, maintain and repair friendly relationships are exhibiting need for affiliation. Individuals with high nAff write TAT stories that emphasize the desire to make friendship and show concern when rejected by friends. People who exhibit high nAff are sensitive to interpersonal relationships; they desire to be with their friends most of the time. Abraham Maslow (1954) viewed love and belongingness as a basic psychological need. According to Baumeister & Leary (1995), desire for interpersonal attachment is a fundamental human motivation. They assert that "the need to belong is a powerful, fundamental and extremely pervasive motivation." Anthropologist Kottak (2000) states that people who affiliate are more likely to survive and reproduce compared with those who are reclusive. There is nothing surprising in these observations. We humans are social beings and we affiliate in many ways. According to McDougall, humans basically are gregarious animals. He believed that there is an instinct of gregariousness. Basically, we affiliate because it provides positive stimulation and emotional support; also, it permits **social comparison**. Social comparison involves comparing our beliefs, feelings and behaviors with those of other people. According to Festinger (1954), social comparison helps us to judge whether we are as good as others in our cognitive and physical abilities. Need for affiliation is not an all or none phenomenon; people with strong nAff sometimes desire to be alone. On the other hand, those with lower nAff may seek periodic social contacts. Therefore, some theorists suggest that for each of us there is an optimal range of social contact. When social contact exceeds that range, we compensate by temporarily seeking more solitude. When social contacts fall below that range, we increase our efforts to be with others. Researches have also found gender differences in the nAff. It appears that women spend more time with their friends and less time alone than men.

Many studies have shown that situational factors influence the tendency to affiliate. People tend to affiliate more under fearful situations. During earthquakes, floods and such other emergencies, people seek the company of others even when they are strangers. People seem to affiliate strongly with others who already have been through the same or similar conditions. For example, people waiting for open-heart surgery like to be with those who already had been through surgery, probably because it provides them with information about what to expect.

Mate selection as a form of affiliation: Seeking a mate is an important and intimate form of expressing affiliation need. People engage in seeking a mate for marriage, but they may also seek mates in other types of relationships, such as companionship. Researches in America have shown that men and women display different mating strategies and preferences. Men typically prefer younger women whereas women prefer somewhat older men than themselves. Men prefer physically attractive women with good domestic skills; on the other hand women place greater value on the mate's physical strength and economic status. One researcher states that women exchange their attractiveness in return for male's earning capacity. But with increase in gender equality these trends are changing. Nowadays, men do not mind marrying elderly women, and women may marry younger men. However, the fact that men value physical attractiveness more than women remains true.

Need for power: The need for power **(nPow)** refers to the human tendency to seek impact, control and influence over others coupled with a desire to be seen as powerful. DG Winter in his book; *The Power Motive* (1973) defines power as "the ability or capacity of a person to produce (consciously or unconsciously) intended effects on the behavior or emotions of another person." People with strong power motive exhibit the tendency to influence, control, persuade, lead others and try to enhance their own reputation in the eyes of other people. Simply put, they enjoy power. Need for power is also measured from the stories people write to TAT-like pictures; the degree of nPow is inferred from the story themes.

People who have high nPow are impulsive and aggressive, especially men coming from lower socioeconomic strata. They prefer to work for huge organizations and seek office of power; they join such organizations in which their nPow could be satisfied. Surprisingly, they also enter soft professions such as teaching, diplomacy or business believing that they can impact people. They associate with people who are not popular with others and who, perhaps, can be more easily controlled. They engage in collecting guns, credit cards, fancy cars, complicated electronic gadgets, and the like. There are some significant gender differences in the display of nPow. Men who have high need for power tend to be aggressive, drink heavily, act in a sexually exploitative manner and participate in competitive games; generally, they tend to exhibit extravagant, flamboyant behavior. On the other hand, women display nPow in a restrained manner. They channel their need for power in socially approved manner, by engaging in nurturing and welfare activities. Women with high nPow seem to engage in building and disciplining their bodies.

Self-actualization

Self-actualization (SA) refers to a powerful tendency among humans to develop, realize and fulfill their potentialities. In other words, it is an urge to become what one is capable of becoming. A good deal has been written about the concept of self-actualization by many psychologists, especially by three eminent personality theorists, Kurt Goldstein, Abraham Maslow & Carl Rogers. Goldstein, the well-known German-American neuropsychiatrist, asserted that self-actualization is the master motive. All other motives, whether biological or psychological, are merely manifestations of the sovereign purpose of life, to actualize oneself. When an individual is hungry, he satisfies himself by eating; when he craves for power, he actualizes himself by acquiring power. Thus, self-actualization is the organic principle by which the human organism becomes more fully developed and more complete; it is the creative trend of human nature. A person's desire to become something important or somebody eminent is converted into actuality by this motive. According to Goldstein, self-actualization is a universal phenomenon, but the specific goals toward which individuals move differ from person to person. It is so because individuals have different innate potentialities; depending on the innate potentiality, one becomes a scientist, musician, painter, sculptor or an actor.

As we have seen earlier while discussing Maslow's theory of motivation, self-actualization occupies the highest level in the hierarchy of needs. According to Maslow (1970), when all four of the basic (deficiency) needs are satisfied, a new discontent or restlessness develops; unless the individual does what he/she is individually fitted for, he/she experiences discomfort. Therefore, "what a man can be, he must be." Maslow borrowed the concept of self-actualization from Goldstein and acknowledged its relationship to constructs such as Jung's archetype of self and Carl Rogers' actualizing tendency. However, he specifically uses the term to refer to "the desire to become more and more what one idiosyncratically is, to become everything that one is capable of becoming." Self-actualization does not mean that the person is lacking something or wants to acquire something that he does not have; rather, it represents the intrinsic growth of what is already there in the organism. Thus, it is not a deficiency motive; it is a growth motive. In his earlier writings, Maslow thought that only selected people like George Washington, Abraham Lincoln, Mahatma Gandhi, Martin Luther King Jr & Albert Einstein have achieved self-actualization. But his later studies convinced him that this tendency can manifest even among ordinary people. For example, a parent who strives hard to raise an excellent family, a teacher who toils to create an environment where the students blossom to realize their full potential and a painter who realizes his creative potential might all be self-actualized. Maslow is well-known for his studies of self-actualizing individuals. He has postulated a list of characteristics that distinguish self-actualizers from others. We shall learn more about his work in the Chapter 11 on Personality.

Carl Rogers, a renowned American psychologist and psychotherapist, also proposed that organisms have a fundamental motive to enhance themselves. He wrote, "the organism has one basic tendency and striving—to actualize, maintain, and enhance the experiencing organism (Rogers, 1951)." The actualizing tendency is selective; it pays attention only to those aspects of the environment that promise to move the person constructively in the direction of fulfillment and wholeness. According to Rogers, the single goal of life is to become self-actualized or a whole person. The actualizing tendency can be thwarted, but it cannot be destroyed without destroying the organism. The organism actualizes itself along the lines laid down by heredity.

There are differences of opinion among psychologists regarding the origin, nature and measurement of self-actualization motive; its utility as a scientific construct and the ways in which it can be measured have been plagued by controversies. These difficulties have been partially faced in recent times. EL Shostrom has developed a test called *Personal Orientation Inventory (POI)* in 1963 to measure several components of self-actualization. It is an inventory of 150 forced-choice items that has been demonstrated to successfully measure some of the important characteristics of self-actualizing people. Whatever the controversies, there is no doubt that the concept has played an important role in the evolution and development of humanistic theories of personality and psychotherapy.

SOME OTHER MOTIVES

Until now we discussed some of the major motives that impel human beings into action. But life is more than eating and sex; it is more than achievement and affiliation. Human behavior is more complex and its motives are many and varied. It is not possible to discuss in one chapter all that has been written about human motives, i.e. it may require a complete book. We may just mention a few of the other important motives about which sufficient literature is available. For example, a great deal has been written about **aggression** motive. People attack, injure and even kill each other. It is reported that approximately 14,000 wars were fought during the last 5,600 years of recorded history. Long ago scientists like Sigmund Freud & William McDougall postulated an instinct of aggression or combative instinct. In recent times, ethologists like Konrad Lorenz have revived the interest in the study of aggressive instincts. They assert that both humans and animals are innately aggressive; animals have learned to control their aggressive tendencies, whereas man has not. Aggression may be physical or verbal, direct or indirect, active or passive. Contemporary psychologists have devoted lots of time and effort to study the origin, development and types of aggressive behavior. They have devised ingenious methods of measuring and controlling human aggression.

Our discussion of motivation will be incomplete if we do not learn something about the motives to seek variety in stimulation, to process information about the world around us, to explore, and to be effective in mastering the challenges of the environment. It is hypothesized that there is a universal "need to know." People spend great amount of time, effort and money to "look at things," traveling, and exploring the environment. They visit new places; watch television, movies, drama and sports; they read books, newspapers, and magazines. People are curious, inquisitive and inquiring about things and events around them. All these activities are triggered by the need to explore (exploratory drive). American psychologist Robert White (1959) has written about a *competence motive*, which encompasses several of these explorative activities.

MOTIVATIONAL CONFLICTS

When there are so many motives, there is a possibility that the expression of one motive interferes with the expression of other motives giving rise to conflicts. **Conflict** is a major source of **frustration**. There may be conflict between aggressiveness and fear of punishment, sex and social disapproval or need for affiliation and need for independence. For that matter, life is full of conflicts and the frustrations arising from motivational conflicts. Therefore, it is not surprising that psychologists have made an extensive study of conflict between motives. In general, three types of motivational conflicts have been identified and researched. These are approach-approach conflict, avoidance-avoidance conflict, and approach-avoidance conflict. When some goal is desirable, it attracts us and we move towards (approach) it; when something is not desirable, it repels us and we move away from (avoid) it.

Approach-approach Conflict

As the name itself implies, it is a conflict between two positive goals—goals that are equally attractive or desirable. When there are two attractive alternatives, selecting one means foregoing the other. For example, there may be **approach-approach conflict** when you have to choose between two equally attractive courses of study, or between two equally paying careers or between two equally attractive partners for life. You must have heard of the donkey standing between two haystacks that died of starvation because it was unable to decide from which one to eat. In reality, no donkey or individual will starve to death because there is a conflict between two positive goals. Such conflicts are easily resolved, maybe after slight vacillation. The organism will choose one of the goals and forego the other. When you are invited to attend two marriages that are equally important and that are being held at the same time, you may decide to attend one of them and let the other go; or you may adjust your time such that you will attend partly one and partly the other. Compared with other conflict situations, approach-approach conflicts do not create serious emotional problems.

Avoidance-avoidance Conflict

The second type of conflict involves two negative or undesirable goals. Suppose you are employed in an institution, which you hate; you want to leave it. You cannot stay in the organization because you hate it. You do not want to leave it because you do not have another source of income. Both alternatives are undesirable. When you choose either of the alternatives, you lose your income. In this case, you have an **avoidance-avoidance conflict**. There are many such situations in life such as you may have to study hard some boring subjects for 2 long weeks or face the possibility of failure in the examination; you may have to work with a detestable coworker or incur the wrath of your boss. In such situations, you are "caught between the devil and the deep sea." Avoidance-avoidance conflicts lead to intense negative emotions such as fear or anger. In such instances, the person may engage in daydreaming—escaping from the situation by running away.

Approach-avoidance Conflict

The most serious form of conflict that is not easy to resolve is approach-avoidance conflict. In **approach-avoidance conflict**, the organism is both attracted and repelled by the same goal object. The best example for this type of conflict is sex. Individuals are strongly motivated to engage in sexual activities, but at the same time, they are repelled by the consequences of such behavior—the fear of pregnancy, the fear of contracting sexually transmitted diseases, or simply the fear of social disapproval. Generally when under these conflicts, people approach the goal until the negative feelings become too strong and then they move away from it. But sometimes the negative feelings are not strong enough to stop the approach behavior. In such situations, people reach the goal, but much more slowly and hesitatingly than they would have in the absence of negative feelings. Even after the goal is reached, the individual may feel discomfort because of the negative feeling associated with it. Whether a person reaches the goal slowly or not reach it at all, the emotional reactions of guilt, fear, anger or resentment commonly accompanies approach-avoidance conflicts.

Multiple Approach-avoidance Conflicts

Many of our decisions in life involve *multiple approach-avoidance conflicts*; that is, we face several goals that have both positive and negative aspects. For example, think of a young woman who is engaged to marry a man whom she loves. Marriage has several positive aspects—provides stability and security in life. At the same time she is working in a satisfying job. Marriage means she has to quit the job. If she continues to work even after marriage, it may create several problems in family life. Thus, both marriage and career have positive and negative components that are conflicting. What should she do? The solution depends on the relative strengths of the approach and avoidance tendencies. She weighs the pros and cons of both the situations. If the sum total of the positive minus the negative components in her career is greater than the sum total of the positive minus the negative aspects in marriage, she may decide not to marry at all. Or if the sum total is greater for marriage than for career, she may resign from the job and decide to get married. Thus, what a person does when faced with multiple approach-avoidance situations depends on the relative strengths of all positive and negative aspects involved.

CURRENT STATUS OF MOTIVATIONAL THEORY AND RESEARCH

The psychologists have analyzed, identified and classified human motives in numerous ways and have developed a variety of theories of motivation to account for a wide range of behavior in both animals and human beings. Each theory has some grain of truth, but no one has completely explained the complexity of human behavior. Biological motives are powerful instigators of behavior because the satisfaction of the organic needs is essential to the survival of the organism and its species. Affluent people living in advanced countries are not worried about their bodily needs; these are easily satisfied. But people living in impoverished countries are dominated by the biological needs. Most of the time, these people are engaged in finding their next meal and a secure environment to live. Unless the biological needs are satisfied, the so called higher needs do not surface. Earlier, drive-reduction theorists attempted to explain all motivated activities in terms of biological needs. They tried to trace the achievement motivation to hunger drive and affiliation motive to sex. This approach could not add much to our understanding of complex motives. Nowadays, the concepts of drive and homeostasis have been replaced by the idea of arousal level.

An organism's arousal or activation level can vary between complete lethargy, high alertness and excitement. Theoretically, there is an optimal level of arousal in terms of internal and external stimuli. Conditions that depart too much from this optimal state in either direction impel the organism to try to restore the equilibrium. We do not like stimuli that are either too boring or too arousing. Arousal state may be affected by internal conditions such as hunger, or by an external stimulus such as the aroma of delicious food or a receptive mate. Too little stimulation may lead to boredom; then the organism seeks novelty and complexity in the environment. Even too intense and sudden changes in the external world may motivate the organism to engage in ways to reduce the intensity of the stimulation since strange and complex situations arouse anxiety. We shall learn more about the concept of arousal in the next chapter on emotion.

Chapter Summary

Motivation refers to the condition within an organism that influences the strength, direction, and persistence of behavior in reaching a goal. There are a number of motives that impel us into action. Some are biological and some others are psychosocial. Psychologists have proposed several theories of motivation. Instinct theorists believe that we are born with some innate tendencies such as sex, called instincts that have an evolutionary basis. Drive theorists propose that tissue deficits

Contd...

Contd...

create drives such as thirst and hunger. Homeostatic models view motivation as an attempt to maintain equilibrium in bodily systems. Incentive theories propose certain environmental stimuli called incentives that pull us toward them. Two models called *expectancy* X *incentive value* theory, and *approach and avoidance motivation* explain why the same incentive attracts some people, but not others. The view that motivation is an aroused state of organism and all individuals try to maintain a state of arousal led some psychologists to propose a theory of motivation around the concept *arousal.* Psychoanalytic theory proposed two forces—life and death instincts—that are believed to underlie most of human behavior. There are some motives, which we have acquired in the social context, such as need for regard, prestige, friendship, achievement, or power. Abraham Maslow proposed a motivational hierarchy that includes most of human needs progressing from deficiency needs (physiological) to growth needs (such as self-actualization). Deci & Ryan proposed the self-determination theory, which emphasizes the importance of three fundamental needs—competence, autonomy and relatedness. Deci's proposition that when an intrinsically motivated task is offered an extrinsic reward the performance suffers has created some controversies in research circles.

Among the major biological motives, hunger, thirst and sex have been extensively studied. Our eating behavior is controlled by both physiological and psychological factors. We eat for pleasure, for nutrition and often as a social activity. Brain senses the lowered level of nutrients in the blood and creates a desire in us to eat; it also tells us that we have taken enough and suggests us to stop eating. The hypothalamus plays a crucial role in hunger and thirst. Overeating can increase the body weight; once it is increased, it is difficult to reduce the body weight. Often cognitive mechanisms override the signals from the hypothalamus and induce people to eat more. There appears to be a set point that determines the weight. The availability, taste and variety of food regulate eating behavior. Obesity is a serious problem and both heredity and environment play an important role in determining whether one is going to become obese or not. Several people, especially women, develop certain eating disorders, such as anorexia nervosa and bulimia nervosa. Water is highly essential for survival. Thirst and drinking water are not as simple as they appear. Thirst is triggered by several complex psychophysiological mechanisms such as cellular dehydration and hypovolemia.

Sex is a powerful motive. With the passage of time people's attitude toward sex has changed enormously. In contemporary society, liberal views are being expressed about sexual behaviors such as homosexuality. The incidences of premarital and extramarital sexual activities have been on the rise, especially in the developed societies. Even same sex marriages are not being disapproved today. Conducting research on sexual behavior among humans has posed several problems. After all, you do not want a researcher to enter your bedroom! During 1950s, Alfred Kinsey pioneered investigations into the sexual behavior of American men and women. His survey research set the stage for later surveys. Master & Johnson undertook groundbreaking studies on the physiology of sex. They have found that during sexual intercourse people go through four stages such as excitement, plateau, orgasm and resolution. Sexual attraction leads to sexual desire, sexual excitement (arousal) and possibly intercourse ending in orgasm. Hormones (androgens in men and estrogen in women) play a key role in sexual development and sexual motivation. Fluctuation in the level of sex hormones affects cognition and emotion. Sexual arousal and desire are triggered by various cues. Visual cues play an important role; visual stimuli activate the hypothalamus in men, but not in women. In women, odor plays an important role.

Among the psychosocial motives, three have been extensively investigated by David McClelland & his coworkers; these are nAch, nAff, and nPow. High need achievers are found to have strong desire for success and low fear of failure; nAch is a stable, learned motive to attain a level of excellence in some chosen field. Need for affiliation is directed toward establishing and maintaining relationships with other people. Humans affiliate in several ways. Seeking close and intimate relationship has several adaptive advantages such as providing positive stimulation, emotional support, and companionship. One of the most important and intimate ways that humans affiliate is by seeking a spouse. Reliable differences have been found between men and women in their mating strategies and preferences. In general, men are found to go for good-looking younger women and women for strong elder men with capacity to earn. Evolutionary psychologists say that these differences are determined by inherited biological factors, but others think that these are due to social factors such as gender inequalities and economic opportunities for women. In short, it is said that mating preferences are influenced, but not determined by evolutionary factors. Need for power is characterized by a strong tendency to control and/or influence other people. It is easily seen among politicians who go to any extent to obtain and retain power.

Often motives conflict with one another. When an individual is faced with two attractive alternatives and finds it difficult to choose between them, he/she is experiencing approach-approach conflict. In approach-avoidance conflict, the individual has a goal that is both attractive as well as threatening. Avoidance-avoidance conflict involves choosing between two undesirable alternatives.

10 CHAPTER
Emotion

PREVIEW

It is difficult to think of any behavioral unit that is not associated with an emotion. You experience joy when you pass your examination in first class or when you land in a good job. You are thrilled to meet your beloved friend or relative. You are sad when you lose someone of your loved ones. We experience several ups and downs in our day-to-day life. Emotions add color and spice to life. Literally you are "red" with anger, "green" with envy or "blue" with sadness. Life without emotions will be drab and boring. However, then, what are emotions? Surprisingly, this question cannot be answered easily. It is very difficult to define an emotion. There are as many definitions as there are writers on the subject. In one review, some 92 definitions were listed (Kleinginna & Kleinginna, 1981).

Any definition of emotion should:

1. Say something about how we feel when we are emotional.
2. Mention about the bodily changes occurring when we are experiencing an emotion.
3. Tell us something about how we perceive the world when we are under the grip of an emotion.
4. Indicate the motivational properties of emotions.
5. Refer to the ways in which emotions are expressed facially and reported in words.

The list must give you an idea of what an emotion is.

Motivation and emotion are closely related. We react emotionally only when our motives and goals are gratified, threatened or frustrated. Some say that both the terms are derived from the Greek root '*emovere*', which means 'to move'. Emotions are also powerful motivators of behavior. Both motives and emotions serve adaptive functions. Emotions such as fear prepare us to run away from dangerous situations thus increasing our chances of survival. Anger helps us to fight in threatening situations. Positive emotions like joy, happiness, love and contentment also have adaptive functions. Happy people tend to attract others and to have richer and supportive relationships. Positive emotions help us form intimate relationships with others and broaden our inner world. Emotions help in social communications. We know when to say what or do what by looking at the emotional state of the others. You do not ask your father or friend help when he/she is angry or sad. Our emotional expressions also influence the behavior of others toward us. When you are sad people try to console you. When you are aggressive people avoid you.

In your profession, reading accurately other's emotions is very crucial. As a nurse, it is extremely important that you understand the emotional expressions of others and also you express appropriate emotions when you are dealing with patients and their relatives. Unless you cultivate the ability to understand the inner feelings of your clients (a process called empathy), it will be difficult to achieve success in your profession. Both in your profession and in your day-to-day life, understanding emotions is an essential social skill. Nowadays, psychologists are talking about emotional quotient (EQ), along with intelligence quotient (IQ). It is not enough if your IQ is high. It is also necessary that you have high EQ. Emotional intelligence is essentially the ability to perceive and understand the emotions of others and to regulate and control your own emotional expressions. Emotional intelligence is believed to be an excellent predictor of success in career and social settings. In fact, some believe that higher level of emotional intelligence is a better predictor of success in life than traditional intelligence. In this chapter, you will be presented with an elementary knowledge about emotions and various factors that influence your emotional life.

Chapter Outline

WHAT ARE EMOTIONS?

Emotions are the affective accompaniments of behavior. Whatever we are doing, it is always accompanied by some or the other emotion. When you eat good food, you are pleased; when you meet the dear and near ones, you are delighted; when hear good music or watch a painting, you are happy; you are angry when you are fighting; you are disgusted when you confront something ugly; you are afraid in the face of a dangerous situation; the list is endless. Life without emotions is unthinkable. It will be dull, dreary and colorless. Life is interesting because we experience varied emotions such as love, joy, fear, anger, hope, disappointment, distress and many other feelings that affect us. But then, what exactly is an emotion? There is no simple answer to this question. The term emotion has proved to be utterly elusive to definitional efforts. Psychologists until today have not produced a single, acceptable definition of emotion. There are as many definitions as there are writers about emotion. One writer who reviewed the definitions of emotion has listed about 100 of them; well, there can be many more. The term itself is derived from the Latin word *'emovere'*, which means *'to move'*, *'to excite'*, *'to stir up* or *to agitate'*. No wonder emotion was defined in early textbooks as "the stirred up state of the organism." The simplest and the easiest way to define the term is that—"It is what we mean when we say that love, wonder, happiness, anger, fear, hate, terror, etc. are emotions."

The reason for the difficulty in defining the term is that emotion has a number of components and any definition should comprise all of them. For instance, emotions and motivations are closely related and it is difficult to distinguish one from the other. We experience emotions only when our motives and goals are fulfilled, obstructed, threatened or frustrated. Emotions have adaptive functions and like motives, they also arouse and energize our behavior. When we are threatened, we run away from the situation; we avoid danger; when we are angry we fight; the fight or flight reactions increase our chances of survival. Similarly, pleasant emotions such as love, joy and contentment also serve adaptive functions. They help us to develop intimate relationships with others, broaden our thinking and enlarge the field of behavior; they help us to examine new ideas, explore alternative ways of living and most importantly, they help us to learn to appreciate what we do and what we have.

In short, we can delineate three functions of emotions:

1. Emotions prepare us for action: when we are threatened, we are physically aroused to move away from the fearful situation.

2. Emotions shape what we do in future: Based on earlier experience, we tend to avoid dangerous situations and approach pleasant ones.
3. Emotions help us to interact more effectively with others. Depending on our interpretation of others' emotions, we plan our interactions with them; similarly, other's behavior toward us is influenced by the emotions we show; thus, emotions promote effective and appropriate social interaction.

It is easier to describe emotions rather than defining them. Emotional states exhibit several common features:

1. They are triggered by stimuli that may be external (events in the environment) or internal (thoughts and images).
2. These stimuli are interpreted by the individual as positive or negative; the process is called cognitive appraisal.
3. They are associated with a number of physiological and neurological changes.
4. They involve motivational properties; emotional arousal is generally viewed as playing a role in impelling activity.
5. They have an expressive dimension; emotions are expressed in words, facial expressions, and/or gestures.
6. They influence the individual's perception, thinking, and behavior.

Any definition of emotion must include all these aspects and it is a difficult task. In short, it can be summarized that emotions are complex feeling states that have three basic components:

1. *Physiological arousal* (neurophysiological activation).
2. *Cognition* (conscious awareness or experience of the feeling as well as the thoughts about the stimuli that evoke the feeling).
3. *Expression* (outward expression of the emotion in the face and through behavior).

TYPES OF EMOTIONS

How many kinds of emotions do we experience? There are about 500 words in the English language that refer to emotions. The range of human emotions is large. We experience love, happiness, delight, awe, wonder, guilt, joy, fear, anger, disgust, sorrow, so on and so forth. Some researchers who have studied emotions argue that the brain produces many gradations and types of emotions by combining sets of simple signals. Just like the three primary colors combine to produce a large array of visible hues, simple sets of neural signals combine to produce different varieties of emotions.

Charles Darwin, who wrote probably the first, scientific treatise on emotion (*The expression of the emotions in man and animal*, 1872), believed that our emotions are innate. He noticed that people from different races and cultures were exhibiting similar facial expressions to signal similar emotional states. Even blind people, who never had opportunities of watching how others look when experiencing a particular emotion, are found to exhibit the same pattern of emotional expression. Therefore, it is often said that we are born with a built-in set of emotions. Thus, emotions are an essential part of human nature. An active researcher in this area Paul Ekman (1972) studied a New Guinea tribe the members of which had not seen White people either in person or photographs. These people were able to identify expressions of happiness, anger, sadness, disgust, fear and surprise in photos of White people. Ekman & his associates have concluded that these are primary emotions, emotions that are innate and shared by all humans. Another researcher (Tomkins, 1991) proposed a slightly different list of primary emotions consisting of surprise, interest, joy, rage, fear, disgust, shame, and anguish. Based on studies of non-human subjects, Panksepp (2005) offered a set of emotional systems, which are believed to guide behaviors such as sexuality-lust, nurturance-care, and joy-play. But whether there is a fixed set of basic emotions, if so, what is their number and nature are questions that have not yet been answered unequivocally.

Emotions are generally classified as positive and negative emotions. In general, approach emotions (such as love and happiness) are positive and withdrawal emotions (such as fear and disgust) are negative. Surprisingly, the positive and negative emotions are opposite sides of the same coin; they can occur at the same time. For example, suppose a young man is enjoying looking at an attractive woman; simultaneously, he is also scared that somebody might be watching him. The idea that positive and negative emotions are independent has found some support in brain studies. Researchers have reported that there are separate systems in the brain for approach and withdrawal emotions. Electroencephalogram (EEG) recordings show that the left frontal lobe tends to be more active than the right when people have approach emotions, whereas the right frontal lobe tends to be more active when people have withdrawal emotions. These reports have to be confirmed by further research.

EXPRESSION AND RECOGNITION OF EMOTIONS

Our expression of emotions has impact on others. When we perceive and identify other's emotional expressions, it will also influence our reactions. When you watch happiness on the face of one of your friends who got first rank in an examination, you may feel happy or sometimes, you may also feel jealous. Based on the emotional expression of people, you may form an idea of their personality. Perceiving other's emotions has important implications in our daily life. Therefore, judging emotional expression of others has been a busy area of research for several years in the past; even today, several workers on emotion are pursuing this area of research.

Several factors operate when we recognize emotional expressions. The voice is an important component of emotional expression. When someone groans, it denotes pain and unhappiness; sobbing denotes sorrow; screaming denotes fear; sharp, loud shout indicates anger. What people say also helps us in judging their emotions; when someone says "get out," you know what emotion the person is experiencing. In addition, bodily movements are powerful clues in perception of emotions. Facial expressions are important components that help in the understanding of emotions. Often the bodily movements including facial expressions are called "body language." In one major study (Izard, 1971), photographs expressing primary emotions (such as joy, excitement, startle, rage, fear, contempt, humiliation, and anguish) were shown to several participants and they were asked to name the emotion portrayed therein. People from various cultures were able to make accurate judgments of the emotions expressed in the photos. Similarity in the ways people express the primary emotions through their faces, both among and within cultures, provides a reliable set of perceptual cues for us in evaluating the emotional state behind the expression. It is interesting to note that women judge emotional expressions more accurately than men (Zuckerman et al, 1976). This ability of women has adaptive significance because woman all over the world are traditionally assigned the task of nursing and taking care of others. It is also worth noting that men engaged in caring and helping professions (such as psychotherapy) are also good judges of emotional expressions.

In addition to facial expression, the situation or the context in which an emotion occurs gives important information for judging that emotion. When facial expressions and the context in which the emotions are experienced are both available, the accuracy of judging emotion increases. Sometimes, the contextual and facial cues conflict; then, we rely more on facial expressions. But one should not conclude that accurate perception of emotions is an easy task. There are several complications. One is that people learn to control their emotions; secondly, many people express the same emotion in different and subtle ways. Some people can be very calm even when they are experiencing anger or fear. Remember, what Shakespeare once said "A man may smile and smile and yet a villain be."

Darwin argued that emotional displays were products of evolution; they helped in the survival of species. There is a good deal of similarity between animals and humans in their expression of emotions. Wild animals as well as humans growl with bare teeth when they are angry. This behavior makes the organism look ferocious and thus decreases its chances of being attacked. According to Darwin, not all emotions were innate, but many of them were. Modern evolutionary theorists (Izard, 1989; Tomkins, 1991; Plutchik, 1994), like Darwin, emphasize the importance of the adaptive value of emotions. They assert that a set of fundamental emotional patterns (also called primary emotions or innate emotional reactions) are built into the nervous system. They have shown that expression of certain emotions such as joy, surprise, disgust, shame, anger and fear are similar across all cultures suggesting a biological basis for them. Other emotions are based on some combination of these innate primary emotions. Of course, evolutionary theorists do not say that all emotions are innate or do they deny the modifiability of emotions by learning.

When people are experiencing an emotion, they would not keep quiet. They become active, energized and respond in ways appropriate to the emotion-arousing situation. These responses are called instrumental behaviors and are directed toward achieving some emotion-relevant goal. For example, anxiety associated with taking an examination makes a student work hard day and night; when you are in love with somebody, you do all that is possible under the sun to catch his/her attention and to evoke affection from your partner. Thus, emotion has motivating properties.

Emotion-eliciting Stimuli

Emotions are responses to external or internal stimuli. We are afraid of something, angry at someone or in love with somebody. Emotions are responses to people, events or things. They can also be triggered by internal thoughts or images. For example, you may be pleased at the thought of meeting a friend; irritated when you imagine the face of a person whom you do not like. Inherited biological factors determine which stimuli trigger which responses. You must have seen newborn infants crying at a loud sound or loss of balance. Adults are more prone to be scared of dizzy heights, gushing water, snakes or spiders, rather than automobiles, electrical transformers or guns (which are more dangerous). Different cultures have different standards regarding what is good, bad and ugly. Physical features that provoke sexual arousal in an African tribe, such as ornamental scars on face or a bone through the nose, may create nausea and revulsion in our society.

COGNITION AND EMOTION

Cognition refers to memories, images, thoughts, and interpretations that are involved in emotions. These inner psychological processes influence what emotion we experience, how we express it, and what actions we undertake under its influence. Any stimulus situation may elicit pleasure or pain, fear or anger, delight or grief depending on how we interpret it. This process of interpreting or attaching meaning to sensory stimuli is called the **cognitive appraisal**.

Cognitive interpretation may be conscious or unconscious; it may occur quickly or gradually. Primary emotions (strong emotions such as fear or anger) are automatically processed because of our previous experience and learning with them. But we may experience some emotions without knowing consciously how they have occurred. Cognitive appraisal process helps us to explain why different people react differently for the same stimulus or even the same person reacts differently for the same stimulus at different times. Cross-cultural researches have shown that people of different cultures employ similar cognitive appraisal processes when experiencing emotions such as joy, fear, anger, sadness, disgust, shame, and guilt. There are instances when people make different types of cognitive appraisal for the same stimulus situation. For many of us, being alone may at times represent a welcome respite from the frantic pace of daily life; the condition may evoke contentment and happiness. But in some cultures, being alone indicates social rejection and isolation, eliciting sadness. People of Tahiti interpret being alone as the opportune time for the evil spirits to visit them and hence they experience fear. So, with regard to cognitive appraisal, there are universals as well as some degree of cultural diversity.

PHYSIOLOGICAL BASES OF EMOTIONS

When you are under the grip of an emotion, you know what is happening within your body. There are changes in the heart rate, blood pressure, blood flow to various parts of the body, activity of the stomach and gastrointestinal system, levels of various substances such as hormones in the blood, breathing rate and depth and several other activities. You may not be aware of all these changes. Psychophysiologists have developed instruments to measure these changes. Most of these bodily changes during emotions are produced by the autonomic nervous system (ANS) and the endocrine system. Before discussing the role of these two systems, let us examine some of the areas in the brain that are involved in the production and control of emotions.

Brain Structures Involved in Emotions

Brain is intimately involved in the perception and evaluation of stimuli that give rise to emotions. It controls the physiological expression of emotion and is also involved in directing behavior driven by the emotional state. Several important parts of the brain, including the limbic system and the cerebral cortex, interact to produce emotional states. Experiments on animals have shown that when a specific area of the limbic system is electrically stimulated, they exhibit violent, aggressive, attacking behavior; destroying the same site produces absence of aggression even when they are provoked. The cerebral cortex has many connections with hypothalamus, amygdala and other parts of the limbic system. The cortex is involved in cognitive appraisal. Regulation of emotion depends on the executive functions of the prefrontal cortex.

Recent research by Joseph LeDoux (2000) has demonstrated that when thalamus receives sensory input, it can send the messages in two independent neural pathways—it can send the messages to the cortex (high road) and also directly to the nearby amygdala (low road). The low road enables amygdala to receive sensory messages and generate emotional reactions even before the cortex has had time to interpret what is causing the reaction. That is probably why we jump aside when we see something that looks like a snake, and later realize that it was after all a rope. It is argued that this primitive mechanism has a survival value because it enables the organism to react quickly before the cortex responds with a more carefully processed cognitive interpretation of the situation. The amygdala also seems to function as an early warning system for threatening social stimulations.

The existence of a dual system of emotional processing may explain the fact that we experience a strong emotion without understanding why. It also explains why people have two simultaneous, but different emotional reactions to the same stimulus, a conscious one mediated by the cortex and unconscious one triggered by the amygdala. Some psychodynamic theorists consider this as an indication that we have unconscious emotions, and it may also explain the concept of ambivalence having two opposing emotions such as love and hate, toward the same person. LeDoux theory is often called *dual-pathway model of emotion*.

Several neuroscientists argue that all of the neural structures underlying emotions have a biochemical basis, and it is the rise and fall of neurotransmitter substances that activate emotional reactions. It is suggested that dopamine and endorphin activities underlie pleasurable feelings, whereas serotonin and norepinephrine play important role in triggering anger and fear. Of course, the last word about the complex interactions between neurotransmitters and neural structures has yet to be written. There are some recent researchers who suggest that emotional reactions depend on which hemisphere of the brain that is activated. They suggest that left-hemisphere activation may underlie certain positive emotions and right-hemisphere activation with negative ones. This hemispheric pattern seems to be innate; infants as old as 3 to 4 days exhibit similar pattern of hemispheric activation.

Role of Autonomic Nervous System

Autonomic nervous system plays an important role in producing the bodily changes associated with emotions. The ANS, which is part of the peripheral nervous system, consists of many nerves leading from the brain and spinal cord out to the smooth muscles of the various organs of the body, to the heart, to certain glands and to the blood vessels serving both the interior and exterior of the body. It has two parts—the sympathetic division and the parasympathetic division. The sympathetic system is active during aroused states preparing the body for extensive action by increasing the heart rate, raising the blood pressure, increasing the blood sugar levels and raising the levels of certain hormones in the blood. The sympathetic system plays a significant role in many strong emotions, especially anger and fear. When you are angry, your face becomes red, blood flows toward upper limbs and your body is ready to fight. When you are afraid, your heart starts beating faster, breathing becomes harder and faster, the blood flows toward the muscles, face becomes pale, digestion is retarded, blood sugar level is increased, the pupils are dilated, the skin perspires and your body is ready to deal with the threatening situations. You will run away from the threatening situation. The pattern of activity is called the *emergency reaction* or the *flight-or-fight response*.

The parasympathetic system tends to be active when the organism is calm and relaxed. It decreases the heart rate, brings down the blood pressure and activates the digestive tract. This pattern of activity is known as the *relaxation response*. The relaxation response is almost the opposite of emergency reaction. When the sympathetic system is active, energy is expended; when the parasympathetic division is active, energy is conserved. Thus, it appears that the effects of the sympathetic and the parasympathetic systems are opposed to each other. In aroused states, sympathetic activity is dominant and in calmer states, the parasympathetic activity. But, both systems can be active in some emotional states. In anger, for example, heart rate is increased (sympathetic effect), so also the stomach activity (parasympathetic effect). Therefore, the pattern of physiological activity that characterizes an emotion can be a blend of both sympathetic and parasympathetic activities.

The hormones from the endocrine system play an important role in the production of flight-or-fight response. The sympathetic system produces arousal within a few seconds by direct stimulation of the organs and muscles of the body. At the same time, the endocrine system pumps epinephrine, cortisol and other stress hormones into the bloodstream. These hormones create physiological effects similar to those triggered by sympathetic activation, but the hormonal effects are long-lasting and keep the body in the state of arousal for a considerable length of time.

The discussion above raises an important question—do different emotions produce different patterns of arousal? The answer to the question is not unambiguous. There are differences of opinion regarding the physiological arousal in specific emotions. One group of researchers (Davidson, 1994; Levenson, 1994; Franks & Smith, 1999) believes that there are specific patterns of biological arousal associated with individual emotions. Others assert that there are only subtle differences among basic emotions as different as fear and anger. Moreover, individuals differ from one another in their pattern of general arousal; they exhibit different patterns of arousal even when they are experiencing the same emotion. Therefore, it is difficult to say, which emotion the person is experiencing based on physiological indicators alone. This finding has led researchers to doubt the credibility of the so called *lie detectors* in detecting crime and deception (Box 10.1).

THEORIES OF EMOTION

We have tried to understand the various factors associated with emotions. But, how are these factors related to each other in the production of distinct emotions? There have been several attempts to answer this question and each of them has developed into a specific theory of emotion. In fact, there are as many theories as there are writers about emotion. Some theories emphasize importance of bodily changes in the production of emotions; some of them emphasize the subjective experience and others, the cognitive components. We shall review here some of the important theories of emotion.

James-Lange Theory

One of the earliest theories of emotion was proposed, more or less at the same time, by two eminent men, the American psychologist William James (1890) & the Danish physiologist Carl Lange (1887) and hence the name **James-Lange theory of emotion**. The basic idea behind the theory is that bodily changes trigger emotion. But the way James presented the theory has ignited a huge controversy and made it very famous in the history of psychology. He wrote, *"Common sense tells us that we meet a bear, are frightened and run; we are insulted by a rival, are angry and strike. The hypothesis here to be defended says that this order of sequence is incorrect and that the more rational statement is that we feel sorry because we cry, angry because we strike and afraid because we tremble."* This is putting the horse behind the cart. Common sense tells us that when we are in a particular situation, the situation induces in us a specific emotion and that emotion leads us to behave in a certain way. James argued that the plausible relation between emotion and behavior is exactly backward. According to him, our perception of the bodily changes is the basis for the emotion we experience. Thus, James-Lange theory

Box 10.1: The Lie Detector Controversy

An instrument called **polygraph** is what has come to be known as a lie detector. Polygraph, as the name suggests, measures simultaneously several physiological responses such as the rate and depth of respiration, blood pressure, heart rate, and galvanic skin response (GSR), which are thought to be indicative of emotional arousal. This instrument is extensively used by police to determine whether a suspect is telling the truth or lying. Because people have less control over physiological responses than over other behaviors, it is assumed that polygraph measures are infallible in determining whether a person is telling the truth. This assumption has been questioned on several grounds.

The police use the services of a trained polygraph examiner who employs a standard procedure of lie detection. The examiner, after obtaining biographical information from each suspect, asks each of them about a dozen or so yes/no, critical and specific questions relating to the alleged crime along with a set of neutral, general questions. The neutral questions are such they evoke emotional responses from almost everyone while the critical questions are designed to evoke emotional responses only from those who are suspects in a crime or those with guilty knowledge. The rationale here is that the innocent person, who knows nothing about the crime, gives larger response to neutral questions than to the critical questions, while the guilty person gives larger responses to the critical questions than to the non-critical questions. Thus, it is assumed that the differential pattern of polygraph recordings gives a clue to lying or truthfulness. The crucial issue here is whether an emotional response to a critical question really means that a person is lying.

An innocent person may appear guilty when doubt, fear, or lack of confidence increases his autonomic activity. The testing situation itself may produce a state of emotional arousal in him. On the other hand, a guilty person may keep his cool and defeat the polygraph test. He might be an expert in producing increased emotional response to general questions while controlling emotional reactions to critical questions. For example, by biting tongue, curling toes, or contracting anal sphincter when critical questions are asked, one can produce an arousal response to those questions that look similar to the arousal that occurs when he/she actually is lying to critical questions. It has been very well demonstrated that several suspects can be trained to fool the polygraph test.

There are several other misgivings about the validity of polygraph tests. When expert polygraph examiners were asked to distinguish between the records of guilty and innocent people, they could identify the records of guilty with an accuracy rate of 80%–98%. However, they were less accurate in identifying the innocent; they judged about 55% of the innocent people as guilty. This error rate shows the possibility of many innocent people being judged as guilty if one goes by the polygraph records only in judging crime. American Psychological Association is opposed to the use of polygraph recordings as the sole proof in identifying the criminal. In spite of research evidence against the validity of polygraph tests, it is unfortunate that several agencies continue to use them in criminal investigation and national security screening.

asserts that our bodily reactions determine the subjective emotion we experience; we experience different emotions because each emotion corresponds to a distinct bodily state. The theory has often been called the *somatic theory of emotion*.

The James-Lange theory has been questioned on several grounds. First, although some types of physiological changes are associated with specific emotional experiences, there is not enough evidence to show that each emotion is associated with distinct bodily change; the range of human emotional experience is so vast that it is difficult to imagine that each subtle emotion is the result of unique physiological change. Second, we experience an emotion instantaneously the moment we face a stimulus and the visceral changes take some time to occur; our emotional experience occurs even before there is time for certain physiological changes to be set in motion. Finally, the physiological arousal may not always produce an emotional state. There are several instances in life when you breathe speedily, you perspire and your heart rate increases, but still you do not experience any emotion; visceral changes by themselves may not be sufficient to induce an emotional state. Further, several emotional states are actually associated with relatively similar sorts of visceral changes. The dominant physiological response during an emotion is arousal. Whether it is anger, happiness, or fear, the pattern of arousal is the same. There are no distinct patterns of physiological changes associated with different emotions. Actually, neither James nor Lange provided any evidence for the theory. They presented it intuitively.

Several attempts have been made to determine whether there is any grain of truth in the theory. For instance, some attempts were made to study the emotional states of people, who because of brain damage, have either lost feelings in major part of their bodies, or at least have reduced sensory feedback. Such people have reported a drop-off in the intensity of their emotional experience. Unfortunately, subsequent studies could not confirm these findings. But in recent times, sophisticated measuring devices have enabled researchers to identify minute changes in body reactions, which may help in finding distinct physiological changes associated with different emotions. Neuroimaging studies have also revealed different patterns of brain reactions when people are experiencing different emotions. We all know that the experience of anger and fear are different and hence it can be speculated that there are different brain activities associated with them. However, it is not correct to conclude that body changes alone produce emotions; emotions are complex experiences involving both body and mind (cognitions). We shall learn more about this line of thinking later in the chapter.

Cannon-Bard Theory

James-Lange theory was challenged by American physiologist Walter B Cannon & his colleague Philip Bard during 1920s. These two have proposed an alternative to James-Lange theory, which to some extent tried to set right some of the difficulties faced by the theory. Based on the research done by Bard, Cannon pointed out that our body does not respond instantaneously to an emotional stimulus and the visceral changes occur several seconds after we experience an emotional state. He asserted that the subjective experience of emotion and physiological arousal do not cause one another, but instead are independent responses to an emotion-arousing situation. It was proposed that both visceral changes and experiencing of emotion are simultaneously produced by the lower centers of the brain (such as the hypothalamus). According to Cannon-Bard theory, an individual first perceives an emotion-producing stimulus in the environment; then the brain centers are activated and the hypothalamus sends information in two directions:

1. The ANS, which produce changes in the internal body organs and the external muscles (the physiological arousal).
2. The cerebral cortex, where the pattern of discharge from the thalamus is perceived as the felt emotion (Cannon thought it was the thalamus that was involved in emotion; it was an error. It is hypothalamus that is involved in emotion).

The James-Lange & Cannon-Bard theories, as you can see, differ on important points. According to the first theory, the feedback from the visceral changes in a situation informs the brain that one is experiencing an emotion. Without visceral changes, there would be no emotional experience. The second theory holds that emotional experience results from neural signals sent from the hypothalamus to the cerebral cortex, and not from the bodily feedback. In fact, Cannon conducted experiments on animals to show that bodily feedback is not necessary to experience emotions. In some animals, he severed the nerves that carry feedback from the internal organs to the brain and still found the animals exhibiting emotional responses. These experiments support his theory that it is the direct sensory messages to the brain that trigger an emotional response. Further evidence for this view comes from human subjects. It is found that people whose spinal cords have been severed in accidents, and as a consequence received no sensory feedback from body areas below the injury, continued to experience emotions. These results appear to cast doubt on the role of arousal feedback on the production of emotions. But the story is not over yet.

Recent researches have shown that feedback from facial muscles involved in emotional displays (at least 20 muscles in the face operate in different facial expression of emotions) also send messages to the brain and these muscles are active even in patients with spinal injuries who received no sensory feedback from below the neck. This is the **facial feedback hypothesis**, which states that feedback from the facial muscles to the brain plays a key role in determining the nature and intensity of emotions that people experience. Remember that facial muscles are part of the body and if the feedback from them is important for production of emotions, James-Lange theory has still a grain of truth in it.

Cognitive Theories of Emotion

However obvious, bodily changes do not tell the whole story about emotions. Bodily sensations are important in the experience of emotions. But, different emotions show pretty much the same pattern of physiological changes. People cannot determine the type of emotion merely based on the heart rate or blood pressure. They are aware that something is going on internally, but they do not define the emotion in terms of their internal changes. When they are asked to describe their emotions, they usually talk about the arousing stimuli; they tell you what angered them, frightened them or pleased them. In short, it is the individual's appraisal of the situation—interpretation of the arousing stimulus—that is the important factor in the experience of emotion. Thus, there is always a psychological component—the cognitive element—operating when you experience an emotion. Thinking and feeling are intimately connected in the domain of emotional experience. Cognitive theorists emphasize the role of higher mental processes such as thinking, memory, perception and information processing in the production of behavior including emotional reactions. The *cognitive theories of emotion* state that an emotional experience is influenced by the way the individual appraises the external situation in terms of memories of past experience. That is, different emotions occur not because of different bodily states, but because of the way one interprets them when they occur. Stanley Schachter & Richard Lazarus are two pioneers in proposing such a view.

The cognitive approach to the understanding of emotion has emerged from an experiment conducted by Schachter & Jerome Singer in 1962, which is now considered a landmark study in psychology. The purpose of the experiment was to show that an emotional experience depends both on the state of physiological arousal and on the cognition appropriate to the state of arousal; that is, when a person was aroused, he would be under pressure to understand his bodily reactions, and he would turn to his immediate surroundings to understand the meaning of his arousal. When aroused, if he were with a beautiful woman, he would interpret it as love or sexual excitement; if he were in confrontation with his wife, he would call it anger; if he were in the company of a group of euphoric friends, he might think he was very happy. Schachter tried to provide evidence for his assumptions through experiments. He produced a state of physiological arousal in a group of participants by injecting epinephrine (adrenalin). The participants were told that they were receiving a vitamin injection for purposes of studying its effect on their visual perception. Four groups participated in the experiment. The first group was given correct information about the physiological changes to be expected from the injection (increased heart rate and trembling of the limbs, etc.). The second group was not informed about any possible effects of the drug. The third group was given wrong information about the effects of the drug; they were told that the drug would cause numbness, itching and headache. The members of the fourth group (the control group) did not receive epinephrine; instead, they were administered a *placebo* (saline solution), which did not produce any physiological change; nor were they told to expect any arousal. Schachter hypothesized that the more misinformed the subjects were about the expected physiological changes the more likely they would be to label their emotions according to what was going on around them. The placebo group should not be influenced by external events because they were not aroused and had no strange feelings to search for a label.

The cognitive states were manipulated using a stooge—a trained confederate of the experimenter, who had presumably been given the same injection and who supposedly, was participating in the experiment just like all other subjects. The stooge acted in two ways creating two opposite conditions, i.e. he either acted euphoric (playful and happy-go-lucky) or angry (complaining about the experiment and resenting about filling the lengthy questionnaire). The design of the experiment and the summary results are shown in Figure 10.1.

The results clearly demonstrated that the participants who had received epinephrine and were either misinformed or informed nothing about its effects were most influenced by the behavior of the stooge. Compared to subjects in the two other groups, they were more euphoric when the stooge behaved in a playful way and angry when the stooge acted in an angry manner. Since they had no idea why they were having bodily changes, they were more influenced by what was occurring around them. Subjects who knew what was happening to them were not influenced by the stooge's behavior. The *placebo* group that was not at all aroused was not influenced by the acting of the stooge. That is, when the participants had an adequate explanation for their aroused state, their emotional states

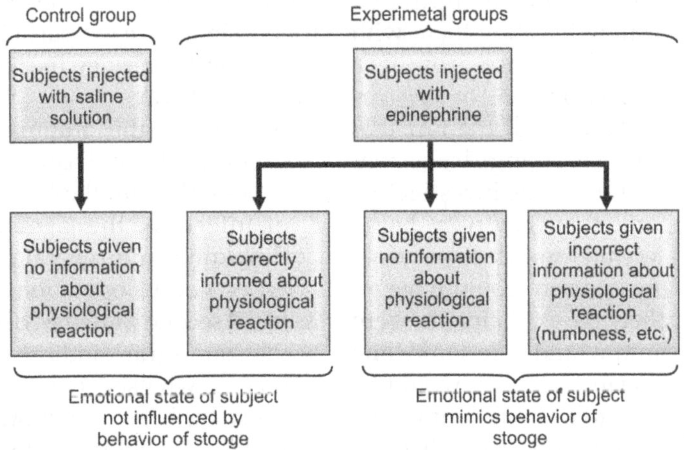

FIGURE 10.1: The design of Schachter and Singer experiment

were not influenced by the behavior of the stooge. Similarly, the unaroused placebo group also was not influenced by the events outside. But, when people were aroused and they did not know why, they were prone to label their emotions based on the environmental cues. Schachter called the theory *cognitive physiological theory of emotion*. In its simplest form, the theory states that emotion is internal physiological arousal in interaction with cognitive processes. The intensity of the physiological arousal tells us how strongly we are feeling about something, but situational cues give us the information necessary to label the arousal as anger, fear, love or some other emotion. Since, the theory emphasizes the role of physiological arousal and the cognitive appraisal of situational cues in producing an emotion, it is often called the **two factor theory of emotion**.

If a cognitive appraisal and physiological arousal are both involved in the production of emotion, how do they affect each other? Researches by Schachter and Wheeler (1962), & Richard Lazarus (2001) have shown that manipulating arousal influences cognitive arousal and vice versa. Schachter & Wheeler have shown that the level of arousal can influence cognitive appraisal. In one of their experiments, they directly manipulated participants arousal by injecting them with either epinephrine to increase arousal, a tranquilizer to decrease arousal, or a *placebo* control substance. To conceal the fact that the participants are receiving drugs that would affect their arousal, the investigators told the participants that they were being given a vitamin to study its effect on visual perception and the vitamin would have no side effects. Further, the participants were told that the vitamin would take some time to act and in the meanwhile they would be shown a short movie to provide continuous black and white stimulation to their eyes. The movie shown was comedy.

While the participants watched the comedy film, they were observed through a one-way mirror by raters. The raters were unaware of which viewers were given which injections. They (raters) recorded how frequently the viewers smiled, laughed, threw up their hands and slapped their legs or grinned. The results indicated that the amount of amusement displayed by the participants depended on the level of arousal. That is, the group that had received epinephrine showed more signs of amusement than the *placebo* group and the tranquilizer group; the *placebo* group was in the middle. Having been told that the vitamin had no side effects the viewers aroused by epinephrine attributed their arousal to the comedy in the film. The group that had received the tranquilizer did not find the film as funny because they experienced a reduced level of arousal. It appears that as long as one's arousal is attributed to the external stimulation, arousal can affect the appraisal.

Richard Lazarus & coworkers (Speisman et al, 1964) manipulated cognitive appraisal to study its effect on arousal. He and his coworkers showed a group of participants a film depicting a puberty rite in an aboriginal tribe. The rite consisted of cutting the genitals (something like circumcision) of aboriginal boys with a crude knife. The investigators tried to influence the participants' cognitive appraisals by varying the sound track of the film in four ways:

1. In one film (the "trauma" condition), the sound track emphasized the intense pain experienced by the boys, the possibility of infection, the jagged nature of the flint knife, and several other unpleasant aspects of the operation.
2. In the second film (the "denial" condition), the sound track indicated that there was no pain whatsoever in the operation, and in fact the boys were showing bravery and were looking forward to enter adulthood by undergoing the rite.

3. The soundtrack in the third film ("intellectualization" condition) downplayed the emotional elements of the scenes and focused on the cultural traditions and history of the tribe as though such a rite was a normal event.
4. The fourth film (the "silent" condition) was shown without any soundtrack at all.

The physiological arousal was measured using **galvanic skin response (GSR)**. The soundtracks produced markedly different levels of arousal to the same visual stimuli. The "trauma" track produced the maximum arousal; the "denial" and "intellectualization" tracks produced lower levels. The silent track produced more arousal than the denial or intellectualization mode, probably because it left participants free to make their own negative appraisal. This and several other studies have shown that what we tell ourselves about external situations influences the level of arousal within us.

Some researchers have tried to develop a new theory of emotion taking the best elements of the available ones. As mentioned earlier, LeDoux tried to modify the cognitive theory in an important way. He claimed that there are different brain systems for different broad categories of emotions; some of these systems operate as reflex pathways do, independent of thought or interpretation, whereas others depend on cognitive processes. Fear relies on amygdala without the need for cognitive interpretation and memories of past experiences. But, other emotions such as shame or guilt, rely on cognitive interpretation of previous occasions when such situations were encountered. Thus, emotions experienced by people at any given moment arise from a mixture of:

1. Brain and body reactions.
2. Interpretation and memories relating to the situation.

Other researchers hold that bodily reactions produce a core affect, which consists of simplest raw feelings. These feelings differ in the degree to which they are positive or/ and the degree to which they are strongly or weakly activated. Changes in core affect are categorized just as we categorize ambiguous stimuli. Context and previous experience help us to categorize the core affect to fit the situation and experience express different emotions.

A Theory of Relationship Among Emotions

Human beings experience a number of emotions. Often these emotional states are indistinct, ill-defined, overlapping and constantly changing. Categorizing emotions has been a challenging task. Psychologists have not agreed on the number and nature of emotions. In order to bring some order into human emotional life, Robert Plutchik (1980, 1994) has proposed a descriptive theory, which tries to identify the basic (primary) emotions and the ways in which they combine to form other secondary emotions. Plutchik uses a wheel to represent how the basic emotions merge to form the more complex secondary emotions. The eight primary emotions (joy, acceptance, fear, surprise, sadness, disgust anger and anticipation) are represented by the segments within the circle (Fig. 10.2). Plutchik maintains that these primary emotions are derived from evolutionary processes and have adaptive value. The adjacent emotions combine to form the secondary emotions that are represented outside the circle. For example, joy and acceptance combine to form love; fear and acceptance combine to form submission; fear and surprise give rise to awe; surprise and sadness form into disappointment, so on and so forth. The primary emotions are arranged in such a way to indicate the polarity among them. Joy and sadness are polar opposites. Similarly, acceptance and disgust, fear and anger, surprise and anticipation are polar opposites. That is,

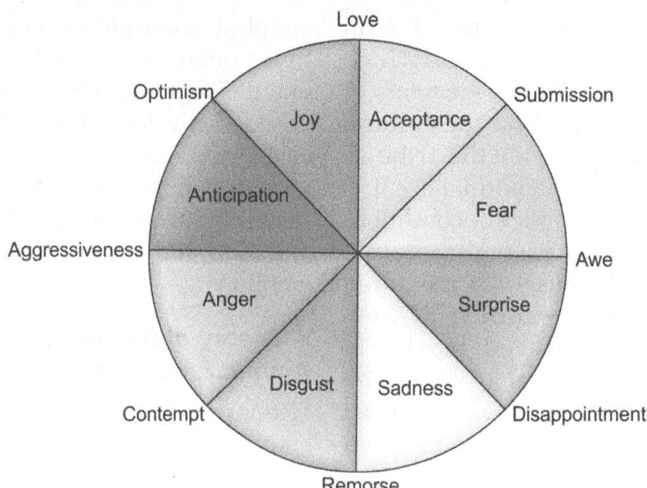

FIGURE 10.2: Plutchik color wheel of emotions

the emotions that are opposite each other conflict, while emotions that are close to each other are complementary. The Plutchik model gives a good description of mixed and conflicting emotions.

Recently, another group of researchers (Fischer, Shaver & Carnochan, 1990) has proposed a classificatory system of emotions; they have organized emotions in the form of a hierarchy, in which emotions are divided into increasingly narrow subcategories (Fig. 10.3). For instance, they divide emotions into positive and negative based on the feeling tone they produce in the individual. Love and joy are positive emotions. Love is further divided into fondness and infatuation. Joy is divided into bliss, contentment, and pride. Negative emotions are those that trigger an unpleasant feeling in us. Anger, fear, and sadness are negative emotions. Anger can be subdivided into annoyance, hostility, contempt, and jealousy. Sadness can be subdivided into agony, grief, guilt and loneliness. Fear can be divided into horror and worry. Other researchers suggest that the list of basic

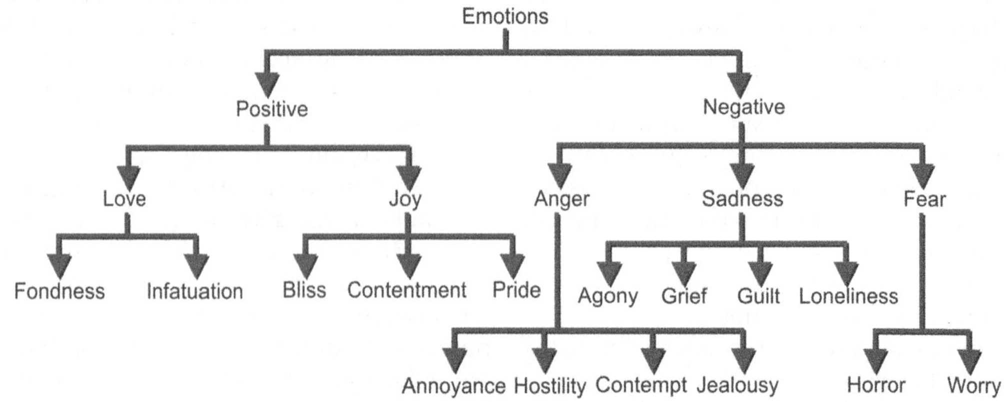

FIGURE 10.3: Hierarchical organization of emotions

emotions would include happiness and surprise. There can be no finality in the naming and classification of emotions. One difficulty in finding a basic set of emotions is that different cultures use different words to indicate different shades of emotions.

SOME MAJOR EMOTIONS

Now that we have learned about some of the important theoretical approaches, it is necessary to understand how the basic emotions develop in our lives. As indicated in the hierarchy of emotions (refer Fig. 10.3), they can be broadly divided into two groups—positive and negative emotion. Love and happiness (joy) are positive emotions; anger, fear, disgust and grief (sadness) are negative emotions. There are other emotions such as pride, contentment, jealousy, guilt, contempt, loneliness, worry, etc. Since, it is not possible to discuss all of them, we have selected some of the major emotions—fear, anger, disgust, love and happiness—that are commonly encountered in everyday life, for slightly more detailed discussion.

Fear

Since it is experienced universally by both animals and humans, fear is one of the best researched emotions in psychology. Think of the things that you are afraid of; the list will be endless. In fact, it is easier to list things that we are not afraid; the list will not be very large. Why we are afraid of so many things—objects, animals, persons, events, and so on and so forth? Are we simply born with a tendency to fear things around us? The answer is not simple. Although some fears appear to be innate, a large number of our fears are acquired. Let us examine the situations that trigger fear in children. Early researchers in the field found (Watson, Sherman & Bridges) that young infants show a startle reaction when they experience a sudden loss of balance. Unless pain is produced by the fall, the fear reaction to falling will generally decrease with increasing age. At about 10 months of age crying was found to be a fairly common reaction to a strange situation. This response was not seen when they were two-month-old (Bayley). Infants between three and six months smiled at nearly all human faces, but at about five to seven months they smiled at familiar faces and would often cry at the sight of strange faces.

Jersild & his coworkers (1935) made a useful study of development of fear in children between the ages of 0 to 12 years. They used four types of stimuli to elicit fear. These were animals, noises, threats and strange things. They found that fear of noises and strange things decreased with age. But the fear of animals and threats increased with age. This is the general trend; there may be some exceptions. But the question is how is it that we come to be afraid of innumerable things, sometimes even harmless ones. One of the first persons who tried to answer this question was JB Watson (1920, 1924).

Watson demonstrated in a classic experiment that we acquire most of our fears through classical conditioning. His experiment with Albert, an 11-month-old boy from a maternity ward in a hospital, has become a landmark study in psychology. Using loud sound as unconditioned stimulus that elicited fear, Watson established in Albert fear of a harmless rat. The experiment goes somewhat as follows:

1. At the beginning, a harmless laboratory rat was placed before Albert, toward which he did not show any fear reaction.
2. Then, a loud sound was produced, to which the child showed fear reactions.
3. Later, the paired stimuli, the rat first and immediately after that the loud sound were presented.
4. After only three such repetitions, the boy cried and crawled away from the rat.

Watson called this conditioned (learned) fear reaction. Still later, the child started showing fear reactions toward other things such as a white fur muff, white beard and other objects that resembled a rat in some remote way; this is what has been called stimulus generalization. Thus, we learn to fear one object by direct contact, but later this fear transfers to similar objects, which may be encountered. One day you encounter a snake in a bush; naturally you experience fear. Next day, the sight of that bush, and later all kinds of bushes trigger fear in you. By virtue of stimulus generalization, we learn to fear harmless snakes, cockroaches, insects, darkness and several other things in the environment. That is, we learn to fear neutral stimuli because these in some way are associated with the original fear-producing stimulus.

Recent researchers have thrown a good deal of light on fear. Fear causes changes in the brain, ANS hormones and behavior. When we are afraid, we tend to freeze, and we have an increased tendency to exhibit startle reaction, a condition called "potentiated startle." Several significant facts about fear have emerged from studying brain systems that produce it:

1. The amygdala plays an important role in the emotional arousal, especially fear. Once we are afraid of an object, later fear can build up as a kind of emotional reflex, without any cognitive appraisal. Amygdala sends signals to other brain areas such as the hypothalamus, which cause autonomic reactions associated with fear. It is now known that conscious awareness is not needed for a stimulus to trigger the amygdala to fear-related responses.
2. Fear is a classically conditioned response, and even after its extinction, the neurons that were linked by conditioning still fire together. Even when emotional expression is blocked by extinction, the neural connections still remain intact. That is why the conditioned fear is reinstated easily. You may not be aware of the association, but it still exists.
3. Although fear is expressed reflexively, it interacts with higher mental processes. For example, even visualizing a fear-producing stimulus or situation can elicit fear reactions; the brain areas involved in cognitive processes activate fear. It is found that when you watch somebody being conditioned to fear, you also acquire fear associations.
4. Although the amygdala regulates fear reactions, it does not have any role in producing emotional experience. Patients whose amygdala is damaged are found to experience fear as often and as strongly as normal people do.

Anger and Aggression

Emotions and motivations are similar in several respects. The motivational (energy-mobilizing) properties of emotions can be clearly seen in the case of anger. Anger releases additional energy in the pursuit of a desired goal. Early theorists considered anger as an instinct—an innate, impulse to fight, attack and destroy (the instinct of pugnacity). Sigmund Freud proposed that humans were impelled by a destructive instinct or death instinct, which he called **Thanatos**. Later, researches on animal behavior by Konrad Lorenz have lent support to such a view. An observation made by Lorenz has created a huge controversy. He emphasized that animals manifest violent tendencies only in the interest of self-preservation and only kill rarely a competing member of the same species; the aggressive activity subsides when the antagonist concedes defeat. But, humans attack and kill their fellow human beings as though by a spontaneous instinct of aggression. Contemporary psychologists do not accept this line of thinking; they do not consider aggression (anger and violence) as an instinct. According to them, aggressiveness is not the product of an instinct of aggression, but instrumental behavior directed towards a goal. Humans seek food, sex, power and prestige "aggressively." The vigor of action is a function of the vigor of the basic motive, not of an instinct of aggression.

Dissatisfied with the instinctive theory of aggression, a group of American psychologists proposed in 1939 the **frustration-aggression hypothesis**, which held that the emotion of anger (and the resulting aggression) was a consequence of the frustration of some goal-directed activity, and the violent behavior followed from frustration, not from an instinct. Blockage of movement (by a barrier) towards a desirable goal induces frustration and the commonest response to frustration is anger, attack on the barrier or some other aggressive behavior.

Murder is an extreme manifestation of aggression. A person may kill another person because the latter blocks the former's path to a desired goal. Killing, in virtually every case, is triggered by frustration of powerful motives such as hunger, sex, wealth, power or prestige. However, later it was found that frustration may produce several other forms of behavior, and anger may result from causes other than frustration. Frustration-aggression theory suggests that anger is built up anew by each frustrating blockage of a powerful drive, but social conditions do not permit the expression of pent up energy underlying the emotion. Under such conditions, *displacement of aggression* takes place. That is, aggression is shown toward objects that are more or less irrelevant instead of those objects that instigated frustration. For example, a wife, frustrated by her husband, may beat the child, slam the door or throw the kitchen vessels. Generally, displacement occurs when:

1. There is a threat to the expression of anger toward the frustrating stimulus.
2. There is some stimulus similar to the originally frustrating one.
3. The substitute is weak and cannot retaliate.
4. The frustrating stimulus is absent.

As is apparent, displacement of aggression is an instance of stimulus generalization. According to psychologist Saul Rosenzweig, when aggression is displaced, it may be focused on one of the following directions:

1. Toward others (*extrapunitive*).
2. Toward oneself (*intropunitive*).
3. Away from the object of frustration (*impunitive*); denying that there was frustration.

By now, it must be clear that anger can function as a motive; it mobilizes energy and facilitates vigorous, sustained activity. It intensifies thought and action. Anger in itself is not a primary drive; it helps in the satisfaction of other needs. But continuous anger may become an impulse demanding an outlet even when the drive it was serving has been satisfied or forgotten.

Anger is a negative emotion and it often leads to undesirable consequences, especially physical or verbal aggression. You may do things in anger that you may regret later. Frequent bouts of anger can impair your health, putting you at increased risk of cardiovascular disorders. It is said that anger is "Danger minus D." Therefore, it is necessary to control your anger. What can you do about it? Here are a few tips to manage anger:

1. To gain control over your anger, you need to identify and control anger-producing thoughts and statements. By doing so you can learn to avoid hostile confrontations, learn to replace such thoughts with calming alternatives.
2. When someone says something unpalatable, do not jump to the conclusion that the other person means you ill. There may be other ways of interpreting the other person's behavior. Review the evidence.
3. Cultivate adaptive thinking. Handle the situation without getting upset. Sit down and think through what you want to say.

4. You can stop becoming angry by engaging in competing thoughts and acts. Try to relax or go for a walk. Count ten before you hit; if you still cannot control, count hundred. While counting, think something other than hitting.
5. Reward yourself when you controlled your anger and handled the situation amicably.
6. Do not expect too much from others. Then, there will not be any disappointments and frustrations and hence no gripe.
7. Do not raise your voice; keep cool even when others fail to do it.
8. Learn to express positive feelings.
9. Remember the proverbial statement—"Keep your temper, nobody wants it."

Appears difficult to execute, is it not? Try to practice, and then it becomes a habit. Nothing is impossible.

Disgust

Disgust is an emotion marked by aversion toward stimuli that are distasteful. Disgust has adaptive value in that it helps in selecting and rejecting the appropriate foods. The sight of a fly in your cup of milk or a cockroach in the soup creates disgust. The facial expression typically accompanied by disgust is itself an adaptive reaction to a potentially harmful food; you wrinkle your nose and your mouth drops open in characteristic gape. Wrinkling of nose closes the air passages, cutting off the offending smell; the gaping expression causes the contents of the mouth to dribble out. Disgust has a psychological component also. Suppose you are given a fresh, sterilized comb to stir sugar in your coffee cup, would you use it? Probably not.

Disgust is experienced universally across all cultures, but the emotion takes time to develop. Children are not disgusted about several dirty things. You must have noticed young children below 4 years putting everything, even disgusting ones, in their mouth. They may play with feces, urine or any other dirty object. They may swallow an insect. Children have no conception of what is good or dirty; they gradually learn what not to put into their mouth.

Love

It is strange that psychologists have done more research on negative emotions like fear and anger than on positive emotions such as love and happiness. Without doubt, love is an important and powerful emotion. Wars have been fought and people killed for the sake of love. Great epic literatures were written on the theme of love. Soldiers have sacrificed their lives to save a loved peer. Children abandon parents and go out of their homes to be with their loved ones. Past and present history reveal the great impact love makes in human lives. There must be some truth in the common adage which says that "love makes the world go round." But, what is love? How can we study this strange emotion, which may be sweet and bitter, quiet and violent, tender and powerful? What are the beginnings and endings of love? How does it manifest and what are its consequences? We do not have clear-cut answers; the mystery surrounding love endures.

Love is called "many splendored thing." Love does not refer only to the passionate attachment between a man and a woman as it is popularly portrayed; it has many facets. Erich Fromm, in his book; *The art of loving* (1956), proposed five major types of love, i.e. parental love, filial love, fraternal love, conjugal love and self-love.

Parental love: It refers to the love towards our parents and other elders, leaders, king, queen and even god.

Filial love: It refers to parents' love for their children, which extends for all other youngsters and helpless beings including animals.

Fraternal love: It is the love between brothers and sisters, neighbors that may in time, extend toward all human beings.

Conjugal love: It refers to the love between the spouses (husband and wife); the special characteristic of conjugal love is that it is focused toward one person, while the first three forms can flow toward a multiplicity of people.

Self-love: It refers to the understanding, acceptance and respect one has toward one self. Self-love does not mean selfishness. A selfish person cannot love himself or others. Self-love is a realistic appreciation of one's own self.

There may be other forms of love, such as love of the motherland, love of nature, so on and so forth.

Till recently, it was thought difficult or even impossible to study love in the laboratory, but an American psychologist Harry F Harlow (Harlow and Zimmerman, 1959) demonstrated that some aspects of love can be studied experimentally. Using monkeys as subjects, he demonstrated that it is **contact comfort** that is at the roots of the development of affectional relationship between the mother and the child. In a series of landmark experiments, Harlow showed how the young ones are touched, held and handled by their caretakers determine the development of love (affectional attachment) between them. Freud had said that touch played the most important part in personality development; Harlow supported and extended the Freudian line of thinking.

In recent years, psychologists have been making attempts to study certain aspects of love relationship between men and women. In the realm of romantic relationship, they have identified two types of love, i.e. **passionate love** and **companionate love**. Passionate love involves intense feeling, arousal and yearning for the member of the opposite sex. There is a sudden feeling of being in love; it involves sexual attraction, a desire for mutual love and physical closeness and the fear that the relation may come to an end. Companionate love is marked by intense affection, deep caring, close friendship, concern for the well-being of the partner and mutual caring, liking, respect and attraction. Compared with companionate love, passionate love is less stable and may decline with the passage of time. It does not mean that the flame of passion will disappear altogether. Both types of love contribute to satisfaction in long-term romantic relationship.

Psychologist Robert Sternberg (1988) has proposed a **triangular model of love**. According to this model, love has three major dimensions such as *passion*, *intimacy* and *commitment*:

1. Passion refers to physical attraction and sexual desire; it is the motivational component.
2. Intimacy involves closeness, connectedness, sharing, warm relationship, and valuing each other; it is the emotional component.
3. Commitment indicates to an intense desire to retain the relationship. It is the decision-making aspect of love and shows how well one sticks to the other in times of trouble.

At any point of time, a love relationship may involve only one, two, or all three dimensions, giving rise in all to seven types of love. The various combinations of Sternberg's dimensions and the resulting types of love are shown in Figure 10.4. For example, when there is intimacy alone, it is liking or friendship. When intimacy is coupled with commitment, it becomes companionate love. When there is only commitment, it is called empty love. When there is only passion, it is infatuation. When intimacy and passion coexist it becomes romantic love. When passion and commitment coexist, it is called fatuous love. When intimacy, passion and commitment are present, it is consummate love, which is an ideal combination.

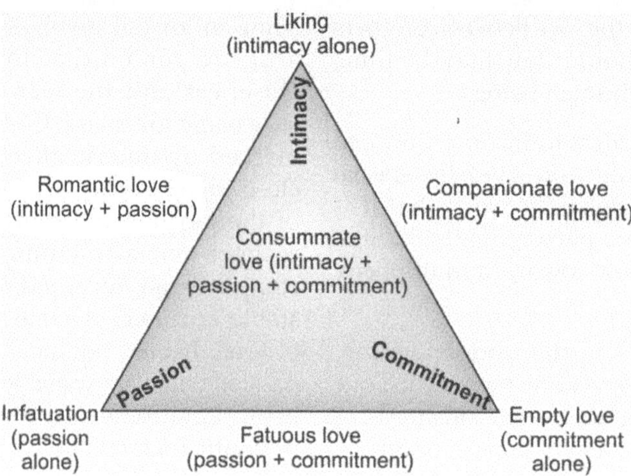

FIGURE 10.4: Sternberg's triangular model of love

Human capacity to love is not genetically determined. Love depends on intimacy and intimacy progresses in stages. How we feel in a relationship influences the relationship itself. A growing feeling of intimacy depends on three factors:

1. A feeling that you are being understood by your partner.
2. A feeling that your emotions and point of view are being respected.
3. A feeling that the other person cares for you.

As the relationship progresses love deepens over time. Your moods can influence love relationship. When you are under positive mood, your relation appears to be good and vice versa. Researches indicate that the following factors determine whether your love is long lasting:

1. ***Similarity between the partners:*** "Similarity breeds content," not contempt!
2. ***Frequency of sex:*** Happy couples have sex more often than they engage in arguments.
3. ***Intimacy:*** Successful couples share their innermost thoughts and feelings with each other.
4. ***Decision making:*** Happily married people consult each other in making important decisions, help each other in housekeeping, and most importantly: "They do not keep an account of mistakes."

Happiness

What makes people happy? Is it health, wealth, power? It is difficult to answer. Happiness is an important human emotion, but like love, it has been a neglected area in psychology. Psychologists were more interested in studying negative emotions such as fear or anger rather than the positive ones such as love and happiness. Research on happiness started very recently. Being happy is one of the conditions studied within an emerging area of psychology called **positive psychology**. Most of the studies have employed self-report techniques to assess the level of happiness under a technical title, **subjective well-being (SWB)**. In one study, ratings were obtained from nearly 1,000 people from 43 countries. The mean rating of personal happiness on a 10-point scale was 6.33, indicating mild happiness. Advanced countries like the United States scored well above the average while India and Dominican Republic fell into the unhappy range. No gender difference was seen in global happiness, but there was an interesting qualifier. Women on average experience both positive and negative emotions more intensely than men. However, the extreme emotions of women balance out, resulting in an average similar to that produced by fewer extremes among men (Diener, 2000).

Some researchers have attempted to identify the factors that contribute to happiness. It was found that money can produce happiness, but only to some extent. Members of the Forbes list (the wealthiest individuals in the world) are only a tiny bit happier than the common man on the whole. Money makes poor people happy, but once they rise above the level of poverty, additional wealth does not contribute to more happiness. Research shows that people in many poor countries (such as Columbia and Costa Rica) are actually happier than those in the wealthy countries (such as Japan, Canada and the United States). Even extreme changes in wealth, such as a big unexpected inheritance or winning a lottery, have a positive but temporary impact on SWB.

Being healthy, wealthy or intelligent does not guarantee happiness. Just as wealth does not bring happiness, misfortune may not make one miserable. People who have suffered a major crisis (loss of wealth, serious illness, death of a loved one) in life recover. However, when multiple crises pile up, a person's outlook may change. According to Martin Seligman, a pioneer in the positive psychology movement, people with a life-threatening disease are not unhappy compared with the rest of the population, but a cascade of minor misfortunes can make a difference. On the whole, people who have satisfying social relationship (having good friends) were found to be happy. Married people remain happier than single and divorced ones. Those who think they are leading a meaningful life were found to be happy. Those who have some sort of religious faith appear to be happy. Personality factors such as optimism, openness to experience, curiosity and altruism were found to correlate with happiness. Identical twins were more similar in SWB, regardless of their life circumstances (Seligman, 2002; Diener & Seligman, 2004).

Perhaps, psychological processes, rather than resources, are the keys to happiness. It appears that people's happiness or unhappiness is based on the comparisons they make with others (**social comparison**) or with experiences from their past. People have some standards for satisfaction (a set point) and they are happy to the extent that these standards are met or surpassed. But these standards are constantly changing. We also do not know how these set points are determined. When you compare yourself with people who are less fortunate than you (downward comparison), you feel comfortable. But when you compare yourself with people who are more fortunate than you (upward comparison), you feel uncomfortable. Some researchers suggest that genetics play an important role in this regard. Happiness is an elusive and fickle phenomenon. A poor man without enough of food and shelter may get up with a smile in the morning and a rich man may be grumbling even when he gets a pot full of money. Further, culture may play a role in determining whether you are happy or not. For example, people living in societies that emphasize collectivism (Asia) are happier than those who live in societies that emphasize individualism (Europe and North America).

Most of the conclusions reached about happiness are based on correlational research; correlation does not mean causation. Research has shown that happiness is associated with several factors. But we do not know whether these factors simply coexist with happiness or cause happiness. Happiness is a complex phenomenon and it may have biological, social and psychological determinants. Some researchers are trying to identify certain brain centers that are believed to control the experience of happiness (Box 10.2).

Box 10.2: Brain and Happiness

In recent times, neuropsychologists like Richard Davidson of Wisconsin University, have made attempts to determine the neurological basis of happiness. It is reported that positive emotions including happiness are associated with increased activity in the prefrontal cortex of the left cerebral hemisphere, whereas negative emotions, such as disgust, are associated with increased activity in the right prefrontal cortex. The prefrontal cortex is the part of the frontal lobe that lies in front of the motor cortex. It is the brain's executive center involved in problem solving, decision making and planning.

Neuropsychologists have also suggested that the ratio between the levels of activation in the two cerebral hemispheres may reveal a person's general disposition. In cases where the ratio shifts in favor of the left hemisphere, people tend to be more enthusiastic and happier, while when the balance shifts further to the right; such people are more likely to suffer from depression or anxiety. Davidson has also suggested certain techniques of shifting the ratio in favor of the left hemisphere. For example, it is said that Buddhist style of mindfulness meditation can produce a leftward shift in the level of activation, making people happy.

It may take a few more years to establish the actual factors that produce SWB. For the time being, psychologists offer the following guidelines to lead a happy life:

1. Have time for social interactions; spend time with others and try to develop close relationships with at least some people. Seligman believes that expressing gratitude to those who impacted your life is a key component of personal happiness.
2. As far as possible, try to help others; doing so will increase self-worth and makes life meaningful.
3. Seek a challenging vocation; enjoyable work is a prime ingredient of happiness.
4. Set some meaningful goals and try to achieve them.
5. Find some time to engage in enjoyable activities outside your occupation.
6. Try to be physically healthy; exercise, practice good dietary habits and sleep well.
7. Be open to new experiences; seek and learn some new things.
8. Be an optimist; be happy with what you have; do not grumble about things you do not possess.
9. Every night, before going to bed, think of three things that went well during the day; write them down and reflect on them you will feel better.
10. Remember, it is not "What you have," but "What you are" that is important for happiness (Erich Fromm).

Researchers have shown that positive states of mind can promote resilience, which is the ability to bounce back from adversity; it can promote personal health and even boost the immune system and help to cope with the disease; it can broaden your field of attention and lead you to become more open and receptive. Positive emotions often promote effective coping strategies and effective coping strategies in turn produce more positive emotions.

Chapter Summary

Emotions are stirred up states of an organism. Like motives, emotions have energizing properties; they prepare the individual to engage in specific types of behavior. You run away when you are afraid; fight when angry and weep when hurt. Emotions have physiological, psychological (cognitive) and behavioral components. They typically involve physiological arousal, a distinctive expression and some kind of subjective experience. Through their physical expression people communicate their feelings to

Contd...

Contd...

others. The arousal prepares for action. Thoughts become focused and muscles are ready to respond. Emotions can be fairly well judged from facial expressions. Research indicates that six primary emotions—anger, fear, disgust, sadness, happiness and surprise—are recognized universally. There are cultural rules that determine how emotions are displayed and how much of expression is appropriate.

The physiological responses are believed to be controlled by the hypothalamus, the cerebral cortex, limbic system structures, endocrines and the ANS. One theory suggests that there are two types of brain activities in processing emotions such as one involving conscious processing by the cortex and the other unconscious processing by the amygdala. Negative emotions seem to reflect greater relative activation of the right hemisphere, whereas positive emotions are related to relatively greater activation in the left hemisphere. The validity of the polygraph as a lie detector has been questioned. It is often difficult to determine the meaning of recorded physiological changes. Also, it is found that several people can learn to control their emotional expressions.

A number of theories of emotion have been proposed over the years. James-Lange theory of emotions asserts that emotions follow bodily reactions to emotion-triggering stimuli. The Cannon-Bard theory proposes that the subjective experience of an emotion and the bodily reactions associated with it occur virtually simultaneously. The Schachter and Singer's cognitive theory proposes that the combination of physiological arousal and cognitive appraisal (labeling) of the source of the arousal produces the specific emotional state. LeDoux's theory suggests that there are two brain pathways for processing fear stimuli; a "high road" leading to the cerebral cortex and a "low road" leading to the amygdala.

Plutchik has proposed a color wheel model of emotions, which says that people experience eight primary emotions—joy, acceptance, fear, surprise, sadness, disgust, anger and anticipation —represented by the segments within the circle and that combination of these primary emotions produce the more complex secondary emotions represented outside the circle (Refer the picture in the text).

The primary emotions such as anger, fear, disgust, love and happiness have been extensively studied. One of the major causes of aggression is frustration. Fear is basically a learned emotion. In the beginning, infants and children are not afraid of the stimuli that scare them when they are adults. Love and happiness have become subjects of investigations only recently. Sternberg has proposed a triangular theory of love. According to him, three basic components of love—passion, intimacy and commitment—give rise to seven forms of love. A new branch of psychology—positive psychology—studies the origins and development of happiness. The subjective experience of emotion of happiness has been found to be relative. Researchers such as Seligman state that whether we feel happy seems to depend on the comparisons we make with others and with our past experiences. In short, emotions are powerful adaptive tools; they increase the likelihood of survival. Remember, emotions can make life colorful and worth living!

Finally remember that motivation and emotions are closely related; both arouse, energize and direct behavior towards a goal; both are highly adaptive. For example, anger is an emotion, but it also drives to action. The two not only increase the likelihood of survival, but also prolong life. According to Leeper (1970), almost all our sustained and goal-directed behavior are emotionally toned, and that it is the emotional tone which provides the motivation for long sequences of behavior. Another theorist Tomkins (1970, 1981) maintains that emotions provide the energy for motives. According to Tomkins, motives simply provide information of some need (need for food, water, sex), but emotions accompany the drives providing energy for the drive and making them motivational forces. The driving properties of motivation and emotion are not easily separated.

11 CHAPTER Personality

PREVIEW

The most important chapter in any textbook of psychology will be on personality and so it is with this book. This chapter is about you, your view of yourself, the person you see when you stand in front of a mirror, your *'personality'*. The most important or the desirable thing in this world is to know "yourself." That is what Socrates, the wisest man ever born in this world, said—*'Know Thyself'*. It is about this concept of self; philosophers all over the world have been talking about over the ages. Although, it is impossible to know either yourself or others fully, an attempt is worth making. Psychologists are not philosophers or religious leaders. They are not interested in the immortal you—yourself or soul. Their aim is to understand your personality—what you think you are and what others think you are—as objectively as possible as scientists do. Psychologists are not interested in the immortal soul. They are interested only in the picture, you have about yourself and how this picture is created within you and how it influences your behavior and mental activities. The personality that psychologists are talking about is born with you and ends with you.

Like all other concepts in psychology, personality is very difficult to define. Way back in 1927, GW Allport, a pioneer in the study of personality, found some 50 definitions of personality and today you may find more of them. There are a number of theories on personality and each theoretical group defines the term in their own way. There are type theories, trait theories, psychodynamic, behavioristic and humanistic theories, each viewing personality from its own perspective. Not attempting to be highly scientific, we may think of personality as the relatively stable set of psychological characteristics and behavior patterns that make individuals unique and account for the consistency of their actions over time. Personality is a composite of the ways in which people relate to others and adapt to the demands placed on them by the environment. Psychologists are interested in the uniqueness and consistency of personality. You are unique; there is nobody in this world just like you. You behave relatively consistently over months and years; your personality does not change easily. Do not fall a prey to the advertisers in the media who promise to change your personality. Courses are popular in the area of personality development. Of course, these courses may teach you how to groom, dress, and speak. It is not that easy to change your personality as psychologists know, although not impossible.

In this chapter, you will learn about the different views that psychologists hold about personality, its structure, dynamics and development. You will learn about what constitutes personality, the energy that activates personality and the way personality develops and changes in the course of your life. You will learn about the biological, psychological and sociocultural factors that shape your personality. You will know how people differ with regard to their behavior patterns. You will be apprised of the attempts made by psychologists to measure personality.

The most fascinating area of psychology is personality. Several psychologists specialize only in studying personality and they have propounded interesting insights in the area. As a nurse, who will be dealing with people, their pains and pleasures, trials and tribulations, it is advisable that you acquire a working knowledge about the various aspects of personality. You will not become an expert personologist by reading this chapter. If it kindles an interest in you to study further the complexities involved in personality, the chapter has served its purpose. There are wonderful books (such as: *Theories of personality* by Hall, Lindzey, and Campbell, 1998), which you must read to enrich your knowledge in the area of personality.

Chapter Outline

WHAT IS PERSONALITY?

All of us talk about personality, make judgments about others' personalities and spend lots of time and effort trying to understand our own and others' personalities. Still we do not know what exactly personality is. There are about 30 to 40 theories of personality, which simply means that even psychologists do not agree with one another in their understanding of personality. But still, they are deeply interested in the study of the enigmatic phenomenon called personality.

When experimental psychology was inaugurated in Leipzig, Wundt or his followers were not interested in the study of personality. For them, psychology was simply the study of the structure of consciousness or immediate experience. In fact, the study of personality emerged not in the laboratories of experimental psychology, but in clinics where people, suffering with some or the other psychological ailments, were being treated. It was the work of clinicians like Charcot, Janet, Freud, and Jung that led to the development of psychology of personality. For that matter, the study of personality has occupied a dissident role in the history of psychology. It was only recently, experimental psychology in general and learning theory in particular has shown interest in the study of personality. However, today personality is a central construct in psychology and almost all theorizing and research in the field of psychology in one way or the other are directed toward understanding and explaining human personality. This is not surprising since every human being including the psychologist is interested in knowing who "he" or "she" is. Some of the best brains in psychology have attempted to unravel the mystery of personality. The study of personality is so important that Henry Murray, an eminent Harvard psychologist, called psychology as "personology" the science of person. But then, what is personality?

DEFINITION

The human personality is probably the most complex construct that is being studied by psychologists. There is no generally accepted definition of the term personality. There are as many definitions as there are writers. One of the difficulties in defining the term is the popularity of the concept itself. Everybody appears to know what personality is. When a physicist talks about the atomic nucleus, nobody claims that he knows better than the physicist does. But, when a psychologist talks about personality, everyone asserts that he knows better than the psychologist about the subject.

When lay people use the term personality, generally, they refer to the impact the person makes on others—his or her social effectiveness. That is what people mean when they say, "He has a personality." They are referring to the person's dress, appearance, the manner of speaking and such other social skills he/she is employing to make a favorable impression on others. This is what the popular courses on "personality development" mean when they advertise in the media. Another way in which common man understands personality is in terms of the dominant feature the person is exhibiting. Thus, we may refer to someone as possessing a dominant, aggressive, shy or submissive personality.

Ross Stagner attempted to analyze the various ways in which the term personality is being used in contemporary psychological literature. He discusses personality under three heads: as *stimulus*, as *response* and as *intervening variable*. Personality as stimulus refers to the social stimulus value of a person—that is, the impression a person makes on others, which may be favorable or unfavorable. For example, when we say that a person has a "personality," we mean that people react positively to that person. This is not a valid definition of personality because the same person makes different impressions on different people at the same time and the same person may make different impressions on the same person at different times. A baby may look ugly to you and me, but for the mother it is the most beautiful object in the world. Hitler was adored by ardent Nazis of Germany, but others all over the world did not perceive him in a similar way. A beautiful young girl of 18 appears differently to men and women. Therefore, we cannot develop a science of personality if we use the stimulus point of view of personality.

The second view—personality as response—concentrates on what a person does. It looks at a person's pattern of behavior. We can objectively observe what a person does over time and based on his or her consistent pattern of behavior, we can develop an idea of personality. We can also ask others to observe his or her behavior and the information given by them can be used to validate our observation. This approach is slightly better, but still it poses certain difficulties. The same behavior is not exhibited by different people for the same reason. A response does not have the same meaning for different persons or even for the same person at different times. For example, when you avoid meeting a person on the street, it may be because he is a dangerous person or because you owe him some money or simply because he is a big bore. Suppose you have money to pay him, then, your behavior will be different. You straight go to him, pay the money you owe him. Does it mean your personality has changed or is it just a change in your economic status?

These difficulties led psychologists to consider personality as intervening variable; it is something that intervenes between the stimulus and the response. That is to say that personality is the inner organization of perceptions, emotions, and motivations of the individual that determines his or her behavior. Thus, personality refers to an inner organization of a number of psychological and even physiological characteristics that a person possesses, which determines his reactions to environmental stimuli. It is an intervening variable between the independent and dependent variable that makes his behavior unique different from all others. An important definition given by Gordon Allport, a Harvard psychologist who wrote the first textbook of personality, fits well with this argument. Allport (1937) wrote: "Personality is the dynamic organization within the individual of those psychophysical systems that determine his unique adjustments to his environment."

Allport's definition of personality is important because it has influenced the thinking and investigations of several psychologists in the field. It has played an important role in the development of several theories of personality. Certain aspects of Allport's definition merit special mention. The term "dynamic organization" implies that personality is constantly developing and changing, but at the same time there is an organization or system that binds together and relates the various components of personality. The term "psychophysical" indicates that personality is neither exclusively psychological nor physiological. The organization involves the operation of both mind and body. The word "determine" implies that personality is made up of determining tendencies that play an active role in the individual's behavior. Allport (1937) wrote: "Personality is something and does something... It is what lies *behind* specific acts and *within* the individual."

In conclusion, it can be said that the concept of personality emerges from the observation of individual differences and consistencies in behavior. We know that people differ meaningfully in the ways they generally think, feel, and act. These distinctive patterns of behavior indicate an individual's identity as a person. But, at the same time we share with others several characteristics. As Kluckhohn & Murray (1953) put it, each of us is in certain respects like *all other* people, like *some other* people, and like *no other* person. The idea of personality also implies that a given person seems to behave consistently over time and across different situations. The consistency is low between childhood personality and adult personality; the consistency becomes greater as one enters adulthood. But, even in adulthood there will be changes in personality. In the light of this, it can be said that personality refers to the distinctive and relatively enduring ways of thinking, feeling, and acting that characterize a person's responses to life situations (Passer and Smith, 2007).

THEORIES

The approaches to the study of personality and the theories developed to explain it are so numerous that it is impossible to review all of them in one chapter. Several books have been written on theories of personality. There are psychodynamic, behavioristic, humanistic, existential, biological, biosocial, sociocultural, and cognitive perspectives that guided the study of personality. Psychodynamic theories, particularly Freud's psychoanalytic theory basically, considered man as an *animal*, at best a domesticated animal. The behaviorists have made man a *machine*, a computer, may be a supercomputer, which can be made to do what you want it to do depending on what you feed into it. The humanists led by Maslow & Rogers look at man as a *human being* with special characteristics that are not to be found either among animals or machines. Personality theorists appear to be not worried very much about the subjective truth of their theories. They are more interested in the usefulness of their theories, especially in stimulating research, and the extent to which the theory provides a comprehensive framework within which known facts can be incorporated allowing them to predict behavior with some precision. We shall review in the following pages some of the major theories of personality.

Freud's Psychoanalytic Theory

Austrian physician Sigmund Freud (Fig. 11.1) expounded the very first and probably the most comprehensive theory of personality in the early years of the 20th century. Freud's theory influenced the development of most other theories of personality in one way or the other. Freud was a genius; his impact on psychology, history, sociology, religion and literature is profound. He is being compared with great people such as Charles Darwin, Albert Einstein & Karl Marx, who have changed the course of human history. Some say that Freud inaugurated the 20th century, because he published his monumental book *'The Interpretation of Dreams'* in 1900 AD. It is also said that he disturbed the sleep of the 20th century man by his views about human nature because he sketched humans as unconscious, irrational, pleasure-seeking, aggressive and amoral, as opposed to the popular view that humans were conscious, rational, altruistic, peace-loving, ethical beings. Freud developed his theory single handedly, without the support of a university position, entirely based on careful clinical observation of his patients over time. His theory known all over the world as **psychoanalysis** is both a theory of personality and a method of treating psychological disorders. Since, the impact of psychoanalytic theory on psychology is immense, it is necessary to deal with its basic tenets in some detail.

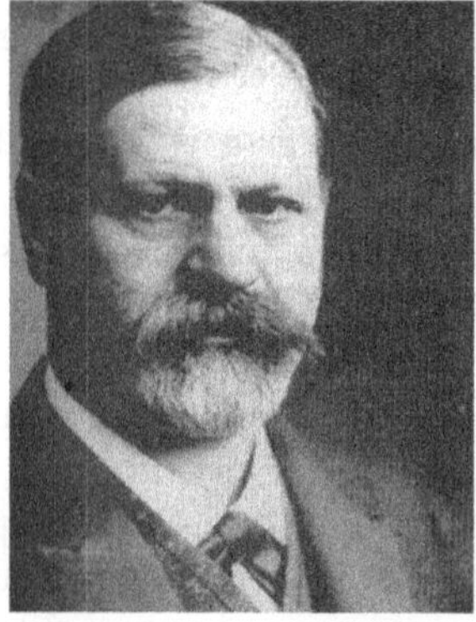

FIGURE 11.1: Sigmund Freud

Topography of Mind

Freud believed that all our mental activities occur at three levels: The ***conscious***, ***preconscious*** and the ***unconscious***. According to him, our conscious experience is just the tip of our psychological makeup. Our conscious mind consists of mental events, which we are currently aware of. The preconscious mind consists of memories, images, thoughts and feelings, which we are unaware at present but can be recalled with some effort. For example, you are not aware now what you ate for your breakfast today; but you can recall it easily. According to Freud, a large part of human behavior is motivated by the unconscious. Conscious and preconscious put together form a small part of human mind. Freud compared the mind to an iceberg: the smaller part visible above the water surface is the conscious while the unseen, huge mass below the level of water is the unconscious. The conscious mind is like a dwarf both in size and importance compared to unconscious. The unconscious is the storehouse of forbidden wishes, amoral impulses, irrational demands, strong passions, emotions and the repressed ideas and feelings, which could not be expressed consciously. It is a great underworld of unseen forces that exercises enormous control over our conscious thoughts and behavior. We come to know about the existence of unconscious only when some of its impulses are discharged in disguise, in the form of dreams, slips of the tongue or in the form of psychological symptoms.

Structure of Personality

According to Freud, personality is made up of three separate, but interacting psychic structures: the **id**, the **ego** and the **superego**. The 'id' is the innermost core and original system of personality out of which both the ego and the superego develop. It consists of everything psychological that is inherited and that is present at birth. It is the reservoir of all the psychic energy. Freud referred to id as "the true psychic reality" and described it as "a chaos, a cauldron of seething excitations." It represents the inner world of subjective experience, is completely unconscious and has no direct contact with objective reality. The id cannot tolerate tension; it needs immediate gratification regardless of rational considerations. The principle of tension reduction by which id operates is called **pleasure principle**. Its slogan is: "I want... I take. "Its main aim is to avoid pain and obtain pleasure and it accomplishes the aim through two processes: **reflex actions** and **primary process**. Reflex actions are innate acts like sneezing, which reduces tension immediately. Primary process refers to the discharging tension through imagination; it is like a hungry person eating an imaginary dish. But, the primary process by itself cannot in the long run reduce tension. A hungry person cannot get satisfaction by eating images of food. In order to set right this anomaly, the second structure, the ego emerges.

Ego: The ego tries to bring about a balance between irrational desires of the id and the realities of the external world. It is guided by the **reality principle**. It tries to find out the real object in the environment that matches the imaginary object held by the id. The realistic thinking of the ego is called **secondary process** and the matching of real object with the image is called *reality testing*. The ego can perform its reality testing because it is endowed with the cognitive capacities such as thinking, reasoning, and problem solving. Thus, the ego takes the role of the executive of the personality. Its role is to mediate between the instinctual desires of the id and prevailing conditions of the external world. It decides what should be done, how and when to satisfy the desires of the id. In a diplomatic way, the ego tries to control the id. It functions like an intelligent minister trying to control the king, who is a tyrant. This is not an easy task because the id is all powerful and the ego has come into existence to satisfy the wishes of the id, not to frustrate it. After all, the ego is an organized portion of the id and come whatever may, it has to serve the wishes of the id, its master. The ego has no existence apart from the id; all its powers are derived from the id and it never becomes completely independent of the id. While describing the lot of the ego, once Freud said that it has to serve "three harsh masters": the id, the external reality and the superego.

Superego: The third system of personality is the superego. It is the moral organ of the individual and represents the traditional social values and ideals. The superego stands for the ideal rather than the real; it strives for perfection rather than pleasure. While the id is guided by the pleasure principle, the ego by the reality principle, the superego is guided by moral principle. The child acquires the social ideals from parents through rewards and punishments he/she receives for the good and bad behavior respectively. The superego has two components: the *conscience* and the *ego-ideal*. Whatever the parents consider bad and the child is punished for indulging in it is incorporated into its conscience. Whatever parents say is good and the child is rewarded for doing it is incorporated into the ego-ideal. The main aims of the superego are to restrain the unbridled fulfillment of the irrational and amoral wishes of the id, persuade the ego to adopt moralistic goals rather than realistic ones and to strive for perfection.

The three structures should not be considered as independent entities operating at cross purposes within the personality. They should not be construed as located at specific sites in the brain. These are mere names given to various psychological processes that follow different system principles. They are not at loggerheads with each other all the time working against each other. Generally, they cooperate with one another and work together as a team under the executive leadership of the ego. The functioning of the three systems can be better understood with the analogy of a passenger bus: the engine of the vehicle, the energy source, is comparable to the id; the driver is the ego and the conductor is the superego. In summary, the id is the biophysical component of personality; the ego is the psychological component and the superego the social component.

Dynamics of Personality

We have examined the structure of personality. For this structure to function there must be energy. The energy that activates the structure is **psychic energy**. The entire energy is stored in the id and it manifests through two groups of instincts called the **life instincts** and the **death instincts**. The purpose of the life instincts is self-preservation and race preservation. The instincts of self-preservation are called *ego instincts*. They are in the service of the individual helping him to get his basic needs (hunger, thirst, safety, etc.). Race preservation through procreation is the aim of the *sex instinct*. The energy behind the sex instinct is known as **libido**. The death instinct is a controversial construct introduced by Freud. It is supposed to lead human beings toward death and destruction. According to Freud, life is a product of living and dying, creation and destruction. Freud asserts that "the goal of life is death. "Every day, we are all moving toward death, the inevitable terminus of life. An important manifestation of the death instinct is aggression. In a nutshell, the major forces that direct most of human behavior are *sex* and *aggression*. When we carefully observe the contents of contemporary movies (filled with sex and violence) and the atrocities occurring around us, we may be tempted to say that Freud was not far from truth.

The life and death instincts and their derivatives may fuse together, neutralize each other or replace each other. In eating, we see the fusion of hunger (life instinct) and destructiveness that is satisfied by biting, chewing and swallowing food (death instinct). Love, a derivative of sex instinct, neutralizes hate, a derivative of the death instinct. Also, love can replace hate and hate can replace love. The life and death instincts were so important in his theory and Freud gave them proper names. He named the life instinct "**Eros**," after the Greek god of love and the death instinct after "**Thanatos**," the Greek god of death.

The dynamics of personality consist of the ways in which the psychic energy is distributed and used by the id, the ego and the superego. The amount of energy in each individual is limited and there is competition among the three systems for the available energy. In the beginning, all energy is in the possession of the id and it uses the same for wish fulfillment by means of primary process. The investment of energy in an object or its image for purposes of gratifying a wish is called *object-choice* or **object-cathexis** (the word object here refers to anything that is required for satisfaction of an instinctual urge. It may be a person, a part of a person or a symbol representative of either). Since, the wishes of the id are unreasonable, they have to be restrained. This has to be done by the ego. The process of restraining the id wishes is called anticathexis. For restraining the id, the ego needs energy, which it must borrow from the id. Since, the ego is engaged in satisfying the id wishes according to the reality principle, the id invests some energy in the ego, a process called **ego cathexis**. Once the ego has trapped enough energy, it can use it for purposes of anticathexes. In the final analysis, the dynamics of personality consist of the interplay of the driving forces (**cathexes**) and the restraining forces (**anticathexes**). All the conflicts and tensions in the personality can be reduced to the opposition of these two sets of forces, cathexes and anticathexes. The entire human mental life can be traced back to the interplay between forces that favor or inhibit one another.

Anxiety, Conflict and Defense

The objects that satisfy the needs of the individual are in the environment and these are not freely available. The environment places certain restrictions on the use of objects. Just because you are hungry, you cannot grab wherever or whatever food is available. When you are driven by sexual urge, you cannot grab whoever is available, and just because you do not like a person, you cannot hit and injure him. Society places restrictions on you as to how you should satisfy your instinctual urges. The environment can offer or withhold objects; it can produce pain and increase tension or reduce tension and bring pleasure. When there is an uncontrollable impulse from within and a concomitant threat from society or the superego about its satisfaction, there will be a strong conflict. If the ego cannot cope up with the conflict and its integrity is threatened, the result is **anxiety**.

Anxiety is an unpleasant state characterized by intense fear and accompanied by physiological arousal and maladaptive behavior.

Freud described three types of anxiety: **reality anxiety**, **neurotic anxiety** and **moral anxiety**. The reality anxiety is what we generally call fear. It is the natural response elicited by real threats or dangers from the external environment and the other two types of anxiety are derived from it. Neurotic anxiety is the fear that instinctual impulses may go out of control and consequent punishment. Moral anxiety is a fear that we may engage in acts that go against the moral code. As you can guess, the source of neurotic anxiety is the id and that of moral anxiety is the superego. Anxiety is a state of tension that warns the individual of impending danger. It is a signal to the ego that unless appropriate actions are taken, its existence will be in danger. When the ego cannot cope up with anxiety by rational methods, it develops some unrealistic measures to protect itself; these are called defense mechanisms of ego or simply mental mechanisms.

Ego Defense Mechanisms

Defense mechanisms are unconscious mental strategies developed by the ego to protect itself from threats from the id, the superego, or/and the external environment. These mechanisms permit the discharge of the id impulses in disguised forms that may not conflict with the injunctions of the superego or the external reality. For example, the major defense mechanism, **repression**, involves the ejection of threatening desires, impulses, and emotionally troubling memories from awareness into the depths of unconscious. It is a type of motivated forgetting. Repression permits people to remain calm and controlled although they harbor lustful or aggressive desires under the surface of awareness. Sometimes repressed memories may enter the conscious in disguise, in the form of dreams or slips of the tongue (Freudian slips). Examine the other defense mechanism called **rationalization** that is most frequently used by all of us. In rationalization, we explain away our undesirable behavior, impulses, or ideas giving probable reasons instead of real reasons. When someone fails in an examination, he may say that the examiners were very strict; the questions were out of the syllabus, etc. He will not mention his own inadequacies, because it is painful or humiliating to do so. When you apply for a job and do not get it, what would you say? You do not say there were better candidates. Generally, you give reasons such as: "The selected candidate had strong recommendations" or "He was relative of one of the ministers." Defense mechanisms are not realistic methods of dealing with problems; mostly, these are irrational operations that deny or distort reality. They are like *"psychological balms"* that relieve pain temporarily, but do not cure the basic malady. The major defense mechanisms are briefly described in Box 11.1.

The theory of ego-defense mechanisms is an important contribution to contemporary psychology. Freud's daughter Anna Freud extended her father's ideas and described many other mental mechanisms such as identification, introjection, intellectualization, compensation and fixation. When we talk of defense mechanisms, what we should remember is that these operate unconsciously and we are totally unaware of their operation and their deceptive nature. These are not realistic ways of dealing with problems. Most of us use defense mechanisms at times, but maladjusted people use them excessively.

Development of Personality

According to Freud, personality develops through a series of dynamically differentiated stages called **psychosexual stages**, which occur during the first few years of a child's life. During the psychosexual stages, the child's pleasure-seeking tendencies are centered on specific pleasure-sensitive areas of the body called **erogenous zones**. Freud was convinced from clinical observations that adult personality characteristics are influenced by experiences occurring during these early years of life. He believed that any deprivation or over-gratification may occur during any of these stages resulting in the

Box 11.1: Defense Mechanisms

Repression: This is the primary mechanism by means of which the ego keeps the unpleasant or traumatic impulses, feelings, thoughts and memories from consciousness. The irrational, immoral and antisocial contents are pushed forcibly into unconscious where they remain active and are waiting for an opportunity to come out. Because of the restraints placed by the ego, they may be expressed indirectly in the form of dreams or often maladaptive symptoms.

Projection: A mechanism through which an unacceptable impulse is repressed and then attributed to external objects, events or persons. For example, a man with loose sexual morals may start suspecting his wife's integrity; a wife who is angry with her husband may punish the child.

Reaction formation: A mechanism, which involves the replacement of an anxiety-producing idea or impulse with its opposite. An extreme example, a person with criminal tendencies becomes a judge in the law court or a wife who hates her husband shows excessive love toward him.

Displacement: Here, an unacceptable impulse is substituted by a safer or less threatening one than the original one. For example, an office worker who is criticized by his superior directs his aggression toward his subordinates.

Rationalization: Giving possible reasons instead of the real reasons for failure is rationalization. When you do not get a job that you applied for, trying to say that the job was uninteresting, not enough remunerative or it was given to influential person, are examples of rationalization. You never say that there were better applicants than you and the deserving ones got the job. To say so would be damaging your self-esteem. We generally explain away undesirable, impulses, ideas and behavior using the mechanism of rationalization.

Denial: In this case, a person refuses to accept the existence of painful events or feelings. For example, a man with a terminal illness, such as cancer, may refuse to accept that he is sick and may even plead that he is perfectly healthy. This is an instance of failure to recognize a threatening event, object or impulse.

Regression: This is a defense mechanism in which an individual, when under stress, reverts to a behavior characteristic of an earlier stage of development. For example, a newly married woman, who finds it difficult to adjust to her new environment, may return to the safety of her parental home or when your father refuses your demand, you start crying like a child.

Sublimation: Here, an attempt is made to redirect the energy behind some frustrated desire toward a socially desirable activity. A woman who could not marry her lover may become a nun in a church or become a novelist. A childless woman may work in an orphanage.

fixation and **regression**. Fixation refers to a concern or conflict that persists beyond a particular psychosexual stage in which it first occurred; it is a state of arrested development in which instinctual desires are focused on a specific theme. Regression is a psychological retreat to an earlier stage of development in the face of an obstacle or a stressful demand, which the individual cannot cope with. Freud proposed five distinct stages of development each having an important function requiring successful completion for the development of a healthy personality.

Psychosexual Stages

Oral stage: The first of the psychosexual stages called the **oral stage** occurs during infancy (birth to 18 months). During this stage, the baby's mouth and lips are the focal points of pleasure. Stimulation of oral zone gives the child immense pleasure. Naturally, the infant gets all his pleasures by sucking on the breast, biting and swallowing. A child who is overly indulged or frustrated in getting oral gratification might become fixated at this stage. Fixation might occur when the baby is fed every time he/she cried or not attended to in spite of his crying. Oral fixation might lead to the development of oral character in adults characterized by excessive mouth-related activities such as kissing, talking, eating and smoking. Freud suggested that orally fixated individuals might become either sarcastic or gullible and either self-indulgent or dependent.

Anal stage: The second stage, called the **anal stage**, occurs between 18 months and 3 years. During this stage, the child derives pleasure through anal stimulation by either excessive elimination or retention (withholding) of the feces. But, the child faces the societal control in the form of toilet training, which is frustrating. Freud suggested that either harshness or laxity in toilet training has important implications for later personality development. Anal fixation might give rise to a set of bipolar personality traits such as *miserliness versus over generosity, stubbornness versus acquiescence* and *orderliness versus sloppiness*. These three sets of polar characteristics are often called **anal triad**. According to Freud, anal fixation may make an adult stingy or spendthrift, excessively concerned with neatness or remaining shabby; he/she may accept everything suggested or vehemently reject all demands.

Phallic stage: At about the age of 3 years, the child enters the third psychosexual stage, called the **phallic stage**. During this stage, the child gets pleasure by fondling his or her genital organs. You must have seen children often touching their sex organs and the parents trying to stop them from doing so. It is natural for children to engage in this type of behavior and they will overcome this tendency over time. Adults need not worry about it. The three stages mentioned above are often called **autoerotic stages**, because the child gets pleasure by the stimulation of his or her body parts. The most important phenomenon that occurs in the phallic stage is the emergence of the Oedipus complex.

Oedipus complex: According to Freud, phallic stage is the most important stage in the personality development because it is in this stage that the well-known **Oedipus complex** surfaces. Oedipus complex refers to an emotional conflict in which the child develops erotic feelings toward the parent of opposite sex along with hatred toward the parent of the same sex. That is, the male child experiences a sexual attraction toward the mother and hatred toward his father; the girl child harbors a sexual attraction toward her father and a dislike of the mother. Freud named this emotional phenomenon Oedipus complex after a character in the Greek tragic drama by Sophocles in which the protagonist Oedipus unknowingly kills his father and marries his mother.

The course of development and resolution of the Oedipus complex occurs differently in boys and girls. In the beginning, both boys and girls are attached to the mother. A little later, the boy is sexually attracted toward the mother and views his father as a rival for the love of his mother. At the same time, he experiences strong feelings of guilt and the fear that his father might punish him. He finds out that his sister is not having a sex organ like his and speculates that she must have been punished by cutting off the penis for harboring feelings like his. The fear that his father might cut off his genital organ is called **castration anxiety**. As a consequence of these complex feelings, the Oedipus complex is resolved and the boy starts identifying with his father. The girl child discovers that she does not possess a penis like her brother (called *penis envy*), blames her mother for the condition and starts hating her. She develops love for the father and a desire to have a child from him as a substitute for her lack of penis. Some writers call the girl's emotional conflict **Electra complex** named after a woman character in another Greek drama, Agamemnon. Electra avenges her father's death by getting his murderers killed—her own mother and her mother's lover. The experience of castration anxiety and penis envy are included under the term **castration complex**. What is important to notice here is that while castration complex resolves Oedipus complex in boys, it starts Electra complex in girls. Freud believed that the girl's Electra complex is not resolved at all and the love of the father is simply transferred to her husband from whom she hopes to derive the satisfactions, which she expected from her father.

Freud considered the phallic stage a landmark in the development of personality because it is here that the children resolve or repress Oedipus/Electra feelings, develop gender identity and attachment to the parents of same sex, a process called *identification*. This identification with the same-sex parent allows the child to possess the opposite-sex parent at least indirectly and also helps the emergence of superego through internalization of the parental values and moral standards. If there are difficulties in crossing the phallic stage and resolving the Oedipal conflicts, one may develop personality problems such as improper sex-role behavior and loss of morals.

Following the resolution of the Oedipus complex, at or around the 5th or 6th year, the child enters into the **latency stage**, which lasts until puberty. During this period, the sexual interests of children remain dormant or remain repressed; they are in the school and engaged in learning and playing; generally, children do not mix with members of the opposite sex. When the children come out of latency period, they are adolescents and their heterosexual interests emerge. Now, they enter the final phase, the **genital stage**, which extends until the end of life.

The first three stages (*pregenital stages*) of development are narcissistic in character. The source of all pleasure is the individual's body. The child gets gratification from the stimulation and manipulation of his or her own bodily organs. During the genital period, some portion of the self-love or **narcissism** becomes channeled into genuine object love. The adolescent starts planning to take up a vocation, becomes interested in a heterosexual relationship and is preparing to marry and settle in life. Gradually, the pleasure-seeking narcissistic infant is transformed into reality-oriented, socialized adult. All these changes occur as a result of the operation of a number of psychological processes such as displacement, identification and sublimation. But this does not mean that all the pregenital impulses are displaced by genital ones; they become fused with the genital impulses. The final organization of adult personality represents contributions from all stages. The psychosexual stages are given in Table 11.1.

Table 11.1: Psychosexual Stages

Psychosexual stage	*Approximate age*	*Erogenous zone*	*Source of pleasure*
Oral	0–18 months	Mouth and lips	Sucking and biting
Anal	18 months to 3 years	Anal region	Retention and expulsion of feces
Phallic	3–5 or 6 years	Penis in boys and clitoris in girls	Self-stimulation
Latency	6 years to puberty	None	Interest in play and school activities
Genital	Puberty to adulthood	Genitals (penis in boys and vagina in girls)	Mature heterosexual relationships

Neo-Freudian Theories

Freud's ideas were so revolutionary that a number of intellectuals from various parts of the world became his followers. Carl Jung from Zurich, Alfred Adler from Vienna, Karl Abraham from Berlin, Sandor Ferenczi, Wilhelm Reich, Otto Rank, Otto Fenichel and Wilhelm Stekel (all from Austria), AA Brill from New York and Ernest Jones from England became Freud's disciples. Karen Horney, HS Sullivan, Erik Erikson, Erich Fromm, Heinz Kohut and several others were influenced by his theory.

Some of the above thinkers did not agree with all the concepts of Freud and tried to modify some of them. Some others rejected outright many of Freud's basic ideas and developed their own theories of personality. These people are generally known as **Neo-Freudians** or neo-analytic theorists. Neo-Freudians believe that Freud gave undue importance to infantile sexuality and did not recognize the role of social and cultural factors in the development of personality. It is not possible to discuss the contributions of all the Neo-Freudians here; only brief summaries of the major theorists are given below.

One of the earliest deviants from Freudian theory was the Swiss psychiatrist **Carl Jung**, (Fig. 11.2) who developed a system called **Analytical Psychology**. Jung disagreed with Freud's *pansexualism*. He expanded the concept of unconscious by incorporating the idea of the **personal unconscious** consisting of a person's life experiences and the **collective unconscious** (*racial unconscious*) that consists of memories accumulated throughout the entire evolutionary history of human race. The memories in the collective unconscious take the form of primordial forces called **archetypes**, which direct human behavior. Jung believed that archetypes are inherited tendencies that allow us to interpret our experiences in certain ways. Archetypes find expressions in the form of symbols, beliefs and myths that are shared by several cultures. For Jung the idea of a god, the mother, the hero, the concept of energy, of wisdom, of good and evil and the search for self-unity and completeness are all manifestations inherited archetypes. Some of

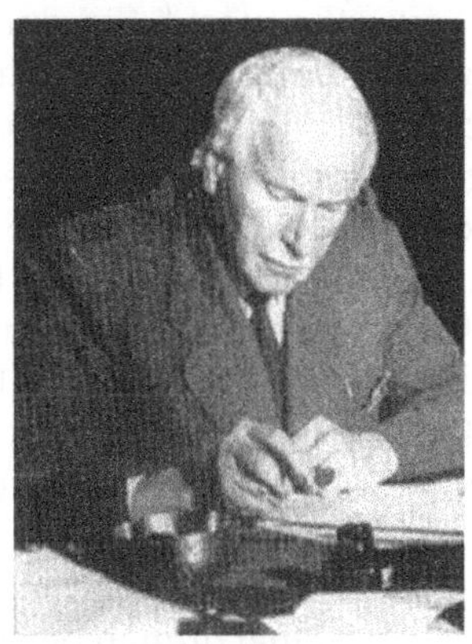

FIGURE 11.2: CG Jung

the ideas of Jung appear to be similar to those of contemporary evolutionary psychologists, who emphasize the role of certain innate cognitive tendencies in the determination of human behavior. Several of Jung's ideas have affected modern psychology. His concept of self-actualization anticipated the work of Abraham Maslow. His emphasis on the role of future (teleology) on personality development was adopted by Alfred Adler. Jung's theory of personality types, *introversion* and *extraversion*, had a colossal influence on the theory, research and assessment of personality. The concept of introversion and extraversion as a dimension of personality has been one of the highly researched topics. An influential psychological test derived from Jung's theory is **Myers-Briggs Type Indicator (MBTI)**, which identifies 16 types of people. Jung's free association test as a tool to unearth unconscious complexes is being used all over the world even today.

Jung was a great thinker and writer. The entire body of his writings is now available in a twenty-volume English-language edition. For 60 years, Jung devoted himself with great energy to analyze the deep processes of human personality. His influence was not confined to psychology and psychiatry. Jung has influenced history, politics, sociology, literature and religion. His impact can be seen among the educated people all over the world. Sigmund Freud had designated Jung as his spiritual heir and had called him "his crown prince." Jung was appointed as the first president of the International Psychoanalytic Association when it was founded in 1910. It was a tragedy for science that Freud and Jung separated within 6 to 7 years after they first met and the two never met again.

The second important dissident theorist to leave the Freudian camp was **Alfred Adler** (Fig. 11.3). Adler did not agree with the Freudian view that human personality is fashioned by biological forces and childhood conflicts only. According to Adler each individual is primarily a social being and people's personality is shaped by their unique social environment and interactions. Adler called his system of psychology, **Individual Psychology**, because it focused on the uniqueness of each person. The central theme of individual psychology is social interest, which is a native tendency among humans. Adler considered humans as social beings who are guided by the desire to help, care for and cooperate with others. According to him, the conscious, not the unconscious was the core of personality. Humans are not simply driven by instincts on which they have no control; they are actively involved in creating their selves and directing their future. Some of Adler's concepts, such as **inferiority complex**, **striving for superiority** and **style of life**, are well known in psychology.

According to Adler, we are all born with a feeling of inferiority and we try to compensate for it. But often we overcompensate for inferiority by developing a superiority complex. Striving for superiority or perfection is the fundamental fact of life. In our attempts to strive for perfection, we develop a style of life, which shapes the development of personality. Adler proposed four basic styles of life: the *dominant type*, the *getting type*, the *avoiding type* and the *socially*

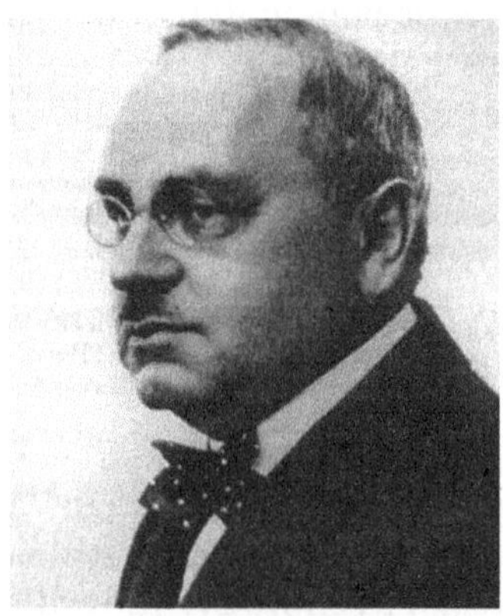

FIGURE 11.3: Alfred Adler

useful type. Those who adopt the first three types generally have adjustment problems. The fourth one fosters the development of healthy personality characterized by social interest. Such people are capable of developing a creative self, which is the ultimate goal of life. Adler believed that parenting styles play a crucial role in the development of healthy (or unhealthy) personality and for raising healthy citizens, guidance was necessary for both parents and children. For this purpose, he started a number of child guidance clinics in Vienna, thus becoming a pioneer in the child guidance movement. Adler also initiated a new line of research that concentrated on the effect of birth order on personality. He proposed that first-borns are high achievers, but dependent, suggestible and anxious, while the last-borns are pampered and more likely to become maladjusted. The only-borns want to be the center of attraction. The research results in this area are not consistent.

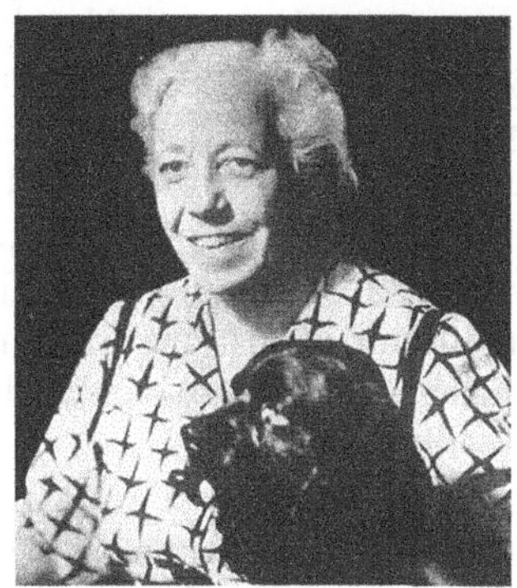

FIGURE 11.4: Karen Horney

Karen Horney (Fig. 11.4) was one of the first psychoanalysts to champion the feminine issues. She was not a disciple or colleague of Freud, but was an officially trained psychoanalyst. She defected from the Freudian camp because of her disagreement with Freud about his views on psychology of women. She was critical of the Freudian concept of penis envy in determining woman's personality development. She asserted that rather than wanting a penis itself, women desire the privileges that go with having a penis (that is, being a male). Horney disagreed with the role and primacy of sexual and aggressive drives in the development of personality. On the other hand, she emphasized the role of parent-child interactions during early childhood. If parents do not provide their children love, warmth and respect, Horney claimed, the children are prone to experience a **basic anxiety**—the feeling of being lonely and helpless in a hostile world. The anxiety produces an excessive need for affection. When this need is not met, the child feels rejected, which in turn results in more anxiety and hostility. These troubled states give rise to a set of neurotic needs, such as need for approval, for power, for perfection, self-sufficiency, for personal admiration, for ambition and achievement, for prestige, and a need to exploit others. These needs create problems. All these problems can be avoided if the child is raised in a home where there is security, trust, love, respect, tolerance and warmth.

Horney's picture of human nature is considerably more optimistic than Freud's. According to her, we are not slaves of biological forces and not cowed down by infantile conflicts. Neurotic behavior results from social anomalies. Parent-child relationship can either satisfy or frustrate the child's need for security. If the need is frustrated the child develops neurotic behavior. Neurotic trends can be prevented if the child is raised with love, acceptance and trust. Each of us has the innate potential for self-realization, which should not be thwarted by social forces. The optimistic theme in Horney's theory is that we can resolve our problems and each of us can shape our personality through *self-analysis*, which is also the title of one of her famous book. Horney was a prolific writer and her books are very popular and widely read all over the world.

Erich Fromm was another Neo-Freudian who is famous through his books that are being read all over the world. Fromm has received considerable attention not only from psychologists, sociologists and philosophers but also from general public. The central theme of all his writings is that in modern society people feel lonely, alienated, homeless and isolated because they have become separated from nature and from other people. This condition of isolation is not found in other animals. It is a distinctly human situation that is at the root of all human problems. The situation can be solved by a suitable social organization based on productive love.

As children grow in society, they gain increasing independence and freedom. But they gain freedom at the expense of security of the primary maternal ties. Children try to escape from this freedom through symbiotic relatedness, withdrawal-destructiveness or love. There is a polarity between the drive for freedom and the drive for security. Six needs result from this polarity: the need for relatedness (to be related to people and nature), rootedness need (to belong to a family, community and society), identity need (to achieve an awareness of uniqueness), transcendence need (to rise above animal nature), excitation and stimulation need (to get stimulating environment to function effectively) and frame-of-orientation need (to have a coherent view of the world). How these needs are satisfied depends on the social conditions. Personality development is the result of compromise between human needs and environment. Depending on how we relate or orient to the real world, we develop certain character types. Fromm distinguished between non-productive and productive orientations. The non-productive orientations are unhealthy ways of relating to the world; these include: receptive orientation (always expecting to get whatever you want from others by being dependent on them); exploitative orientation (taking from others by force or cunning), hoarding orientation (amassing and preserving material possessions); marketing orientation (how well one sells oneself; a person for whom superficial qualities are more important than genuine knowledge or skills). Fromm's productive orientation is characterized by ideal self-development. Any given individual is a blend of these two types of orientations. Later in his theory, Fromm included other character types such as biophilous (being in love with life), necrophilous (attracted towards death), having orientation (concerned with possessing and consuming resources) and being orientation (concerned with what one is rather than what one has). Fromm was sincerely concerned with the problem of humans and their relation to society. This concern can be summarized in the following propositions (Hall, Lindzey and Campbell, 1998):

- Humans have an essential, inborn nature
- Society is created by humans in order to fulfill this essential nature
- No society that has been devised meets the basic needs of human existence
- It is possible to create such a society.

Fromm called such an ideal society: '*Humanistic Communitarian Socialism*'. It is a society in which people relate to each other lovingly and are rooted in the bonds of brotherhood and solidarity; it is a society in which people transcend nature by creating rather than destroying; in which everyone gains a sense of self by experiencing himself as the subject of his powers rather than by conformity.

Another important Neo-Freudian was the American psychiatrist, Harry Stack Sullivan, who made '*interpersonal relations*' the focal theme in his theory. He advocated that personality develops in the social context and the type of relationships the individual establishes with important people around him (often called *significant others*). After Freud's death, a number of his followers emphasized the role of the ego in the development of personality. For them, the ego was not a slave of the id; it is autonomous and develops independently of the id. They are often called ego psychologists. Important among them were Anna Freud, Heinz Kohut, George Klein, Robert White and Erik Eriksson. A summary of the Neo-Freudian theories is given in Table 11.2.

Evaluation of Psychoanalytic Theory

Freud is probably the most criticized person in the history of human thought. Although his theory has had a profound impact on contemporary psychology, psychiatry and several other fields, it has been severely criticized on scientific grounds. Many of his concepts have not stood the test of scientific scrutiny. His concepts are so nebulous that it is very difficult to measure them. For example, how can one measure psychic energy, the id impulses, penis envy, castration complex or the Oedipus complex? Science demands operational definitions and assessment of concepts used in the theory. Freud's concepts were not and are not amenable to measurement. How can one study the processes that are by definition unconscious and not available to the person?

Freud based most of his theoretical constructs on the observation of his patients and his own self-observation. He was the only person who underwent self-analysis and incorporated data from it in his theory. Some critics are of the opinion that Freud's own needs and expectations have influenced his observations and theorizing. A very important lacuna is that there was no controlled observation of the data and his patients did not represent the general population.

Another major criticism leveled against Freud is about his overemphasis on sexual motivation. Several critics assert that human behavior can be better explained in terms of motives other than sex; for several of them psychoanalytic theory seems to be more a science fiction than objective scientific discipline and it can never be tested scientifically. One important characteristic of a good

Table 11.2: Neo-Freudian Theories

Neo-Freudian theorist	*Key concepts*	*Brief summary*
Carl Jung	Personal unconscious and collective unconscious; complexes and archetypes; introversion and extraversion	Complexes and archetypes express in the form of dreams, religious and artistic symbols
Alfred Adler	Inferiority, compensation, style of life and creative self and social interest	People compensate for the sense of inadequacy, develop a style of life, and social interest
Karen Horney	Basic anxiety, neurotic needs	Insecure childhood, feeling of helplessness leading to neurotic needs
Harry Stack Sullivan	Interpersonal relations	Personality to be studied in the interpersonal situations
Erick Fromm	Human need for relatedness, rootedness, transcendence, identity and the need for a frame of reference	Humans have to develop a satisfying relationship based upon productive love. What you are is more important than what you have?
Anna Freud	Emphasis ego and defense mechanisms	Ego psychology
Heinz Kohut	Object relations	
Erik Erikson	Psychosocial theory of personality development	

theory, according to the eminent philosopher of science Karl Popper, is falsifiability. That is, for a theory to be scientific, it must specify some observations that if made would refute the theory. Freud's theory explains virtually everything people do, and hence it is not a scientific theory.

Despite the criticisms, many believe that Freud made important contributions to psychology and psychiatry. May be the theory has not withstood the rigors of scientific scrutiny, but scientific methodology is not the only criterion by which a theory has to be judged. In the history of psychology, Wundt's structuralism was built using rigorous scientific principles, but still it failed while psychoanalysis survived. "A theory that, among other things, makes sense personally may survive longer than one that develops and is tested within the realm of science (Hergenhahn, 2001)." That is exactly what has happened to psychoanalytic theory. Human behavior is so complex that it may have to be studied differently apart from the modern scientific method; it may need altogether a different kind of science, a human science, to study human phenomena.

BEHAVIORAL THEORIES

Behaviorists led by Pavlov, Watson, and Skinner were more interested in discovering universal laws of learning than in the notion of an internal personality that directs behavior. Nonetheless, the laws of learning that they discovered have great relevance for understanding personality. According to behaviorists, many of the behavioral patterns used to describe personality are acquired through classical and operant conditioning, in addition to life experiences. Behaviorists consider personality as an organized pattern of learned responses. For behaviorists, internal events such as thoughts, emotions and motivations are irrelevant. The individual is an empty organism and the environmental stimuli determine what he/she does or becomes. Behaviorists, thus, were radical environmentalists. According to Watson, the founder of behaviorism, learning and life experiences make people what they are; when experiences change, the personality changes. Careful upbringing of a healthy baby born of a longline of crooks, murderers, thieves and prostitutes can be made into a perfect gentleman. Watson made the following statement that has become a landmark in the history of psychology:

> *"Give me a dozen healthy infants, well-formed and my own specified world to bring them up in and I'll guarantee to take any one at random and train him to become any type of specialist I might select—a doctor, lawyer, artist, merchant-chief and yes, even into beggarman and thief, regardless of his talents, penchants, tendencies, abilities, vocations and race of his ancestors."*

Similarly, **Skinner** held that personality is a collection of reinforced responses—learned behavior patterns. According to him, we are the persons that we are because we behave in certain ways; we behave in certain ways because of the reinforcement contingencies we experience. Similarities in responses across different situations are caused by similar patterns of reinforcement that have been received in such situations in the past. If you take a friend to a party or a movie, it is because you have been reinforced previously for doing so and not because you are fulfilling a repressed unconscious wish based on some early childhood experience, or because you have an internal trait of sociability. In Skinner's view, there is really no need for a concept of personality, let alone a theory of personality. He generated a "personality less" view of personality. Many psychologists are offended by Skinner's efforts to reduce the seeming richness of personality to nothing more than a set of responses strengthened by reinforcers and punishers. Of course, there are also others who consider Skinner's work as refreshing because it is an effort to be clear, precise and parsimonious, explaining personality in terms of the smallest number of theoretical constructs and assumptions.

One of the most elegant and economical theories of personality within the behavioristic mold was proposed by sociologist John Dollard and experimental psychologist Neal Miller. They have integrated into their theory (Dollard & Miller, 1950) the insights derived from learning theory, psychoanalysis and sociology. They explained learning in terms of four conceptual elements: *drive, cue, response* and *reinforcement*. According to these researchers, personality is made up of habits. Habits are formed by stimulus (cue) and response linkage when a drive is reduced by reinforcement under the social context. An interesting feature of the theory is its attempt to explain several psychoanalytic and psychopathological concepts in terms of learning principles.

It is true that *behavioral theories* (also known as *learning theories* or *stimulus-response [S-R] theories*) of personality typify experimental, objective approaches to the study of human behavior. But, an adequate understanding of human behavior must involve more than the slavish application of the experimental methods borrowed from the physical sciences. The bulk of the investigations carried out by S-R theorists are concerned with simple, elementary pieces of behavior instead of complex human behaviors. Their investigations have been carried out on animals such as rats and pigeons that are phylogenetically different in many crucial respects from the human organism. The findings of the S-R theories, obtained in restricted and controlled settings, may not be applicable to the human organism that operates in the real-world environment. The rigor and formal adequacy of S-R theories appear to be illusory. These theories have nothing to say about the structural organization and acquisition of personality. The S-R theories are segmental, fragmented, atomistic and molecular, and there is no appreciation of the molar, holistic nature of personality. These theories are minimally concerned with the subjective and intuitive side of human behavior. In the light of these criticisms, some behavioristic psychologists have viewed personality from a modified perspective, the social-cognitive perspective. These theorists combine behavioral and cognitive perspectives that stress the interaction of thinking humans with a social environment that provides them learning experiences.

SOCIAL COGNITIVE THEORIES

Social cognitive theorists such as **Julian B Rotter** (Fig. 11.5), **Albert Bandura**, and Walter Mischel believe that purely behavioral accounts cannot capture the complex functioning of human personality. They are of the opinion that the learner is not simply a passive reactor to environmental stimuli and that internal processes cannot be excluded from an understanding of personality. According to them, humans are perceivers, thinkers and planners, who mentally interpret events, think about the past, anticipate the future, and decide how to behave in a given situation. Social-cognitive theorists consider the debate whether behavior

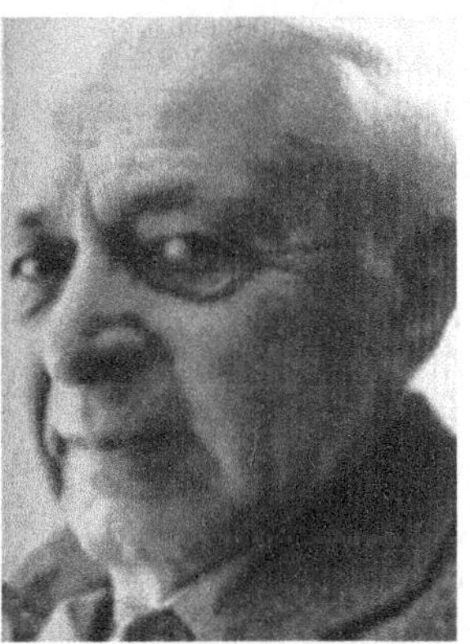

FIGURE 11.5: JB Rotter

is more strongly influenced by personal factors or by the person's environment as meaningless. Instead, they averred that the person, the person's behavior, and the environment all influence one another in a pattern of two-way causal links. Bandura calls this interactive relationship **reciprocal determinism**. Human behavior is part of an interactive process involving psychological and social forces. Our thoughts, emotions, expectations and personal factors influence both the environment and behavior; in turn, the environmental and personal factors influence and are influenced by behavior.

According to Rotter, who laid the foundation for social-cognitive approaches, the likelihood that a particular behavior occurs in a given situation is influenced by two factors: *expectancy* and *reinforcement value*. Expectancy refers to an individual's perception of the likelihood that a consequence will follow if he/she engages in a particular behavior. Reinforcement value refers to the extent to which we desire or dread the outcome that we expect the behavior to produce (Rotter, 1954). For example, when you value a profession and expect that the profession will bring you name and fame, you are more likely to enter into that profession. Note that social-cognitive perspective makes use of reinforcement, a central concept in behavior theory, but view it within the cognitive framework—how we think about our behavior and its expected outcome.

An important expectancy construct in Rotter's theory, '**locus of control**,' has proved to be highly influential in personality research. Locus of control refers to the source an individual perceives as exerting control over his or her life's events. People who think that the locus (source) of control is within them are called *internals*; those who perceive it to be outside are *externals*. Internals are more likely to believe that their life outcomes are largely under their personal control and depend on what they do. On the other hand, externals are prone to think that what they achieve is largely determined by outside forces such as luck, chance, or influential others. Rotter (1966) developed a tool to measure individual differences in locus of control: **Internal-External (I-E) Scale**—which has initiated large-scale research. Studies using the scale have shown that generally internals behave in a more self-determined manner, achieve better grades in college, resist social influence and tend to cope with stress effectively in comparison to externals. Internals exhibit high self-esteem, feelings of personal effectiveness and suffer less from psychological maladjustment.

Major contributions have also been made by the distinguished psychologist of Stanford University, Albert Bandura (1999) (Fig. 11.6) to the **social-cognitive theory** of personality. Bandura's studies of modeling, social learning analysis of aggression, moral behavior and behavioral self-control have demonstrated the wide applicability of the social-cognitive approach. His most important contribution, however, is his theory and research on **self-efficacy**. According to Bandura (1997), people regulate their lives through their sense of self-efficacy, which refers to their belief that they have the ability to follow through and produce desired behaviors. People with high self-efficacy have confidence in their ability to do what they want to do and to overcome the obstacles in their path. Self-efficacy beliefs are always specific to particular situations; one may have high self-efficacy in one situation and not in another. Bandura believes that four factors affect self-efficacy:

1. *Previous performance experiences in similar situations:* These experiences shape your beliefs about your capabilities.
2. *Observational learning:* When you watch someone similar to you accomplishing a task, you are likely to think that if you perform the same behaviors, you will also succeed.

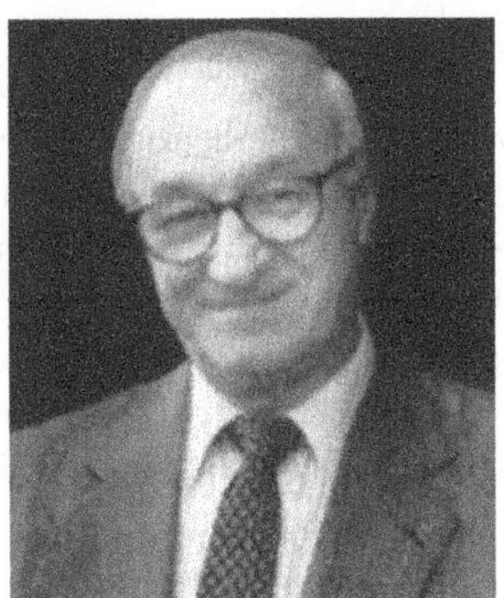

FIGURE 11.6: Albert Bandura

3. *Verbal persuasion:* When others praise or criticize your performance, these messages influence your self-efficacy belief.
4. *Emotional arousal:* When you experience anxiety, it may bring down the experience of efficacy, but if you can control the arousal and be relaxed, it increases your self-efficacy.

Bandura thinks that strong efficacy beliefs are good predictors of performance. These beliefs operate like **self-fulfilling prophecy**. If you strongly believe that you can achieve something, you will do so; if you think you cannot, you will not do.

The third key researcher who made significant contributions to social-cognitive theory is Mischel, who was a student of Rotter and a colleague of Bandura. Mischel along with his former student Yuichi Shoda has developed an approach to personality known as **cognitive-affective personality system (CAPS)**. According to Mischel (1999), CAPS is an organized system of five variables that continuously interact with one another and with the environment, generating a distinctive pattern of behavior that characterizes a person. The five variables are:

1. ***Encoding strategies:*** The way we perceive, categorize and interpret stimuli (objects, persons and events) coming from the external world; our encoding or mentally representing of the stimuli determine how we respond emotionally and behaviorally to situations.
2. ***Expectancies and beliefs:*** What we expect will happen when we behave in a particular way determines our behavioral choices. These *behavior-outcome expectancies* represent the 'if-then' links between alternative behaviors and possible outcomes. In addition, beliefs about our competencies and about the degree of personal control we have, also influence our behavior.
3. ***Goals and values:*** These motivational elements guide our behavior, cause us to persist in the face of obstacles and determine the outcomes we desire and our reactions to them. People with different goals and values may behave differently in the same situation.
4. ***Affects:*** Any behavioral consequence (whether good or bad) triggers an emotional response. Emotions color our perceptions and influence behavior. For example, anxiety lowers outcome expectancies in any of the performance situations.
5. ***Personal competencies and self-regulatory processes:*** Some competencies allow people to develop cognitive problem-solving strategies to adapt to life successfully and pursue important goals. Other competencies involve the ability to exert personal control over thoughts, emotions and behaviors. It is found that people who score high on measures of self-esteem are capable of regulating their behavior and experiencing positive outcomes. Some people regulate their own behavior through self-administered consequences, a process called self-reinforcement. That is, we may evaluate our behavior positively and feel proud or evaluate negatively and experience guilt and shame. *Self-reinforcement processes* often override external consequences, making us more autonomous and self-directed.

Social-cognitive theories combine the insights of behavioral and cognitive approaches in conceptualizing personality dynamics. The constructs used in the theory are well-defined, measured and researched, giving us an understanding of how the person and situational factors interact with each other to influence behavior. A significant feature of social-cognitive theories is their attempt to resolve a persistent problem in personality theory: *the issue of stability versus variability of personality*. Several researchers argue that since behavior varies from situation to situation, the concept of a stable personality is meaningless. Can there be a personality that is stable and coherent and yet exhibiting variability and inconsistency across situations? The ongoing research in social-cognitive theory may provide an answer to this paradox of *personality coherence and inconsistent behavior*.

According to CAPS theory, personality is defined in terms of cognitive-affective-person variables and interactions among them. The CAPS system is believed to be stable and consistent although it can be changed by significant experiences. For these theorists, behavior need not be consistent. The behavior depends on many factors such as the characteristics of stimuli, how these characteristics are encoded, the expectancies and beliefs that are activated, the goals that are relevant, the emotions that are experienced and the plans and self-regulatory processes that help determine behavior. Therefore, it is entirely possible for people to behave inconsistently across situations that appear very similar to outside observers. People will behave similarly in situations that, to them, have important characteristics in common, but they may behave inconsistently in situations that differ in ways that evoke different responses from the CAPS.

As the interactions between personality systems and situations continue to operate, people develop certain consistent patterns of behavior in particular classes of situations. This outward manifestation of personality that gives a person a unique identity is called **behavioral signature**. Researchers have shown that people can have very distinctive behavioral signatures. According to Mischel and Shoda, even the inconsistency of a person's behavior across situations is actually a manifestation of a stable underlying cognitive-affective personality structure that reacts to certain features of situations.

HUMANISTIC THEORIES

Humanistic approach to personality is often referred to as the '*third force*' in psychology in contrast to the two others, the psychoanalytic view, which considers human beings as animals driven by sex and aggression and the behavioristic view that humans are empty organisms that can be trained to do what you want them to do. According to humanists, people's behaviors are neither controlled by irrational impulses emerging from the unconscious nor are their behavior patterns acquired mechanically under reinforcing conditions; humans are conscious individuals who are aware of what they are doing and why. A person's behavior is determined by his or her conscious experience of self and environment. Since humanistic theorists emphasize the primacy of immediate experience as a determinant of behavior, their approach is called *phenomenological approach*. Humanists affirm the inherent dignity and goodness of the human spirit as well as the creative potential and the capacity for personal growth. The works of two eminent psychologists, Abraham Maslow and Carl Rogers, represent the humanistic tradition in psychology. Both of them viewed the **self-concept**, the picture a person has about himself, the self-image, as the core determiner of personality.

Maslow's Theory of Self-actualization

The personality theory proposed by Abraham Maslow (Fig. 11.7) is based on his theory of motivation (the hierarchy of needs), which we discussed earlier in the chapter on motivation. He believed that each person has an essential nature that presses him to become what he can become; this he called the need for **self-actualization**, the need that occupies the top position in the hierarchy of needs. The need for self-actualization becomes salient only when the other primitive deficiency needs are satisfied. Self-actualization refers to "the desire to become more and more what one idiosyncratically is, to become everything that one is capable of becoming (Maslow, 1970)." It does not entail a deficiency or a lack of something external; rather, it represents intrinsic growth of what is already in the person. It is this growth need that makes an individual distinctly human. According to Maslow, the human being is not a white rat; he has a higher and transcendent nature (Maslow, 1971).

In order to understand the transcendent nature, Maslow thought, we should study transcendent people and he undertook such a study that is considered a milestone in psychology. In his research, Maslow studied people who have fulfilled their basic potentialities, models of self-actualized people, such as Abraham Lincoln, Thomas Jefferson, Eleanor Roosevelt, Albert Einstein, Mahatma Gandhi, Walt Whitman, Thoreau, Beethoven and several others who had excelled in their chosen fields including business, sports, arts, science and literature. As you can see, some of his subjects were historical personages and others his contemporaries. His investigation led him to propose that these "optimal" people share some distinguishing characteristics that are not found among ordinary people. A list of the characteristics of the self-actualizers is given below:

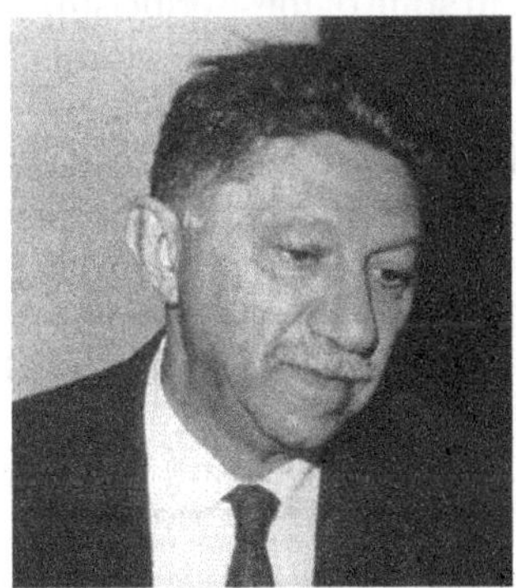

FIGURE 11.7: Abraham Maslow

1. Self-actualized people are realistically oriented. They are open to experience, perceive reality accurately and efficiently; they see people, themselves and things as they are, not as they should be or as they want them to be and have cordial relations with them; their perceptions are not distorted by personal expectations and prejudices.
2. They accept themselves, other people and the natural world for what they are along with their assets and liabilities (good and bad characteristics); they appreciate what is and do not worry about what is not there. Self-acceptance (not selfishness) is a special characteristic of self-actualizers.
3. They are spontaneous, autonomous and independent. Their behavior is self-initiated, not forced by external pressures; they do what they think is right; they are honest and genuine, and do not pretend to please others. They do not wear façades.
4. They are problem-centered, not self-centered. They have a goal; it may be big or small. They try sincerely to reach the goal. The goal, however, is not self-aggrandizement.
5. Most of the time they are detached; they may not be popular with people. They need and enjoy privacy, but do not suffer from loneliness.

6. Their appreciation of people, events and things is fresh rather than stereotyped. They enjoy even small and ordinary things. They are thrilled by everyday events such as a sunrise, birth of a baby and the budding flower more than a nightclub dance or an extravagant dinner party.
7. Most of them have had profound mystical or spiritual experiences; these experiences do not have to be religious in character; they often come from ordinary events such as the singing of a bird or a passing cloud. They are totally immersed in these experiences and often forget themselves when enjoying them.
8. They identify with and love mankind in general. They help others—in spite of their shortcomings—when necessary. In fact, their love is not restricted to only humans; it extends toward all living beings.
9. Although they love all living beings, they have intimate relationships with a few specially loved people; the relationship tends to be profound and deeply emotional rather than being superficial.
10. Self-actualizers cherish democratic values and attitudes. They fight against divisive tendencies based on religion, race or social class and fight against exploitation.
11. They do not confuse between means and ends. They do not want to somehow reach the goal. For them means are as important as ends. For that matter, means themselves are goals for them.
12. They have a healthy sense of humor, but it is devoid of hostile sarcasm. They see humor even in the problems they face. Their sense of humor is more philosophical rather than hostile.
13. They have a great fund of creative skill. They do not consider creativity as an extraordinary talent. They exhibit creativity in their speech, work, social interactions and in whatever they do.
14. They resist conformity to culture. They do not blindly follow traditions and cultural mores. On the other hand, they fight them if and when necessary. They refuse to be road-rolled by socialization forces.
15. They transcend the environment rather than just coping with it. They do not try to adjust somehow to changing circumstances; they try to go beyond and change the environment.
16. Some of them are capable of what Maslow called "oceanic feelings" or "**peak experiences**." These are the moments with intense clarity of perception, a suspended sense of time, and a feeling of wonderment at the experience.

Self-actualizers are fully human; they are guided by intrinsic values, not by the quest for goal objects. They are not driven by basic primary needs; they are motivated by metaneeds or '**being-values**'. The metaneeds are instinctoid or biological necessities, just as the primary needs in the hierarchy.

Maslow's views are highly appealing, but it is difficult to validate them. Many of his concepts are not amenable to objective scientific scrutiny. His theory appears to be more inspirational than scientific. Some critics accuse Maslow and other humanists "of accepting as true that which is still hypothetical, of confusing theory with ideology and of substituting rhetoric for research. In spite of these criticisms of the sort of psychology that Maslow stands for, there are a large number of psychologists who are attracted to his viewpoint because it tries to deal with vital and contemporary human concerns (Hall, Lindzey & Campbell, 1998)." Maslow's theory may appear unscientific, but it is useful and has influenced a large group of psychologists.

Rogers' Theory of Personality

Carl Ransom Rogers (Fig. 11.8) was one of the most influential scientist among the

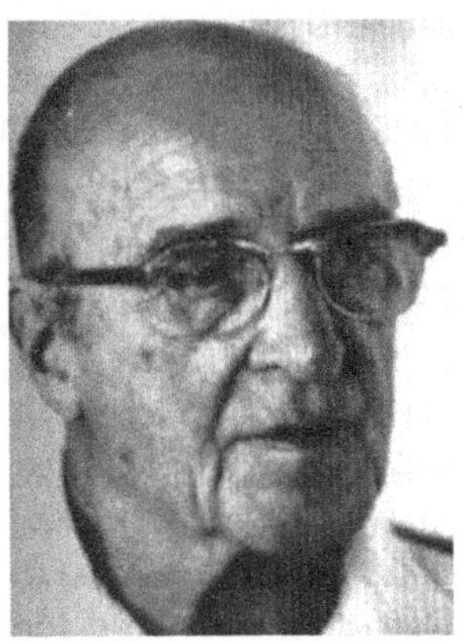

FIGURE 11.8: Carl Rogers

humanistic psychologists. Like all other humanists, Rogers opposed the bleak pessimism and despair inherent in the psychoanalytic view of humans on the one hand and the robot conception of humans portrayed by behaviorists on the other. Rogers was more hopeful and optimistic about humans. According to him "the basic nature of the human being, when functioning freely, is constructive and trustworthy. Man's behavior is exquisitely rational, moving with subtle and ordered complexity toward the goals, his 'organism' is endeavoring to achieve (Rogers, 1961)." Thus, Rogers was less pessimistic than Freud and less mechanistic than Skinner. His theory, like that of Freud, developed within the clinical setting. In the eyes of the psychologists all over the world, Rogers is the founder of a psychotherapeutic procedure called non-directive or '**client-centered therapy**' (or person-centered counseling). This form of therapy has enjoyed considerable popularity among practitioners and it was out of his clinical experience as a client-centered therapist that Rogers' theory of personality evolved. In fact, the theory of psychotherapy appeared first and later the personality theory. Rogers' personality theory has an existential flavor in that it stresses the importance of freedom of choice among humans. It is basically phenomenological in that Rogers placed strong emphasis on the conscious experiences of the persons, their feelings and values and all that could be included under the term inner life. Since, Rogers' theory occupies an important position among personality theories, it is necessary that we examine it in some detail.

Structure of Personality

Two important structural constructs used in Rogers' theory are the *'organism'* and the *'self'* or the **self-concept**. The organism is the whole individual—a living, growing, holistic system, the basic psychological reality. It is the locus of all experience; all that happens to the individual, happens here. Experience includes everything potentially (need not be actually) available to awareness (consciousness) that is going on within the organism at any given moment. The totality of experience constitutes the *phenomenal field*. The phenomenal field is the individual's frame of reference that can only be known to the person. "It can never be known to another except through empathic inference and then can never be perfectly known (Rogers, 1959)." How the individual behaves depends upon the phenomenal field (inner or subjective reality) and not upon the environmental stimulating conditions (external or objective reality).

The phenomenal field is not the same as the field of consciousness (awareness). Consciousness is the symbolization (representation) of some of our experience. The phenomenal field at any given moment is made up of conscious (symbolized) and unconscious (unsymbolized) experiences. The organism may, however, perceive (discriminate) and react to an experience that is not symbolized. This phenomenon is called *subception* (discrimination without awareness). When the experience is not accurately perceived (symbolized), the person will behave inappropriately.

However, people check their perceived experiences against reality. This reality testing gives people dependable knowledge helping them to behave realistically. But, they may not be able to test all perceptions adequately and these untested experiences may cause them to behave unrealistically, creating problems.

The second important structural construct of Rogers' theory is the self. The self is the differentiated portion of the phenomenal field. Rogers (1959) defines self as *the organized, consistent conceptual gestalt composed of perceptions of the characteristics of the "I" or "me" and the perceptions of the relationships of the "I" or "me" to others and to various aspects of life, together with the values attached to these perceptions. It is a gestalt available to awareness though not necessarily in awareness. It is a fluid and changing gestalt, a process, but at any given moment, it is a specific entity.*

During the early years of his work, Rogers was hesitant to use the concept of self in his theoretical formulation since the term was vague, ambiguous, philosophical and scientifically meaningless. But, when his clients during therapy had opportunities to express their problems and their attitudes in their own words, they invariably used the term self. The self was ultimately found to be an important element in the experience of the client and in some strange way the client's important goal was to become his *'real self'*. These clinical observations induced Rogers to develop his theory of personality around the concept of self (often Rogers' theory is called *self-theory of personality*). In addition to self, Rogers uses another construct, the '**ideal self**,' which is what the person ideally would like or aspire to be.

The importance of the structural constructs of organism and self becomes clear when we learn about Rogers' use of **congruence** between self as perceived and the actual experience of the organism. If the perceived self truly represents organismic experience, the individual is well adjusted, mature and fully functioning. Such an individual accepts his organismic experience without threat or anxiety. When there is *incongruence* between the self and organism, the individual feels threatened and anxious; he/she behaves defensively and thinking will be rigid and constricted. Therefore, the incongruence or congruence between the self and organism could be construed as a measure of adjustment. Since, it was difficult to operationalize the organism, Rogers in his research studied the congruence or incongruence between self and ideal self. He and his students have made extensive use of self-ideal-self discrepancy as a measure of adjustment. The self-ideal self-discrepancy was assessed using various techniques, especially a statistical procedure called '*Q-technique*' or simply '**Q-sort**'.

Dynamics of Personality

The motivational construct in Rogers' theory is self-actualization or **actualizing tendency**. According to him, "the organism has one basic tendency and striving—to actualize, maintain, and enhance the experiencing organism (Rogers, 1951)." It is the basic tendency of growth. The actualizing tendency is selective; it pays attention to only those aspects of the environment that promise to move the person toward fulfillment and wholeness. The actualizing tendency of the organism expresses itself also in the actualizing of that portion of the experience of the organism, which is symbolized in the self. This is the self-actualizing tendency. In a healthy person, actualizing tendency and self-actualizing tendency are congruent. In Rogers' theory, the single motivating force is the self-actualizing drive and the single goal of life is to become self-actualized or a whole person. The organism actualizes itself along the lines laid down by heredity. The actualizing tendency may be prevented from accomplishing its goal, but it cannot be destroyed without destroying the individual. Rogers (1951) maintained that "behavior is basically the goal-directed attempt of the organism to satisfy its needs as experienced, in the field as perceived."

In addition to the single basic growth need (actualizing tendency), Rogers also mentioned about two learned needs: **need for positive regard** and **need for self-regard**. The former develops during infancy because of the baby's being loved and cared for by parents and the latter by virtue of the baby's receiving positive regard from others. The two needs may work at cross purposes with the actualizing tendency by distorting the experiences of the organism.

Development of Personality

Both the organism and the self possess inborn tendency to actualize themselves. The expression of these tendencies is influenced by the environmental forces, especially the parental evaluations during childhood. If these evaluations were positive, then there would be no incongruence between self and organism. Rogers (1959) wrote: "if an individual should *experience* only *unconditional positive regard*, then no *conditions of worth* would develop, *self-regard* would be unconditional, the needs for *positive regard* and *self-regard* would never be at variance with *organismic evaluation* and the individual would continue to be *psychologically adjusted* and would be fully functioning."

But, the parental evaluations of child's behavior are sometimes positive and sometimes negative. As a result, the child learns to differentiate between behaviors that are worthy and those that are unworthy. Unworthy experiences, tend to become excluded from the self-concept even though they are organismically valid. This leads to the development of a self-concept that is not in tune with organismic experience. The child tries to be what others want it to be instead of trying to be what it really is. As Rogers (1959) put it: "he values an experience positively or negatively solely because of these conditions of worth which he has taken over from others, not because the experience enhances or fails to enhance his organism." For example, an adolescent boy may be drawn toward a girl, which is organismically normal. But, when his parents disapprove this behavior and even punish him for that, he may start avoiding the company of all girls. He may even start thinking that his behavior is bad. This way he starts denying his real feelings. But, denial does not mean that his feelings cease to exist; they will still influence his behavior in various ways even though they are not conscious. This may lead to a conflict between the interjected conscious values and the genuine unconscious values. If such conflicts between genuine feelings and borrowed spurious ones accumulate, the individual develops a distorted self-concept that is at war with itself. Such an individual will feel tense, defensive, and uncomfortable; he starts feeling as if he does not know what he is and what he wants. The breach between self and organism not only distorts the self-concept but also affects interpersonal relations.

In order to heal the breach between organismic experience and self, Rogers suggests that a therapist creates the following conditions, which are the basic components of client-centered or person-centered therapy:

- Provide the individual (client) *unconditional positive regard* and accept him as he is and all that he says without any qualifications
- Try to have an *empathic understanding* of the person's internal frame of reference
- Communicate, at least minimally, the empathic understanding and acceptance to the person (client).

Rogers called these conditions as *necessary* and *sufficient* for personality change. The first one, unconditional positive regard implies that the person is cared for, accepted and valued as he is. The caring is unconditional; there is no evaluation or judgment of the person's thoughts, feelings and behavior as good or bad. Acceptance is the recognition of client's rights to have his own beliefs and feelings. Research has shown that the greater the degree of caring, prizing, accepting and valuing of the person in a non-possessive way, the greater the chance that constructive personality change occurs.

The second condition, empathic understanding, implies that the therapist understands the client's experience and feelings sensitively and accurately as they are revealed during therapeutic interaction. The therapist senses the client's feelings *"as if"* they were his own without becoming lost in those feelings. The third and the most important condition is the therapist's ability to reflect (communicate) the empathic understanding to the client. Reflection encourages and enables the client to become more reflective about his inner self. Therapist's empathy results in the client's self-understanding and clarification of his beliefs and world views. **Empathy**, especially emotional empathy, helps clients to pay attention to and value their experiencing, process their experience cognitively, see old experience in new ways, modify their self-perceptions and their worldview, increase their confidence in their perceptions in making decisions, and in following a course of action.

In short, maladjustment occurs when an individual is exposed to *conditional positive regard*. The associated *conditions of worth* lead to self-experience incongruence. The incongruence generates anxiety as it approaches awareness. The individual responds with denial or distortion, because awareness of incongruence would jeopardize receipt of positive regard from self and others. The individual maintains an inaccurate or artificial self-concept. On the other hand, individuals who experience unconditional positive regard maintain or reinstate congruence between self and experience. Because of the absence of conflict or incongruence, such individuals have no need to rely on defenses. Rogers called such healthy people '**fully functioning persons**.' The fully functioning persons (self-actualizing persons) have three characteristics. First, because there is no need to defend against any experience, the person develops an increasing openness to experience; that is, there is no defensiveness and the person is able to acknowledge and express all his feelings. Second, such people exhibit increasingly existential living. There is no rigidity and no preconceptions about what he should do or be; rather, the person lives fully in each moment. Finally, fully functioning people have increasing trust in the organism. Such people make and rely on their own decisions. They develop a sense that doing what feels right proves to be a competent and trustworthy guide to behavior, which is truly satisfying. As they become more open to all of their experiences, they are able to do what they feel like doing, not in a hostile or arrogant way, but in a confident way. In essence, such people are open to their feelings and free of defenses. They are free to act on their inclinations, because they can accept the consequences and can correct them if they are not satisfying.

Evaluation of Rogers' Theory

The chief criticism leveled against Rogers' theory is that it is based upon a naïve type of **phenomenology**. Rogers gave importance to what people say about themselves and the world. According to him, the person is revealed in what he says about himself. But, there is enough evidence to say that what people say about themselves is distorted by defenses and deceptions of various kinds. Self-reports lack reliability because people try to deceive listeners. People do not know the whole truth about themselves and several factors that are not available to consciousness influence their behavior. Psychoanalysts criticize Rogers for ignoring the role of unconscious in determining behavior.

This criticism need not be taken too seriously because Rogers never denied the role of factors that are unavailable to conscious. According to him, the organism has many experiences that are not symbolized and denied entry into consciousness because they are inconsistent with the self-image. The difference between this process and repression is negligible. But the real difference is in Rogers' belief that repression can be prevented by giving a child unconditional positive regard, and if repression has occurred, it can be corrected by therapeutic intervention. In fact, in his later writings Rogers accommodated unconscious in his theory and said that unconscious organismic processes do in fact and should, guide much of human behavior. He asserted that these unconscious processes are not irrational, immoral or antisocial impulses, but dependable guides for the development of the person. Rogers seems to be saying: "trust your unconscious."

Although Rogers' humanistic approach appears to some psychologists as non-scientific, it is noteworthy that he developed a theory the concepts of which could be measured and tested. His groundbreaking studies of self-growth that can occur during therapy (Rogers & Dymond, 1954) have opened new pathways and stimulated substantial amount of therapeutic research. Rogers and his followers measured the discrepancy between client's ideal self and actual self (operationally considered a measure of self-esteem) using the Q-sort methodology and found that the discrepancy becomes gradually smaller and smaller as therapy progressed. The assessment of **self-esteem** as an indicator of psychological adjustment has led to innumerable studies of mental health, and extended the usefulness of self-concept in personality research (Box 11.2). Heuristically, Rogers' theory has been extremely powerful and a pervasive force.

Box 11.2: Building Self-esteem

Several psychologists including humanistic psychologists recognize the importance of self-esteem in people's life. It is reported that the need to feel a sense of self-worth is a universal phenomenon (Sheldon, 2004). Several studies have shown that self-esteem is associated with better health and psychological well-being. People with high self-esteem were found to do well in their academic pursuits. Self-esteem is not a fixed quality; it goes through ups and downs throughout life. It develops naturally as we pursue and achieve the goals we set for ourselves. Achievement depends on an individual's competencies such as intellectual abilities and social skills. Social-cognitive theorists like Bandura have emphasized the role of self-efficacy in the development of self-esteem. When you set for yourself reasonable goals and succeed in them, your feeling of self-confidence increases, which in turn will increase your self-worth. But when you put up highly challenging and perfectionist goals in which you fail, your self-esteem may go down. One who sets realistic, achievable goals, is prone to develop better self-esteem. You know that success leads to success. Avoid perfectionist expectations and do not expect approval of everybody. You will have a better view of yourself.

TYPE AND TRAIT THEORIES

Personality Types

Early thinkers in the field of personality classified people into categories called *personality types* based on their physical, psychological and behavioral characteristics. One of the earliest theorist Hippocrates (ca. 460–377 BC), who is recognized as the Father of Medicine, classified people into four categories based on certain body humors. Some 500 years later, Galen (ca. 130–200 AD) extended Hippocrites' typology, which played an important role in the evolution of personality theory and continues to be influential even today. The theory is summarized in Table 11.3.

Ernst Kretschmer, a German psychiatrist, proposed a personality typology based on

Table 11.3: Galen's Typology

Humor	*Temperament*	*Characteristic*
Phlegm	Phlegmatic	Sluggish, unemotional
Blood	Sanguine	Cheerful
Yellow bile	Choleric	Quick-tempered, fiery
Black bile	Melancholic	Sad

the body build. He proposed that there were three basic body types, the **asthenic** (thin, lean), the **athletic** (muscular), and the **pyknic** (fat and thick set) each of which was associated with specific psychological characteristics. The asthenics were believed to exhibit schizophrenic characteristics, the pyknics the manic-depressive characteristics, and athletics the normal characteristics. William Sheldon developed a complete personality theory based on the constitution. According to him there are three basic body types namely, **endomorphic**, **mesomorphic** and **ectomorphic** and each of them is associated respectively with a specific temperament namely, **viscerotonic**, **somatotonic** and **cerebrotonic**. The endomorph is short and plump, and is said to be sociable, relaxed and even-tempered (viscerotonic). The ectomorph is tall, lean and thin, and is said to be restrained, self-conscious and likes solitude (cerebrotonic). The mesomorph is muscular and heavily set; he is described as noisy, callous and likes physical activities (somatotonic).

A type theory of personality that was purely based on psychological characteristics was proposed by Jung. Jung divided people into two types called introverts and *extraverts*. Introversion and extraversion are considered as attitudes by Jung. The extraverted individual is oriented toward external, objective world. The psychic energy in him is directed outward. When under stress, the extravert seeks the company of others. He is likely to be highly sociable and tends to choose occupations that permit him to deal directly with people. The introvert is oriented toward the inner, subjective world. He tends to withdraw into himself, particularly in times of emotional stress and conflict; he tends to be shy and prefers to work alone. These two opposing attitudes are both present in the personality, but ordinarily one of them is dominant and conscious, while the other is subordinate and unconscious. In actuality, there is no one who is a total introvert or complete extravert. Most people fall somewhere between the two extremes (these are often called ambiverts). In fact, this is one of the major problems of type theories. Most typologies, whether they are based on physical or psychological characteristics, involve a continuum of individual differences rather than discrete types. Type theories are appealing because they provide a simple way of classifying people in well-defined categories, but in actuality personality is far more complex to be categorized into distinct types.

Personality Traits

Suppose you are asked to describe another person; in all probability, you will come out with a list of characteristics such as intelligent, smart, sociable, helpful, curious, creative, so on and so forth. Psychologists call these personal qualities **traits**. A trait refers to any characteristic on which one individual differs from another in a relatively permanent and consistent manner. When we describe people using adjectives such as intelligent, sociable, cautious, friendly or anxious, we are employing trait terms. We abstract trait terms from behavior. When we observe a person behaving in a careless, disorganized and messy manner on several occasions, we may call him a sloppy individual. A person's personality, then, can easily be described by his position on a number of continuous trait dimensions.

Several psychologists have attempted to develop models of personality around the concept of trait and they are called trait theorists. They have tried in their respective theories to define the term trait and determine the number and nature of traits. Although theorists differ in the ways they define the term, they all agree that trait refers to a relatively stable characteristic that defines an individual's identity and distinguishes him/her from others. The theorists assume that traits exist on a continuum. For example, a person may be placed somewhere between "most sociable" to" least sociable." Among the psychologists who believed that personality is built on traits, the names of GW Allport and RB Cattell stand out. Let us briefly review their approaches.

Allport's Trait Theory

Gordon Allport (Fig. 11.9) is an important name in the field of personality. He wrote and researched extensively about personality emphasizing the uniqueness and individuality of every person. As we noted earlier, he wrote the first text on personality in 1937 (*Personality: A psychological interpretation*). Scanning through dictionaries, Allport found nearly 18,000 separate words that were being used to describe personality. After eliminating words with the same meaning, he was left with 4,500 words referring to personal characteristics. Obviously, the list was too big to handle and therefore he came out with a classification of traits into three groups: **cardinal traits**, **central traits**, and **secondary traits** (Allport used the term trait in 1937 and changed it as personal disposition in 1961. Since, he is well known as a trait theorist only, the former term is retained here). Allport defined a trait as a "neuropsychic structure having the capacity to render many stimuli functionally equivalent and to initiate and guide equivalent (meaningfully consistent) forms of adaptive and expressive behavior (Allport, 1937)." A cardinal trait (disposition) is a single characteristic that influences all of an individual's behavior. It is so general that almost every act of an individual who possesses it can be traced to its influence. For example, a totally altruistic person might give away his entire property in the service of society. Cardinal trait is relatively unusual and cannot be seen in many individuals. Central traits are a bunch of major characteristics, such as honesty and sociability that make up the core of personality. An individual may possess five to ten central traits that can be easily inferred from his or her behavior. Secondary, traits are more limited in their occurrence, less crucial to a description of the personality and more focalized in the responses they lead to as well as the stimuli to which they are appropriate. They affect behavior in fewer occasions and are less influential than cardinal or central traits. Love of music and dislike of alcohol are examples of secondary traits.

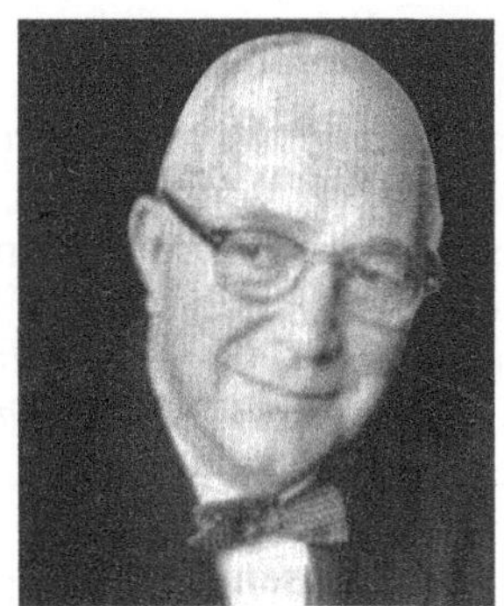

FIGURE 11.9: Gordon Allport

Although trait is an important construct, Allport has proposed a few interesting (often controversial) concepts in his theory of personality. His definition of personality, which we discussed in the beginning of this chapter ("personality is the dynamic organization within the individual of those psychophysical systems that determine his unique adjustments to his environment,") is well known. The psychophysical system includes constructs such as intentions, proprium and functional autonomy. Intentions refer to what the individual intends or striving for in the future. Allport includes an individual's hopes, wishes, ambitions, aspirations and plans under intentions. It is important to note here that Allport turned to the intended *future* while most others emphasized the *past* as an essential determinant of behavior.

Through the introduction of the term **proprium** in his theoretical writings, Allport has been often referred to as an "ego" or "self" psychologist. In order to avoid the confusion and special connotations associated with the terms ego and self, he proposed that all of the ego- or self-functions be included under appropriate functions of the personality. These functions—bodily sense, self-identity, self-esteem, self-extension, and sense of selfhood, rational thinking, self-image, propriate striving, cognitive style and the function of knowing—are all true and vital portions of personality and together they comprise the proprium. In proprium we find the root of the consistency that marks attitudes, intentions and evaluations. People are not born with proprium; it is acquired in time.

Allport's approach to the complex and controversial problem of human motivation is unique. He insisted that any theory of motivation should emphasize:

1. The *contemporaneity of human motives*—whatever motivates an individual must motivate him here and now.
2. *Plurality of motives*—there must be motives of many types.
3. The *dynamic force* behind cognitive processes such as planning and intention.
4. Allowance for the concrete *uniqueness of motives* within an individual.

He thought such a theory could be built around the concept of **functional autonomy**. According to Allport (1961), "functional autonomy regards adult motives as varied and self-sustaining contemporary systems, growing out of antecedent systems, but functionally independent of them." Any behavior, although it may originally have derived from organic or segmental tensions, may be capable of sustaining itself indefinitely in the absence of any biological reinforcement. That is, a given behavior may become an end or goal in itself, in spite of the fact that it was originally engaged in for some other reason. An example will make the concept of functional autonomy easy to understand: A postman walks several miles a day because he has to deliver letters in different parts of a town. After his retirement, he goes for long walks although there is no need for this act. The walking has become self-sustaining; he simply "likes" walking. The act of walking has become an end or goal in itself. It has become functionally autonomous from the original cause. Of course, all adult motives are not functionally autonomous.

Allport emphasized the importance of conscious determinants of behavior; asserted that the individual is more a creature of the present than the past; believed that there is a discontinuity between normal and abnormal, child and adult, animal and human. By making these assertions, he was opposing several greats in psychology. No wonder he was the target of vehement criticisms. But, Allport has raised some questions that are of general concern to psychologists, and that is why he is well known within psychology.

FACTOR THEORIES

Cattell's Factor-analytic Theory

Raymond Cattell (Fig. 11.10), a British-American psychologist, employed a different approach called the factor analytic approach to the study of traits. We have seen in an earlier chapter (on intelligence) how **factor analysis** was used by Spearman, Thurstone, Guilford and several others to determine the basic dimensions of intelligence. Cattell was a student of Spearman before he came to the USA. He applied factor analysis to determine

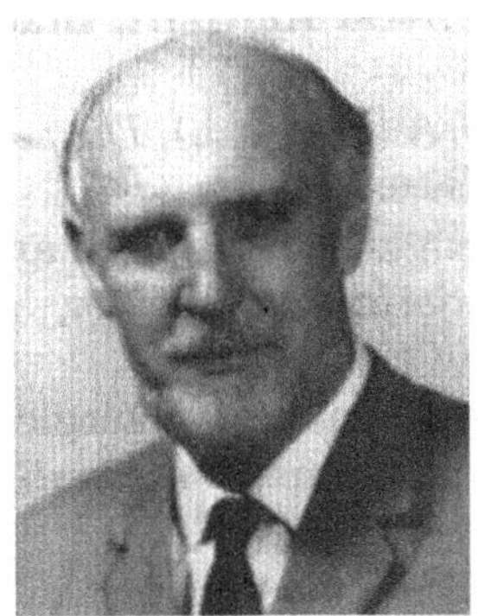

FIGURE 11.10: RB Cattell

the basic dimensions of personality and derived 16 factors or dimensions that constitute human personality. He developed a test to measure these factors, which is very well known as '**Sixteen Personality Factor Test (16 PF)**'. The 16 PF test measures the individual differences on each of the factors and provides a comprehensive picture of personality. Based on the scores of the test, an individual's profile or a profile for groups of people (artists, athletes, lawyers, etc.) can be drawn. The 16 factors along with their technical names and a brief description of each of them are given in Table 11.4.

There is more to Cattell's theory than the 16 factors mentioned above and all of it cannot be discussed here. He viewed personality as a complex and differentiated structure of traits. For him a trait is a mental structure or inference made from observed behavior. It accounts for the regularity or consistency of behavior. Cattell has distinguished between '**surface traits**' and '**source traits**'. Surface traits refer to what we see from outside in an individual, a person's manifest characteristics that seem to go together. Source traits represent the underlying variables that produce the multiple surface traits. Surface traits are the products of interaction of source traits and are less stable than the latter. Traits are further divided into *dynamic traits, ability traits,* and *temperamental traits.* Dynamic traits motivate the individual toward some goal. But the effectiveness with which

Table 11.4: Summary of Cattell's 16 Factors

Description of low scorers	*Description of high scorers*
Sizia: reserved, detached, aloof	*Affectia:* outgoing, easygoing, participating
Low intelligence: dull	*High intelligence:* bright
Low ego strength: emotionally unstable, easily upset	*High ego strength:* emotionally stable, mature, calm
Submissiveness: docile, mild, humble	*Dominance:* assertive, stubborn, aggressive
Desurgency: serious, sober, talking less	*Surgency:* happy-go-lucky, carefree, enthusiastic
Weaker superego strength: expedient	*Stronger superego strength:* moralistic,
Threctia: shy, timid	*Parmia:* venturesome, uninhibited, bold
Harria: tough-minded, realistic	*Premsia:* tender-minded, sensitive
Alaxia: trusting, accepting	*Protension:* suspicious, hard to fool
Praxernia: practical, down to earth	*Autia:* imaginative, absent-minded
Artlessness: forthright, genuine	*Shrewdness:* polished, astute
Untroubled adequacy: self-assured, secure	*Guilt proneness:* apprehensive, insecure, worrying
Conservativism: respecting traditional values	*Radicalism:* liberal, experimenting
Group-dependency: sound follower	*Self-sufficiency:* prefers own decisions
Low self-control: lax, careless	*High self-control:* socially precise, high will power
Low ergic tension: composed, relaxed	*High ergic tension:* tense, driven

he/she reaches the goal is determined by the ability traits. When traits are concerned with constitutional aspects of behavior such as speed of response, energy available, or emotional reactivity, these are called *temperamental traits*. According to Cattell, ability and temperamental traits are more stable than dynamic traits. Cattell (1950) defined personality as "that which permits a prediction of what a person will do in a given situation," and believed that the goal of personality research is "to establish laws about what different people will do in all kinds of social and general environmental situations." For purposes of predicting an individual's response in some particular situation, Cattell has suggested an equation called *specification equation*, which can be written as follows:

$$P_j = b_1T_1 + b_2T_2 + \dots b_nT_n,$$

where, P_j is the performance j, the response predicted in a given situation; T_1, T_2, ... , T_n are the traits of the individual and b_1, b_2, ..., b_n are the weights determined by factor analysis.

Five-factor Model

In recent times, other trait researchers started arguing that 16 is too big a number and personality can very well be explained in terms lesser number of higher-order factors. These theorists have proposed that five factors called "Big Five" are sufficient to understand human personality The **Big Five factors**, obtained through factor analysis, have been found to occur quite consistently in different populations all over the world. The **five-factor model** is not really new. Several early researchers, including Cattell, had proposed such a point of view. There are several versions of the five-factor model. One version of polar factors popularly known as OCEAN (an acronym developed using the first letter of each factor) is shown in the Table 11.5.

Two active researchers of the Five-factor Model, McCrae Costa (2003), have developed a test called '*NEO Personality Inventory* **(NEO-PI)**' to assess the five factors. Although the big five factors appear adequate to describe important aspects of personality, it was surmised later that a larger number of specific traits such as Cattell's would provide a better knowledge of behavior within particular situations and make prediction more precise. It was also noticed that the Big Five factors never correlated above 0.20 to 0.30 with real-life behavioral outcomes. In the light of these observations, certain modifications were made in the Big Five model by adding six subcategories, or facets, under each of the five super factors. For example, the six underlying facets for extraversion are warmth, gregariousness, assertiveness, activity, excitement-seeking and positive emotions. The six facets of conscientiousness include competence, order, dutifulness, achievement-striving, self-discipline, and deliberation. The Revised NEO-PI (NEO-PI-R) provides measures of personality at both levels (major traits as well as the subcategories).

The Big Five factor model has been vastly successful in stimulating research in the area of personality. Researchers have demonstrated that NEO-PI measures of extraversion correlate positively and neuroticism negatively with self-esteem. People who are happy and satisfied with life tend to be high on extraversion and low on neuroticism. It is proposed that the Big Five approach can be useful in helping people to select appropriate forms of psychotherapy. It is also suggested that the five-factor model can be used to help understand distinctions among various personality disorders.

Eysenck's Dimensions

British psychologist **Hans Eysenck** (1985) (Fig. 11.11), another factor theorist, contended

Table 11.5: Big Five Personality Factors

Big five factors	*Underlying behavior characteristics*
Openness	Artistically sensitive vs artistically insensitive Intellectual vs unreflective, narrow interests Polished vs crude, boorish Imaginative vs direct, simple
Conscientiousness	Tidy, organized vs careless Responsible, efficient vs irresponsible, undependable Scrupulous, thorough vs unscrupulous, unfair Persevering vs fickle, quitting
Extraversion	Talkative vs quiet, silent Cheerful, elated vs gloomy, depressed Adventurous vs cautious Sociable vs reclusive
Agreeableness	Good-natured vs irritable Not jealous vs jealous Gentle vs headstrong Cooperative vs negativistic
Neuroticism	Nervous vs poised, balanced, confident Anxious vs calm Excitable vs composed Moody vs emotionally stable

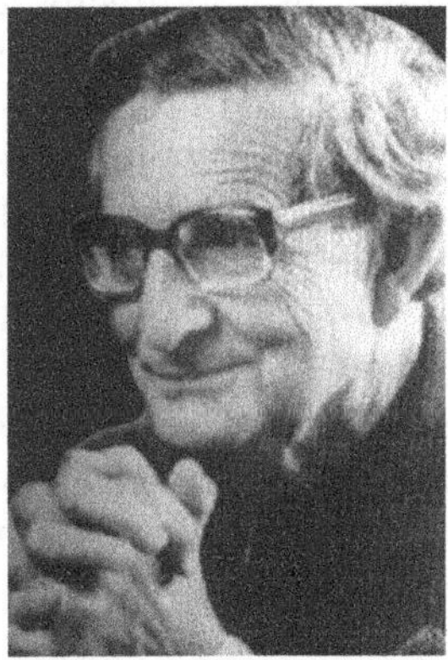

FIGURE 11.11: HJ Eysenck

that only three factors (or dimensions) were enough to explain individual differences in personality. Using factor analysis, Eysenck identified the three factors as **extraversion**, **neuroticism** and **psychoticism** (often abbreviated as PEN). Each of these is a bipolar factor, representing opposite ends of a single dimension. In terms of bipolarity, the first factor (E) varies between extraversion and introversion, the second factor (N) varies between neuroticism and stability and the third factor (P) varies between psychotic behavior and normality. Eysenck and Eysenck (1975) developed a test called Eysenck Personality Questionnaire (EPQ) to measure these factors. High scorers on factor E are extraverts and low scorers introverts. As described in the manual of EPQ: "The typical extravert is sociable, likes parties, has many friends, needs to have people to talk to and does not like reading or studying by himself." "The typical introvert is quiet, retiring sort of person, introspective, fond of books rather than people; he is reserved and distant except to intimate friends." The typical high N scorer is anxious, highly emotional, moody, worrying and often depressed. The stable individual, on the other hand, tends to respond emotionally only slowly and generally weakly and returns to baseline quickly after emotional arousal. He is usually calm, even-tempered, controlled, and unworried.

Eysenck's three-dimensional model provides a system for describing different types of individuals in terms of their characteristic behavior patterns. But, why a particular person is predisposed to exhibit a particular set of behaviors? Psychoticism, neuroticism and extraversion refer to observed (phenotypic) components of personality. But what are the underlying (genotypic) components that are responsible for observed variations in behavior? Eysenck has proposed two explanations in terms of physiological differences that covary with high or low status on these factors. The first model accounts for differences between extraverts and introverts in terms of central nervous system in its levels of inhibitory and excitatory neural processes. The second model accounts for differences between:

1. Introverts and extraverts in terms of cortical arousal.
2. Neurotics and stables in terms of levels of visceral brain activation.

Eysenck believed that the cortex of extraverts is less easily aroused than in introverts. His view was that, it takes more stimulation to arouse extraverts. Because of this higher threshold, extraverts seek out activities that are more stimulating. Introverts and extraverts have different biological responses to caffeine, nicotine, and sedatives. There are also differences in their skin conductance and electroencephalographic recordings. High scorers on neuroticism are easily and intensely aroused and so they are more likely to experience conditioned emotional responses, that is, they learn to show emotional responses to previously neutral stimuli easily and quickly. For example, a person who is high on neuroticism, when stuck in an elevator, is more likely to develop a fear of elevators than the one who is low on this dimension.

Neuroimaging data indicate that extraversion and neuroticism exhibit different types of brain activation. These findings show that the two personality factors are distinct and are related to different brain systems. Those who are high on psychoticism have less control over their emotions and therefore are more likely to be aggressive or impulsive. They have difficulty in learning not to engage in particular behaviors. Both these tendencies could lead to criminal and antisocial behavior. Eysenck claimed that these tendencies are inherited largely (50%–60%). It does not mean that some are born criminals, but rather that some are born with autonomic and central nervous systems whose under-arousal indirectly leads them to engage in risky behavior, especially when exposed to certain environmental influences. Eysenck thus follows a biosocial model in explaining behavior. Biology leads all of us to a need to eat, but how, what and when we eat are determined largely by the way we are brought up. Environment plays a role in the development of criminality and such other psychotic and antisocial behavior. The summary of trait approaches to personality is given in Table 11.6.

Table 11.6: Summary of Trait Approaches to Personality

Approach	*Key concepts*	*Brief summary*
Gordon Allport	Cardinal traits, central traits and secondary traits	Traits are neuropsychic structures that influence behavior; cardinal, central and secondary traits are used to describe people
Raymond Cattell	Source traits and surface traits; traits are factor analytically derived	Underlying source traits produce observed surface traits
Five-factor model	Openness, conscientiousness extraversion, agreeableness, neuroticism (OCEAN)	The five broad factors have most consistently emerged in personality research
Hans Eysenck	Psychoticism, extraversion and neuroticism	Three dimensions explain all variations in personality

BIOLOGICAL APPROACHES

In one way, we can consider Eysenck's dimensional approach as biologically based. But, there are other researchers who attempted to explain personality in biological terms more explicitly. We mentioned the work of Jeffrey Gray (1991) in the chapter on motivation. Gray proposes two biological systems that underlie motivation as well as differing aspects of personality. One of them is the behavioral activation system (BAS), which is a mechanism based on activation, or reward. The BAS can be thought of as the "go" system that initiates the approach behavior and is similar to the extraversion dimension of the Big Five factors and also the dimension proposed by Eysenck. People in whom BAS is easily activated are more sensitive to and more easily conditioned by, reward. On the other hand, introverts are more sensitive to, and more easily conditioned by, punishment. The BAS triggers positive emotions, such as elation or hope and approach behaviors. It also underlies impulsivity. People with an easily activated BAS tend to respond readily to even minor rewards. Such people have a predisposition toward substance abuse.

The other system proposed by Gray is behavioral inhibition system (BIS). This is a mechanism based on inhibition, or punishment. BIS can be thought of as the "stop" system that initiates avoidance behaviors. This system is similar to the neuroticism dimension of the Big Five factors model and that of Eysenck. The BIS is activated by threat-related stimuli, which produce anxiety and inhibit behavior. People with easily activated BIS become distressed in the face of minor threats. Many of these people are anxious and depressed.

Gray and others argue that the properties of these systems arise from characteristics of specific brain structures, neurotransmitters and neuromodulators. It is found that introverts and extraverts exhibit different patterns of electroencephalogram (EEG) activation, while they play a card game in which money is lost (punishment) or won (reward). Neuroimaging and EEG studies have shown that the right frontal lobe is involved in withdrawal from aversive stimuli (BIS), whereas the left frontal lobe is involved more in approaching rewarding stimuli (BAS).

Cloninger and his associates have postulated the following four basic personality dimensions on which people differ:

- Reward dependence (motivated by warm attachment to others as opposed to pragmatism and tough-mindedness)
- Harm avoidance (pessimism, shyness, and fear of uncertainty, inhibition of approach behaviors and increase in escape behaviors)
- Novelty seeking (excited response to new situations; this is related to Gray's BAS)
- Persistence (the tendency to continue to seek a goal in the face of obstacles or resistance).

Cloninger argues that each of these dimensions corresponds to some combination of Big Five factors and is associated with a distinct biological system. For example, novelty seeking is similar to sensation seeking and it corresponds to a combination of high score on extraversion and a low score on conscientiousness in the Big Five model. People who score high on novelty seeking are found to be impulsive, exploratory, fickle, excitable, quick-tempered and extravagant, whereas low scorers are rigid, reflective, loyal, stoic, slow-tempered and frugal. Cloninger has hypothesized that the novelty-seeking dimension is related to the dopamine-based reward pathway, and harm avoidance to the neurotransmitter serotonin. The biological mechanisms of the remaining dimensions of Cloninger's theory have not yet been established.

Like Cloninger, Zuckerman has proposed five personality dimensions that are based on biological mechanisms. The system is known as alternative five:

1. Sociability (similar to extroversion).
2. Neuroticism-anxiety (similar to neuroticism).
3. Impulsive sensation seeking (a tendency to act impulsively; this dimension is a reconceptualization of Eysenck's psychoticism and is related to sensation seeking and Gray's BAS; it is the opposite of the Big Five's conscientiousness and has a high heritability estimate).
4. Activity (need for activity, high energy level, preference for challenges and difficulty in relaxing).
5. Aggression-hostility (tendency toward antisocial behavior, verbal aggressiveness and vengefulness.

Biologically based inclinations to engage in certain style of behavior are generally referred to as temperament. According to Arnold Buss, temperament influences behavior more than personality traits or factors. Temperament affects not only what people do, think and feel, but also how they act, think and feel. These inherited tendencies can appear at an early age and persist throughout adulthood. Studies have shown that temperamental factors at age three are correlated with their personalities at age 18. Temperament is also found to be linked to behaviors such as unsafe sex, alcohol dependence, violent crime and rash driving. Arnold Buss & Robert Plomin (1975; 1984) have identified four dimensions of temperament. These are:

1. Sociability (preference to be in the company of others rather than alone; similar to Big Five's extraversion).
2. Emotionality (tendency to become aroused in emotional situations, but only when the emotion of distress, fear or anger is involved; similar to neuroticism).
3. Activity (general expenditure of energy; it has two dimensions: vigor referring to the intensity of activity and tempo referring to speed of activity).
4. Impulsivity (tendency to respond to stimuli immediately, without reflection or concern for consequences).

Studies have shown that emotionality (neuroticism), activity level and sociability are partly inherited. Rothbart & Derryberry on the other hand have proposed only two fundamental temperament dimensions such as reactivity and self-regulation. Reactivity pertains to the ways in which people respond to novel or challenging situations. For example, some people consistently respond in situations with negative emotions such as fear or distress. Reactivity includes both the intensity and the time delay of response. Self-regulation pertains to the ability to control attention and inhibit responses, and it is affected by reactivity.

Two specific temperamental traits, shyness and sensation seeking, have been well studied by psychologists. Jerome Kagan and his colleagues (1988) have found that some babies are more reactive or sensitive to environmental stimuli. These high-reactive babies tend to have faster heart rates and higher levels of stress hormone cortisol. When they grow up, they become inhibited, fearful children who startle more easily. Their sympathetic nervous system is more easily aroused. Some of these inhibited children become shy teenagers and adults. They will become extremely self-conscious and self-critical and tend to avoid social interactions. They become preoccupied with their shyness and its effects and experience fear and distress in social situations. On the other hand, uninhibited children respond positively to new situations and people and seem to enjoy novelty. Kagan has estimated that about 20 percent of infants are inhibited and about 40 percent are uninhibited. These temperamental patterns can be identified during the first 4 months of life and these patterns persist into later childhood in many children (but not all). Kagan has suggested that the amygdala was involved in the physiological over reactivity in inhibited children. Although having an easily aroused autonomic nervous system (ANS) and certain brain structures predispose some people toward shyness, the view taken by the family and culture toward this type of behavior has a greater role in the determination of shyness.

Sensation seeking—the pursuit of novelty, seeking of high-stimulation situations such as sky diving, fast driving, using of drugs or alcohol, working in challenging occupations (espionage, in emergency room in hospitals)—has been investigated by Zuckerman and several others. Sensation seeking has been found to be associated with lower levels of the chemical monoamine oxidase-B (MAO-B) in the blood. This chemical helps in the breakdown of neurotransmitters for storage, affecting the amounts of those neurotransmitters that are available, at least in males.

Genetic Factors: Is Personality Inherited?

We all know that several of our physical features, such as eye color, are inherited. But, what about personality traits, are they also inherited from our parents? Inheritance of personality is a hotly debated issue in personality research. The most preferred method of studying the effect of genetic factors on personality is to compare the degree of personality resemblance between monozygotic (identical) twins, who have identical genetic makeup and dizygotic (fraternal) twins, who do not. On a number of personality characteristics, identical twins are found to be more similar to each other than fraternal twins, suggesting the importance of genetic influence on personality. But, the issue is complicated by the possibility that identical twins may also have more similar family environment than fraternal twins because the parents are inclined to treat them more similarly.

This problem was solved by comparing personality traits of identical and fraternal twins who were raised together and those who were reared apart. If the identical twins reared apart in different families were as similar as the ones reared together, then there is a case for the importance of genetics. The most comprehensive study of twins was conducted by Auke Tellegen and his associates (1988) at the University of Minnesota (known as the Minnesota Study of Twins Reared Apart, MISTRA). Four groups of twins (identical and fraternal twins reared apart and reared together) were tested on 14 personality traits and the personality variation due to genetic, familial environment and unique environment was determined for each trait. It was found that genetic factors accounted for approximately 40 to 50 percent of the variance among the subjects in trait scores. On the other hand, the degree of resemblance did not differ much whether the twin pairs were raised together or apart, indicating that the general features of the family environment, such as its emotional climate and degree of affluence, accounted for little variance in any of the traits. This does not mean that an individual's unique experience is of no consequence. Rather than the family environment, it was the individual's unique environmental experiences, such as his or her school climate and social interactions with friends that accounted for considerable personality variance. It means that even when individuals grow up in the same family, they may have different experiences and it is these experiences that help mould personality. Other researchers have studied the heritability of the Big Five super factors, Eysenck's three dimensions, psychological interests and social attitudes. They found more or less similar results.

Evaluation of Biological Theories of Personality

Researchers are trying to identify some of the genes that affect personality. Although a few studies found that a particular gene is associated with a particular trait, variations of a single gene account for less than 10 percent of the genetic influence. Also, the studies attempting to find the relationship between a particular gene and a particular trait have come out with inconsistent results. It is believed that unlike eye color, personality traits are not affected by a single gene. Rather, sets of genes exert their influence in concert. Also, variations in a single gene may affect more than one personality characteristic. Further, we are not sure about the mechanism by which genes affect personality. Recent studies have focused on the activities of neurotransmitters. Discovering of the relationships of genes to neurotransmitters and neurotransmitters to personality has just begun and it may take several years before we know the exact genetic basis of personality.

Recent technical advances in measuring neural activities and in evaluating genetic influence have helped us in several ways to understand the biological bases of personality. But, biology is not destiny; biological functions are affected by developmental experiences and these two interact with situational factors. Genetic factors interact with environmental factors. So, it is believed that nature and nurture are two inseparable factors and separating them is simply an academic abstraction.

INFLUENCE OF CULTURAL FACTORS ON PERSONALITY

It can easily be seen that personality is a product of interaction between biological and environmental factors. Among the several environmental factors that influence personality, the one whose impact has not been sufficiently appreciated is the culture in which the individuals are raised. Often, we are unaware of cultural influences because of its amorphous nature. Culture refers to our shared beliefs, customs, values, traditions and expectations about the appropriate ways of behaving in certain situations in society. It includes the intellectual aspects of life such as art, science and religion. Culture encompasses unstated assumptions, social norms, sex roles and habitual ways of behaving that are shared by members of a social group and passed on from one generation to the next. It influences what people perceive, how they perceive, how they relate to others and in short, how they behave. Cultural determinism asserts that behavior patterns are influenced more by culture than by biological or genetic factors.

Cultures differ along a number of dimensions that can influence personality development. A society may be highly complex, tightly knit, individualistic or collectivistic. For example, the contemporary mobile-phone culture we witness in Indian cities is totally different from the one prevalent in an underdeveloped tribal society. There is immense scope for diversity and conflict of values and behavioral norms in complex cultures. But, several societies are organized so tightly that even a minor deviation from a social norm is likely to be severely punished. In some societies, youngsters are not permitted to use alcohol, smoke or engage in sexual behaviors. So, people in tight cultures differ less from one another than they do in loosely organized society. In loose cultures, people are not highly dependent on one another and diversity is tolerated if not encouraged. Important personality differences are found between individualistic and collectivistic cultures. Collectivistic cultures rank the needs of the group as more important than those of the individual. People raised in collectivistic cultures appear to value humility, family honor and maintenance of social order; they care for others, even strangers. Asian, African, Latin American and Arab cultures belong to this group. In contrast, individualistic cultures emphasize equality, individual freedom and enjoyment—even at the expense of others. The United States, Great Britain, Canada and Australia belong to this group. Collectivistic cultures exert more social control over the individuals. As a consequence, it appears that the crime rate is higher in individualistic cultures than in the collectivistic cultures. It is sometimes said that with the transition from collectivistic orientation to individualistic one because of urbanization, industrialization and globalization, crime rates and social evils will increase.

Several personality differences have been found between people in individualistic and collectivistic cultures. People from an individualistic culture characterize their 'self-concept' as a composite of traits independent of the group, while people from the collectivistic culture see their self-concept in the social context. In one recent study, such differences were found between American and Japanese college students. The social embeddedness of the collectivistic Japanese culture was reflected in their self-perceptions as was the cultural individualism in the self-concepts of Americans. In this context, it is interesting to note that personality trait measures do not predict behavior as well in collectivistic cultures as they do in individualistic cultures, probably because of the stronger influence of the environmental factors in determining the behavior of people in collectivistic cultures.

Self-enhancement needs are strong in both individualistic and collectivistic cultures, but these are satisfied in different ways. Individualists enhance the self through personal successes, whereas collectivists feel better about themselves when their group succeeds. Personal success increases motivation among members of individualistic cultures whereas in collectivistic cultures, motivation increases after personal failure as the person attempts to change the self and conform to the demands of the situation. Studies have shown difference between collectivistic Japanese and individualistic Americans regarding their emotional lives and self-esteem. Americans reported more self-oriented positive emotions, such as self-pride and personal happiness, whereas Japanese reported more interpersonally oriented positive emotions, such as closeness, friendship and respect. Japanese scored lower than Americans on measures of self-esteem. This is said to be because self-criticism is not considered bad among Japanese (in fact, it is believed to encourage self-improvement), while in Western cultures, self-criticism is indicative of depression. In addition, individualists were found to use more often the first person pronoun 'I,' whereas the collectivists use the third person pronouns such as "he/she."

It should also be noted that personality changes occur within a culture over time. It is reported that the number of college students reporting external locus of control, anxiety and neuroticism have increased significantly from 1963 to 1993; the degree of extraversion has increased and personality traits typically considered consistent with gender roles have decreased in both the sexes. Such changes are believed to reflect certain cultural shifts over the second half of the 20th century. For example, increasing fear of crime, terrorism and other dangers might have lead to increased anxiety, neuroticism and external locus of control. Similarly, increasing valuation of traits related to extraversion and decreasing emphasis on personality traits related to sex role standards are supposed to be the products of cultural shift.

GENDER DIFFERENCES IN PERSONALITY

In general, personality differences between men and women are not as great as the differences found among people within each sex. Some researchers think it is counterproductive to search for sex differences in personality, for the differences in personality occur because of the context in which behavior develops. Studies have shown that there are no notable sex differences in self-esteem, social anxiety and locus of control, impulsiveness or reflectiveness. However, some consistent sex differences have been found. Women tend to score higher on traits reflecting social relationships, kindness and helping others. Men tend to score higher on traits reflecting individuality, separateness, emotional strength, autonomy, achievement and self-sufficiency. Women tend to be more empathic than men, report more nurturing tendencies and can assess emotions in others better than men. It is found that women can easily detect when their partners are deceiving them. In making moral judgments, women are a bit emotional; they pay more attention to the interpersonal context, to whether and how it will hurt others, whereas men are more likely to make a moral decision based on laws or abstract principles. Women score higher on neuroticism than men, but score lower than men on anger and aggression and on assertiveness. Women feel more anxiety and guilt about their aggressiveness and are more concerned about its effect on their victims. Men and women differ regarding estimation of their abilities and the probability of future success. In one study of college students, it was found that more men than women considered themselves above average in overall scholastic ability. In general, women evaluate themselves more critically and harshly than men do. Men and women differ in their verbal and non-verbal communication styles. The content of men's and women's speech also differs. These findings are consistent with stereotypes about men and women, but the fact that sex differences exist does not tell us why they exist. Are these differences caused by biological or cultural factors? Although sex differences in personality have been observed, they do not necessarily hold in all situations. An extensive 26 country meta-analysis of gender difference using results from the NEO-PI-R found that, in general, differences between men and women are not as large as differences within each sex.

What Causes Gender Differences?

Some sociocultural theories have tried to explain sex differences in personality in terms of sex typing. Social role theory asserts that boys and girls learn different skills and beliefs. In most of our families, there are differences in the socialization process itself. Parents treat boys and girls differently. Boys and girls are given different kinds of toys; they engage in different types of games, watch different TV programs and read different types of story books. Boys and girls come to have different expectancies about likely responses when they exhibit behaviors that are seen as appropriate or inappropriate for typical sex roles; they are rewarded for performing behaviors that are perceived by society as being appropriate for men and for women respectively. Culture assigns girls the role of primary caretakers of children. Children between the ages three and five years realize that they belong to different sexes and this will have an important influence on their personality. Even our educational system treats boys and girls differently. According to Sandra Bem, an expert in the field of gender differences, socialization produces a gender schema, a mental framework that organizes and guides a child's understanding of information relevant to gender. Based on their schemas for appropriate and inappropriate behavior for men and women, children begin to behave in ways that reflect society's gender roles.

As you might have easily guessed by now, personality is a product of interaction between biological, sociocultural and situational factors. Biology plays a significant role in the determination of gender differences. Every cell in the female body is different from those of the male. Several biologists attribute the sex difference to the effects of male hormone testosterone. Exposure to the male hormones during the fetal stage (by pregnant mothers taking a drug containing male hormones) affects the brains of girls in such ways that they favor certain masculine traits when they become adults. It is also suggested that men and women have evolved differently because of differences in mate selection and parenting strategies. According to evolutionary theory, women have a greater investment in their children than men because they cannot have many of them as men can. This greater investment, along with their nurturing role, is believed to cause women to become more strongly attached to their offspring, which is believed to have an evolutionary advantage. Highly attached mothers are more likely to have children who survive into adulthood and have children themselves. Evolutionary psychologist, David Buss has proposed an interesting but controversial explanation for the differences in the nature of jealousy between men and women. Buss and his colleagues found that men were more jealous when they found sexual infidelity in their partners, as opposed to emotional infidelity in which there was an emotional attachment to another man, but no actual sexual infidelity. In contrast, women were more jealous in cases of their partners' emotional infidelity rather than sexual infidelity. According to Buss, the root cause for the differences in jealousy lies in the evolutionary implications of sexual versus emotional infidelity in men and women. He argues that for males, sexual infidelity represents a threat to their belief that their children are actually their own. They do not want to expend the scarce resources on others' children. That is why they are more upset over sexual as opposed to emotional infidelity. On the other hand, the woman has no doubt that the child is her own. Her major concern is in keeping the male involved in child rearing. Therefore maintaining her man's emotional attachment is more crucial than his sexual fidelity.

Many critics do not agree with this explanation. Some have proposed that differences in jealousy depend on the meaning attached to the concept of infidelity. For instance, men are prone to believe that women have sex only when they are in love with the other person; therefore, they see sexual infidelity as an indication that the woman is in love with some other man, which they cannot tolerate. On the other hand, women believe that men can have sex without being in love, and therefore, they do not bother about man's sexual infidelity so long as he is not in love with some other woman. For women, sexual infidelity of her partner is less bothersome than his emotional infidelity. In the final analysis, we are not sure about the extent to which biological or evolutionary factors underlie sex differences. At most, they explain, only partly, some of the differences in behavior between men and women. The summary of personality theories is given in Table 11.7.

ASSESSMENT OF PERSONALITY

By now, you must have realized that personality is a complex phenomenon, which is difficult to understand. But, it is necessary to understand people around you and yourself for successful living. It is essential to understand the person you want to marry, employ and make friendship with. You must understand your parents, brothers and sisters, your teachers, your peers, your tailor, barber, washerman; for that matter, virtually everyone with whom you want to interact. How do you do it? Probably you meet the person, talk to him, observe his or her behavior in varying situations and collect information about the person from others. Well, that is what psychologists also do when assessing personality. But, there is a difference. When you interpret the information collected, there is a possibility

Table 11.7: Summary of Personality Theories

Approaches	*Key theorists*	*Major concepts*	*Assessment methods*
Psychoanalytic	Sigmund Freud	Unconscious; id, ego and superego; life and death instincts; psychosexual stages; anxiety and defense mechanisms	Interview; case study; projective techniques
Neo-Freudian	Jung, Adler, Horney Sullivan, Erikson	Racial or collective unconscious, archetypes; life style, creative self; basic anxiety; interpersonal relations; psychosocial development	Interview; case study projective techniques
Trait	Allport, Cattell; Eysenck	Personality traits and factors	Personality inventories such as MMPI*, 16 PF†, EPQ‡, NEO-PI§
Behavioristic	Skinner; Dollard & Miller	Classical and operant conditioning	Behavioral techniques
Social-cognitive	Rotter; Bandura; Mischel & Shoda	Social learning; locus of control CAPS‖; self-efficacy	Behavior observation; cognitive skills, self-report inventories
Humanistic	Maslow; Rogers	Phenomenology; self-actualization	Interview; Q-sort; adjective check list
Biological	Gray, Cloninger, Buss	BAS¶ BIS** Temperament	EEG††, Neuroimaging

*MMPI, Minnesota Multiphasic Personality Inventory; †16PF, sixteen personality factor; ‡EPQ, Eysenck Personality Questionnaire;§NEO-PINEO, Personality Inventory; ‖CAPS, cognitive-affective personality system; ¶BAS, behavioral activation system;**BIS, behavioral inhibition system; ††EEG, electroencephalogram. +The results are tentative.

that your interests, attitudes, expectations, philosophy of life, your world view and several other factors color your interpretation of the data. That is, there is chance for the operation of subjective or personal bias. You assess people not as they actually are but as you think they are. This tendency is meticulously avoided when psychologists observe people, collect and interpret the data; that is, they try to be as objective as possible in the collection and interpretation of data. They achieve this goal of objectivity using of certain standard tests devised to assess behavior objectively. These tests are based on the definition and the theoretical orientation of the personality psychologist. There are a number of methods currently in use for assessing personality, such as questionnaires, rating scales, adjective checklists, semantic differential, Q-sort technique, projective tests, interview, behavioral assessment, physiological measures and remote behavior sampling.

The task of devising useful personality measures is not an easy one. To be useful from theoretical and practical perspective, personality tests, like all other tests, must conform to certain standard criteria, such as reliability and validity. You may recall that reliability refers to the consistency of measurement. A reliable test yields the same results each time it is used on the same group or different groups and whoever uses it. Tests have validity when they actually measure what they are designed to measure. Only valid tests yield results from which meaningful conclusions can be drawn. Psychological tests must also have norms that permit an individual score to be compared with the scores of similar others who have taken the same test. Psychologists have developed several standardized tests of personality. We discuss below briefly some of the major tests used to assess personality.

Personality Inventories

Personality tests (also called questionnaires, inventories or scales), are the most commonly used tools in the assessment of personality. These are paper-and-pencil tests that require the person being assessed to read each of the statements and indicate whether it is "true" or "false" about him, or how much he agrees or disagrees with each statement along a multipoint rating scale. As you can see, these are self-report measures. Personality inventories generally assess many different traits and contain a number of statements to cover different aspects of each trait. The personality scales are objective measures; they include standard sets of statements that are scored using an agreed-on scoring key. An important advantage of personality inventories is that they can be administered to a number of people at the same time and their performance scored easily and quickly.

Psychologists follow two approaches in selecting the statements for the tests. One is called the rational theoretical approach, in which items are selected based on theorist's conception of personality trait to be measured. For example, to develop a measure of introversion-extraversion, he may ask himself what introverts and extraverts often say about themselves and then, write items that capture those kinds of self-descriptions (e.g. "I want to be in the company of others" or "I want to be left alone"). Several scales have been developed according to this approach, for example, NEO-PI, locus of control, ascendance-submission, self-monitoring, optimism-pessimism, etc. The second approach is the empirical approach, in which items are chosen based on how different groups of people answered the items. A widely used personality test, Minnesota Multiphasic Personality Inventory (MMPI), has been developed following the empirical approach. Let us examine how that test was constructed and is being used.

Minnesota Multiphasic Personality Inventory

In the development of MMPI, groups of psychiatric patients with a specific diagnosis, such as hysteria, depression or schizophrenia, were asked to answer a large number of items. Then the authors of the MMPI (SR Hathaway & JC McKinley, clinical psychologist and neuropsychiatrist respectively) determined the best items that differentiated members of these psychiatric groups from a comparison group of normal participants and included those items in the final version of the test. By systematically carrying out this procedure on groups with different psychiatric diagnosis, the authors developed a number of subscales that identified different forms of abnormal behavior. Although MMPI was originally designed to provide an objective basis for psychiatric diagnosis (measuring severe personality deviations such as schizophrenia, depression, psychopathic tendencies and so on), later it was found to be useful in the study of certain personality features of normal people also. Nowadays, the test is being used for various purposes such as a screening device in industrial and military setting. MMPI has gone through several modifications since its publication in 1942 and the recent version, Minnesota Multiphasic Personality Inventory-2 (MMPI-2) has 567 items and has three validity scales and 10 clinical scales (Table 11.8). There is also a short version of the MMPI consisting of 370 items.

Table 11.8: Validity and Clinical Scales of MMPI-2

Scale	*Symbol*	*Interpretation of high scores*
Validity Scales		
Lie	L	Lies to present a favorable image of self
Frequency	F	Exaggerates complaints; answers haphazardly
Correction	K	Denies problems; sees oneself in positive ways
Clinical Scales		
Hypochondriasis	Hs	Expresses bodily concerns and complaints
Depression	D	Is depressed, pessimistic, guilty
Hysteria	Hy	Reacts to stress with physical symptoms
Psychopathic deviate	Pd	Is impulsive, in conflict with law, involved in stormy relationships
Masculinity, femininity	Mf	Has interests in characteristics of opposite sex
Paranoia	Pa	Is suspicious, resentful, paranoid
Psychasthenia	Pt	Is anxious, worried, high-strung
Schizophrenia	Sc	Is confused, disorganized, and withdrawn from others
Hypomania	Ma	Is energetic, elated, active, restless
Social introversion	Si	Is withdrawn, introverted, with little social contacts

The validity scales are designed to assess a test taker's frankness and thoroughness in answering the items and to check for defensiveness or other attitudes that might influence the answers. Validity scales can detect tendencies to present either an overly positive picture or exaggerate the degree of psychological disturbance.

Whether MMPI is used as an aid in psychiatric diagnosis or to study personality characteristics of normal people, the psychologist looks at the total profile, not just the separate scales. The features, such as overall elevation of the profile above the average level, the highest, the lowest scores and their relationship to one another, along with the scores on validity scales, are all taken into consideration. It requires considerable training and skill to interpret MMPI scores.

MMPI is the most widely used personality test. The test is cost effective, objective and reliable. It has already been used in over 6,000 studies and is likely to be used in several thousands more. Several other self-report inventories have been constructed using items from MMPI. One of these is the famous 'Manifest Anxiety Scale' developed by Taylor (1953). Another is the 'California Psychological Inventory (CPI) developed by Gough (1975). The CPI is designed to assess several normal personality traits such as dominance, sociability, self-control, flexibility and femininity. It also includes several validity scales to determine response sets. Some special scales to assess addiction proneness, addiction acknowledgment, and marital distress have been derived from the MMPI items in recent times. The other popular personality tests are Cattell's 16 PF questionnaire, and NEO-PI.

Projective Tests

Freud and other psychodynamic theorists believed that people's behavior and personality are determined by forces unknown to them—unconscious determinants. The personality tests such as MMPI, 16 PFT or NEO-PI tap only conscious determinants and hence, our knowledge of personality is incomplete. Therefore, they suggest the use of certain tests that tap unconscious determinants. For this purpose, psychodynamic theorists advocate the use of projective tests. Projective tests call for the test taker to respond to unstructured stimuli such as inkblots or vague pictures, in which there are no guidelines as to what the response should be, thus providing an opportunity to give highly individual responses. The projective testing is based on the projective hypothesis derived from Freud's personality theory, which states that people, while responding to vague or ambiguous stimuli, project their underlying unconscious motives and feelings. That is, when test takers respond to the relatively unstructured test stimuli, they attribute meaning to the stimuli and in doing, so they are revealing their inner world. The participants are unaware of the underlying meaning in their responses, but the people trained to interpret projective tests are taught ways of inferring such meanings and judging personality characteristics accordingly. Thus, projective tests are designed to provide information about unconscious impulses, desires, inclinations and unfulfilled wishes about which the test taker does not have any knowledge. There are several types of projective tests. Some require the participant to complete an incomplete story, a picture or a sentence. Others may require them to express themselves via a play, drawing or drama. But, we focus here on the two of the well-known projective tests: the Rorschach Inkblot Test and the Thematic Apperception Test (TAT).

Rorschach Inkblot Test

Developed by a Swiss psychiatrist Hermann Rorschach (1924), the test consists of ten cards each with a different inkblot. Some are colored and others are in black and white. The participants are presented with the cards, one at a time and asked questions such as: "What might it be?" or "What does this remind you of?" After recording the participant's responses for all the cards, the test giver inquires the participant about what it was in the blot that determined the response: its shape, color or other features. The interpretation of Rorschach response is a specialized task and needs extensive training. Personality characteristics are inferred based on the location of the response (whether based on the whole inkblot or a part of it), its determinants (whether based on form, color, texture, movement), its content (human, animal, nature, art, anatomical, botanical, landscape) and whether it is a popular response or original response. Examiners categorize and score responses in terms of the kinds of objects reported and their characteristics, based on which an inference is made about the personality. Rorschach inkblot test is extensively being used in clinical practice. One drawback of the Rorschach is that different examiners may interpret the same response very differently, producing unreliability among examiners. Recently, attempts have been made to minimize subjectivity in interpreting responses by introducing specific coding categories and scoring criteria.

Thematic Apperception Test

A different projective test was developed by Christina Morgan & Henry Murray (1938), which is based on Murray's theory of needs. The TAT makes use of a standard set of 30 pictures derived from paintings, drawings and magazine illustrations. One may not use all the pictures. Based on specific research interest, 10 to 20 of them may be used. These pictures are also vague, but not as ambiguous as the Rorschach inkblots. The pictures are shown one by one and the participant is asked to make a story, keeping the following questions in mind:

- What is happening? Who are the people involved?
- What has led up to this situation?
- What is being thought, felt, wanted and by whom?
- What will happen?

The stories told in response to the pictures are analyzed for recurrent themes that are assumed to reflect important aspects of the participant's personality. These may refer to personal relationships mentioned in the story, the types of needs and emotions attributed to the characters, whether the outcome is positive or negative and factors that produce these outcomes such as personal weakness or environmental barriers. The TAT suffers from the same drawback as Rorschach, the subjectivity in interpretation. Therefore, it is necessary to be cautious in making interpretations about personality based on the stories. However, TAT approach has been found to be useful in inferring certain motives such as need for achievement (nAch), need for affiliation (nAff) and need for power as we have seen in the studies made by McClelland and his followers (see the chapter on Motivation).

INTERVIEWING

Interviewing is probably the oldest and the most popular method of assessing personality. Interviews are held to select people for jobs, students for various courses and even to choose one's life partner. Interviews are held for diagnosis of physical and psychological disorders. Interview is a face-to-face encounter where judgments are made about others by observing them and talking with them. It is possible to obtain information about a person's thoughts, feelings, and other psychological features during an interview.

Interview is a valuable method because it provides an opportunity to have personal contact with the person being tested. In spite of its popularity, it should be noted that interview is one of the highly fallible methods. There are several limitations. The first one is that there is no guarantee that the interviewee is telling the truth. If the interviewee is dishonest, uncooperative and is not reporting accurately the required information, the interview becomes an exercise in futility. In addition, there is immense scope for interpersonal influence; the influence of the interviewer on the interviewee and vice versa.

Several attempts have been made to improve reliability and validity of the interview. One such is to make the interview structured by asking a set of specific questions to all interviewees. Here an attempt is made to create a standardized situation in which all participants respond to identical stimuli making it easy to compare the people. But in most interviews the questions are tailored to suit the particular individual and the situation. Despite the limitations, interviews are extensively used by clinical psychologists, especially those who follow psychodynamic or humanistic approaches. Interviewing is a special skill; it needs extensive training. The challenge is to learn to design and conduct interviews in ways that minimize subjectivity and maximize reliability and validity of the information obtained from the respondent. Interview data pertains to one specific individual and the results cannot be generalized.

BEHAVIORAL ASSESSMENT

Often, psychologists, especially those who subscribe to the learning theory approach, observe the behavior of an individual to infer his or her personality. For this purpose, they devise an explicit coding system that contains behavioral categories of interest. Then they train observers until they show a high degree of agreement (interjudge reliability) in using the coding categories to record behavior. This type of behavior assessment may be made in the natural setting where the behavior occurs: at home, in school, during play, in the workplace or in the laboratory. Regardless of the settings, an attempt is made to ensure objectivity is maintained and the behavior is quantified as much as possible. For example, one may be interested in the study of aggression among school children. For this purpose, the observer may note down what triggers aggression in a child, how often the behavior occurs, the intensity of aggressive acts and the consequences of such acts.

Behavioral assessment is very useful in identifying behavioral problems, such as cheating, stealing, aggressiveness and eventually remedying these activities using appropriate intervention techniques. Behavioral assessment techniques based on learning theories of personality have made important contributions to the treatment of certain kinds of psychological as well as physical disorders.

Remote Behavior Sampling

It may not be possible or even practical to make behavioral assessment of people in all situations on a daily basis. Sometimes, the personality assessor may be interested in unobservable events, such as emotional reactions and thinking patterns that may throw light on personality functioning. For this purpose, a technique called **remote behavior sampling** has been developed. In this method, the researchers and clinical psychologists make an attempt to collect self-reported samples of behavior from participants as they go on with their day-to-day activities. For this purpose, a tiny computerized device resembling a mobile phone is used. The device pages participants at randomly determined times of the day. When the beeper sounds, respondents rate or record their current thoughts, feelings or behaviors, depending on what the researcher or therapist is assessing. Respondents may also report on aspects of the situation they are in so that situation-behavior interactions can be examined. Remote behavior sampling procedures can be used over weeks or even months to collect a large sample of behavior across several situations. Thus, the method provides an opportunity to detect personality functioning that is not revealed by other methods.

CONCLUDING THOUGHT

The topic of personality has captured the imagination of psychologists, litterateurs, religious leaders and philosophers throughout history. From the 5th century Greek physician, Hippocrates to modern psychologist Albert Bandura, several thinkers have proposed differing theories of personality. The field of personality within psychology draws the insights developed in diverse subfields such as developmental, physiological, evolutionary, cognitive and social psychology. In the years to come, it is expected that scientists will shed more light on this elusive concept.

Chapter Summary

The term personality refers to a relatively stable organization of psychophysical characteristics within an individual, which determines his or her unique ways of thinking, feeling, acting and relating to people around him/her. Since, the study of personality is a fascinating area and central to psychology (it is often said that the study of personality is the beginning and the end of psychology), a number of theories have been proposed to explain its structure, dynamics and development.

One of the first and the best-known theories of personality was proposed by Sigmund Freud. According to him, personality is shaped by unconscious conflicts between opposing forces within the mind. Freud thought that mind consisted of three levels of consciousness: the conscious, the preconscious and the unconscious. He believed that personality consisted of three psychological components: the id, the ego and the superego. The id is the unconscious psychological structure containing the instinctual impulses that are craving for unbridled immediate satisfaction. It works according to the pleasure principle—seeking pleasure and avoiding pain. The ego, a differentiated portion of the id, is the executive wing of personality that balances between instinctual demands of the id and the environmental and social reality. Its functioning is governed

Contd...

Contd...

by the reality principle. The superego is the custodian of morality. The ego uses defense mechanisms when threatened by disturbing id impulses. Personality develops through five psychosexual stages; the oral, anal, phallic, latency and genital stages. The important driving forces in personality functioning are sex and aggression. Often Freud's theory has been criticized as pansexualism because of its overemphasis on sex.

Some of the followers of Freud did not agree with several of his ideas, especially his overemphasis on sexuality and developed rival models of personality. These are called Neo-Freudians. Carl Jung, Alfred Adler, Karen Horney, Erich Fromm and HS Sullivan are important Neo-Freudians. Jung emphasized the role of racial unconscious and archetypes in the development of personality. Adler emphasized the role of social forces in shaping personality. Horney's was an early voice in feminine psychology. Erich Fromm wrote extensively about the state of contemporary humans and the problems they encounter.

Behaviorists led by Watson, Skinner, and Hull considered personality as an acquired pattern of behavior. Skinner constructed a model of personality in terms of reinforced responses called operants. Dollard and Miller developed an elegant theory of personality in terms of a set of habits developed in the context of drive reduction. Social-cognitive theorists Rotter, Bandura, Mischel and Shoda tried to show how social relationships, learning experiences and cognitive processes jointly contribute to personality development. Rotter believed that personality was influenced by expectancies a person has and the reinforcement value of potential outcomes. Rotter's concept on locus of control generated a great deal of interest among personologist. Bandura developed a theory in terms of observational learning or modeling. His concept of self-efficacy stimulated a good deal of research in the area of personality. According to Mischel & Shoda, situational features activate the person's cognitive-affective personality system (CAPS). The CAPS involves individual differences in encoding strategies, expectancies, beliefs, goals, values, affects, competencies and self-regulatory processes. The CAPS interacts with features of environment, helping to explain why people have specific behavioral signatures and so not necessarily behave consistently across situations.

Humanistic theories of Abraham Maslow and Carl Rogers emphasized the subjective experience of the individual and dealt with perceptual and cognitive processes. These theorists viewed humans as having an innate capacity to actualize themselves (self-actualization) and asserted that a person will become fully functional when given appropriate environmental support. Rogers built his theory around the concept of self and the congruence or incongruence between self and organismic experience. When self and experience are congruent, the person becomes fully functioning. Rogers' theory stimulated a great deal of research on self-concept, self-esteem and therapeutic change in self-concept.

Trait theorists like GW Allport have proposed a theory of personality in terms of basic components of personality called traits. RB Cattell used factor analysis to identify traits and came out with 16 personality traits. Theorists do not agree on the number and nature of traits needed to describe personality. Eysenck said three bipolar factors were enough. Recent researches have come to the conclusion that five big factors called OCEAN (openness, conscientiousness, extraversion, agreeableness and neuroticism) are sufficient to describe personality. Traits have not proved to be consistent across situations and over time.

Biological approaches to personality focused on differences in the functioning of the nervous system, contributions of genetic factors and the possible role of evolution in the shaping of personality. Studies of twins indicate that genetic factors may account for as much as half of the variance in personality test scores, while individual experiences accounting for the remainder. Differences in temperament appear early in life and are assumed to have a biological basis. There is evidence to show that temperamental behavior tendencies remain stable during an individual's life. Culture can affect personality development. Whether one belongs to a culture that emphasizes individualistic or collectivistic orientation determines his or her self-concept. There are gender differences in certain personality traits. Men tend to value achievement, emotional strength and self-sufficiency, whereas women prize interpersonal skills, kindness, nurturance and helpfulness to others.

Psychologists have used several methods to assess personality including interview, behavioral assessment, remote behavior sampling, objective personality inventories and projective tests. Personality inventories are developed in two ways: in the rational approach, the items are selected on an intuitive basis, while in the empirical approach items that discriminate between groups known to differ on the trait of interest (such as extraverts and introverts) are selected. The NEO-PI built according to the rational approach is used to measure individual differences in the Big Five factors. The MMPI–2 constructed according to empirical approach is the most popular test of personality. It measures several components of personality and is being used all over the world. Projective tests, such as Rorschach Inkblot Test and TAT, are most commonly used in clinical practice. These tests present ambiguous stimuli to people and it is assumed that responses given to these stimuli can be scored to infer certain personality traits. Humanists use special techniques, such as adjective checklist, Q-sort and semantic differential, to assess changes in self-concept, especially during psychotherapy.

12 CHAPTER

Developmental Psychology

PREVIEW

Were you ever surprised how you came to be what you are today? When you were born, you were a helpless bundle of muscles, bones and nerves. Today, you are a well formed mature individual. You can walk, talk, read, write, think, plan, solve problems, laugh, weep, make love and do several other things. How did you acquire all these skills? That is the subject matter of developmental psychology. This branch of psychology started as study of childhood during the 19th century and gradually evolved into lifespan development, which includes study of children, adolescents, adults, middle aged and the elderly people. Nowadays, development is studied during periods such as: prenatal period, infancy, childhood, adolescence, early adulthood, middle adulthood and late adulthood. From the time of conception, human beings undergo a continuous process of growth and development. Developmental psychologists study these processes. They are interested in the change and stability in various domains of behavior. They study physical development, motor development and psychosocial development. They are engaged in understanding the complex processes involved in the development of language, intelligence, thinking, problem solving and the sense of morality; in short human personality.

The major goal of developmental psychology is description, explanation, prediction and modification of behavior. Although development is a universal process, people differ in the course of development. They differ in sex, height, weight, motivational level, emotional reactions, energy level, intelligence and personality. Several factors influence the developmental outcomes in these areas. Most of the differences are explained in terms of heredity, environment and maturation. A major portion of the differences can be explained in terms of genetic endowment inherited from parents. The environmental influences may emerge from the family into which one is born, the socioeconomic status of the family, the area in which the house is located and the school to which one goes. Many typical changes are intimately tied to maturation of the body and the brain. The unfolding of a natural sequence of physical changes and behavior patterns such as walking, eruption of teeth, acquisition of language are all determined by maturation.

Contemporary American developmental psychologist, Paul Baltes and his colleagues have identified six key principles of development which help you to understand the concepts discussed in this chapter:

1. Development is a lifelong process of change in the ability to adapt to the situations one encounters in life. Each period of development has its unique characteristics and each period is influenced by the previous period and influences the next period. Development does not end at a certain period as it was held earlier. Even death is an essential developmental experience without which life would be incomplete.
2. Development is multidimensional; it is a product of multiple forces such as psychological, biological and sociocultural, interacting with each other. Development proceeds in more than one direction. There will be losses and gains in each developmental stage.
3. The relative influence of nature and nurture shifts over the lifespan.
4. Development involves changing allocation of resources (time, money, energy, social support); during childhood, bulk of resources goes for growth, and in old age, to regulation of loss.
5. Development is modifiable; many abilities such as memory and endurance can be improved with training even in old age.
6. Development is influenced by the historical and cultural context; your development depends on the historical period in which you live (war, depression, famine) and the society and culture to which you belong.

Now that you have had a brief preview of the field of human development, proceed to look more closely in this chapter at some of the important issues that developmental psychologists are thinking and working about. In your profession, knowledge of the developmental tasks—what people are expected to do, what they can do and what they cannot do—at various periods is very crucial. It enables you to understand and appreciate your patients better, especially in pediatric and geriatric wards.

Chapter Outline

WHAT IS PERSONALITY?

If someone asks me to name the most wonderful thing in the world, I shall say it is "You." Remember, "You" started your life as a tiny cell in your mother's womb and today, you are a full-blown individual with a beautiful body and marvelous mind. How did this happen? Part of the answer to this question is provided by developmental psychologists. Developmental psychology studies the kind of changes that occur in your body and mind over the years. It is the study of the changes in the structure and functions of human organism over the life span. It is often called lifespan psychology. Starting with conception, developmental psychology examines the pattern and course of development during the prenatal period, infancy, childhood, adolescence, adulthood, middle age and finally, old age. As you see, the scope of this division of psychology is very vast and each of the areas mentioned above is the subject of independent study. In this chapter, we examine briefly the major areas of developmental psychology. We begin our discussion with some of the special issues that confront the developmental psychologists and the specific research procedures they have developed to deal with these problems.

MAJOR ISSUES IN DEVELOPMENTAL PSYCHOLOGY

Nature Versus Nurture

The nature-nurture issue is concerned with the relative impact of heredity and environment on the development of humans and other organisms. There has been a long-standing debate over the relative contributions of nurture (environment, experience and learning) and nature (heredity or genetic predisposition) to the development of the human organism. Philosophers have discussed this issue under the general title, **empiricism** versus **nativism**. Hereditarians assert that we are what we are because of our inherited biological characteristics and environmentalists believe that we are molded by the sociocultural environment in which we live. An early researcher in developmental psychology, Arnold Gesell (1880–1961), emphasized the role of biological processes in the development. Environmentalists like Watson maintained that behavior is determined by learning and experience. Modern psychologists follow the middle path. Today, no one believes that nature alone or nurture alone completely determines the course of our development. Most of them agree that development is shaped by the interaction of heredity and environment and they are interested in determining how much of development can be attributed to heredity and how much to environment instead of quarreling over the issue. The contemporary version of the controversy is therefore more about the relative contributions of nature and nurture to particular behavior than about nature or nurture per se. However, resolution of nature-nurture controversy is far from over; the debate is very much alive even today. You will face this problem frequently when we discuss the various aspects of the development later in this chapter.

Passivity Versus Activity

When we accept that heredity interacts with the environment, another question creeps up: How much of this interaction is triggered by heredity and how much is initiated by the environment? Do we passively yield to environmental pressures or do we actively manipulate the environment to suit our purposes? Again there is no unequivocal answer to this question. As you know, Watson asserted that the child is the raw material waiting to be molded by parents and other elders. Similarly, Skinner declared that human behavior is shaped by the rewards and punishments emanating from the environment. On the other hand, Jean Piaget argued that a developing human being does not passively submit to the environmental influences; people do not copy or learn the reality, they actively construct their own reality. People manipulate the objects and events around them. The issue whether humans are active or passive has important implications in the field of child rearing and education; it cannot be brushed aside lightly.

Continuity Versus Discontinuity

Several psychologists believe that development is a continuous progression. A child first lifts its head, then sits, stands up and finally starts walking. People develop gradually; they accumulate knowledge and skills and slowly reach maturity. Thus, development can be seen as a smooth curve without breaks. But there are others who consider development as occurring in discreet steps; it is a discontinuous progression. According to them, individuals develop in steps or stages that are qualitatively different from one another. What one can do at a particular stage is not more than the previous stage or less than the next stage. What they do in each stage is qualitatively different from what they do in other stages; the difference is not quantitative but qualitative. The crawling caterpillar is qualitatively different from the flying butterfly. You will appreciate this point of view better when we examine later in this chapter the Piaget's stage theory of cognitive development.

Universality of Developmental Sequence

Does development follow the same course all over the world or does it differ from culture to culture depending on the specific experience of the developing individual? This is another hotly debated issue in developmental psychology. Developmental psychologists differ with regard to the universality issue. Some believe that development occurs in the same way all over the world; others think that it is an culture-specific. But most thinkers take the middle of the road. They assume that there is an interaction between biology, environment and the person in determining the course of development. We will see later in the chapter that some of the developments such as cognitive development are invariant all over the world, while certain other developments depend on the culture, ethnicity, socioeconomic status, lifestyle and diet.

Stability Versus Change

Do human characteristics remain stable as people grow? Some traits remain stable, while others may change. For example, after maturity many physical characteristics such as height do not change. Psychological characteristics such as intelligence do not change after reaching an upper limit. Psychologists talk of constancy of intelligence quotient (IQ). Some researchers have found consistencies across time in certain characteristics such as temperament. Several personality characteristics change as an individual grows. Some believe that nothing remains stable in the universe, including human beings. It is said that "change is the only constant in life." Even stable characteristics are found to change under environmental pressure. Change versus stability is a hotly debated issue in developmental psychology.

Critical Periods

Closely related to stage concept is the notion that there are critical periods in the course of development of an organism. A **critical period** is a biologically determined period of time during which an organism is optimally ready for the acquisition of certain responses. The organism must go through certain experiences during this time period for development to proceed normally along a certain path. If the appropriate experiences do not occur during this period, then the behavior can be learned later only with great difficulty, if at all. The existence of critical periods has been established in animals. The best known example is the critical period for **imprinting**. Here, imprinting refers to the formation of a strong bond of a newborn animal to the first moving object seen after birth. Imprinting takes place rapidly within a relatively compressed time span and is exceedingly resistant to extinction. Konrad Lorenz (1903–1989) studied imprinting in geese. The geese tend to form a strong bond of attachment to the first moving object seen after birth. A gosling will instinctively follow its mother wherever she goes. But goslings hatched in the laboratory will imprint on objects that happen to be present at the time of their birth, including humans and even mechanical toys. The goslings that imprinted on Lorenz followed him everywhere, even to the point of ignoring adult female geese (Fig. 12.1). If imprinting does not occur in the critical period, it can never be learned and the organism may not develop normally.

It is harder, although not impossible, to demonstrate the existence of such a phenomenon (critical period) among humans. For example, the British psychoanalyst, John Bowlby (1969) suggested that a child must form a satisfactory emotional attachment

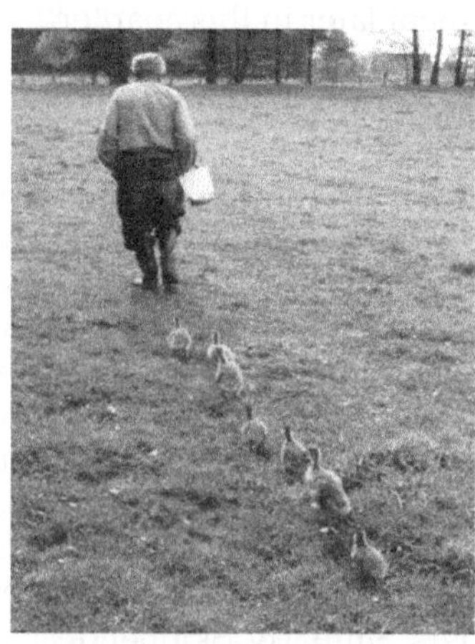

FIGURE 12.1: Imprinting

to an adult during the first 3 years of life in order to be capable of normal affectional relationships in later life. Mary Ainsworth (1978) shared with Bowlby the view that the parent-infant relationship is crucial to the development of secure attachment. If this is true, the first 3 years of a child's life constitute a critical period for the development of social relations.

METHODS OF STUDY

Developmental psychologists face special issues and they have developed specific research procedures to tackle them. In order to study the relative importance of heredity and environment, they take recourse to animal experiments. By selective breeding, they can produce a strain of animals with similar heredity and observe how they develop in different environments to determine the effect of nurture over nature. Of course, such experiments cannot be conducted on human beings. But nature provides us with an opportunity to study the effects of similar heredity in the form of identical (or monozygotic) twins. Development at psychologists study identical twins reared under the same roof (heredity same and environment same) and compare them with those that were reared apart (same heredity and different environment). If there are differences between the two groups, these have to be attributed to variations in the environment. Similarly, they study children with dissimilar heredity that were raised in the same family (heredity different and environment same) to determine the relative contribution of heredity and environment on development.

In order to study behavioral changes across different ages, developmental psychologists have devised three unique procedures. The most widely used one among them is the **cross-sectional method**. In this procedure, groups of people belonging to different ages are studied at one point of time and the results compared. Suppose we are interested in determining the changes in intelligence from age 15 to 65 years. We administer a test of intelligence to groups of 15-, 25-, 35-, 45-, 55-, and 65-year-olds at the same time. Now we can calculate the average score for each group and compare the averages to determine how people's intelligence changes with age. But the cross-sectional method has some limitations. The variation in scores between different age groups, called **cohorts** (a group of people who grew up at similar times, in similar places and under similar conditions), may not reflect the actual difference in intelligence. They grew up in different historical periods when conditions were different. The 15-year-olds today are living in a stimulating environment, while the 65-year-olds grew up in a world that was different; they had no computers, microwave ovens, mobile phones or even TVs. Therefore, if they scored poorly on an intelligence test compared to 15-year-olds, it may be due to poor environmental conditions at that time; they might have been denied of adequate educational facilities, nutritive diet, hygienic environment and medical facilities.

For purposes of obviating this difficulty, developmental psychologists have devised another procedure known as **longitudinal method** in which the same cohort is tested repeatedly at different intervals of time. We can test a sample of 15-year-olds today and retest them every 10 years, up to the age of 65. With this procedure, we can be sure that all the participants were exposed to similar environmental conditions. But this procedure is awfully time-consuming and costly. With the passing of years, the sample may become smaller and smaller because participants may drop out of the study or move away from the place, or even die. Further, suppose intelligence declines at age 65. Is this due to aging or some developmental experience unique to the cohort tested? To answer these questions, researchers have developed a new procedure, called *cross-sequential method*, which combines the cross-sectional and longitudinal approaches. For example, we can test 15- through 65-year-olds now, repeat the test after every 10 years and examine whether the developmental pattern occurring is the same for all the cohorts. As you can guess, this is the most comprehensive procedure, but also the costliest and the most time-consuming.

STAGES OF DEVELOPMENT THROUGH THE LIFESPAN

Now that we have examined the issues confronting developmental psychologists and the research methods they use, we may proceed to the study of developmental processes through the lifespan. We shall examine the course of various psychophysiological developmental processes during the prenatal period (conception to birth), infancy (birth to 12 months), childhood (1–12 years), adolescence (13–19 years), early adulthood 20–44 year), middle adulthood (45–65 years) and late adulthood (65 and onwards). We begin with the prenatal period, which spans from conception to birth, roughly 266 days during which a tiny cell, barely larger than a pinhead, transforms into a wondrously complex newborn baby.

PRENATAL PERIOD—FROM CONCEPTION TO BIRTH

Genetics and Sex Determination

During conception, a male reproductive cell, **sperm**, combines with a female reproductive cell, the **ovum** or egg, to produce a fertilized cell called **zygote**. The scientific term for the reproductive cell, either a sperm or an egg cell, is **gamete**. The gametes are formed from specialized cells that, while themselves containing the full 23 pairs of **chromosomes**, in the course of cell division called *meiotic division*, produce cells with half that number. That is, a female's sex cells and a male's sperm cells each have 23 chromosomes. At conception, the egg and sperm unite to form the zygote, which now contains the full set of 23 pairs of chromosomes found in other human cells. The genetic heritage of every normal human being is determined by these 23 pairs of chromosomes and the **genes** they carry. The 23rd pair, the sex chromosome, determines the baby's sex. A female's 23rd pair contains two X chromosomes (XX). Because women carry only X chromosomes, the 23rd chromosome in the ovum is always an X. A male's 23rd pair contains an X and a Y chromosome (XY). Therefore, the 23rd chromosome in the sperm is either an X or Y. The child's sex depends upon the specific combination of sex chromosomes. The union of an ovum (always containing only an X chromosome) with a sperm having a Y chromosome results in an XY combination and hence the baby will be a boy. If the sperm contains an X chromosome, it results in XX combination and therefore the baby will be a girl. Therefore, it is foolish to blame a woman for not giving birth to a male child! It is man's genetic contribution that determines the sex of the baby (Box 12.1 and Fig. 12.2 for more information about chromosomes and sex determination).

Stages of Prenatal Development

Prenatal development takes place in three stages.

Germinal Stage

The first one called the **germinal stage** starts with the formation of a zygote and lasts for approximately 2 weeks. The zygote is a one-celled entity and within 3 days it increases to about 32 cells and within a week, it grows up to 100 to 150 cells. Thus, through repeated cell division, called *mitotic division*, the zygote becomes a mass of cells and attaches to the mother's uterus at about 10 to 14 days after conception.

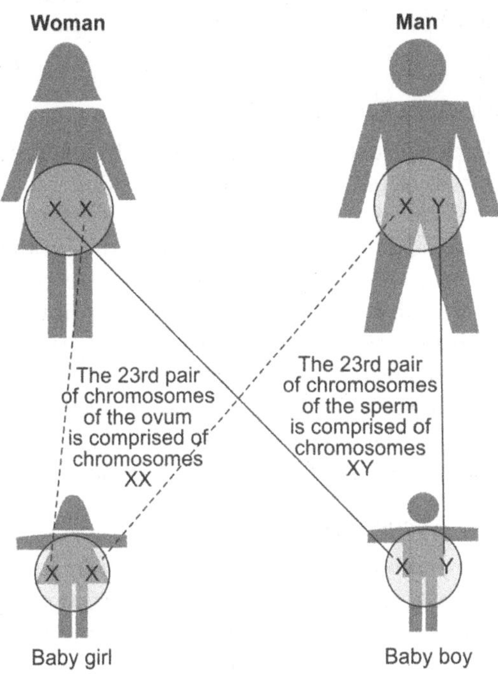

FIGURE 12.2: Sex determination

Embryonic Stage

The second stage, called **embryonic stage**, spans 2 to 8 weeks. Now the mass of cells is called the **embryo**. The embryo develops through a complex, preprogrammed process of cell division and becomes 10,000 times larger by 4 weeks, attaining a length of about one fifth of an inch. By about 8 weeks, the embryo is about an inch long and has arms, legs and face that can be recognized. A rudimentary heart starts beating, the brain is developing and the intestines are formed. At the beginning of this stage, two life-support structures, the placenta and the umbilical cord, develop. The *placenta* allows nutrients to pass from the mother's blood to the umbilical cord. In turn, the blood vessels in the *umbilical cord* carry these nutrients and oxygen to the embryo and transport waste products back from the embryo to the mother.

Fetal Stage

The third stage, which lasts from the 8th week to birth, is called the **fetal stage**. Now, the embryo is called the **fetus**. During fetal stage, muscles become stronger and

Box 12.1: Chromosomes and Sex Determination

Chromosomes are microscopic bodies found in the nucleus of a cell. These are strands of DNA (deoxyribonucleic acid). Chromosomes carry genes, the ultimate carriers of heredity. Each species has a constant normal number of chromosomes. There are 46 chromosomes in human somatic cells arranged in 23 pairs. The ovum and sperm contain one from each pair of chromosomes. Of the 23 chromosomes, 22 are **autosomes** and one is the **sex chromosome** (either X or Y). In fertilization, the 23 chromosomes from the male unite with the 23 from female. The X chromosome is the female determining chromosome and the Y, male determining. Normal female somatic cells are XX, normal male are XY; normal female ova are X, normal male sperm either X or Y. An XX embryo will be female and an XY male (refer Fig. 12.2). The Y chromosome contains a specific gene, called the **testis-determining factor gene (TDF)**, which triggers male sexual development. At roughly 6 to 8 weeks after conception, the TDF gene initiates the development of the testes. Once formed, the testes secrete sex hormones called **androgens** that continue to direct a male pattern of organ development. If the TDF gene is not present, as happens with an XX combination in the 23rd pair, testes do not form and in the absence of sufficient androgen activity during this prenatal critical period, an inherent female pattern of organ development ensues.

Each chromosome contains thousands of genes, which transmit genetic information. Genes, either singly or in combination produce specific human traits, both physical and psychological. For example, researchers have identified a gene that determines, at least partly, human novelty-seeking behavior. It is estimated that there are some 30,000 genes in humans. Recently, scientists have succeeded in mapping these genes as part of a huge enterprise known as "Human Genome Project." This project is likely to produce a revolution in health care, as scientists identify particular genes that are responsible for different disorders.

other bodily organs develop. The fetus can respond to touch. At about 16 to 18 weeks the fetal movements become strong enough for the mother to sense the baby's movements. Around the 27th week, the fetus reaches the *age of viability*; that is, it can survive outside the womb in case of premature birth. It is reported that fetuses several weeks younger also can survive with top medical care. At about 28 weeks, the fetus weighs about 3 pounds and is 16 inches long. It is believed that the fetus is capable of some rudimentary forms of learning (remember the story of Abhimanyu in Mahabharata). In the final weeks of pregnancy, the fetus continues to gain weight and grow. At the end of the normal 38 weeks of pregnancy, the fetus typically weighs around 7 pounds and is about 20 inches in length.

Genetic Influences on the Fetus

Just because the zygote is formed there is no guarantee that it will be born as a normal baby. The journey from zygote to birth is not smooth. It is reported that half of all fertilized eggs contain some kind of abnormality in their chromosomes. Most of these eggs are aborted; thirty percent of zygotes do not reach the embryonic stage. More male embryos than female embryos end in abortion. One in 250 babies is born with some abnormality that is obvious and probably more are born with some abnormalities that are not easily detected. Fortunately, normal fetal growth occurs in 95 to 98 percent of all pregnancies. The remaining 2 to 5 percent of cases are born with some serious birth defects. These are generally caused by defects in chromosomes or genes. The following are some of the major genetic or chromosomal difficulties.

Phenylketonuria

Phenylketonuria (PKU) is a genetic disorder in which an enzyme necessary for normal development is missing. The result is a severe type of mental retardation known as phenylpyruvic oligophrenia. Fortunately, if detected early, the untoward effects can be prevented by placing the affected children on a special type of diet that allows them to develop normally.

Sickle-cell Anemia

Sickle-cell anemia is a hereditary disease that destroys red blood cells by causing them to take on a rigid sickle shape. Children with sickle-cell anemia suffer from chronic anemia, shortness of breath, severe pain in the abdomen as well as susceptibility to infection. A large number of African-Americans (about 10%) and a few from the Middle East including India suffer from this disease. There is no known cure for sickle-cell anemia and most of the afflicted die.

Tay-Sachs Disease

Tay-Sachs disease is another inherited disease marked by severe neurological deterioration, which is accompanied by mental and physical retardation. The deterioration is the result of a lack of a single enzyme necessary for proper metabolism. It occurs more frequently among Jewish children than among other racial and ethnic groups. Many of the afflicted children die within the first 18 months of life.

Down Syndrome

Down syndrome is a congenital condition marked by a flat skull, stubby fingers, and skin folds on the palms of hands and soles of the feet, a fissured tongue and often severe mental retardation. In 90 percent of the cases there is an extra 21st chromosome and hence it is sometimes called **trisomy 21**. It was called *mongolism* by Langdon Down, who first described it and after whom the condition is now named. Down syndrome is believed to be related to the mother's age at pregnancy. It is reported that among mothers under 30 years of age, the incidence is 1 per

1,000 and among those over 45, the incidence is as high as 1 per 40.

Environmental Influences

Much of the early development is determined by **maturation**, the process that produces genetically programmed changes with increasing age. But from the very beginning, genes (nature) and the environment (nurture) interact. Although the genes from the ovum and sperm determine the characteristics the person eventually develops, the environment plays a crucial role in whether the sperm ever reaches the ovum. The subtle muscle contractions in the uterus direct the movement of the sperm. The waves produced by the contraction move in correct direction in fertile woman. They may be wrong or weak in infertile women and impede the movement of the sperm toward the egg. Further, the consistency and chemical composition of the intrauterine fluid must be right for the sperm to complete the journey.

Several other environmental conditions and external agents can have deleterious effects during the prenatal development. Environmental agents, such as chemicals, drugs, viruses or certain types of radiations that can cause damage to the fetus, are called **teratogens**. The damage caused by teratogens depends upon the stage at which they affect the organism and the damage caused may be physical or psychological or both. Generally, the placenta prevents many harmful substances from reaching the embryo and fetus, but some harmful agents can pass through. Some of the major environmental factors that may cause damage to the developing fetus are mentioned below.

Maternal Illness

Several diseases that the mother suffers during the early parts of pregnancy can cause serious damages to the fetus. For example, if the mother contracts German measles (rubella), especially when the embryo's eyes, ears, heart and central nervous system are developing, it can cause blindness, deafness, heart defects and mental retardation in the infant. Mothers with untreated sexually transmitted diseases may give birth to children with brain damage, blindness and deafness. Among mothers suffering from syphilis, 25 percent of babies are born dead. A mother who is human immunodeficiency virus (HIV) positive can pass the virus on to the baby during gestation or birth in one third of the cases. The HIV virus can cause brain damage leading to several cognitive impairments such as defects in attention, concentration, memory and reasoning.

Alcohol and Smoking

Alcohol and nicotine are dangerous to the development of the fetus. If the mother is an alcoholic, the baby is likely to be born with **fetal alcohol syndrome (FAS)** in at least 50 to 65 percent of cases. Children born with FAS are found to have malformed brains leading to mental retardation and certain cognitive deficits. In addition, they may exhibit irritability and impulsivity. Although there is disagreement about the threshold level of alcohol exposure needed to produce FAS, pregnant women and those who are trying to have a baby are advised to be away from alcohol altogether. Maternal smoking (even passive smoking) during the gestation period affects both mother and fetus; it may lead to premature delivery, miscarriage, respiratory infections and low birth weight. Recently, it is reported that maternal smoking may even damage genes, alter the functioning of the autonomic nervous system, and can be one of the causes of **sudden infant death syndrome (SIDS)**.

Use of Drugs

Using heroin or cocaine during pregnancy can cause a number of problems such as irritability, sleep disturbances, attentional problems and certain physical defects in the newborn. The children may be born with a tendency toward drug addiction and experiencing **withdrawal symptoms**. In addition, the children's ability to regulate their arousal and attention may be impaired. Even legal drugs taken by pregnant women (without knowing they are pregnant) can have devastating effects. It is reported that a drug (Accutane) prescribed to control acne has produced fetal abnormalities.

Mother's Diet

Needless to say that mothers who are undernourished during pregnancy do not provide adequate nutrients to the growing fetus and they give birth to underweight babies. A mother's poor diet can lead her infant to have fewer brain cells than normal. The lack of certain important vitamins and minerals can have significant effects. It is reported that insufficient folic acid can disrupt the early development of the brain and spinal cord. Folic acid is essential for the production of the iron-containing protein needed in the formation of red blood cells. Mothers who eat fish with high levels of methylmercury are likely to give birth to babies with auditory and visual problems.

Maternal Stressors

Severe stress in the pregnant mother's life can endanger the developing fetus. Stress hormones can pass through placenta. Prolonged stress is associated with increased risk of premature birth. There is evidence that stressed mothers give birth to babies with smaller heads. Mothers who are anxious and tense during the last months of their pregnancies are more likely to give birth to babies who will be irritable and who eat and sleep poorly. Don't panic! There is also evidence that mild stress may actually be good for the developing fetus.

A number of other environmental factors may affect the development during the prenatal period. For example, radiation from X-rays may produce physical deformities and even mental retardation. Mother's age is an important factor; mothers under the age of 18 and above 40 may give birth to children with Down syndrome. In spite of all these negative genetic and environmental factors, fortunately, the vast majority of pregnancies develop normally without much difficulty.

Prenatal Testing

Several techniques are used to detect fetal abnormalities during the prenatal period. One of them is **amniocentesis**, in which a syringe is inserted into the amniotic sac to take out the fluid containing fetal cells and analyze fluid to detect biochemical and chromosomal abnormalities. Amniocentesis is performed between 16 and 18 weeks of pregnancy. Another technique, *chorionic villus sampling* (CVS), may be performed several weeks earlier than amniocentesis. In CVS, a small amount of tissue from the *chorion*, the membrane that holds the amniotic sac and fetus, is analyzed. Both these techniques can detect a wide range of abnormalities, including Down syndrome. Often *ultrasound imaging* is also used to detect fetal abnormalities. Here, sound waves are bounced off the fetus, revealing an image of the fetus and amniotic sac that can be displayed on a TV-type monitor.

INFANCY AND CHILDHOOD

A newborn baby is called **neonate** and the period from birth to 12 months is referred to as **infancy**. Although the parents consider their baby as the most beautiful thing in the world, it does not meet the standard of beauty in the real sense of the term. The strange appearance of the newborn is the result of several factors. The incompletely formed skull might have been compressed and the nose flattened during the journey from womb to the external world. The eyelids may look puffy with accumulation of fluids because of its upside-down position during birth. Some people call the neonate, a bundle of muscles and bones. But within 2 weeks, the neonate takes on the appearance with which we are familiar. The infant appears to be utterly incompetent, capable of only eating, sleeping, emptying (bowels and bladder) and crying; that is not true. The baby is not an empty box. The baby's brain is not a blank sheet of paper waiting for something to be written on it either through learning or maturation. The world is not a 'buzzing, blooming confusion' for the baby as William James had remarked. Babies come into the world equipped with a surprising array of abilities, both physical and psychological.

Reflexes in the Newborn

The neonate is born with a number of reflexes. Reflexes are inborn, unlearned, automatic responses to specific stimuli. Many of these reflexes are necessary for the survival of the baby. The following are some of the major reflexes exhibited by a newborn baby.

Sucking reflex: When something is put into the child's mouth, it automatically starts sucking.

Rooting reflex: When the baby's cheek is touched, it turns its head and opens the mouth.

Startle (Moro) reflex: When there is a sudden loud sound, the baby makes a series of movements such as flinging out of arms, fanning of the fingers arching of its back; also starts crying.

Gag reflex: Clearing of its throat.

Palmer reflex: When the palm is pressed, the baby grasps the object that is pressing the palm.

Babinski reflex: When the sole of the foot is stroked, the big two flexes and the other toes fan out.

Eye blink reflex: Automatic blinking of the eyes when there is a bright light.

Many of these reflexes disappear within 6 months to 1 year. It is believed that these reflexes were useful to our ancestral human beings or they are simpler versions of later behaviors, such as walking or swimming. The presence of these reflexes and their disappearance at known periods of time are considered normal neurological development.

Physical Development

The physical growth of the neonate in the next few months is astounding. The human body and the motor (movement) skills are programmed to develop in an orderly fashion by the biological process of **maturation**. By about one year the body weight triples and the height increases by 50 percent. This rapid growth slows down as the child gets older. The average rate of growth from age 3 to 13 is a gain of about 5 pounds in weight and 3 inches in height per year. The comparative sizes of the various parts of body also change dramatically with age. For example, the head of the neonate is disproportionately large, about 1/4th of the body size; it will be 1/5th at 2 years, 1/6th at 6 years, 1/7th at 12 years and 1/8th at 25 years. Developmental psychologists have spent many years studying the precise ways in which motor development takes place. Arnold Gesell (1948) has described that all babies, all over the world, pass through a series of milestones in an orderly fashion. In general, the motor control progresses from the head down the trunk to the arms, and finally to the legs—the **cephalocaudal sequence**. At the same time, control extends out from the center of the body toward the periphery (hands, fingers, toes)—the **proximodistal sequence**. By about 2 years, the child develops better control over all limbs. Motor abilities emerge at different times. The Table 12.1 shows the average age ranges for important motor developments.

Table 12.1: Typical Ages for Early Motor Development

Age	Development
5 months	Follows movements with eyes; lifts head and chest while lying on stomach; holds head steady; holds an object placed in hand
6–9 months	Rolls over; sits upright; picks up small objects with thumb and fingers; shifts objects between hands; crawls
10–12 months	Pulls to upright standing; walks with support; turns pages of book
13–18 months	Walks alone easily and unaided; feeds self; points to pictures when asked; throws a ball

Development of Brain

Needless to say that the brain is the single most important structure in the human body; it is not fully matured at birth and has reached only about 25 percent of its eventual adult weight. Much of its development takes place after birth; luckily, brain overtakes all other organs of the body in the speed of development. By about 6 months, the brain reaches 50 percent of its adult weight. Neural networks, which are the basic structures for cognitive and motor functions, develop rapidly. The brain structures that regulate vital survival functions such as heartbeat and respiration are the first to mature. These structures lie deep within the brain. The frontal cortical areas, which regulate the higher cognitive functions, are among the last to mature. The development of the brain slows down during later childhood. But, even after reaching 90 percent of its adult size by about 5 years of age, the maturation process of the brain continues. New synapses are formed, unnecessary synapses are pruned back, association areas are put in place, and the cerebral hemispheres become highly sophisticated.

We must carefully note the role of heredity and environment in physical development. Biology (nature) sets limits on environmental (nurture) influences. For example, you cannot train a child to walk alone before 11 months, because his/her neuromuscular coordination has not yet matured. Similarly, without proper environmental support physical development can be delayed. Severe malnutrition stunts general growth and brain development. Enriched environment, in which the infant has opportunities to interact with others and manipulate objects (such as attractive toys), fosters physical and psychological development. Enriched environment also enhances the brain development; in turn, brain development facilitates the ability to learn several skills and profit from the experience. Motor development also allows the child to go around and explore the environment, which helps visual search and depth perception. Thus, 'travel broadens the mind'.

Sensory and Perceptual Capacities

Along with physical development, the sense organs also develop. In the beginning, the infant's visual system is not well developed. Still, babies can scan their environment, see and follow moving objects within their field of vision. They also show the rudiments of depth perception. Within hours after birth, infants can distinguish the familiar face of their mother from that of a familiar stranger and they prefer to gaze at the face of the mother. Babies prefer human voices to other sounds and they can distinguish mother's voice from that of a female stranger. They respond to touch and can distinguish different odors. Their facial expressions after tasting sweet, sour or bitter substances indicate that they have a fairly well developed sense of taste.

Investigating infants' sensory and perceptual skills is a tough task because they cannot answer your questions. But psychologists working in this field have developed a number of ingenious techniques to study these processes. For example, Eleanor Gibson and her students (Gibson and Walk, 1960) constructed an apparatus called "visual cliff" (Fig. 12.3A) to study depth perception in infants and animals. She placed infants on a level sheet of glass that at first lies directly on the floor, but then extends over a part of the floor that has been stepped down. The mother called the child from the cliff side and the shallow side successively. Almost all infants crawled off on the shallow side, but refused to crawl on the deep side. They frequently peered through the glass on the deep side and then backed away. Some of the infants patted the glass with their hands, but still remained unassured that it was solid and refused to cross. The researchers tested infants ranging in age from 6 to 14 months and all of them exhibited the ability to perceive depth. The results with other organisms indicate that depth perception is present at least as soon as the animal is able to walk (see the goat in the Fig. 12.3B).

Other experiments have shown that babies under 6 months can also perceive depth. In one study, researchers measured the heart rate of infants when they were placed on the shallow or deep side of the visual cliff and found that 2-month-old babies had slower heart rates on the deep side; slower heart rates indicate that someone is paying closer attention, which suggests that the infants could in fact differentiate between two depths.

Another way of studying perceptual processes is known as looking time technique or habituation technique. This is based on the fact that all animals, including human beings, habituate to a stimulus. If a baby continuously looks at a particular shape long enough, he/she will no longer find it interesting and thus will prefer to look at something new. Suppose a baby is shown a circle over an extended period of time and then shown a circle along with a square, he prefers to look at the square rather than the circle. This technique can be used to determine what shape differences babies see and whether they see depth or other physical properties. Habituation techniques have shown that babies can detect depth between 2 and 3 months of age.

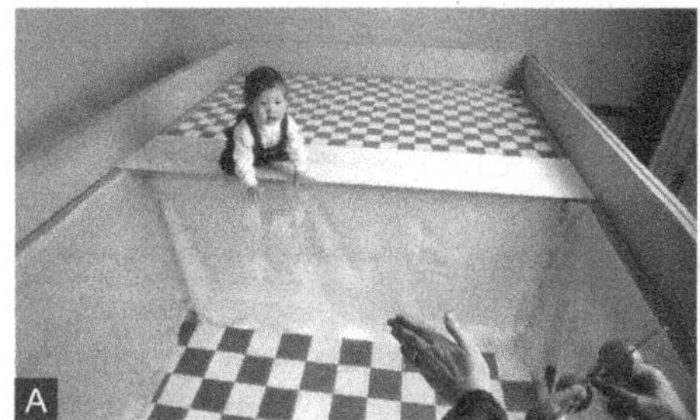

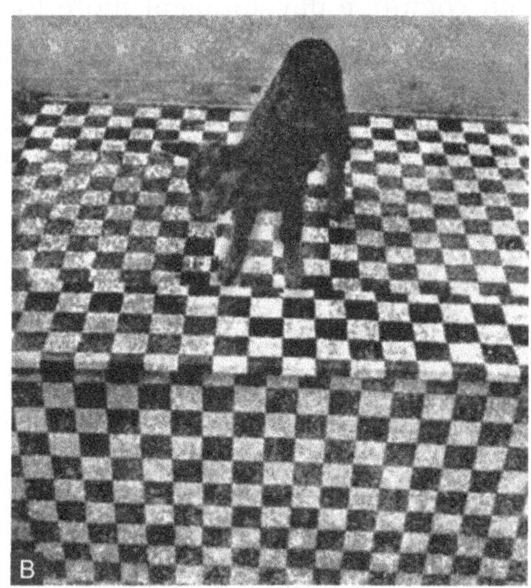

FIGURES 12.3A and B: Visual cliff

Compared to visual perception, auditory perception appears to be more fully developed in an earlier age. Using 4-month-olds researchers have found that they prefer consonant tones rather than dissonant ones. Perceptual development is a continuing process and it is found to develop steadily until late adolescence.

Cognitive Development

The term cognition broadly refers to complex higher mental activities such as thinking, conceiving, reasoning, problem solving and information processing. Obviously these mental capacities are not well-developed at birth. The attention span of infants is short; they understand very few concepts and about the relationships between objects and events in their surroundings. For example, they do not know that fire hurts and water wets them. Children cannot understand problems let alone solve them. They acquire these capacities gradually and this process is called *cognitive development*. Psychologists owe a great deal to a Swiss psychologist **Jean Piaget** (1970) for their knowledge about cognitive development more than to anyone else. Piaget (Fig. 12.4) proposed a far reaching and comprehensive theory of cognitive development, which helped generate several lines of research in the field. Someone called him a "giant with a giant theory."

Piaget's Theory of Cognitive Development

After his early training in biology, Piaget worked with Theodore Simon, one of the pioneers in intelligence testing. When he was testing the intelligence of children, including his own children, he noticed that children of the same age made similar errors on test items. Intrigued by this phenomenon, he started observing children's problem-solving procedure and came to the conclusion that they think differently at different ages. According to Piaget, thinking changes qualitatively with age and it is different from the way adults think. Cognitive development is the result of interaction between biological maturation and personal experience. Piaget's biological background had a great impact on his theorizing about cognitive development. He called his system "genetic epistemology." Epistemology is the study of the nature and acquisition of knowledge. Piaget's approach to the study was "genetic" in the sense that it focused on the origins (genesis) of cognitive development. The term reflects his interest in the process of how children acquire knowledge and how the process changes as they develop.

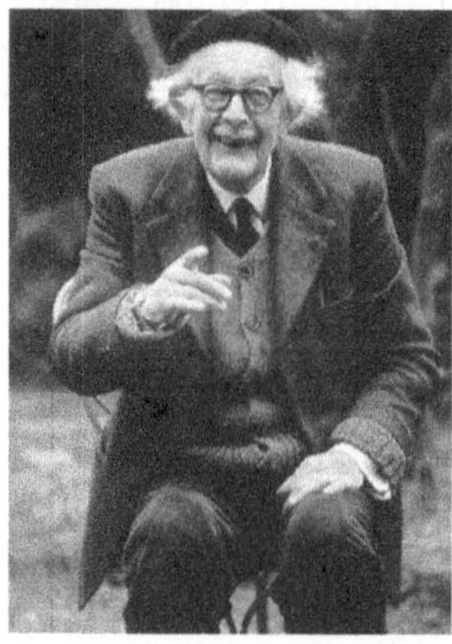

FIGURE 12.4: Jean Piaget

The child tries to understand the world in terms of simple innate schemas. **Schema** is a mental structure that organizes thought and action. For example, the child's response of sucking the nipple when hungry is an innate schema; it is an action sequence guided by thought. To say metaphorically, the child comes to "know" the world through his mouth (sucking). Cognitive development takes place as the child acquires new and more complex schemas and incorporates new experiences into the existing schemas. Piaget called the process of incorporating new experience into the existing schema as **assimilation**. When the infant sees a toy, it puts the toy into the mouth; thus, the baby is fitting a new experience (seeing a toy) to an existing schema (objects are suckable). This is assimilation. As the child tries to suck whatever comes his way, he realizes that certain things cannot be sucked, may be because they are too big to suck, or they are bitter. Now, he changes his schema. The process of changing the existing schema in the light of new experience, Piaget called **accommodation**. Thus, cognitive development involves attempts to understand new experience in terms of what is already known (assimilation) and modifying the old thought when new experience does not fit into it (accommodation). The two processes are the engines that drive cognitive development and the child's thinking changes systematically with age as new schemas develop. Piaget also uses the term **equilibration** to refer to the process of self-regulation (balancing) in which there is constant interplay between assimilation and accommodation.

According to Piaget, the processes of assimilation, accommodation and equilibration operate in different ways at different ages. As a consequence, our ways of thinking about or knowing the world, pass through certain predictable stages. Piaget proposed four stages (or periods) of cognitive development, namely, **sensorimotor**, **preoperational**, **concrete operational** and **formal operational**. Each stage is governed by different principles and includes several substages. The age at which the children reach the four stages may slightly vary, but the sequence of the stages never varies. Thus, Piaget's theory of cognitive development may be age variant, but it is stage invariant. Although Piaget's theory is discussed under the section on Infancy and Childhood, it should be noted that cognitive development is an ongoing process that occurs throughout life. Let us take a closer look at Piaget's four stages of cognitive development.

Sensorimotor Stage (Birth to 2 Years)

During the **sensorimotor stage**, infants try to understand the world through their sensory experiences and physical contact (motor activities) with the objects, hence the label sensorimotor. Infants and toddlers deal with objects and events around them using mouth, hands, eyes and other sensorimotor instruments in a predictable, organized, and often adaptive ways. Their understanding of the world is primarily based on sucking, chewing, touching, shaking and manipulating objects. But they cannot represent (in their mind) objects or people in the form of images, words or any other symbols. Initially, they lack the idea of **object permanence**; that is, they are not aware that an object continues to exist even if it is out of sight. For young infants "out of sight" means "out of mind." Suppose a toy that they were playing with is hidden under a blanket; children under 8 months will make no attempt to search for it. For them, it is just not there. Only around 10th month will they begin to search for it, indicating that they have developed a mental representation of the toy. Thus, object permanence is an important development during sensorimotor stage. Sensorimotor stage consists of six substages. As children pass through these stages, they progress from reliance on reflex actions to a basic understanding of the world around them. We see here the beginnings of the ability to represent the world symbolically through words.

Preoperational Stage (2–7 Years)

The word operation (as used in the term preoperational) refers to actions we perform mentally to gain knowledge. To know an object is to act upon it. That is, you mentally compare it, change it and bring it back to its original state. Knowledge is not just a mental image of an object or event. You do something to it mentally. **Preoperational stage** then refers to a period in which the children can use symbols (such as words) to represent objects and events, but cannot operate or mentally manipulate them; they cannot apply basic principles of logic to their experiences. For example, a child who cannot take something apart and put it together again is passing through preoperational stage. Piaget has identified several features of preoperational thinking such as realism, animism, artificialism and transductive reasoning.

Realism: Refers to the child's growing tendency to distinguish and accept the real world that exists apart from him. Youngsters initially confuse between internal and external world. They confuse between thought and matter. This confusion disappears at about age seven.

Animism: Refers to a child's tendency to attribute life to inert objects. When it rains a child may say: "The sky is crying." In the beginning, children think that all things are alive and conscious. A little later, they think only those things that can move are alive; still later, only things that move spontaneously are alive; finally, they think only animals are conscious. Comparing one's own thoughts with those of others helps in conquering animism.

Artificialism: Piaget used the term artificialism to refer to a preoperational child's tendency to assume that everything is the product of human creation. For example, if you ask a child, "Why the sun rises?" he may say, "Because we rise." Only at about 9th year, the child realizes that human activity has nothing to do with the rising of the sun. The decline of artificialism parallels the development of realism.

Transductive thinking: Piaget used the term transductive thinking to the kind of illogical thinking that is neither deductive nor inductive. Here the thinking moves from particular to particular. For example, the child might say, "The sun won't fall down because it is hot," or "The sun stays there because it is yellow."

During both sensorimotor and preoperational periods a child's thinking reflects **egocentrism**, a tendency to see things as he wants them to be. His/Her universe is entirely centered on self. Egocentric children are simply unaware of other's viewpoints; they lack the cognitive ability to take another person's point of view. For example, when a child wants to play with his mother, he does not understand that mother is tired and needs rest. Children also exhibit **centering** (**centration**), a tendency to concentrate on only one aspect of an object or event at a time to the exclusion of all other aspects. They cannot also reverse their thinking; they may say 2 + 2 = 4 but cannot understand 4 – 2 = 2. This inability of children to reverse their thinking is called **irreversibility**.

Concrete Operational Stage (7–12 Years)

During the **concrete operational stage**, children overcome the limitations of preoperational thinking. Now, they can accomplish true mental operations, but only on concrete (tangible) objects or events. Their thinking is concrete (not abstract) and bound by reality. For example, if they are shown three blocks of varying size, they can say, "A is larger than B, B is larger than C and therefore, A is the largest block." But if you tell them, "Rama is taller than Krishna; Krishna is taller than Govinda; then, who is the tallest of them?" They cannot answer the question because the three persons are not present in front of them.

Notable accomplishments during this period are: conservation, seriation, classification and number concept.

Conservation is the realization that essence of something remains constant although surface features may change. As adults we take the conservation principle for granted. We know that the amount of substance (mass) in an object is not changed when its shape changes, or when it is divided into two parts; the total weight of a set of objects will remain the same no matter how they are packaged together; liquids do not change in amount when they are poured from a container of one shape to that of another. For children, attainment of these concepts takes several years. For example, in one of the famous experiments children saw two identical jars filled with water to the same height. While they watch, water from one jar was poured into a thinner and taller jar, so that the liquid reaches to a higher level. When asked which jar has more water, children around 4 years of age said that the taller and thinner jar had more water. Only when they were around 7th year, they could say that both the jars have the same amount of liquid. They conserved the idea of equal amounts of water by **decentering**; that is, by focusing on more than one aspect of the problem. Now they can reverse their thinking; they can mentally pour the water back into the original container; they have acquired the concept of **reversibility**. Different types of conservation appear at different ages: number conservation occurs between 6 and 7 years; liquids, length, substance, and area between 7 and 8, weight between 9 and 10 and volume between 11 and 12 years.

Seriation is the ability to arrange objects in a serial order, either increasing or decreasing, say according to size. As we have mentioned in the beginning of this section, children in this period can arrange the concrete blocks according to their size and say, which is the largest among them. But when the problem is presented verbally as in determining the heights of three persons (mentioned in page no. 314), they fail to give the correct answer. *Classification* refers to the ability to group objects with some similarities within a larger category. Suppose children at preoperational stage are shown six oranges and six apples, they will correctly answer questions about the number of oranges and apples, but when asked, "Are there more oranges or fruits?" they will say oranges. Concrete operational children, however, are able to classify both oranges and apples as fruits.

Number concept is not the same as the ability to count; it involves understanding the meaning of numbers, such as the "oneness" of one. In one experiment, Piaget showed preoperational children two rows of tokens (checkers), six in each row; the preoperational children were able to count. But when the tokens in one row were spread out, the child answered that it contained more than six tokens; for him "one" is not always "one." Only after acquiring the concept of seriation and classification (that is, during concrete operational stage), children will be able to understand the "oneness of one;" now one boy, one girl, one apple, and one orange are all one of something. The thought systems of the concrete operational child gets well organized into what Piaget called *cognitive operations*. When children reach this phase, they are on the threshold of adult thinking or formal operations (refer examples of conservation in Table 12.2).

Formal Operational Stage (12 Years and Onwards)

In Piaget's model, **formal operational stage** is the final stage of cognitive development in which children (adolescents) are capable of thinking about both concrete and abstract objects logically and in a systematic manner. Now, they are thinking like adults. They can distinguish between the real and imaginary, mentally experiment, analyze logically and discern all possible relations in a problem. They are capable of producing novel and creative solutions to problems in school and at home. They can form hypotheses and evaluate them in a thoughtful manner. In fact, they seek problems and enjoy solving them. In problem solving, they follow the scientific method: first, they collect necessary information (data), classify and organize data; second, form statements or propositions (hypotheses) about the relationships among the variables and finally, test the propositions to determine whether they are true. The most important feature of thinking during this period is that adolescents can conceive of possibilities beyond what is present in reality, to think of alternatives to the way things are and question the ways in which adults run the world.

Piaget devised an experiment called "pendulum problem" to illustrate how children think during the formal operational period. He gave children a set of weights, strings that could be attached to the weights and a bar to which the string could be tied. Using these materials a pendulum was constructed allowing the weight to swing. Then, he asked children to find out

Table 12.2: Piaget's Problems on Conservation

Type of conservation	Initial presentation	Transformation	Question	Preoperational child's answer
Liquids	Two equal glasses of liquid	Pour one into a taller, narrower glass	Which glass contains more?	The taller one
Number	Two equal lines of checkers	Increase spacing of checkers in one line	Which line has more checkers?	The longer one
Mass	Two equal balls of clay	Squeeze one ball into a long thin shape	Which piece has more clay?	The long one
Length	Two sticks of equal length	Move one stick	Which stick is longer?	The one that is farther to the right

the factors that determine the speed with which the pendulum swings: Is it the length of the string, the weight of the pendulum or the force with which the pendulum is pushed? Concrete operational children approached the problem in a haphazard manner: they changed the length of the string, the weight of the pendulum and the force of push simultaneously. Since they varied all factors at the same time, they were not able to solve the problem. On the other hand, formal operational children varied the factors one by one like scientists and found that it was the length of the string that determines the speed with which the pendulum swings. The ability to eliminate competing possibilities is the crucial characteristic of formal operational thought. The adolescents have grasped the essential points of scientific experimentation, varying systematically one variable at a time holding all other variables constant. That means all the ingredients for scientific thinking have developed during the formal operational period.

Although, formal operational thought appears to emerge during adolescence, it does not happen universally. Studies have shown that only 40 to 60 percent of American college students and adults reach this stage. Many people do not reach this stage at all. It is also reported that in certain societies, which are educationally and technologically backward, almost no one reaches the formal operational level of thinking. A summary of Piaget's stages of cognitive development is shown in Table 12.3.

Evaluation of Piaget's Theory

Piaget's theory, no doubt, has revolutionized our thinking about children's cognitive development. Several researchers all over the world have confirmed that generally cognitive abilities develop in the same order across cultures as proposed by Piaget in four stages; children apprehend object

Table 12.3: Summary of Piaget's Stages of Cognitive Development

Stage	*Average age*	*Important characteristics*
Sensorimotor	Birth to 2 years	Knowledge comes from sensory and motor experiences. Object permanence develops. Symbolic thought is emerging, but it is primitive.
Preoperational	2–7 years	Language develops; representation of objects in words and images. Thought is self-centered, animistic and reasoning is faulty. There is confusion between reality and fantasy.
Concrete operational	7–12 years	Logical thinking develops, but at concrete level conservation concepts emerge, concept of reversibility develops classification and serial ordering of objects is possible.
Formal operational	12 years onwards	Logical thinking at abstract level is possible. Capable of forming and testing of hypothesis. Concern for future and ideological issues emerge.

permanence, before they are capable of symbolic thinking, and concrete reasoning occurs before abstract reasoning. But the theory has not gone on unchallenged. Other researchers, using techniques and materials different from Piaget and making use of subtle measurements, have come up with results that differ from his; they have produced evidence to show that children often can acquire certain competences well before they have reached the appropriate Piagetian stage. For example, Andrew Meltzoff and colleagues (2002) have found that 2- to 3- week old infants can show imitation and others have found that even 2-day-old infants can imitate happy and sad facial expressions. There is evidence that 3-month-olds can exhibit object permanence, 4-month-olds are aware of temporal intervals, 9-month-olds can add and subtract, and 3-year-old children can understand the conservation of mass. Thus, researchers claim that the capacities of infants often far exceed those proposed by Piaget and that he has underestimated the cognitive sophistication of babies. It is also found that cognitive development within each stage proceeds inconsistently. A child may perform at the preoperational level on most tasks yet solve some problems at a concrete operational level. This cannot happen if development proceeds in distinct stages. Some developmental psychologists believe that cognitive development proceeds in a more continuous manner than Piaget's stage theory implies and suggest that it is primarily quantitative in nature rather than qualitative. Therefore, it has to be concluded that cognitive development is more complex and variable than what Piaget proposed.

Despite all criticisms, the fact remains that Piaget's theory has had a tremendous influence on our understanding of cognitive development. He has provided a fairly accurate account of age-related changes in children's thinking. The influence of his theory has been enormous in the field of curriculum development in educating children. Some researchers called neo-Piagetians have modified certain aspects Piaget's theory to account for the issues mentioned above.

Vygotsky's Sociocultural Theory

Russian psychologist **Lev Vygotsky** emphasized the importance of social interaction in the development of cognitive abilities. Not that Piaget ignored the role of social environment in cognitive development; his main focus was on children's independent exploration of the world around them. While Piaget believed that the child constructs representations of the world through first-hand experience, Vygotsky (1978) proposed that the child constructs representations of the world under the influence of the culture in which he lives. For him, the culture as represented in the child's mind guides his behavior. According to Vygotsky, the sociocultural context interacts with biological maturation of the brain in determining cognitive development. The guidance from parents, teachers and elder siblings assists the development of child's cognitive problem solving skills. More specifically, children's cognitive abilities increase when they are exposed to information that falls within their **zone of proximal development (ZPD)**. The ZPD is the distance between a child's actual developmental level and a higher level, which he is capable of reaching with adult guidance; that is, the distance between what children can do by themselves and what they can do with help from others. When the information falls within the ZPD, they can master the task. Thus, by presenting information that falls within ZPD, others can facilitate the child's cognitive development. The support provided by elders in learning and problem solving is called **scaffolding**.

According to Vygotsky, cultural creations, especially language, play a crucial role in development. Once children learn a language, they begin to use what he called inner speech to plan and guide behavior. In the beginning, children speak aloud to themselves; later the speech turns inward and becomes silent inner speech or private speech. Researchers have found that young children use inner speech when trying to perform difficult tasks. They also use inner speech during free play (as compared with structured play) and after they have made an error.

Finally, we must remember that culture and biology do not act independently; the two interact. Culture affects the brain and brain affects culture. For example, culture determines which language we speak, which in turn affects how the brain processes sound. Similarly, brain affects culture in that we do not have customs that require more working memory capacity than the brain provides. The conclusion is that nature and nurture interact.

Information-processing Approaches

Many developmental psychologists have proposed an alternative to Piaget's stage theory that is known as **information processing approach**. This approach assumes that cognitive development is a continuous, gradual process in which the same kinds of information processing skills become more and more effective over time. The ability to process information depends on a host of distinct processes and these, in turn, depend on the development of the brain. If younger children perform more poorly than older children on several tasks, it is because they cannot attend to the task effectively, are unable to formulate and follow plans efficiently, and they do not have enough stored information to organize the input. More importantly, younger children's working memory is not as good as that of the older children. Young children are simply slower in mental processing than older children and adults. The speed of processing increases with age as some abilities become automatic. The speed at which stimuli can be scanned, recognized and compared with other stimuli increases with age. With increasing age, children can pay attention to stimuli longer and discriminate between different stimuli more readily and they are less easily distracted. Thus, the information-processing approach asserts that it is the quantitative changes in these skills that are at the root of children's improved understanding of the world.

In the beginning, children's memory is not well developed. The immediate memory span of preschoolers is only 2 or 3 chunks of information; 5-year-olds can hold four chunks; 7-year-olds can hold 5 and adults can keep 7, plus or minus 2 chunks. Researchers have demonstrated that the capacity of working memory increases with age. The size of the chunk also increases with age. As the working memory capacity increases, the child can solve several problems that were previously beyond his reach. That is why Piaget's subjects failed to solve problems involving object permanence. Therefore, what produced the realization that "out of sight" objects continue to exist are quantitative changes in capacity and not qualitative changes in performance. A quantitative change in the amount of memory produces a qualitative change in performance.

Before concluding our discussion of cognitive development, it is necessary to mention briefly about two interesting concepts that are believed to play a crucial role in improving children's thought processes. These are metacognition and theory of mind.

Metacognition and Theory of Mind

Metacognition refers to awareness and understanding of one's own cognitive processes; it involves the planning, monitoring and revising cognitive strategies. Younger children who cannot monitor their cognitive processes often fail to recognize their own errors and incapabilities in solving problems. Older children, in contrast, can better judge how well they understand or test the problem presented to them. When the metacognitive capacities are well developed, they are in a position to know what they do not know. This knowledge helps them in deciding whether they need to study more or seek help from elders. Such increasing sophistication reflects a change in children's **theory of mind**. The term theory of mind refers to a person's idea about the mind and the ability to understand other people's mental states—their beliefs, desires, expectations and feelings. In children, the theory of mind enables them to predict what other people are thinking and how they will react in a given situation. Remember, even Piaget believed that children below the age of 6 or 7 years cannot understand what other people are thinking.

One of the ways to assess the theory of mind is to tell children a story and see whether they draw proper inferences about the mental state of the leading character in the story. The story used for this purpose may be as follows: "A boy named Ram hides his candy bar in a drawer and leaves the room. Then, his mother takes the candy bar out of the drawer and puts it in a cupboard. Ram has not seen his mother doing this. A little later, Ram returns to the room and wants to get his candy bar because he is hungry. Where will Ram look for his candy bar?" For questions like this, children about 2 or 3 years of age indicate that Ram will look for his candy in the *cupboard* as if he had the same knowledge that they have. But many 4-year-olds say that Ram will look up in the *drawer* recognizing that he does not have the knowledge that they have. Thus, they recognize that Ram's mental state (his mind) is different from theirs. Studies conducted in China, Japan, Africa, the United Kingdom and the United States yielded similar results. So, it appears that children begin to understand some aspects of other people's thinking by about 4 years, well before Piaget thought they could.

In this context, a word about cognition is in order. Psychologists, for a long time, were not always receptive to the study of higher mental processes such as cognition. Throughout much of the 20th century, the behaviorism of Watson and Skinner dominated psychology and discouraged studies of mental activities that could not be observed. Studying mind and mental processes was considered the business of speculative philosophy, not of respectable experimental psychology. It was not until 1960s that cognitive psychology made inroads into the broader domain of psychology. It was during the second half of the 20th century, many experimental psychologists who had been trained to conduct experiments on learning in animals shifted their interests to the study of higher mental processes in humans. By the 1970s, this movement has become so strong to be called "cognitive revolution." The study of cognition is now a respectable area of inquiry, which draws upon experimental psychology, computer science, mathematics, neuroscience and linguistics. Surprisingly, modern cognitive psychology is turning toward Wundtian psychology whose subject matter was the analysis of immediate experience.

Social and Emotional Development

The development of children is not mere physical growth, acquisition of motor skills and cognitive competencies; it includes development of emotional regulation, social relations, moral values and ultimately a unique personality. We have seen in earlier chapters the emotional development in children, the importance of social interactions and the development of personality. Study of emotional development in children is difficult because they cannot describe their feelings. Still, their facial expressions, vocalizations and other behaviors indicate that they are experiencing some emotions. You can see the distress in the face of the child when it cries and the contentment when it is well fed. Around 6 months after birth, rudiments of surprise and joy can be seen in the face. Gradually, the expression of distress branches out into separate emotions of disgust, anger fear and sadness. Just as emotional expressions become diversified, children also learn to regulate their emotional expressions. Emotional development is influenced by the reactions of parents, teachers and peers. The children generally model their expressions after the people around them.

Temperamental Differences

An important aspect of an individual make-up characterized by dispositions towards particular patterns of emotional reactions to stimulation is called **temperament**.

Temperament in its simplest sense refers to a child's general level of emotional reactivity, a characteristic style of behavior or disposition. For instance, one child may display a cheerful temperament in approaching new situations, whereas another may exhibit fearful temperament. There are suggestions that temperament has a significant genetic basis because striking differences are seen in children's reactivity to stimuli such as bright light, loud noise, sudden movement and physical contact. Psychologists Chess & Thomas in 1996, conducted a study on middle and upper-middle class children from the New York City area (the New York Longitudinal Study–NYLS) and based on the data have categorized infants into three temperamental groups.

Easy children: These are children who are playful and respond positively to new stimuli. They adapt to changes easily, are generally happy, and develop food and sleeping schedules quickly. About 40 percent of NYLS children belonged to this category.

Difficult children: Those who react negatively to new situations or people belong to this category. They were generally irritable and could not develop eating and sleeping schedules easily. About 10 percent of the children fell into this group.

Slow-to-warm-up children: These were inhibited infants who avoided novel stimuli, have a low activity level and took more time to adjust to new situations. In fact, they were subdued, distressed and withdrawn while facing unfamiliar situations. About 15 percent of NYLS children were put into this group.

The remaining 35 percent of children belonged to a mixed group who could not be easily classified. Latest, researchers have shown that these distinct types of temperament predict future differences in adjustment. The easy children became well-adjusted adults, slow-to-warm-up children were more anxious and depressed and the difficult children exhibited problems of adjustment.

Temperament has been found to be related to interaction with others in play situations. Children with flexible temperament were more cooperative than inflexible ones. Children with difficult temperament became more aggressive; and had difficulties in language acquisition. Developmental psychologists believe that temperament is shaped by both genetics (nature) and environment (nurture). Although the question whether the basic temperament could be changed is difficult to answer, it is found that parents, teachers and other care givers can use suitable techniques (gentle encouragement) to mellow down temperamental difficulties.

Attachment

You must have seen a child smiling at the sight of its mother's face; it is an indication that the child is socializing. The most significant form of social development that occurs during infancy is **attachment**, the strong, positive emotional bond, between the children and their primary care givers. We are attached strongly to someone or the other. We are happy to be with people to whom we are emotionally bonded. We miss them when we are separated from them. Attachment thus, is a fundamental form of social behavior. What are the roots of attachment behavior? The earliest studies of attachment were conducted on animals by Konrad Lorenz. He first observed that ducklings follow instinctively their mother, the first moving object, to which they were exposed immediately after birth. Later, he found that ducklings whose eggs were raised in an incubator and who saw Lorenz immediately after hatching would follow him as if he were their mother. He named this behavior as **imprinting** (refer Fig. 12.1), a sudden, biologically primed form of attachment. Imprinting occurs in some bird species including ducks and geese. Imprinting involves a critical period. In ducklings, only those that were exposed to the mother or any other moving object within one day after birth exhibited this behavior and by two and half days the capacity to imprint was lost. Thus, among some animals the young ones must be exposed to their parents within a known interval of time after birth for attachment to occur. Ethologists believe that getting attached to someone is an instinctive form of behavior.

What about human children? Earlier, people thought that the emotional bonding between a child and the mother or other adults results primarily from the care giver's role in satisfying children's need for nourishment. This assumption was tested by Harry Harlow (1958, 1959) in one of the classical experiments in psychology. Harlow separated monkeys from their biological mothers shortly after birth. Each of the infant monkeys was raised in a cage with two artificial surrogate mothers. One of them was a *hardwire mother* with a milk bottle attached to its chest; the other was a *soft mother* covered with terry cloth, but without milk bottle. When faced with a choice like this, the infant monkeys developed attachment with the soft mother (Fig. 12.5). When they were hungry, they drank milk from the bottle attached to the hard mother, but returned to soft mother to rest and relax. When they were frightened, they ran to the soft mother and clung tightly to it. They often maintained contact with the soft mother even while feeding from the bottle attached to the hard wire mother. From these observations, Harlow came to the

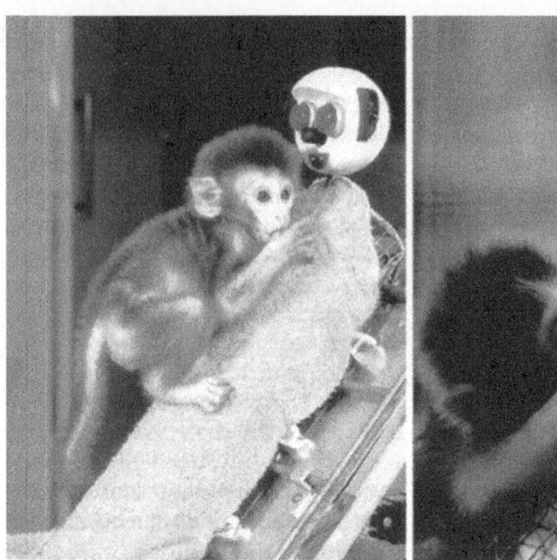
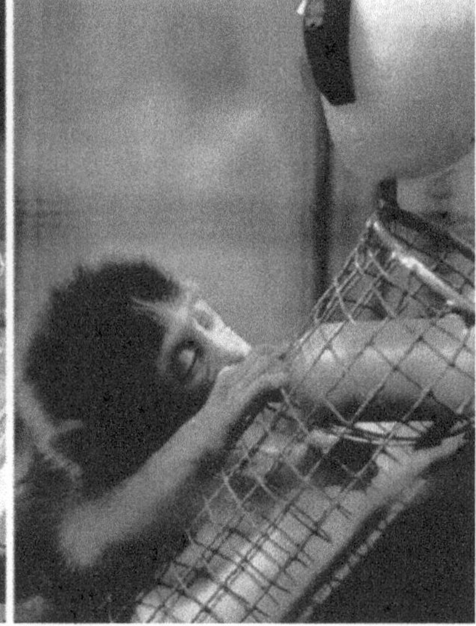

FIGURE 12.5: Harlow's monkeys

conclusion that it was the "contact comfort" that helped the development of attachment and not merely feeding.

But Harlow's studies were on animals. What about human children? Several researchers, inspired by the pioneering work of Harlow, started studying attachment among humans. As we mentioned earlier, British psychoanalyst John Bowlby (1969) studied attachment in human children. Based on his observation, he proposed a theory of attachment that has been widely accepted by developmental psychologists. According to him, children go through three biologically determined phases in developing attachment:

1. ***Indiscriminate attachment:*** In the beginning, infants cry and smile at everyone and these behaviors evoke care-giving behaviors from others.
2. ***Discriminate attachment:*** The 3-month-old infants tend to develop more attachment toward caregivers than toward strangers.
3. ***Specific attachment:*** At or about 8th month, infants develop genuine attachment to specific care givers. The care giver now becomes the center around which the baby crawls and explores the surroundings.

As attachment is well established, children start experiencing two kinds of anxiety, especially during the latter half of the first year. One is **stranger anxiety**, which is distress expressed in front of unfamiliar people or when they are left in strange places. When strangers approach, touch, or handle the baby or when the baby is handed over to strangers, the baby starts crying and reaches towards the mother. This behavior starts around 7th month and disappears by about 18th month. The other is **separation anxiety**, a form of distress expressed by the child when he/she is separated from the primary care giver. For example, when the mother is out of sight, the child starts crying. Children aged between 1 and 2 years, experience separation anxiety that lasts up to the age of 2 to 3 years. These two forms of behavior are observed all over the world in all cultures.

Mary Ainsworth and coworkers (1978) tried to determine various types of attachment behaviors using a standardized procedure, a scenario, called **strange situation**. The setup involved a staged sequence of events designed to discover how children would react when left with a stranger or alone in an unfamiliar situation. The procedure was somewhat as follows: First, the infant plays with toys in the presence of the mother. Then a stranger enters the room and starts interacting with the child. Soon the mother leaves the room leaving the child with the stranger. Later, the stranger leaves the room and the child is left alone. Finally, the mother returns. The children's behavior was observed throughout this procedure. The studies using American children (about 12–18 months old) revealed four types of attachment.

Secure attachment: In the presence of the mother, the babies explore the playroom; react positively to the stranger; upset when the mother leaves the room; not easily comforted by the stranger, and when the mother returns, the babies greet the mother with joy. About 60 to 70 percent of American babies exhibit this type of attachment.

Avoidant attachment: Babies do not seem to care very much whether the mother is present or absent; they are equally comfortable with both mother and stranger; do not cry when the mother leaves the room, and remain indifferent when the mother returns. About 15 to 20 percent exhibit this type of attachment.

Resistant attachment: Babies do not use their mothers as the base of operation; but they stay close to her demanding attention from her; become angry when mother leaves the room and may even hit her when she returns; it is difficult to calm them down easily thereafter. This type of insecure attachment was exhibited by about 10 to 15 percent of children.

Disorganized/disoriented attachment: Babies show inconsistent and often contradictory behavior; they may become depressed and remain unresponsive, or show spurts of sudden emotional outbursts during the strange situation. About 5 to 10 percent of babies exhibited this type of attachment.

How do children behave when they are deprived of stable, secure attachment and what are the long-term effects of such deprivation? Harlow has some answers to this question based on studies of monkeys. When young monkeys raised in isolation for 6 months were later returned to the monkey colony and exposed to other monkeys, the isolates were found to be indifferent, aggressive or terrified. When some female isolates became adults, they were artificially inseminated and gave birth. They were highly abusive towards their firstborns. Harlow concluded that monkeys raised without secure attachment to a real interactive caregiver, develop behavioral problems. But what about human babies reared in isolation? As you can guess, such studies are difficult to undertake on human children. Still there are some indications that lack of attachment has lasting effects on humans; they may suffer from behavioral problems. Researchers have observed the behavior of **feral children** (children raised in isolation by animals) and behavior of children in orphanages. For example, Victor, the Wild Boy of Aveyron, was severely impaired after his isolation and showed only limited recovery after intensive remedial training (Victor, a feral child, was found in the early 1880s near the town of Aveyron in France. He was about 7-year-old at that time. Victor was trained and extensively studied by a French physician Jean Itard). The studies of orphanage children have yielded mixed results. Some of them who were adopted by decent people recovered and developed a healthy attachment, while a large majority was not that lucky.

The type of early attachment can have long-lasting effects. In one study, babies who had experienced a secure attachment were observed at age 11. When compared with others who had disturbed attachment, the children who had developed secure attachment were found to be more socially and emotionally competent, more cooperative, capable and playful. They had closer relationships with friends, acquired better social skills. They could learn things easily and establish more intimate love relationships in later life; more important, they had fewer psychological difficulties. But it does not mean that children who lack secure attachment will always have difficulties in later life. Also, being securely attached at an early age does not ensure good adjustment in later life. Several researchers have focused on the impact of culture on attachment. Some cultures foster higher levels of secure attachment than others. Therefore, attachment style may be related to the social environment in which the children grow. However, we have to accept the conclusion that infancy is a sensitive (not critical) period during which an initial stable attachment to caregivers forms most easily and facilitates subsequent development. Prolonged deprivation of attachment may create developmental problems, but when deprived children are placed in a nurturing environment at a young enough age, many, if not most, become attached and grow into well-adjusted adults.

Day-care Controversy

In modern society, in several families, both the parents are employed for one reason or the other and leave the child in someone else's care, most likely in a day-care home. It is reported that in the United States more than 80 percent of infants are cared for by people other than their parents for part of the day during their first year of life. Almost 30 percent of preschool children, whose mothers work outside their home, spend their time in day-care centers. Most of these infants begin day-care before the age of 4 months and stay there almost 30 hours per week. This has raised the issue of the consequences of day-care on children's development. Is it beneficial or harmful? The researches indicate that the impact depends on the quality of the facilities provided by the day-care centers.

According to the results of a large scale study, supported by the US National Institute of Child Health and Development (NICHD), children who attend high quality childcare centers might not only do as well as children who stay at home with their parents, but in some respects might do better. Superior quality day-care centers offer a stimulating environment: the caretakers are well trained; they cater to children's needs; only a few children are allotted to each caretaker; the caretakers are looked after well and as a consequence, the staff turnover is low. Psychologists working with NICHD Early Child Care Research Network have studied some 1,400 children from birth through third grade and reported the following results:

1. Attachment was optimal in children who resided in high quality day-care centers, while the risk of insecure attachment was high among those from poor centers.
2. Children with high day-care experience exhibited better social skills compared with those with less day-care experience.
3. Children who spent more time in day-care centers showed better cognitive and language skills and these gains persist for a longer duration.

But it should also be noted that the outcomes from day-care experience are not always positive. Often some kids felt less secure when left in day-care institutions for more than 20 hours a week during their 1st year of life. However, for children from impoverished homes, day-care experience has been found to be very helpful; the enriched environment (toys, books, good food, active companions and high quality caregivers) seems to stimulate social and intellectual development. In short, the key to improved social, emotional, and intellectual development is the quality of the day-care service.

Styles of Parenting

All parents do not treat their children in the same way. Some parents show excessive love and concern (overprotection) for their children, some others may neglect them and there may be some others who are indifferent toward raising their children. Researches have shown that child-rearing practices used by parents play a significant role in social development. Psychologist Diana Baumrind (1967) has identified two key dimensions on which parents vary regarding their interactions with children. The first is ***warmth versus hostility*** and the second, ***restrictiveness versus permissiveness***. Warm parents exhibit love and care toward children; hostile ones are not caring and they may even reject their children. Permissive parents are liberal, while restrictive ones are strict in enforcing discipline. Baumrind has proposed three styles of parenting: authoritative, authoritarian and permissive. Later researchers, with slight modification, have identified the following four styles of parenting.

Authoritative parents (warm-restrictive) set goals for their children and reward them when the goals are reached; they establish clear rules and enforce them firmly and consistently; they are demanding, but also caring and supporting; they encourage autonomy and are reasonably warm in dealing with children; there is good parent-child communication. Children who grow up under this climate are believed to develop high self-esteem, achieve good grades in school and do not show behavior problems.

Authoritarian parents (hostile-restrictive) are hostile, restrictive, cold, rigid, rejecting and punitive. They put up strict standards, apply pressure for compliance and do not show warmth. They expect unquestioning obedience from their children. Such children tend to be immature, withdrawn, unsociable and fail to develop high self-esteem. Their academic performance will be poor and they are unpopular with friends.

Indulgent parents (warm-permissive) have a warm relationship with their children, but are lax in setting standards and disciplining them. They are highly permissive, do not guide their children properly and instill the sense of responsibility. Such children tend to be self-centered, immature and spoiled.

Neglecting parents cater to the needs of their children in a routine manner, but are indifferent and detached in their attitude. They neither show love or dislike. Children brought up under such climate tend to be insecurely attached to their parents; their academic performance will be poor and they will have a disturbed relationship with friends. Often, they are impulsive and aggressive. Neglectful parenting generally leads to negative development.

This classification should not be taken too seriously; there are exceptions. The findings apply primarily to the US society. Further, we must not forget the role of heredity in determining behavior. Several children are born with a temperament (an innate biological disposition) that determines whether they become easy-going and cheerful or irritable and fussy. As in several other domains, it is safe to accept an interactionist view here also. For example, biology may make a child irritable; then, the parents find it difficult to deal with the child and treat him/her harshly; this in turn may promote behavior problems in the child.

Development of Self-concept and Gender Identity

An important component of social development is the emerging sense of who one is and what his/her relationship to others is. The picture one has about himself or herself is referred to as **self-concept**. It is what children mean when they use the word "I" or "me." It consists of an organized set of perceptions and beliefs people have about themselves. We have seen in Chapter 11, the importance of self-concept in explaining human behavior, and how Carl Rogers (1959) developed a theory of personality around this construct. Naturally, developmental psychologists are interested in the origins and development of self-concept. When and how a child recognizes that he/she has certain characteristics and an identity as a separate individual? Emergence of a sense of self occurs gradually and depends on the development of cognitive capacities such as reasoning and development of language. A clear idea of self therefore occurs during what Piaget described as the period of formal operations. However, researchers have hinted that children have rudiments of self-concept as early as 3 months.

Preschool children think of themselves in very concrete terms of physical appearance. For example, when one researcher placed a dab of red paint on 15-month-old children's nose and allowed them to look into a mirror, he saw them rubbing it off. By about 2 years all children responded in this way. Others found that 3-month-old children prefer to look at the face of another child of the same age rather than at their own face, suggesting that they are already familiar with their faces. It is also reported that newborn babies can distinguish between touching themselves and being touched by someone else. When they are 3-year-old, some children report that they are happy in certain situations and not in certain others. These observations suggest that children have some rudimentary experience of their body (what William James called material self), but this is not the awareness of self as it is being understood. Real sense of self develops only later, at about 11 to 12 years, when children can describe themselves in terms of self-perceptions and social relationships. The development of self-concept depends on the capacity to think and understand language. One theory of self proposes that we develop an understanding of what we are from what others say about us. This is known as the 'looking glass theory of self'. When people tell you that you are a 'good girl', you think of yourself as a 'good girl'. You see yourself as mirrored by others.

A crucial component of self-concept is **gender identity**, a child's belief that he/she is a boy or a girl. The knowledge that you are a boy or girl comes partly from biology and partly from upbringing. Most children develop gender identity between 2 and 3 years, but their understanding of gender is fragile. Some children believe that a boy may grow to be a girl and vice versa. **Gender constancy**, an understanding that a boy remains a male and a girl remains a female permanently, appears around age 6 to 7 years. Along with the development of gender identity, children also acquire **sex-role stereotypes** or **gender roles**, which are beliefs concerning behaviors considered appropriate for boys and girls. All societies, all over the world, have **social norms** that prescribe certain types of behavior for boys and other types for girls. Parents, teachers and other elders expect and accept different kinds of behavior from boys and from girls. We internalize these social norms and they become part of our identity. Still later, children develop **sex-typing**, which is a tendency to treat others differently based on their gender. All over the world, boys and girls are treated differently by their parents, teachers and society in general. When a boy cries we say, "You are crying like a girl," We prohibit a girl from climbing a tree or jumping over a compound, although both boys and girls can perform these activities equally well. Parents believe that boys will do well in science and mathematics and girls in fine arts and humanities, although there is no evidence that such a difference exists between the sexes. By about 7 or 8 years, sex stereotypes are well established in the minds of children. The idea that boys and girls possess different personality traits and are meant for different professions is entrenched in the minds of children.

Social development is a continuing, lifelong process. We have discussed here certain primary forms of social behavior. More complex forms of social behavior emerge during adolescence and adulthood. How psychological and social developments evolve throughout life was presented by the renowned psychologist, Erik Erikson in his theory of psychosocial development. We shall discuss Erikson's theory a little later under the section on adolescence.

Moral Development

As children mature, they need to develop character and a sense of morality. Acquiring a sense of morality is at the heart of human development. We all know what is right and proper and what is wrong and improper. The development of morality, the process whereby people, particularly children, acquire and internalize the standards of right and wrong of their society, has been an interesting area of study in developmental psychology. In fact, it was Piaget (1932) who pioneered the study of moral development. His studies involved telling children stories in which the intentions of the characters and the results of their actions were varied and the children were asked to make moral judgments about the outcome. Based on his observations, he proposed that moral development, like cognitive development, occurs in stages and proposed a two-stage theory. The first one occurring during early childhood is called the **heteronomous morality stage** or the stage of *moral realism*; in this stage, the child accepts as right and proper the rules set by elders and other authority figures. The second one emerging during later childhood is called the **autonomous morality stage** or the stage of *moral independence*; at this stage, the child's determination of what is right and proper is modified to suit the particular circumstances. American psychologist and educationist, Lawrence Kohlberg took the clue from Piaget, extended and elaborated Piaget's stage model of moral development and developed an influential theory of moral reasoning. Morality is an abstract concept and it cannot be handled until the child enters the teens. In fact, most of the work on moral development has been conducted with adolescents and adults. Therefore, we should have included discussion of morality in the next section on adolescence and adulthood. But because the foundation for moral development is already laid during childhood, we discuss this topic under the section on childhood.

Kohlberg's Theory of Moral Development

Kohlberg (1963, 1981), like Piaget, believed that the sense of morality develops in stages. But he was more interested in the process by which children make a moral judgment, that is, how they distinguish between right and wrong. Kohlberg decided to study the active thinking (cognitive process) involved in making decisions when one faces a moral dilemma. For this purpose, he presented children, adolescents and adults with stories containing hypothetical moral dilemmas, and asked them what they would do and why they would do it under such circumstances. The dilemmas were imaginary conflicts that forced participants to make decisions based on their moral reasoning.

The following is one of the famous stories, used by Kohlberg in his research, containing moral dilemma:

A woman, wife of a man called Heinz, was suffering from a severe form of cancer and was nearing death. There was one recently discovered drug that could save her life. The druggist is charging $2,000 for the *drug whose actual cost is only $400. Heinz does not have that much money. With some difficulty he raised somehow $1,000. Heinz came to the drugstore with $1,000 and told the druggist that his wife is dying and needs the drug urgently and asked him to lower the cost or let him pay the remaining amount later. But the druggist flatly refused saying "I discovered the drug, and I am going to make money from it." Heinz got desperate and that night broke into the drugstore to steal the drug to save his wife. What do you think? Should Heinz have stolen the drug? Should he have broken the law? Why or Why not?*

For this and similar stories Kohlberg obtained answers from his participants and probed their replies trying to get at their level of moral reasoning. He was not interested in whether people approved or disapproved Heinz's behavior in the story, but rather in the reasons and intellectual justification for their judgment. He conducted in-depth interviews with all the participants to discover how their thinking affected their ideas about moral reasoning and how these ideas changed with age. From his exhaustive study of the participant's responses, Kohlberg identified three general levels of moral judgment with two substages in each level. The three primary levels and the six stages (two under each level) are briefly described below.

The Preconventional level (about 4–10 years): This is the premoral level in which behavior is evaluated only on the basis of personal outcomes or perceived consequences of behavior without any regard for right or wrong. The stage 1 of preconventional level is characterized by *obedience and punishment orientation*; children tend to obey rules just to avoid punishment. For example, in the above story the respondent might say: "Heinz should steal the drug because if he lets his wife die he will be blamed for her death;" or "He should not steal the drug because he could get caught and sent to jail." Stage 2 represents an *instrumental purpose orientation*; an act is judged good when it serves the person's needs and interests. Here, self-interest and desire to be rewarded are important. The response to the dilemma might be: "Heinz should steal the drug because that way he will still have his wife to serve him, meet his needs for companionship, love and support." Notice that the rationale is based on the immediate external consequences of the action rather than on some abstract principle.

The conventional level (about 10–13 years): In this level, the focus is on conformity to social expectations, laws and duties. Children not only conform, but actively support social codes; an action is right or wrong because it maintains or disrupts the social order. They justify their actions based on internalized rules. Thus, stage 3, is characterized by *"good boy—good girl" orientation*. Conformity stems from the desire to gain people's approval. They value the need to do the right thing in the eye of others. The response to the Heinz dilemma might be: "People will think that Heinz is bad if he does not steal the drug to save his wife," or "Heinz should not steal the drug because he might get caught and punished." In stage 4, the focus is on adherence to strong, legitimate authority. It represents *law-and-order orientation*. Children believe that rules must be obeyed because they are meant to be followed. The correct behavior is: "Doing one's duty." Thus, they might say: "Heinz should steal the drug because it is his duty to take care of his wife," or "Heinz should not steal because people cannot be permitted to break the law even when they are in difficult situations."

Postconventional level (about 13 years and over): In postconventional level, children's judgments are based on well thought out general moral principles. A true sense of morality emerges during adolescent years. A person adopts moral standards not to seek approval from others or an authority figure but to follow some universal ethical principle. Now, the person thinks that when laws are unjust, one is bound to disobey them. As a consequence, his moral reasoning may even conflict with accepted social standards. Thus, Kohlberg's stage 5 represents the ***social contract orientation***, which involves the belief that laws are based on mutual agreement among members of the society and they are not infallible. One does not have to blindly follow the laws out of respect for authority. Laws must be open to question. Stage 5 children recognize the importance of societal laws; but at the same time, they also take into consideration rights of individuals. They may argue protection of life is more important than the protection of property. The answer to the dilemma might be: "Stealing breaks the law, but what Heinz did was reasonable because he saved his wife's life." On the other hand, they may also argue that individuals must obey the laws because the common good takes precedence over the individual good, and the ends, no matter how noble they may be, do not justify the means. Stage 6 of Kohlberg's model involves the adoption of ***universal ethical principle***. Here the moral reasoning is based on abstract, ethical principles of justice that is universal. People's acts are not guided by fear of punishment, desire for approval or the dictates of social law, but by their own internalized standards of right and wrong. They may believe that if laws devalue the sanctity of human life, it is immoral to obey them. So, the response to the dilemma might be: "Saving life comes before financial gain, even if the person is a stranger," or "An individual human life is more important than society's dictum against stealing." Kohlberg believed that very few people reach stage 6.

Evaluation of Kohlberg's Theory

Despite its far reaching influence on our understanding of moral development, Kohlberg's theory did not go uncontested. Researchers questioned several aspects of the theory. Some assert that moral reasoning does not always dictate moral behavior. Do people who exhibit high levels of moral reasoning in Kohlberg's model actually practice what they preach? It is argued that situational factors are more likely to determine how people act when faced with a moral dilemma (Bandura, 1986).

Several cross-cultural studies have shown that people generally progress through stages suggested by Kohlberg. A review of 44 studies conducted in 27 countries supports the universality of Kohlberg's first four stages (Snarey, 1985). But several other researchers have argued that Kohlberg's theory holds good for Western societies and not so well for other cultures. For example, studies in India revealed striking differences in moral decision making from those found in Western countries. A study by Richard Shweder and colleagues (1990) found that both Hindu children and adults are likely to think that it is perfectly all right for a husband to beat his disobedient wife, an act which would be condemned in the United States. Punishing disobedient family members by elders is considered a moral obligation in India.

Familial upbringing of children has been found to play a major role in children's moral development. For example, when parents listen to their children and discuss moral issues with them, such children reach higher levels of moral reasoning than when parents yell at and threaten their children (Walker and Taylor, 1991). Length of schooling appears to influence moral reasoning; individuals who have higher levels of education demonstrate greater moral maturity. People from industrially advanced countries seem to move through Kohlberg's stages more quickly and to higher levels than those from underdeveloped societies. Moral reasoning also appears to be related to self-esteem. Children with higher levels of self-esteem were found to make correct choices when faced with morally challenging situations.

An important criticism relates to gender bias in Kohlberg's study. All the participants in Kohlberg's study were American males. Carol Gilligan (1982) has questioned the applicability of Kohlberg's conclusions to women. She argues that women have different self-concepts that lead them to different interpretations of moral behavior. Girls are generally raised with an emphasis on attachment and dependence, while boys are raised with an emphasis on separation and independence. Girls' moral decisions are based on the ***ethic of caring***, a concern and responsibility for the well-being of others, while boys are encouraged to follow the path of ***morality of justice***. Kohlberg's higher levels of morality emphasize the concepts of rights and justice, which are male-oriented perspectives. Hence, the test is more applicable to males rather than females. But later studies have shown that males and females do not differ that much in their moral reasoning and both sexes reveal concern for caring and justice. Women use justice reasoning when the situation demands and men's morality is based on caring when it is necessary.

It has been noticed that high levels of moral reasoning can be based on values other than justice. Further, as we said earlier, moral reasoning has to be distinguished from moral behavior. The fact that one reasons in a particular way does not guarantee that his/her behavior is triggered by the thinking and reasoning. Moral behavior may not completely be determined by moral reasoning; possibly, it is guided by certain aspects of character such as, conscience and empathy. There are indications that conscience develops much earlier than sophisticated moral reasoning. The other personality trait that facilitates moral behavior is empathy, the ability to experience another person's inner feelings as your own. In short, it is believed that moral behavior is guided by a set of complex personality factors that develop much earlier than the ability to think and act logically. Behavior is not just the result of how people reason, but also of who basically they are. So it is with moral behavior.

ADOLESCENCE

Adolescence is the period of development between childhood and adulthood. It is what we popularly call teenage. It is a crucial period in human development during which profound changes, both physiological and psychological, occur. According to GS Hall (1904), the pioneer in the study of adolescence, it is a period of "storm and stress." In the 20th century, a great deal has been written about the "crisis" that adolescents face during the teenage period. It is said to be a period of transition from childhood to adulthood, during which the person is neither a child nor an adult. It is said that the adolescent is confused and trying hard to know who he/she is. The person is supposed to be searching for an identity. Is this a true picture of adolescence? The question is difficult to answer. Actually, the period called adolescence is largely an invention of 18th to 20th century Western culture. During the times prior to the Industrial Revolution, when an individual attained **puberty**, a period in which a person becomes sexually mature and capable of reproduction, he/she was considered to have reached adulthood. In several cultures both boys and girls, definitely girls, were married off when they reached the reproductive stage. The same condition continued for several years in non-industrialized countries and exists even today in some backward countries. But Industrial Revolution changed all this in Western societies. Emergence of technology created a need for more schooling, higher education and acquisition of new skills. Thus, bestowing of adulthood was delayed and a long period of adolescence was created. This has initiated a great deal of thinking and research about the issues pertaining to the period of adolescence in Western countries.

However, we should not lose sight of the fact that adolescence is a period of enormous change in the individual. The young men's physical appearance changes as a result of hormonal events of puberty. They take on the bodies of adults. There is a change in their style of thinking. Adolescents can think abstractly and hypothetically. There are changes in their social and emotional life. They are trying to become independent of parents, discover their identity, develop a value system, and form social relationships. More importantly they become sexually aroused, which may create several social, emotional and adjustment problems. Let us review briefly the developmental history of adolescents in contemporary society.

Physical Development

The biological changes that signal the end of childhood bring about rapid growth in height, weight, body shape and sexual maturity. These dramatic changes have important psychological ramifications, which continue into adulthood. The most significant change that occurs during adolescence is sexual maturity. The hypothalamus in the brain signals the pituitary to increase its hormonal secretions. Pituitary hormones stimulate other glands accelerating the maturation of reproductive organs (primary sex characteristics) as well as secondary sex characteristics (non-reproductive physical features such as growth of facial hair in boys and breasts in girls). In girls the landmark change is the occurrence of **menarche**, the first menstruation. In boys, it is the production of sperms and the first ejaculation. Menarche starts typically between 12 and 13 years of age today. In the mid 19th century girls were having their first menstruation at about 17 years of age (even today, girls in several backward countries, such as New Guinea, reach menarche at 17 years).

In recent times, the age of puberty for both sexes has declined throughout the developed and developing countries; this may be because modern-day children receive better nutrition and good health care.

Physical changes during puberty can have important implications for the way the adolescents think and feel about themselves as well as how others view them. Most teenagers are more concerned about their looks than about any other aspect of themselves; many of them do not like what they see in the mirror. Girls tend to be more dissatisfied with their appearance than boys. The age at which puberty sets in itself can impact psychological processes. For example, it has been found that early-maturing boys have certain advantages over late-maturing ones. Those who mature early do well in schools, have more friends, become successful athletes, and have positive body image. Of course, there is also a chance that they come under the influence of elderly boys with antisocial tendencies and as a consequence, may get introduced to drugs and engage in some delinquent activities. But such possibilities are rare and generally they grow to be responsible citizens in later life.

The consequences of early maturity on girls are slightly different. Many of them welcome their changed appearance because they are being sought after by boys. But for some, the weight gain may result in a negative body image. They are more likely to become self-conscious about their bodies and eventually develop eating disorders. Often their physical development (especially breast development) may become a source of ridicule and embarrassment among their peers. Moreover, early-maturing girls are exposed to greater social and sexual pressures from the boys.

Late maturation has some problems for both boys and girls. Boys may be branded as lean and lanky weaklings and looked upon as less attractive kids by their peers. In course of time, these boys might come to view themselves in the same way. Late-maturing girls hold low social status among peers and may be overlooked by boys. But later, at least for some of them, their small size turns out to be an advantage. Now, they might be looked upon as relatively tall and slim—the social ideal of feminine beauty in contemporary society. Overall, early maturation tends to be associated with fewer negative outcomes for boys than girls. Pubertal changes in boys and girls are shown in Table 12.4.

Physical development during adolescence also includes growth of various body parts. During infancy and childhood, the body grows from the trunk outward (proximodistal sequence); the upper arm grows before the lower arms and the lower arms grow before the hands. At puberty the trend is reversed. Rapid growth of the hands, feet and legs is followed by the growth of the trunk. Under the influence of sex hormones, the shoulders of young boys grow large relative to their hips and vice versa for girls. At age 11 to 12, girls typically are taller and heavier than boys because their major growth spurt starts about 2 years earlier than that of boys. By age 14, however, boys' height and weight start increasing, whereas girls have stopped growing or have begun to grow more slowly.

Brain Development

Compared to infancy and early childhood, overall brain development slows from late childhood to adolescence. But within the brain several changes start occurring. In fact, the adolescent brain is said to be a brain in flux. New neural connections are formed, and a number of excessive synaptic connections, formed during the earlier years of explosive brain growth, are pruned. Neural networks are streamlined to permit more efficient communication between various regions of the brain. It is speculated that these changes may explain why, when adolescents are engaged in problem-solving tasks, neural activity within the regions is more highly focused than it was during childhood.

Neural restructuring is especially prominent in the prefrontal cortex and the limbic system, regions that are involved in planning and coordinating behaviors that lead to the satisfaction of motives and emotional urges. Moreover, restructuring in the prefrontal cortex includes an upsurge in activity of

Table 12.4: Pubertal Changes in Boys and Girls

Approximate age in years	*Boys*	*Girls*
8–9		Appearance of breast buds
10–11		Appearance of pubic hair Rapid growth of vagina, ovaries, uterus and labia Enlargement of breasts
12–13	Growth of testes and scrotum Growth of pubic hair	Onset of menarche Growth of underarm hair
14–16	Voice change, penis growth First ejaculation of semen Growth of hair at underarm and on upper lips	Breasts become bigger Ovaries mature Girl is capable of conception Voice deepens
17–18	Growth of hair on cheeks and growth of hair on body Marked change in voice	

dopamine, a neurotransmitter involved in regulating emotional arousal, pleasure, reward and learning. Psychologists are actively exploring how these brain changes provide a biological basis for the increase in drug abuse, risk-taking, sensation-seeking and aggression displayed by many adolescents.

Cognitive Development

Cognitive skills improve dramatically during adolescence. Among some adolescents, but not all of them, abstract reasoning shows marked improvement. In Piaget's terms, adolescents have reached the formal operational stage during which they can think systematically using abstract concepts. As we have mentioned earlier, Piaget demonstrated the working of the adolescent mind through his well-known pendulum experiment, which has become a landmark in developmental psychology. Adolescents can contemplate on hypothetical issues, ranging from scientific problems to questions about social relationships, political problems, justice, causes of human behavior and even the meaning of life. Many of them can decipher the rules underlying algebra and geometry. There is evidence that adolescents can understand algebra better than adults.

It is assumed that adolescents reach the higher level of thinking and reasoning because of the development of their working memory, which in turn depends on the maturation of the brain. The improved working memory enables the adolescents to process information speedily. They can ignore distracting information, suppress irrelevant responses and keep focused on the problem at hand. But thinking is more than using logic; it must be guided by emotion. This ability is controlled by ventromedial frontal lobes, which are not fully mature in adolescence. This may be the reason why sometimes adolescents appear to lack "common sense." Often adolescent thinking becomes distorted because of certain self-serving bias. They are self-absorbed and think more about their uniqueness and importance than anything else; this phenomenon is often referred to as *adolescent egocentrism*.

David Elkind (1967), who studied several immature characteristics of adolescent thought, believes that such behavior stems from adolescents' inexperienced venture into formal operational thought. According to Elkind, adolescent egocentrism has two components. One is their exaggerated feeling of self-importance and uniqueness called **personal fable**. It is a story in which the adolescents believe that they are stars, and as stars, have extraordinary abilities and privileges. For example, one may say, "My parents can't possibly understand how I really feel," and "Nobody ever felt love as deeply as me." The second is their feeling that they are always "on stage" and that "everybody is going to notice." Elkind calls this oversensitivity to social evaluation, the **imaginary audience**. Adolescents view themselves as actors and everyone else as audience. As a consequence, they become extremely self-conscious and easily embarrassed. The egocentrism and the sense of invulnerability may lead adolescents to engage in risky behaviors, such as reckless driving and unprotected sex, especially when they are under the influence of peer groups. Fortunately, in the majority of cases such things do not happen because they are under the influence of their families when it comes to basic values and goals.

Social, Emotional and Personality Development

Adolescence may be full of storms and stresses because adolescents grapple with several problems when crossing the bridge between childhood and adulthood. Although the period poses several conflicting issues, some adolescents find it to be a positive period of life. As Jeffrey Arnett (1999) puts it, "not all adolescents experience storm and stress, but storm and stress are more likely during adolescence than at other ages." The major concern of adolescents is the **search for identity**, which is the search for an answer to the question, "Who am I?" According to Erikson, the chief task of adolescence is to resolve the crisis of ***identity versus identity confusion*** and to become an unique adult with a coherent sense of self and to play a valued role in society. Search for identity is a pivotal issue in the adolescent's life, and it has been extensively studied by Erikson (1968) in his theory of psychosocial development. The theory covers psychosocial development that occurs throughout the lifespan (from childhood to old age) and it is necessary to have a look at the theory before we proceed further.

Erikson's Theory of Psychosocial Development

Erikson (Fig. 12.6), a renowned psychoanalytically-oriented psychologist, proposed a theory of human development, which passes through eight stages throughout the human lifespan from infancy to old age. The theory is an extension of Freud's psychosexual development with an added emphasis on the influence of society on the developing personality. While Freud thought that childhood experiences permanently shape personality, Erikson contended that personality development was a lifelong process. The first four stages occur during infancy and childhood, the fifth stage during adolescence and the last three stages during adulthood and old age. Erikson believed that personality emerges from a series of conflicts (crises), which if resolved, result in a mature sense of self. These crises occur at each of eight stages of life. Each crisis results in an increased state of either vulnerability or heightened potential for growth, which can lead to either maladjustment or better psychological health respectively. Erikson's eight stages, the crises in each stage and the positive or negative outcome resulting from each of the crises are described below and a summary of the same is given in Table 12.5.

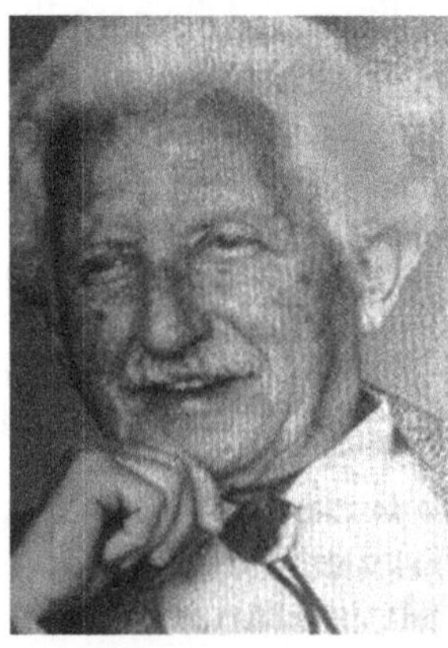

FIGURE 12.6: Erik Erikson

Erikson presented his theory in his book, *Childhood and Society* in 1950. In his later writings, he made some minor changes, but the basic structure of the theory remains the same. The stages he enumerated do not occur in a strict chronological order; each child has its own timetable. Each stage may not be passed through successfully. However, each stage contributes to the formation of the total personality.

Personality develops according to a plan carrying the essential features of the previous stages while entering into the next stage. This is called the ***epigenetic principle***, a term borrowed from embryology. At each stage, the individual faces a crisis or a conflict. If the crisis is resolved successfully, the result will be a positive outcome, a basic strength (also called *ego strength* or ***virtue***); if the crisis is not handled properly, the result is some kind of maladjustment or core *pathology*.

Basic trust versus basic mistrust: Healthy personality must be built upon a strong sense of trust and the sense of trust or mistrust develops during the first year of infants' life. Infants derive security and comfort from a warm relationship with their parents. When the infants are well cared for, treated properly and their needs are satisfied, they interpret

Table 12.5: Summary of Erikson's Psychosocial Stages

Stages	*Approximate age in years*	*Crises (psychological conflict)*	*Virtue (positive development)*	*Pathology (negative development)*
Infancy	First year	Basic trust vs basic mistrust	Hope	Withdrawal
Early childhood	1–2	Autonomy vs shame, doubt	Will	Compulsion
Play age	3–5	Initiative vs guilt	Purpose	Inhibition
School age	6–12	Industry vs inferiority	Competence	Inertia
Adolescence	13–19	Identity vs identity confusion	Fidelity	Repudiation
Early adulthood	20–39	Intimacy vs isolation	Love	Exclusivity
Middle adulthood (middle age)	40–64	Generativity vs stagnation	Care	Rejectivity
Late adulthood (old age)	65 onwards	Integrity vs despair	Wisdom	Disdain

the world as safe, orderly and trustworthy. On the contrary, if their needs are frustrated and they are exposed to cold parental care and rejection, the result is mistrust, which affects later development. Such babies feel insecure, anxious and unsafe. If infants are attended to with love, they trust people, objects and events. The resulting virtue that develops out of basic trust is ***hope***, a belief that they can fulfill their needs. On the other hand, if mistrust predominates, it will lead to ***withdrawal***, a pathological condition in which the child views the world as unfriendly and unpredictable. Wholesome parental attachment is the basis for the development of trust. The critical element in developing trust is sensitive, responsive, consistent care giving by parents.

Autonomy versus shame and doubt: The second and third years are decisive for establishing proper balance between standing on one's own feet and dependency on others and the feeling of being protected. During these years children learn the meaning of self-control without loss of self-esteem; they are now ready to exercise their individuality. They become autonomous. Parental treatment is crucial during this stage. If parents are unduly restrictive or make harsh demands during toilet training, children develop self-doubt and shame; they start doubting their abilities and do not acquire the courage to be independent. The positive outcome at this stage is ***will*** and the pathology is ***compulsion***. Parents who view children's expression of will as normal healthy striving for autonomy, not as stubbornness, can help them learn self-control, contribute to their sense of competence and avoid excessive conflicts.

Initiative versus guilt: During the third stage (4–5 years), children acquire freedom of movement, mastery over language and expanded imagination. They display curiosity, explore the environment and test their world. Preschool children want to do several things. At the same time, they come to realize that some of the things they want to do are approved by elders and some are not. This creates a conflict. If children are given freedom to probe and their queries are answered, they develop a sense of initiative. If they are snubbed or punished, they develop guilt about their needs and suppress their curiosity. The positive outcome, when the crisis is resolved, is the development of ***purpose***; the courage to pursue goals without being unduly inhibited by guilt or fear of punishment. The negative outcome is *inhibition*.

Industry versus inferiority: During the fourth stage (6–11 years), children control their exuberant imagination and settle down to formal education. They develop a sense of industry and learn the rewards of continued hard work. Now they possess a sense of being able to do things well; they want to win recognition by doing things. The virtue that develops during this stage is *competence,* a view of self as capable of mastering skills valued in the society. According to Erikson, a major determinant of self-esteem is children's view of their capacity to do productive work. If the children cannot (or made to feel they cannot) master the tasks they undertake or the tasks set by their parents or teachers, they develop a sense of inferiority. The core pathology that develops because of inferiority is *inertia* or lack of interest in anything.

Identity versus identity confusion: In Erikson's theory, special emphasis is placed on the adolescent period, because this is the time during which the individual is going through a transition from childhood to adulthood. What happens during adolescence will have immense impact on the person's later life. Through his writings about adolescence, Erikson has made terms such as **identity** and **identity crisis** popular in psychological literature. As mentioned earlier, adolescence is the period during which the individuals are in search of their own identity. Erikson uses the term identity crisis to refer to the adolescents' necessity to resolve the transitory failure to form a stable identity. Several factors cause the adolescents make major decisions about their identity. This is the time of life in which adolescents try to define what they are and what they want to be in future. They are not clear about all these things. Faced with immense changes taking place in their body and mind (physical, sexual and cognitive changes), coupled with expectations from elders in the family and peers outside, the individuals experience doubt and uncertainty about their identity. This condition is called *identity confusion.* Those who resolve their personal crises successfully are said to have achieved a sense of identity and those who fail to do so develop a negative identity. Those who resolve their identity crises develop the virtue of *fidelity.* Despite difficulties they face during adolescence, individuals seek an inner knowledge and understanding of themselves and attempt to formulate a set of values. These particular sets of values are what Erikson called fidelity. Fidelity is believed to be the foundation upon which a continuous sense of identity is formed. Those who develop a negative identity think that they possess a set of undesirable traits and project these traits onto others. They start saying, "Others are bad, not me," and such projections may lead to a form of social pathology (repudiation) such as racism, prejudice and crime.

James Marcia Extension of Erikson's Theory

Erikson's views on identity have been extended by James Marcia (1966). His studies of the **identity statuses** of adolescents and young adults yielded four ways in which the identity crises are resolved (in the fields of religion, politics, vocation or sexuality). These are includes the following.

Identity diffusion characterized by an inability to commit oneself and the lack of sense of direction, concern or ideology.

Identity foreclosure in which persons make a commitment only because someone else has made the particular choice for them; these are outer-directed people.

Identity moratorium marked by the desire to make a choice at some time in the future but being unable to do so.

Identity achievement characterized by the ability to commit oneself to choices about identity and maintaining that commitment under all circumstances.

Marcia found that most adolescents are in identity diffusion or foreclosure; they have not yet experienced an identity crisis. But during teen years, they begin to think more deeply about who they are, or reconsider values they have embraced earlier. This leads to an identity crisis and over time, the adolescents successfully resolve it by early adulthood. Latest, researchers have identified various correlates of differences in identity status. Achievement and moratorium subjects showed more cognitive complexity compared to the other two types of people. High identity people were more open, cooperative and more at ease when facing controversial issues. Foreclosure and diffusion subjects tended to be rigid, concrete and impulsive. Foreclosure subjects tended to use antagonism or acquiescence in their interactions as means of protecting themselves from opposite points of view; they also exhibit the closest relationships with parents. Identity diffusion people exhibit the greatest distance from parents. Several other studies have confirmed Marcia's suggestions regarding the development of identity formation.

Identity is not a simple concept; it has several components. These include:

1. Individuals' gender, ethnicity or other attributes by which they define themselves as members of social groups (sons, daughters, students).
2. How people view their personal traits (aggressive, submissive, friendly, shy).
3. People's goals and values relating to family, friends, career and so forth.

Some people achieve a stable identity about some components before others and changing situations may trigger fresh crises and cause them to re-evaluate prior goals and values. Culture influences identity formation. Individuals who grow up in an individualistic culture develop an autonomous self-concept with clear boundaries separating them from others. But people who are brought up in collectivistic cultures develop self-concepts that are based on social relationships. Therefore the question "Who am I?" may have to be answered in ways that reflect an individual's relationship with family members, friends and relatives.

Intimacy versus isolation: During this stage, young adults are capable of forming intimate social relationships. Intimacy is the ability to open oneself to another individual and to form close relationship without loss of self-identity. Young adults seek partnerships and affiliations and are in a position to fulfill commitments and make sacrifices to maintain the relationships. The most important relationship they make now is with a loved one. Young adults require someone to love, to marry and to have sexual relations with and with whom they can share in a trusting relationship. Erikson believed that intimacy goes beyond sexual involvement; it includes the capacity to develop sincere and mutual psychosocial intimacy with friends, and the ability to care for others without losing one's self-identity. The negative outcome during this stage, *exclusivity*, is the development of a sense of isolation, the avoidance of relationships because of one's inability or unwillingness to commit oneself to intimacy. The virtue that develops during this stage is ***love***.

Love is a dominant virtue that is expressed in several forms at various stages of human development. During infancy and childhood, it is the love of parents; during adolescence love manifests as infatuation. Young adults are capable of committing themselves to a mature love relationship with an intimate partner. People during this stage continue to develop their identity by close relationships with others.

Generativity versus stagnation: By now, people are middle aged and they start thinking about the future of their progeny and the society at large. Erikson used the term generativity to refer to an individual's productive and creative responsibility for the next generation; generativity implies an obligation to guide the next generation by passing on desirable social and human values. The transmission of values is a necessity for both the psychosexual and psychosocial aspects of personality enrichment. If generativity is lacking, individuals may stagnate, regress, become impoverished and suffer from a morbid self-concern.

The virtue that develops during this stage is *care*. It is expressed by one's concern for others, through a desire to help those who are in need, and sharing one's knowledge and experience with others. The best way to accomplish this is by child-rearing, teaching, demonstrating and supervising. It is believed that humans have a need to teach and this is achieved by teaching children, adults and even animals. Facts, knowledge, wisdom and logic are preserved throughout the generations because people have a passion to teach and impart information. Caring and teaching are responsible for the survival of culture; this way customs, rituals, mythologies and legends are preserved. During their lifetime, individuals accumulate knowledge and experience about education, vocation, love, style of life and philosophy; these are passed on to the next generation through caring and teaching.

Integrity versus Despair: This is the last stage in the Erikson's theory of development during which the elderly think about the achievements and failures in their life. The older people reflect and review their past and evaluate its meaning. If they feel that they have resolved the crises of the earlier stages successfully, taken care of people and products, they experience integrity. Their accomplishments of the first seven stages make them perceive that they have lived their life meaningfully. Their life appears to have some order and meaning within a larger order. The elderly who feel that they have not achieved positive outcomes in the earlier stages, experience despair, which is an essential counterpart of integrity. They may regret that they have not lived their life in a more fulfilling manner. The feeling that life is meaningless may be aggravated in the face of impending death. Since, the time is now too short to develop alternate forms of living, they may even wish for death. The feeling of despair may give rise to a basic antipathy, *disdain*—the feeling that someone is unworthy of consideration. According to Erikson, the virtue that develops out of the experience of integrity is *wisdom*. He describes wisdom as a detached concern with life in the face of death. People who have reached the stage of wisdom can represent to youngsters a style of life marked by a feeling of wholeness and fullness. The wholeness the elderly people experience may alleviate their feelings of despair, helplessness, and dependence that are common during terminal periods of life.

Although we discussed Erikson's theory of psychosocial development to highlight the concerns of adolescents, especially their search for identity, it should be remembered that the theory encompasses development throughout the lifespan, from infancy to old age. You have to consult this theory when you discuss psychosocial changes during infancy, childhood, adulthood and old age in addition to adolescence.

Relationship with Parents

Popular opinion is that adolescents have "uneasy" relationships with their parents. Research findings are unequivocal in this regard. One report says that adolescents have conflicts with their parents; the *frequency* of the conflicts is greatest during early adolescence, whereas the *intensity* of conflicts is greatest during midadolescence. Conflicts are most frequent between mothers and daughters who are in the early stages of adolescence. Conflicts are found to be severe when there is discord between the father and mother. In a national survey, conducted by the Gallup organization during 1970s, 56 percent of American adolescents reported getting along very well with their parents. Similar findings are reported by studies conducted on Dutch and Chinese adolescents. Even when conflicts were frequent, their intensity was low. Andrew Fuligni (1998) studied 1,341 male and female American students in 6th, 8th and 10th grades coming from immigrant and native families of Mexican, Chinese, Filipino and European ancestry. Among all the four ethnic group adolescents agreed that their parents have a right to make rules on some issues, but older adolescents did not feel that it was appropriate for parents to make the rules.

In another study of 600 teenagers of 7th and 8th grades coming from American, Taiwanese, and Chinese origin, Chuansheng Chen and coworkers (1998) found low conflict between parents and children in each cultural group, but those who exhibited higher levels of conflict showed misconduct (fighting and damaging property) in school. Other studies found a sense of hopelessness and low self-esteem correlating with high conflicts between children and parents. In short, we may conclude that some parents and adolescents do struggle a lot and parent-adolescent conflict is correlated with other signs of distress.

Peer Relationships

Relationship with peers is important in adolescence. It is found that adolescents spend more time with peers than doing almost anything else. They tend to identify more with peers than with any others. This tendency is seen more in North America than Europe and Asia, where everybody including teenagers rally around the family. Generally, adolescents develop intimate friendship and share their concerns with their age mates. Peer relationships also facilitate the process of separating from parents and developing one's own identity. There is also a negative side to peer relationship. Under the influence of the peer group, teenagers may engage in improper behaviors such as absenting from schools, damaging property or disobeying parents. Fortunately, peer pressure is even stronger in helping the adolescents resist the temptation to engage in misdeeds. Although teenagers are influenced by their friends regarding dress, hair style, attitudes toward others, parental influence remains high on issues of politics, religion, morality and career decisions.

Emotional Life of Adolescents

The popular picture of teenagers is that they are moody and troubled. In fact, Anna Freud (1946) not only believed that adolescent "angst" (anxiety) was inevitable, but also that "normal" behavior during adolescence was in itself evidence of deep abnormalities in the individual. A strong reaction to this view soon followed and many psychologists have dismissed this idea as another popular misconception. However, later researches have shown that there is, in fact, a tendency for normal adolescents to have several types of emotional problems.

Adolescents are found to experience mood swings and around mid-teen years about one third of them are seriously depressed. They also experience feelings of nervousness and loneliness. Teenagers are prone to take risks and often exhibit increased levels of delinquency. Hall (1904) wrote that adolescents go through a "period of semi-criminality." They have problems in regulating their emotions and as a consequence, may engage in crimes, reckless driving and unprotected sex. Teenage pregnancy is a serious problem among American youngsters.

Reed Larson and coworkers (2002) made an important study of changes in adolescent emotions using a sequential research design combining both cross-sectional and longitudinal procedures. They studied the emotional states of 328 students of 5th through 8th grades (ages 10–14) and repeated the study 4 years later when the students were in 9th through 12th grades (ages 13–18). They were able to repeat the study on the 220 students who were still living in that area and able to complete the study. According to them, the daily emotional experience of boys and girls became less positive as they move into and through early adolescence and their emotional life leveled off and became stable during late adolescence. Girls at all ages experienced slightly more positive emotions than boys and both sexes showed a similar downward trend between early and late adolescence.

ADULTHOOD

Becoming an adult appears to be an aim for youngsters because they can engage in several activities, which they could not till now. True, you can vote, drink, drive, make independent decisions without consulting your parents, and marry when you have become an adult. But when do you become an adult? In most societies, when one is 18 to 20 years old, he/she is considered an adult. But this is not accepted universally. In fact, your achievement of adult status depends on the cultural group to which you belong. In some societies, an individual becomes an adult immediately after the death of the father. In others, you are considered an adult when you reach puberty or when you are sexually matured, are fit for marriage and capable of reproduction. In some societies, you become an adult just when you marry, irrespective of your age. Sometimes, becoming an adult depends on certain distinct *rites of passage* (initiation rites) associated with sexual maturity such as the ceremonies held when a girl reaches her menarche or during circumcision. Therefore, it is difficult to say when one is an adult.

In an interesting study, Jeffrey Arnett (2001) asked 519 Americans when they have reached adulthood. Among adolescents (average age 16 years), less than fifth reported that they are already adults. Among those whose average age was 24 years, almost half of them said they have reached adulthood. Only those who were around 42 years unanimously said they had attained adulthood. Arnett asked the participants, which are the characteristics that must be taken into account (among 38 characteristics) to be considered an adult. For example, "reaching age 19," "employed full time," or "marriage" was endorsed by 47, 32 and 13 percent of participants respectively. In contrast, irrespective of age, 90 percent endorsed "accept responsibility for the consequences of your actions" as the important characteristic. Becoming a responsible and independent person (individualism) appears to be the single most important criterion of adulthood.

Developmental psychologists study adulthood under three heads: ***early adulthood*** (between 20 and 40 years of age), ***middle adulthood** or **middle age*** (40–65 years) and ***late adulthood** or **old age*** (over 65 years). Surprisingly, researchers were not interested in the study of adulthood for a long time; they concentrated only on childhood and adolescence and occasionally on old age. It is only recently there has been an increase in the study of adulthood. In the following section, important developmental changes during early adulthood, middle age and old age are summarized.

Physical Development

Physical health is at its peak during early adulthood. Legs, arms and several other parts of the body are well developed.

Sensory acuity, reaction time and muscular coordination are at their peak during the mid-20s. They are strong, their reflexes are at their quickest, ill health is an exception, reproductive capacity is at its best and the chances of dying are very slim during this period.

Around the 25th year, body becomes slightly less efficient, but it is not noticeable. After 40, the decline starts in most of the areas. Muscles become weaker, sensory acuities decline and rate of basal metabolism becomes slow. Middle age people put on weight because of their sedentary habits.

There is decreased fertility among middle-aged women due to hormonal changes, especially decrease in the secretion of estrogen and finally they reach menopause, the cessation of menstruation (around age 50). Once, a great deal was written about post-menopausal symptoms. True, some women sometimes experience hot flashes, sudden sensations of heat and slight reduction in the sexual drive. They may also pass through a state of depression. These difficulties are more a reflection of a woman's feeling that she is becoming infertile and expectations of old age. In a society where youthfulness is highly valued, the feeling that one is losing youthful appearance can be really frustrating. Often, these feelings may affect a woman's self-concept and her level of self-esteem. Women's reactions to menopause differ from culture to culture. In some societies, where old age is valued, women welcome menopause. They are happy they do not have to go through the ordeals of childbirth and nursing.

Changes among men during middle age are subtle. There is no such thing as male menopause. Male fertility persists throughout the lifespan, although there is a decline after middle age. There is a decrease in sperm production and the frequency of orgasm comes down.

In spite of these changes, many middle aged people remain generally active and maintain excellent health. It is only during old age, physical changes become more noticeable; bones become brittle, muscular agility is reduced, vision and hearing become poor. But with good food, regular exercise and a positive attitude toward life, many people can remain healthy during old age.

Brain works more efficiently during early adulthood, but like all other parts of the body, brain functions also decline during later years. In one longitudinal study of brain changes among 92 healthy men and women over a 4-year period, Susan Resnick and coworkers (2003) found brain tissue loss at the rate of 5.4 percent per year. The changes in the brain may cause certain cognitive difficulties such as memory loss. Aging is not the only cause of death of neurons, but aging impairs communication among neurons, possibly because of disruption in the functioning of neurotransmitters or because of degradation of white matter, which provides the connections among neurons.

Cognitive Development

The picture of cognitive changes over the life-span is complex. Cognitive and intellectual abilities remain relatively stable throughout adulthood, but signs of slow but steady decline can be easily noticed, especially, around the age of 50 years. Again, this trend is not universal; it occurs in most of the cases, but not among all. The decline is slow in the beginning and increases with advancing age. In some abilities, the decline is more than in others. The reaction time (perceptual speed) declines steadily after the 20th year.

Sensory Abilities

The ability to visually identify and evaluate stimuli gradually decline. In later years, more serious visual difficulties will emerge. More than 50 percent of people above 60 years have cataract (clouding of the lenses in the eye). Hearing impairments are also common among people above 50 years. However, the decline in visual perception has nothing to do with the defective vision; it reflects the changes in the brain functioning. Unlike vision and audition, taste is not affected with advancing age, but the sense of smell declines. When the elderly say that they have lost the sense of taste, they are confusing taste with the smell. They have difficulty noticing if the food has gone bad. In general, the ability to comprehend ideas, objects, events and persons is slower in the late adulthood than in early adulthood.

Memory Changes

It is popularly believed that as one grows older he/she becomes more and more forgetful. True, memory appears to decline with age. But memory comes in many forms and not all of them decline in the same way if they decline at all. Aging affects some aspects of memory more than others. ***Immediate memory span*** (the number of discrete items one can comprehend when presented once) decreases gradually. Memory for recent information (materials learnt just now) is lost sooner than the memory for the items learnt long ago (remote memory). For example, elderly people may recognize the name and the face of a high school friend, but they may not remember the person who they met in the morning today. They can easily remember the phone number of a friend, but they cannot remember the number of the person who called just now. They take relatively more time to accomplish difficult tasks. The harder the task, the larger is the difference in the time taken by young adults and the elderly. For some, this time difference is more, while for others it may just be a second. **Semantic memory** (memory for words, meanings and facts) and **episodic memory** (memory for specific events) remain fairly intact even during late adulthood. Elderly people also exhibit good **implicit memory** at least as well as younger people. Although older people cannot recall, they can recognize information (names, objects, words, etc.) better. **Prospective memory** (ability to remember things to do in future) declines, but it depends on the task. Laboratory studies indicate that performance of elderly is inferior to those of younger ones. But outside the laboratory, the difference becomes insignificant.

Several factors contribute to memory impairment, but the most important one is the changes in the brain. The production of acetylcholine, the neurotransmitter, which is essential for proper functioning of the hippocampus, is impaired. Hippocampus affects the ability to recall. Recall of specific information is believed to depend on the frontal lobes. This area is found to decrease in size with age. The elderly show ***source amnesia*** (forgetting the source of a learned fact) just like patients who have frontal lobe damage. They have difficulties with their **working memory** which is also traced to frontal lobe impairment. Generally, they cannot keep some information in mind when they are doing something else. The other fact that is sometimes observed is ***confabulation***—fabricating information to hide the memory loss.

Intellectual Functions

Early researches indicated that growth of intelligence more or less stops after about the 16th year and starts declining after the 30th year onwards. But later, it was found that there are various types of intelligence and not all of them decline with age. You have learnt that there are two types of intelligence: **fluid intelligence**, which involves flexibility in abstract thinking, reasoning, and problem solving in novel situations, and **crystallized intelligence**, which involves the ability to use accumulated factual knowledge and verbal skills. Crystallized intelligence relies on experience and it is less likely to decline with age. Studies have shown that fluid intelligence begins to decline as early as the late 20s, whereas crystallized intelligence may actually grow with age and decline only during the later years. There are doubts whether the decline of fluid intelligence, as measured by intelligence tests, is the result of aging. It is argued that this fall is a result of different types of experiences faced by different generations. The older people of today may have had less exposure to tasks involving abstract reasoning and scientific problem solving in their school days and that could be the reason why they score low on tests of fluid intelligence.

Older people are considered wise, because they have knowledge and experience, which are used in solving problems. Wisdom is the ability to draw from stored information, which in short is effective use of crystallized intelligence. Senior citizens are highly skilled in telling more interesting, highly informative, better quality stories than younger adults. Laboratory studies show that in certain respects (especially in the use of accumulated facts) older people can reason more logically and consistently than the younger adults. We are grateful to Warner Schaie (1994), an eminent gerontologist and his coworkers for enlightening us on the changes that occur during late adulthood. Schaie's longitudinal studies have shown that most abilities are relatively stable throughout early and middle adulthood and do not show reliable decline until late adulthood. He has also shown that certain special abilities, apart from general intelligence, do not decline with age. He examined the effect of aging on five measures of special abilities including the ability to recognize and understand words and the ability to rotate shapes mentally. It was found that by age 60, about three-fourths of the participants maintained their level of performance from the previous 7 years on at least four of the five abilities tested. It was also found that for a given person, some aspects of intelligence were affected by aging more than others. On the whole, several studies have indicated that fluid intelligence declines at an earlier age than crystallized intelligence.

Age-related intellectual decline (as measured by intelligence tests) is partly the result of lowered perceptual speed, poor memory, and disruption in visual and auditory functions. Therefore, the fall in scores on intelligence tests may be due to the fact that many of them are speed tests (timed tests), which call for quick responses. On the other hand, when power tests (untimed tests) are used, the decline in score is minimal. Is it possible to maintain intellectual efficiency even during late adulthood? Schaie observes that people who have had above average education, are engaged in stimulating activities and have married a spouse, who is more intelligent than they, can maintain their intellectual functions the longest. He has found that spatial and reasoning skills could be improved with training even among people who were 65 to 95-year-old. The important point that is highlighted in several studies seems to be: "**use it or lose it.**" When you are physically fit, exercise regularly and engage in perceptual-motor activities (requiring quick responses), it is possible to retain your cognitive abilities even when you are passing through 70s and 80s.

Cognitive Impairment in Old Age

Gradual loss of cognitive abilities that is associated with abnormal brain deterioration is called dementia, and when this condition occurs in old age (after 65 years), it is known as **senile dementia**. The most common cause of senile dementia is Alzheimer's disease. **Parkinson's disease** and **Huntington's disease** are other common causes. Sometimes, complications arising from high blood pressure and stroke can lead to senile dementia. The first symptom of senile dementia is impairment of memory for recent events. Poor judgment, language problems and deterioration appear gradually or sporadically. People with dementia are distressed, confused and exhibit a lack of inhibition. They may not be able to engage in familiar tasks. There will be physical decline along with cognitive disturbances. Nearly half of those diagnosed with senile dementia show symptoms such as depression, anxiety, agitation, and thought disorders that resemble schizophrenia. In the end, the condition may become so bad that the person will not be able to walk, talk or recognize friends and even the members of the family.

A large Canadian study reports that the overall rate of senile dementia is about 8 percent and a female to male ratio of about two to one. The rate of dementia is estimated to be 2 percent among 65- to 74-year olds, which increases to 11 percent for 75- to 84-year olds and 34 percent for those above 85 and older. Studies in Finland, Germany and the United States report that among adults over the age of 65 who do not suffer from dementia, 20 to 25 percent exhibit mild cognitive impairment. On the whole, expert estimates indicate that 79 percent of 65- to 74-year olds and 45 percent of 85 and older remain cognitively normal. It is also reported that cognitive impairment is not inevitable during old age, and in spite of the decline, people can still accumulate knowledge that leads to wisdom. There are always exceptions; some people who are 80 and above display greater wisdom than many young adults.

Social, Emotional and Personality Development

Psychological development is a continuous process and it becomes more diversified and complex during adulthood. As we have seen earlier, adulthood passes through the last three of Erikson's stages. During young adulthood, an individual develops deep intimate relationships with others or remains isolated. Of course, the former is more common than the latter. To be successful in life, people have to develop cordial relations with several others. The first thing that young adults do is entering into an occupation, where they have to develop working relationships with fellow workers, subordinates and superiors. The second important relationship is with a person one is going to marry and an amicable relationship with parents and other members of the family. If these are not achieved, the individual becomes isolated. In short every adult, as Freud and Adler once said, faces three challenges in life: vocation, love and society. A healthy and mature person is one who has a satisfying vocation, a loving spouse and cordial relations with society.

Career Development

According to Donald Super (1957), a leader in vocational psychology, an individual goes through several stages in his/her vocational development. During childhood and adolescence, individuals enter into the *growth stage* in which they come in contact with some jobs they may like or dislike. Next, they enter into an *exploration **stage*** in which they form tentative ideas about preferred jobs and try to acquire the necessary education and training to get into them. During mid-20s to mid-40s, people enter into *establishment stage*, during which they begin to make their mark. In the beginning, they experiment and may change jobs, at least once. Eventually, they enter into a ***maintenance stage***, when their careers become more stable. Finally, people enter into the ***decline stage*** during which their engagement in their job decreases and eventually they retire. Super considers career development as a continuing process of **self-actualization**.

Work is an important aspect of life. When you ask a person, "What do you want to be when you grow up?" the answer will be in terms of a vocation—"I want to be an engineer, a doctor, nurse, lawyer, or an artist." People are identified by their vocations. We have prepared, educated and trained ourselves to enter some work. Work is more than a source of income; it is tied up with a person's sense of identity, self-image and sense of worth. People are devoted to work and spend most of their time and energy for it. It is also a testing ground for their accumulated information and skills. Jobs are a major source of many lasting friendships. When you have job satisfaction, you are most often contented with your life. On the other hand, when you are not engaged in meaningful work, you feel lonely, depressed, anxious and problem ridden. When you fail to develop a vocational identity, you feel unappreciated or underestimated and your future becomes bleak and life directionless.

Marriage and Family

Marriage is a universal social institution. Most people all over the world marry at some time or the other during their adulthood. Marital satisfaction does not come automatically; one has to work hard to achieve it. Successful marriage is characterized by intimate emotional involvement, positive communication, agreement on basic issues, willingness to care, share, respect and accept the partner. The institution of marriage has changed during the last few decades and the changes have not always been favorable, especially in the light of rapid urbanization and industrialization. It is reported that on average, marital satisfaction declines over the first few years after the marriage. For many couples, marital satisfaction declines within a year or two after the arrival of the first child. In fact, the birth of the first child brings in dramatic changes in the family. Compared to husbands, wives are more likely to resign from their jobs to spend more time in parenting. There is a concomitant feeling that the husband is not helping enough in running the family. Disagreements over the division of labor and parenting add to familial discord. Once a cynic said, "Today, 90 percent of married people are unhappy; the other 10 percent are lying!" This may not be completely true. There are quite a few couples who are still satisfied, just less than what they were in a way, the honeymoon is over.

Despite the stresses and strains of married life, research reports indicate that married people experience greater subjective well-being than unmarried adults. Married people tend to be happier, live longer and have lower rates of diseases, both mental and physical. Although raising children entails stress, it can be construed as one of the best things that could have ever happened in the life of the couple. It is also reported that newly-weds who take advice from other married people, and expect a decline in marital satisfaction over time, may develop a more realistic expectation of married life and take a more active role in maintaining the relationship.

Midlife Crisis

During middle adulthood, individuals are engaged in raising children, establishing in a vocation, providing for the family and contributing to the welfare of society. This is what Erikson called generativity; developing a sense of contributing something to the family, vocation, community and society. When people feel that their activities are trivial, insignificant and inconsequential, they experience the feeling of stagnation, a feeling that they have done nothing important in life, especially for the future generation. Generally, people who have not established an identity during adolescence will also flounder in middle adulthood. Several writers have found some similarities between adolescence and middle age. Just as adolescents are passing from childhood to adulthood, middle aged people are passing from adulthood to old age. They are said to experience a **midlife crisis** during which people face issues such as failing physical stamina, the feeling that time is running out and redefinition of life goals.

Daniel Levinson (1978, 1986) and his coworkers conducted a longitudinal study of 85 men and women and found that many of the participants experienced a turbulent *midlife transition* between the ages of 40 and 45. A commonly held belief is that people in their 40s and 50s, especially women, are likely to experience depression and lack of direction in life when children leave home. This is called **empty nest syndrome** which is disappearing with changing times. There are some researchers who consider the notion of an inevitable, full-blown midlife crisis a myth. In fact, this may be the time for a second honeymoon for couples who have discharged their parental duties successfully. In short, people during middle adulthood, experience some important conflicts, frustrations, and disappointments, but such experiences are common in all stages. There are important problems to solve, tasks to accomplish, goals to achieve, rewards to enjoy, and crises to resolve at all stages.

Changes During Late Adulthood

During late adulthood (old age), people start reviewing and evaluating their past, the type of life they lived, the problems they encountered and the solutions they discovered. If they feel they have resolved the crises of earlier stages successfully, they experience a sense of integrity, a sense of wholeness and fulfillment. On the other hand, if they start regretting that they have not lived their lives satisfactorily, they experience a sense of despair. They experience a feeling of having not achieved positive outcomes in resolving the crises during the earlier stages. An important event during late adulthood is retirement, a reminder that one is growing old. The effect of retirement varies with several factors, such as a person's feelings about the job, physical health and family income. There is often a role change within the family after retirement and increased marital stress after a spouse retires, especially when the other spouse is still in service. Some people seek voluntary retirement so that they may engage in more satisfying work and others are forced to retire for one reason or the other. People who are working or retired voluntarily report higher life satisfaction and better physical and mental health than those who are either forced to work or retire.

Personality Changes

Available evidence suggests that personality does not change substantially during adulthood. Studies using the "Big Five personality" factors—openness to experience, conscientiousness, extraversion, agreeableness and neuroticism—(OCEAN), on thousands of men and women, revealed that personality was stable over time for both men and women. Aging appears to have little effect on personality (Costa & McCrae, 1988). Changes in personality over time do not reflect the changes in the person as much as the changes in the challenges of life a person confronts at the time. All of us face changes in vocation, love and social relations. These changes become less frequent and less severe as a person grows older, which explains why people become increasingly consistent in their personal dealings.

It is also reported that people, as they enter old age, tend to experience a more extended period of positive emotions and less enduring spells of negative emotions than do younger people. Older people are more mature in their emotional expressions; they can regulate emotions better. As people age, they come to value emotionally fulfilling relationships. They interact with less number of people, but with the few they interact, they establish intimate relationships. During earlier years, people spend more time with friends than relatives; with age, this trend is reversed. The elderly spend more time with relatives than friends.

Death and Dying

Humans are mortals. One day we will all die. All that starts must also end. Death is an inevitable biological process. Elisabeth Kübler-Ross, an influential writer, in her well known book *On Death and Dying* (1969), has described five broad stages that terminally ill patients experience.

Denial

At first, people facing impending death refuse to accept that the illness is terminal; even when told that their chances of survival are bleak, they refuse to admit they are going to die.

Anger

Denial gives rise to anger; they are angry at the people around them—those who are in good health, the medical people who were unable to cure their illness, and God.

Bargaining

Anger leads to bargaining. They think of ways of postponing death, may become religious and decide to dedicate their remaining life in the service of religion. They may plead with God to keep them alive till they get their daughter married or till the birth of a grandchild.

Depression

When they realize that bargaining is of no use, people become depressed. Now, they are convinced that their life is coming to an end, and begin to grieve. Kübler-Ross called this state "preparatory grief."

Acceptance

During this final stage, people accept the impending death as a reality. Now, they become uncommunicative and unemotional. They come to terms with death and try to accept it without bitterness.

These stages may not occur in the same order and not all people may experience them in the same way. There are individual differences. Further, participants in Kübler-Ross's study were all suffering from terminal illnesses and they knew they were going to die soon. We do not know how others, who are not suffering from a specific illness, would react to death. Several variables, such as the kind of illness and its causes, the time left before death, gender, age, personality traits of the individuals, the social support available to them from family, friends and relatives, all are found to influence the way people react to death and dying. Limitations apart, Kübler-Ross's pioneering work has spurred great interest in understanding and helping people cope with death.

Concern about our own death apparently does not increase with age. Death anxiety remains the same throughout the lifespan. In fact, some believe that it decreases toward the end of life. Women report death anxiety more frequently than men. Even culture determines reactions toward death. Some invite death with the hope of going to the heaven soon. In some religions, people announce their death in advance and prepare themselves to die by refusing food and water and by not allowing others to talk to them.

We have seen how people may react to death. This is one side of the picture; the other side concerns the effect of death on members of family, friends and relatives. Generally, people experience ***grief***, the emotion of distress that follows the loss of a loved one, and **bereavement**, the experience of missing a loved one and longing for his/her company. American researchers have found that grieving process passes through three stages (at least among people of the United States):

1. During the first three weeks after death, the bereaved person is in a state of shock. He/She feels empty and disoriented and may not believe that the beloved person is dead. Gradually, they pass on to a state of deep sorrow.
2. From 3 weeks to 12 months, the bereaved persons experience emotional upheavals —anger, guilt and loneliness. People may review their relationship with the deceased; wonder whether the death was inevitable, whether they have done all that should have been done and whether they should have done things differently. During this stage, some people may report that they have seen the face or heard the voice of the deceased in a crowd.
3. During the 2nd year, the grief lessens. The bereaved persons may stop thinking of the deceased and start living their life. If it is the death of a wife, the man may think of marrying again; the same is true about women (where widow remarriage is socially accepted). On several occasions, the grief may continue indefinitely; especially in the case of parents who have lost an adult son or daughter. Often the death of a child may make the parents to become close. The objects belonging to the deceased persons, memory of places they visited, the things they were saying and the birth and death anniversaries may contribute to the continuance of grief.

For several years, clinicians believed that the bereaved persons "work through" their loss for purposes of recovering from the loss. Working through the grief involved talking to others about their feelings and gradually forgetting their attachment to the decreased person. Later, it was found that such activities have no effect on alleviating grief. Nowadays clinicians, in fact, recommend suppressing or avoiding negative emotions and maintaining an internal relationship with the departed person. The effect of the death of a person depends on several factors such as the age of the deceased, dependence of the bereaved on the departed person and the nature of the illness the person was suffering from.

Death is an inevitable biological phenomenon. As one grows older, there is a gradual deterioration on all fronts—biological, social and psychological. With advancing age, the blood vessels become smaller in size and the supply of blood and nutrients to the brain decreases. The neurons do not work effectively because they do not receive sufficient blood-borne nutrients and oxygen. Sociologically, the elderly may incorporate negative conceptions of old age prevalent in the society and these stereotypes may reduce their desire to live. There may be decreased social support and lack of opportunities for social interaction, which in turn may result in cognitive degradation. Put together, all these may hasten the desire to die early.

Successful Aging

Despite all the handicaps associated with aging, several people in their 70s report that they have had a satisfying life both physically and psychologically. There are several things that the elderly and the young together can do to make life comfortable. First of all, the elderly should stop worrying about what they have lost and concentrate on what they are left with. They must learn to use the available resources to compensate for the loss of physical energy, memory or fluid intelligence. They do not have to compete with young people in athletics or entrepreneurship. Instead they must focus on more important and meaningful activities such as helping the family, looking after grandchildren, giving tuition, visiting friends and attending social and religious functions.

The elderly must be helped to look at life from a positive angle and to cultivate an optimistic outlook. They must be convinced that they have done all that they could do. Optimism gives them a feeling that they can face the challenges of life and teaches them to live with insurmountable obstacles. The key to successful aging is to do things that matter. They should learn "not to add years to life, but to add life to years." Not surprisingly, material assets and income levels are associated with psychological well-being in late adulthood. A practical advice to the elderly therefore is: "Don't part from your property, bequeath it."

There are several things we can do to make the life of the elderly a bit more tolerable and pleasant. We can talk to them, listen to them and spend some time with them. If the elderly are provided with opportunities for social interactions and to engage in challenging activities, research has shown that the blood supply to the brain improves and the thought processes become more effective. The brain generally becomes smaller in size with age, but among people with more education, the size decrease is found to be less. The *cerebral reserve hypothesis* states that education either strengthens the brain itself or helps people develop multiple strategies. When some part of their brain is damaged, educated people can draw on the reserves from other parts and continue to function reasonably well. The moral therefore is to keep the elderly stimulated and socially active; they will retain a healthy self-concept for some more time and lead a comfortable life. Then, when the death comes they can face it with a sense of stoicism.

Chapter Summary

Developmental psychology is the branch of psychology that is engaged in studying lifespan development. It explores physical, emotional, cognitive, moral and social development of people. The study of human development has been shaped by major issues, such as heredity versus environment (nature versus nurture), continuity versus discontinuity, stability versus change, the universality of developmental sequence, and activity versus passivity. The concept of critical period and imprinting are other intriguing issues of development. Developmental psychology uses different research methods to study developmental processes, most commonly cross-sectional and longitudinal methods. In cross-sectional study, individuals belonging to different age groups or developmental levels are compared at the same point of time. In longitudinal procedure, the same individuals are compared at varying intervals over an extended period of time.

Development passes through several stages. The first is prenatal stage, which consists of three substages: the germinal stage (first 2 weeks) spans the time from fertilization to implantation; during the embryonic stage, from implantation to about the 8th week of pregnancy, major organ systems begin to form; during the fetal stage, from 9th week to birth, the size of the fetus increases and its organ systems mature. The developing fetus faces many risks due to maternal malnutrition and teratogens. Maternal stress, illness, drug use and environmental toxins can cause abnormalities in the fetus.

Infants enter the world with some motor reflexes that may have had survival value among ancestral humans. Most of these reflexes disappear within the first 6 months of life. Physical development in the infant is controlled by the process of maturation.

Maturation is the biological unfolding of the organism according to a genetic program. Shortly after birth, infants are capable of discerning many different stimuli including the mother's odor, face and voice. They can also distinguish between different visual patterns, sounds, odors and tastes. They display primitive perceptual and learning skills. Motor development

Contd...

Contd...

in infancy progresses rapidly through a series of steps from near immobility to coordinated running around by about 18 months of age. Biology and environment jointly steer physical and psychological development.

According to Piaget, cognitive development depends on the processes of assimilation and accommodation. He proposed that children progress at about the same ages through a series of four stages of cognitive development: the sensorimotor, preoperational, concrete operational and formal operational stages. Though Piaget continues to have significant impact on the area of cognitive development, it is now held that cognitive development is more complex and variable than what Piaget believed. Vygotsky for instance proposed that sociocultural factors affect cognitive development. According to Vygotsky, each child has a zone of proximal development, reflecting the difference between what a child can do independently and what the child can do with assistance from others. It is also found that information processing capacities improve with age; older children search for information more systematically, process it more quickly and display better memory.

Children exhibit varied emotional expressions as they age. They employ complex strategies to regulate their emotions. Temperament is a biologically based pattern of reacting emotionally and behaviorally to the environment. It is believed that children differ in their basic temperament and that these differences are at least partially determined by genetic factors. Extreme temperamental styles in infancy and childhood can predict some aspects of behaving in later years. Attachment is the enduring emotional bond that infants and children form with their caregivers. Using a laboratory method for measuring attachment, Mary Ainsworth has classified infants as exhibiting basic attachment styles such as secure type, insecure-avoidant type, and insecure-resistant type. The quality of parenting is an important determiner of children's emotional, social and intellectual development. Baumrind has identified three basic parenting styles: authoritative, authoritarian and permissive styles. Gender identity begins to form early in childhood and socialization influences children's sex-role stereotypes.

Kohlberg proposed an influential theory of moral development, according to which children's moral reasoning proceeds through three stages: preconventional, conventional and postconventional levels. In preconventional level, decisions about right and wrong are made primarily in terms of external consequences, that is based on whether the behavior will lead directly to some reward or punishment. In the conventional level, actions are judged to be right or wrong based on whether they maintain or disrupt social order; that is, based on whether the act conforms to the rules and conventions prevailing in society. In postconventional level, actions are judged on the basis of a personal code of ethics; that is, general and abstract and that may not agree with social norms; that is, one behaves morally not to get a reward or social approval, but to follow some universal ethical principle. The development of moral behavior is closely related to children's cognitive, emotional and social development. There is a criticism that Kohlberg's stages were derived from the study of male participants and they do not apply to women. Men and women are socialized differently and they view morality from different perspectives.

Adolescence, the transition period between childhood and adulthood, has been portrayed as a stressful time. Several thinkers today believe that adolescence is a social construct, a myth and most developing individuals pass through adolescence without any important turmoil. It does not mean that adolescence is completely trouble free and calm. There is bickering and argument in the family. The occurrence of puberty is a major event in adolescence. Sexual maturation occurs during puberty leading to reproductive capability, whether or not adolescents are psychologically prepared for it. Generally, early maturation produces more positive experiences among boys than among girls.

Abstract thinking blossoms and information-processing abilities improve during adolescence; they enter Piaget's stage of formal operations. Adolescent egocentrism, a state of self-absorption, in which adolescents view the world from their own point of view, is another source of strife with parents. They believe that every other person is thinking about them. They may also have an exaggerated sense of uniqueness and perceptions of personal invulnerability (personal fables).

Erikson's theory of psychosocial development is considered a major contribution to developmental psychology. According to the theory, personality development proceeds through eight major psychosocial stages. Each stage involves a major crisis, and how a person resolves it affects his/her ability to meet the challenges of the next stage. During infancy and childhood, children pass through the first four stages—*trust versus mistrust, autonomy versus shame and doubt, initiative versus guilt* and *industry versus inferiority.* Although Erikson's theory applies to all stages of development, it has special relevance to

Contd...

Contd...

adolescents. According to this theory, the major life challenge adolescents face is the development of a sense of ego identity (*identity versus role-confusion*), a coming to terms with the fundamental question: "Who am I?" Until now, teens have not experienced an identity crisis, a serious soul searching and self-examination of issues relating to personal values and direction in life. Now, they face such a crisis. Fortunately, most of them resolve the crisis successfully. Peer pressure is an important influence in the social and emotional development of adolescents. Issues relating to independence come to the fore in the adolescent's social and personality development. These issues often bring adolescents into conflict with their parents and friends. Though there are conflicts, adolescents report that they have good relationships with their parents. In general, the emotional experience of both boys and girls are less positive during early adolescence, but as time passes emotions tend to become positive and remain stable during late adulthood.

Developmental psychologists include under adulthood three stages—early adulthood (20–40 years) middle adulthood (40–65 years), and late adulthood (65 years and after). Important events occur during adulthood. Physically, people will be at the peak of health during early adulthood. Brain functioning undergoes a general decline later in adulthood. Beginning with early adulthood, speed of information processing slows down gradually. But many intellectual abilities do not decline reliably until late adulthood. Wisdom appears to increase steadily from early adolescence through the mid-20s and then levels off through the mid-70s. Major biological changes take place during middle age and old age. An important event occurring during middle-aged women is menopause. Social developmental changes during adulthood are profound. According to Erikson, entry into early adulthood is marked by the crisis of *intimacy versus isolation*. During this stage, people typically enter into a career, get married, have children and raise families. For many couples, satisfaction in married life tends to decline in the years following the birth of children; but surprisingly for many people it is found to increase later in adulthood. With the establishment of career and family, as one enters the middle age, arrives the Erikson's crisis, *generativity versus stagnation*. For some people, this period is marked by soul searching questions about personal identity reminiscent of those faced by adolescents. It is often called "midlife crisis" (or *midadolescence*). But it is reported that most adults do not experience a full-blown midlife crisis. Similarly, most retired people do not become more anxious, depressed or lonely due to retirement.

The final stage in Erikson's theory, *integrity versus despair*, occurs during late adulthood. Older people undertake a life review to find ultimate meaning in their achievements. If successful in this search for meaning, they acquire wisdom; if unsuccessful they experience despair. A number of physical and cognitive changes take place during late adulthood. The skin wrinkles, hair grays and the senses become less acute; there will be a decline in body mass, bone density and physical strength. Several physiological processes, including immune system functioning, decline. There is a decline in psychological functions such as learning, memory and intelligence. Elderly people have difficulty in recalling words and names. But crystallized intelligence remains relatively intact. Negative emotions tend to decline and positive emotions remain fairly stable; still, many elderly people suffer from emotional problems, especially depression.

A few elderly people are prone to suffer from Alzheimer's disease, a form of progressive and irreversible dementia (loss of mental abilities). The disorder is characterized by memory problems, confusion and eventual death. One of the important problems the elderly encounter is to face death. Elisabeth Kübler-Ross described the psychological experience of dying (of people suffering from a terminal disease) in terms of five identifiable stages: denial, bargaining, anger, depression and finally acceptance. However, not all dying people experience these stages, and those who do may experience them in different order. Successful aging is associated with the ability to focus on what is important and meaningful, to maintain a positive outlook and to continue to challenge oneself.

13 CHAPTER
Social Psychology

PREVIEW

Stop for a while; think about the extent to which your thoughts, actions and feelings are influenced by people around you, your father, mother, friends, relatives and even strangers. We are social beings and spend most of our time in the company of others, interacting with them. These others have a powerful influence on our behavior. They determine what we do, how we do and why we do. We dress in a particular way because of others; we walk, sit, talk, work, earn and do several other things in certain ways because of others. Sometimes, we wonder how many things we do for our own sake! not much. Most of what we do is for the sake of others. In short, do not be surprised, we work for the sake of others; we live for the sake of others. Such is the influence of social environment on our behavior. Social psychology is the branch of psychology that studies how people perceive, think about, influence, and relate to others as well as how they are being influenced by others.

Since, we will be interacting with people most of the time, it is essential to know what these people are like and why they behave as they do. We form an impression of the people the moment we meet them. You must have heard about what is called the 'first impression'. Often we say 'the first impression is the best impression'. Is it true? When we see someone, we do not keep quiet. We would like to know what type of person he/she is. We would like to know why he is doing what he is doing. We try to interpret people's behavior and develop certain opinions about these people. How do we engage in these activities? These processes are studied by social psychologists under the headings: impression formation, attribution and attitude formation.

How are we influenced by the presence of others? Why we follow some people and not others? Why sometimes we agree with others even when we know they are wrong? Why do we yield to other's requests even when it is not comfortable to do so? Why do we obey certain orders in spite of our conviction that doing so is wrong? These issues are studied under the titles, social conformity, compliance and obedience. Another fascinating area of social psychology is about establishing social relations. Why do we like some people and not others? What are the factors that make other people attractive to us? Social psychologists will surprise you by their researches in these areas. They have collected evidence to show how familiarity, similarity, proximity and reciprocity lead to your being drawn toward other people. In recent times, social psychologists are trying to unearth the factors underlying the deep and intimate emotional relationship called love. They tell us that love is a complex phenomenon involving intimacy, passion and commitment.

In your profession and in your life, you will come across several varieties of people. It is necessary for you to understand them as accurately as possible. You must be aware of the type of errors you make in understanding people. Remember, your success or failure in life depends on interpersonal relationships; your relationship with your parents, siblings, spouse, friends, relatives and employers. Whether your interpersonal relationships are positive or negative is the crucial determiner of your life-satisfaction. Social psychology is a huge area. This chapter is only a small introduction to the subject. You will profit a great deal if you study extensively the fascinating themes that social psychologists are researching.

Chapter Outline

Human beings are social animals. Rarely one lives alone in this world. Most of the time we live with others: our spouses, children, parents, uncles, relatives, friends and so many others. We spend a large part of our time dealing with these people, understanding them, interacting with them and thinking about them. Ours is a social world; we are born into and live in a social world—a world of people. People around us play a very important role in our lives. They influence our thoughts, behaviors and actions. Our relations with others constitute a very important part of our lives. Our success or failure in life depends on our relationships with "others". At various times and on different occasions, the "others" provide us with some of the satisfying experiences (praise, love, reward and help); on the other hand, there are others who cause painful experiences (rejection, criticism, insult, and irritation). We try to value some people and dislike some others. People influence us and often we engage in influencing others. We often help people in distress; sometimes we do not. We do innumerable things when we are in the company of others, things we would not dream of doing had we been alone. For example, when we are in a crowd, we throw stones at cars; we damage public property and shout slogans.

Since others are important in our lives, we spend a lot of time and energy trying to understand them, thinking about them and trying to get at the basic principles that govern our social behavior with the hope that this knowledge will help us predict people's behavior in our future interactions with them. In doing so, we are often guided by traditional wisdom, the collective knowledge of our society or by what has generally been called 'common sense.' This informal knowledge is quite appealing and appears to be true on the face. Consider the following pairs of statements:

1. a. Birds of the same feather flock together.
   b. Opposites attract.
2. a. Absence makes the heart grow fonder.
   b. Out of sight, out of mind.

We accept each of these statements as true. But, are the pairs not contradictory? So, our age-old wisdom offers no clear-cut answer. Speculation, intuition or intelligent guesses will not help; only science helps us. Accurate and useful information about complex aspects of social thought and social behavior can be obtained only through the application of the basic methods of science. One of the fascinating branches of psychology, social psychology, is trying to do this.

WHAT IS SOCIAL PSYCHOLOGY?

Giving a formal definition of any field of study is a difficult job. It is so with social psychology. It is a complex field covering varied aspects of social thought and behavior, which is changing rapidly. Contemporary social psychology studies a wide variety of topics and with changing times new topics are included; but most social psychologists seem to focus their attention on one central task: Understanding how and why people behave, think and feel as they do in situations involving other individuals. Having this in view, we can define social psychology as the scientific field that studies the manner in which the behavior, feelings, and thoughts of one individual are influenced or determined by the actual, imagined or implied presence of others. In short, social psychology seeks to understand the nature and causes of individual thought and behavior in social situations. An important point in the definition has to be taken note of that the influencing others need not actually be present, their presence may be imagined or implied. Remember; whatever you do and wherever you do it, the others are always present at the back of your mind influencing your behavior and thought. When you are talking to a person over the phone, he/she is not present in front of you, but still the influence is there. You must have witnessed the expressions on the face of a young man or woman who is engaged in telephonic conversation, while walking in the road. When you are writing a letter, the person to whom you are addressing it is not there, but is definitely influencing your letter writing behavior. Imagine for a while how you would have behaved if nobody was around you. But such a situation will never occur. People are always present around you or in some corner of your mind, and are influencing your behavior. Social influence is so pervasive that often we do not take note of it.

In short, social psychology is concerned with understanding the causes and determinants of social thought and social behavior. It is engaged in identifying the factors that shape human feelings, thoughts and behavior in social situations. If psychology studies behavior, social psychology studies behavior in social situations, or simply, social behavior. Social psychologists try to study social thought and behavior through the use of scientific methods. Social thought and behavior are influenced by a wide range of social, environmental, cultural, physiological and cognitive factors. The subject matter of social psychology is vast. Under social thinking it includes areas such as social perception (our understanding of others) and social cognition (what and how we think about people). Under social behavior (how we act in the presence of others), it studies social influence, social relationships, and behavior in groups. Thus, social psychologists are engaged in studying complex processes involved in attribution (how we determine the causes of other's behavior), impression making and impression management, attitudes, stereotypes, prejudice, social influence (how we conform to social forces, comply with social pressures and obey orders from others), social relationships (liking and disliking and intimate relationships), positive social behavior (helping others) and negative social behaviors (aggression, prejudice and discrimination) and related issues. As you can see, all these areas cannot be covered in detail in a single chapter. What follows in the remaining part of this chapter is a brief summary of the important findings of social psychology. The subject of social psychology is a fascinating subject. It is full of surprises that may challenge some of our ideas about people and the relations between them.

SOCIAL PERCEPTION

Social thought is studied under two broad heads: **social perception** (understanding others) and **social cognition** (thinking about people). Social perception (often called person perception) is a central topic of research in social psychology. It refers to the processes involved in our understanding of other people and the social world in general. Social perception and social cognition do not focus on the objective social world, but instead on how we perceive our social world and how we attend to, store, remember and use information about other people and the social world. Be warned. Understanding other people is not easy; people are often puzzling. They say and do things that we do not expect, have motives we do not comprehend, and appear to see the world through eyes very different from our own. But we cannot afford to leave the mystery of other people unresolved because they play a highly important role in our lives. Accordingly, we engage in efforts to understand their motives, intentions and characteristics. On the basis of this knowledge, we try to determine the best ways of interacting with them. The process through which we seek such information is what is known as social perception.

We make use of several sources of information in understanding others. Two of them are important: One is non-verbal cues obtained from people's facial expressions, eye contact, body posture and movements. The other is **attribution**, a complex process in which we observe samples of others' behavior and then attempt to infer causes behind it, using various cues. In addition to non-verbal communication and attribution, social perception is also concerned with attempts to get at a unified impression of other persons. Remember, when we meet a person, especially for the first time, we try to combine diverse information about him/her (appearance, language, and behavior) into a consistent overall impression. You know how important the first impressions are (first impression is the best impression). At the same time, we also try to make a favorable impression on others, a process known as impression management. Therefore, **impression formation** and **impression management** are two important aspects of social perception. Let us discuss these processes—non-verbal communication, attribution, impression formation and impression management—briefly.

Non-verbal Communication

When we want to interact with somebody, we do not do it abruptly. We wait for an opportune moment or condition. You watch carefully his/her current emotional state. For example, suppose you want to ask your father some extra money. You watch his current mental state and wait until he is in a good mood. But how do you know he is in a good mood? One way of knowing people's current feelings, intentions, motives, emotional states, or moods is through their non-verbal behavior. Such behavior is relatively irrepressible; that is, difficult to control. Even when one tries to conceal them, the inner feelings leak out in many ways through non-verbal cues. In a sense, non-verbal behaviors constitute a silent, but eloquent language. For this reason, non-verbal communication has become an important area of research in social perception. Researchers have identified some basic channels of non-verbal communication that transmit information about people's inner emotional and mood states. These are facial expressions, eye contact, body movements, posture and touching.

Facial Expressions

You must have heard of the statement: "The face is the index of the mind". About 2000-years-ago, the Roman orator Cicero stated: "The face is the image of the soul". It means that human feelings and emotions are reflected on the face. Modern research suggests that Cicero was correct in this regard; it is possible to learn about others current emotional states from their facial expressions. It appears that six different basic emotions such as anger, fear, sadness, disgust, happiness and surprise are expressed universally in similar ways on the face from a very early age. Therefore, these emotional states can be recognized. But do facial expressions really reflect underlying emotions? People learn to regulate their facial expressions, so that they smile, frown, or show surprise only in situations defined by their particular culture as appropriate for such expressions. Still, it is true that at least part of the time facial expressions are guides to inner feelings.

Language of the Eyes

Did you not feel uncomfortable when interacting with a person who is wearing dark glasses? This is because you cannot see the person's eyes and are not sure about how he/she is reacting. When poets stated that "eyes are windows to the soul", they were probably right. When a person is gazing at us, it is an indication that he/she likes us. When someone avoids eye contact with us, we may conclude that the person does not like us. He/She is unfriendly, or is shy. If a person gazes at us continuously regardless of our reactions, he/she is said to be ***staring*** at us. Staring is often interpreted as a sign of hostility (remember the phrase ***cold stare***) and we tend to avoid such staring. So, we can infer the emotional states of other people by looking at their eyes.

Body Language

People's current moods are often reflected in the position, posture, gesture and movement of the body. Together, these non-verbal expressions are called '**body language**' and these too give us useful information about the person's inner states. You must have heard of the statements such as: "He was uncomfortable in his seat;" "He greeted us with open arms;" "He adopted a threatening posture". Large number of movements, such as touching, scratching and rubbing reveal an individual's internal conditions. Gait (the manner in which one walks) is also an important source of non-verbal information.

Touching

One of the most intimate non-verbal cues is touching. Touch can suggest affection, sexual interest, caring, dominance or aggression depending upon who touches whom and when. Touch is strongly influenced by social norms and cultural context. Age and gender are important determiners of who touches whom. In Western societies, it was found that men touched women more often than vice versa. In several conservative societies, touching a member of the other sex is almost forbidden.

In short, body language communicates a good deal about others' feelings, reactions and traits and we use them frequently in understanding the people around us.

ATTRIBUTION

Understanding other's current emotional states is only the first step in social perception. But the important thing is to know the other person's stable emotional state, to know what type of person one is and why he acts the way he does. That is, for effective social interaction, we must be able to infer the causes behind the behavior of others. The process through, which we obtain such information is called **attribution**. Formally, we may define attribution as the process through which we seek to identify the causes of people's behavior and obtain knowledge about their stable traits and dispositions. On some occasions, the term is also used to the processes involved in understanding the causes behind our own behavior.

As you might have guessed by now, attribution is based on the observation of the target person's behavior. Suppose your friend does not answer your phone call. Has he lost interest in you? Is he busy in a meeting? Or is something wrong with his phone? What exactly is the cause? Difficult to conclude; is it not? Social psychologists have suggested certain guidelines, which we follow in making attribution. Attribution is a complex process; books have been written about it and several theories are proposed to explain its operation. These theories offer us frameworks for understanding how we try to make sense out of the social world. We shall consider two of the theories, one by Jones and Davis and the other by Kelley.

Theory of Correspondent Inference

The theory of correspondent inference, proposed by Edward Jones and Keith Davis (1965), explains how we use information about other's behavior as a basis for inferring their enduring personality traits. For example, in the example above, why your friend did not answer your phone call? The theory suggests that we accomplish this difficult task by focusing our attention on certain types of behaviors—those that are most likely to be useful. First, we take into consideration only those behaviors, which seem to have been ***freely chosen*** by the person, not those that were forced upon him. Second, we focus on behaviors that produce **non-common effects**—outcomes that can be achieved by one specific act, but not by others. For example, let us say that one of your friends has chosen to marry a man who is good-looking, friendly and profusely rich, has good manners, and comes from a decent family. Why did she agree to marry him? All these are good reasons and anybody would marry such a person. Your friend's decision to marry him does not say anything special about her disposition. On the other hand, suppose she chose to marry one who is very handsome, short-tempered, ill-mannered, and unemployed. Now you can say something about her; she values physical attractiveness more than anything else. So, we can generally learn more about others from actions or decisions on their part that yield non-common effects than from ones that do not. The third factor the theorists suggest is that we pay more attention to actions by others that are low in **social desirability** than to actions that are high on this factor. Social desirability refers to actions one engages in that are in line with social expectations rather than what he wants to say or do? Then, we learn more about others' characteristics from actions they engage in that are somehow out of the ordinary than from actions that are similar to those performed by most other people. For example, suppose a sales girl in a shop packs your things neatly and smiles at you, nothing extraordinary is expressed in her behavior; that is, she is doing what she is expected to do and paid for. But on the other hand, suppose she tells you to go to a nearby shop where the same product is available for a cheaper rate, this behavior will definitely tell you something special about her. Such behavior is not part of her regular duties. Her behavior is characterized by low level of social desirability, which is useful in inferring her personality.

So, according to Jones and Davis's theory of correspondent inference, we are most likely to infer that others' behavior reflects their enduring traits and dispositions when the behavior is ***freely chosen, yields distinctive and non-common effects, and is low in social desirability***.

Kelley's Theory of Causal Attribution

According to Austrian-American psychologist Fritz Heider (1958), our attempts to understand why people behave as they do typically depends on two factors: (1) Whether others' behavior stems from internal or personal causes (their own characteristics, motives) or (2) From external or situational causes (some aspect of the social or physical environment). Personal attributions indicate that people's behavior is caused by their own characteristics (internal causes). For example, suppose one of your friends got a first class in his degree examination. If you think that his success was due to his superior intelligence and hard work, you are making personal attribution (internal causes). On the other hand, if you think that he got a first class because the question papers were easy or the examiners were very liberal, then you are making situational attributions (external causes).

How do we decide whether a behavior is caused by internal or external factors? One of the answers is provided by Harold Kelley (1972). According to Kelley's theory, our attributions are based on three factors: **consistency, distinctiveness** and **consensus**. Consistency refers to the extent to which the person whose behavior we are interested reacts to the stimulus or event in the same manner on different occasions; that is, the extent to which the person's behavior is unvarying over time. Distinctiveness is the extent to which the person reacts to different stimuli or events in the same way. Consistency and distinctiveness should not be confused with each other. Note that consistency refers to similar reactions to a given stimulus or event at different times; distinctiveness refers to similar reactions to different stimuli or events; if an individual reacts in the same way to a large number of stimuli, the distinctiveness is considered low. Consensus refers to the extent to which people react to same stimulus or event in the same way as the person we are considering. The higher the number of people who react in the same manner, the higher is the consensus.

According to Kelley, under conditions in which consensus and distinctiveness are low, but consistency is high, we are likely to attribute another's behavior to internal causes. On the other hand, under conditions in which consensus, consistency and distinctiveness are all high, we are more likely to attribute the person's behavior to external causes. A concrete example may make the theory clearer.

Suppose you are watching a group problem-solving situation in which one member (call him Mr Y) offers a solution to the problem that is being discussed. One of the participants (call him Mr X) opposes the solution vehemently, he is highly critical about the solution and even goes to the extent of ridiculing Mr Y publicly for suggesting such a solution. Now, why did he act that way? Is it because of internal causes or because of external causes? In other words, is he generally a critical or intolerant person or was the solution to the problem really ridiculous? According to Kelley, your attribution (your decision as an outside observer) depends on three factors mentioned above. Let us say the following conditions are present:

1. No other member in the group, apart from Mr X, expressed disagreement with Mr Y's solution (consensus is low).
2. You have seen Mr X behaving in a similar way during other group discussions in response to suggested solutions (consistency is high).
3. You have seen Mr X behaving critically in response to several other different stimuli too (distinctiveness is low).

In this case, Kelley's theory suggests that Mr X behaves critically because of internal causes (personal attribution). He is critical of everything.

Now compare what happens when the following conditions prevail:

1. Several other participants in the group also behaved in the same way at Mr Y's solution (consensus is high).
2. You have seen Mr X behave critically during other group-discussion sessions in response to this kind of solution (consistency is high).
3. You have not seen Mr X behaving critically in other situations (distinctiveness is high).

In this case, you would attribute Mr X's behavior to external causes (situational attribution)—the suggested solution really was a ridiculous one.

Kelley's theory appears reasonable and can be applied to a wide range of social situations. Many different studies have confirmed the assumptions made in the theory and some researchers have also suggested certain modifications to the theory.

Bias in Attribution

On the face of it, attribution appears to be a rational process; that is, we follow orderly cognitive steps in identifying causes for others' behavior. Generally, it is so. However, there are instances in which we commit several types of errors in identifying the causes for others' behavior. These are called 'attributional biases'—tendencies that can lead us into serious errors in inferring the causes for others' behavior. Some such errors are mentioned below.

Fundamental attribution error: There is a strong tendency in us to explain others' actions in terms of internal (personal, dispositional) causes rather than external (situational) causes. Generally, we overestimate the impact of personal factors and underestimate the role of situational factors in explaining other's behavior. This bias is known as the **fundamental attribution error**. For example, when someone spills coffee on your table, you are generally prone to think that he/she is clumsy; you ordinarily do not think that the person did so because the coffee was very hot. Although robust, research evidence suggests that the fundamental attribution error weakens over time. When you have time to reflect on your judgments or are highly motivated to be careful, the fundamental error is reduced.

Actor-observer effect: The second bias, called **actor-observer effect**, refers to the tendency to attribute our own behavior (especially undesirable ones) to external causes and behavior of others to internal causes. For example, when you see someone in the street slips and falls while walking, you say he is careless or his movements are clumsy. But, when you slip and fall, you are prone to say that the ground was uneven, slippery and so on. When someone is driving fast, you say he is very rash and careless. When you do so, you are on an urgent work. Thus, we tend to perceive our own behavior as arising largely from situational factors, but the behavior of others as emanating mainly from their dispositions.

Self-serving bias: The third attribution bias is known as **self-serving bias**, which refers to the tendency to attribute positive outcomes to internal causes, but negative ones to external causes. When you pass your examination in first class, it is due to your hard work. When you fail, it is because the examiner was very strict or the questions were very hard or out of syllabus. The self-serving bias is quite general in its occurrence and powerful in its effects. There is a general tendency to take credit for our accomplishments and explain away our failures. Often, self-serving bias is the cause of much interpersonal friction. It leads people working together in a joint venture to think that "they", not their associates, who have made the major contributions.

Cultural Influence on Attribution

Many studies suggest that there are cultural influences in the operation of the fundamental attribution error. It has been found that Indians generally use more situational (external) attributions than dispositional (internal) attributions because of prevailing social norms and value orientations. Indians emphasize societal obligations more than others do. They tend to believe that society or government owes them their living (Miller, 1984). Americans and Westerners, who emphasize individualism, use more internal (personal) attributions (Triandis, 2001). Asians living in their homeland are less likely to display a self-serving attributional bias than are Americans or other Westerners. Chinese college students take less personal credit for successful social interactions and accept more responsibility for their families than Americans because modesty is highly valued in China's collectivistic culture.

Self-attribution

Up to this point we have talked about attributions we make about the characteristics of other people. But, how do we attribute certain qualities to ourselves? An attempt was made by Daryl Bem (1972) to answer this question in his self-perception theory. According to Bem, we make inferences about the causes of our behavior (self-attribution) in much the same way as we do with other-attribution. Bem suggests that when we want to make inferences (attributions) about our own behavior, we act as observers of that behavior and make attributions much as if we were observing someone else. Even here, we determine whether the behavior is due to some environmental force (external cause) or due to some personal disposition (internal cause). Thus, people come to know about their own intentions only by observing and making inferences from their own behavior. Internal states are inferred by ruling out external forces. Although the processes may be similar, self and other attributions are different in some ways. According to Jones and Nisbett (1971), we tend to see our behavior as controlled more by the situational forces (external causes), while we see the behavior of others as caused more by internal forces (personal disposition)—actor observer effect.

IMPRESSION FORMATION

You are familiar with the statement: "First impression is the best impression". People believe that initial impressions we make of others will determine our future interactions with them. Also, we believe that first impressions are difficult to change. That is the reason why we make elaborate preparations when we want to attend job interviews, marriage interviews and other situations in which we meet people for the first time. Are these common sense assumptions about the nature of first impressions true? Research evidence suggests that to some extent they are true. For example, social psychologist Solomon Asch (1946) conducted a simple experiment in which participants in two different groups were shown one of the following descriptions of an imaginary person:

Intelligent—industrious—impulsive—critical—stubborn—envious
Envious—stubborn—critical—impulsive—industrious—intelligent

Note that the two lists are identical in content except the order in which the adjectives are presented. The first list starts with desirable qualities followed by negative ones and in the second list the opposite is true. The participants who read the first list rated the hypothetical person as more sociable, humorous and happy than those who read the second list. Why did this difference occur? Asch suggests that the impressions we form of others are more strongly affected by information we receive first—a phenomenon called '**primacy effect**'. There is a strong tendency among us to attach more importance to the initial information that we learn about a person, thing or event. In the Asch's experiment, the order in which the adjectives were presented played an important role in that the first words read changed the meaning of the ones that were read later. Having noticed that someone was intelligent and industrious (as given in the first list), the participants interpreted the later, negative adjectives within this favorable framework; that is, the fact that the imaginary person was 'critical'—implied that this person made good use of his intelligence. On the other hand, having learnt that the person is envious and stubborn (as given in the second list), participants interpreted the fact that the imaginary person was intelligent as suggestive of calculating shrewdness.

Kelley (1950) made a more striking demonstration of the primacy effect. He used two groups in an experiment. Both groups were told that they were about to hear a guest lecturer. The members of the first group were told that the lecturer was "a rather a warm person, industrious, critical, practical and determined". The second group was told that he was "a rather cold person—industrious, critical, practical and determined." The simple substitution of the word "cold" for "warm" brought about huge difference in the way the participants perceived the lecturer, even though the lecturer gave the same talk in the same style in each condition. Participants who were told he was "warm" rated him more positively than those who had been told he was "cold".

These primacy effects occur because when once we have some initial information at our disposal, do not bother to pay a lot of attention to additional input. This tendency, to minimize the amount of cognitive work we do while thinking about others, is a strong one and plays a key crucial role in many forms of social thought.

Asch's and Kelley's findings were later researched and elaborated over a decade using more sophisticated methods. Today we have a comprehensive model of impression formation. According to this model, in forming impressions of others, we seem to combine available information about them into a kind of cognitive weighted average. The following factors influence the relative weight, we place on various pieces of information about others.

Source of the input: Information from reliable sources (sources we trust and admire) is weighed more heavily than information from sources we do not trust.

Nature of information: Whether the information is positive or negative; we tend to weigh negative information about others more heavily than positive information, probably because it is more novel and distinctive.

Atypical or extreme nature of behavior: If the behavior is more unusual, it is given more weight.

Primacy factor: We often assign greater weight to information received first than to information received the later.

We are not always influenced by primacy effect. Often primacy effects decrease, especially when we are asked not to make snap judgments, reminded to consider the evidence carefully and made to feel responsible for our judgments. Sometimes we are influenced by **recency effect**—giving greater weight to the most recent information.

IMPRESSION MANAGEMENT

Impression management is the fine art of looking good in the eyes of others. All of us have a strong desire to make a favorable impression on others. For this purpose, we engage in innumerable activities to appear in the most favorable light to others. This process is known as **impression management** and studies have shown that those who can perform it successfully will have several advantages in social interactions. But how do people go about making favorable impressions? Let us see a few tactics people use in impression management.

One of the tactics most people use in impression management is to alter their own appearance in specific ways. For example, people may dress in ways that they believe will be evaluated favorably. Other aspects of personal appearance include hair style, cosmetics and even eyeglasses. These tactics may appear as an exhibition of vanity, but they are not harmful and often have produced good results.

Another important tactic in impression management is "other-enhancement", which includes efforts to induce favorable reactions in target persons by specific actions toward them. One such method is heaping undeserved praise on target persons. Flattery may appear crude and artificial, but it works; people like to be flattered. Expressing agreement with the target persons, appreciating their views, and showing a high degree of interest in them verbally or non-verbally, usually endear you to them. Offering some small, but useful favor works sometimes. There is evidence that ***asking advice*** or ***feedback*** from the target person works wonders in creating a good impression. People feel flattered when you ask for their advice, and no doubt they will form a good opinion about you.

But the important question concerning the impression management is: Does it work? Although there is no definite answer to this question, there is growing evidence that if used with skill and care, the techniques mentioned above can indeed be helpful to the person who uses them.

SOCIAL COGNITION

Social perception and social cognition are two limbs of social thought and it is difficult to differentiate between the two. The differentiation is just academic. There is a good deal of overlap between the two processes. Social perception is about understanding people and social cognition is thinking about people, and as you can see, it is very difficult to distinguish between the two.

Thinking about people and the social world in general is one of life's major activities. We want to understand the people around us, know why they do and say the things they do; we want to make judgments about them, decide whether we like them, trust them, and can work for them and with them. We also like to know whether others like us or not. For doing all these, we must somehow notice, sort, remember and use a great deal of social information. Social cognition thus, refers to the manner in which we notice, interpret, analyze, store, retrieve and later use information about the social world; this is a major area of research in contemporary social psychology. As you can guess, this is a complex process and a large volume of current research focuses on how we think about the social world. In the next few paragraphs, we summarize some of the major processes involved in social cognition.

Mental Shortcuts in Social Cognition

At any given moment, we are bombarded with a huge amount of information about the social world, and it is difficult handle all of it. In order to deal with this so called ***information overload***, people develop certain shortcuts to minimize the cognitive effort. One group of the shortcuts used in social cognition is called **heuristics**. Heuristics are simple decision-making rules people often use to make inferences or draw conclusions about social stimuli quickly and easily. Two of the frequently used heuristics are representativeness and availability. Suppose a person has come to occupy a vacant house in front of yours. He looks very smart, well dressed, owns a costly car, leaves home early in the morning and comes back a bit late in the night. You wonder what he does for a living; a teacher, a businessman, an advocate or an IT professional. You compare him with people in all these professions and finally you conclude that he is an information technology (IT) man. In this case, you are using **representativeness heuristic**. You are using the rule, which states that the more similar the person is to typical members of a given group, the more likely he/she belongs to that group. Often, we judge a person to be an advocate, a physician, a professor or a medical representative using representativeness heuristic.

When you make your judgment based on the ease with which you can recall some information, you are making use of the **availability heuristic**. It refers to the tendency to judge events as more likely to occur when information pertaining to them comes readily to mind. Suppose you are asked to name six people who are friendly with you, you do so easily; under such a condition you rate yourself friendly. On the other hand, suppose you are asked to recall 12 people who are friendly with you, it is a bit difficult. Under such circumstance, your rating of yourself as friendly gets reduced. Several researchers have demonstrated that information, which can be brought to mind readily, is judged to be more frequent than information that is harder to bring to mind. In short, in making social judgments, it is not only that we remember what is important, the ease or difficulty with which we remember it is also crucial. Remember that although we use heuristics to make social judgments, there is no guarantee that these judgments will be correct.

An important tendency in social thought is to assume that others agree with you to a greater extent than they actually do. For example, in one study a group of students was asked to estimate the number of students who smoked. Among them, those who smoked estimated that 51 percent smoked. But the non-smoker's estimate was only 38 percent. This is known as the **false consensus effect**, and it has been observed in many different contexts. It is comforting to think that others are like us and that they share our attitudes. The false consensus effect enhances our self-esteem, so we engage in such thoughts. The effect seems to stem from the availability heuristic. After all, we notice and remember more instances in which people agreed with us than when they disagreed. We choose as friends those who agree with us, and as a result, we are exposed to more instances of agreement than disagreement. But, while the false consensus effect is common, it is not universal. For highly desirable attributes, we would be motivated to think that we are unique and unlike the others; "I'm honest and not many are."

Other Aspects of Social Thought

Our efforts to understand the social world is subject to several biases and tendencies, which together lead us into serious errors.

While resulting in errors, they may also help us in deciphering the world of people. Let us examine some of them.

One of the tendencies in social cognition is that we pay greater attention to information that is inconsistent with our expectation. Suppose one of your young professors suddenly decides to resign from his job and goes to the Himalayas to meditate. This is totally unexpected information; you pay more attention to it and store it in long-term memory. Such information has greater potential to influence your later social judgment. Many research studies have shown that individuals often allocate more attention to actions by others that do not fit with their expectations than to actions that do match such expectations. Again do not generalize the conclusion; there are exceptions.

The second tendency that has been well researched is known as ***automatic vigilance***—a powerful tendency to notice undesirable or negative stimuli or information. In fact, it is said that humans are exquisitely sensitive to negative social information. Suppose your friend—mentions 25 positive traits and one negative quality in a third person, you remember better the negative quality rather than the positive ones. When you read a newspaper, you notice the news about theft, murder, suicide, rape and ragging more easily than other positive items such as art, music, religion or science.

A third important principle in social cognition is that we are skeptical about information, which is inconsistent with our initial preferences, but quite open to information that supports our views. That is, we examine information that supports our preferred conclusions much less carefully (and less skeptically) than information that is inconsistent with our preferred conclusions. This tendency is known as ***motivated skepticism***. We require relatively little supporting evidence to arrive at the conclusions we want to reach, but a great deal of disconfirming information to arrive at conclusions opposite to our initial inclinations. When someone tells you that your friend is a likable person, you do not have to scrutinize the statement; you know your friend is nice. It is your initial view, and you accept the statement without examining it. On the other hand, if your friend is referred to as unreliable, you examine the statement more carefully. You need more information before you conclude that he is unreliable because this is contrary to your earlier view.

The processes mentioned above—heuristics, automatic vigilance, motivated skepticism—can be seen as efforts that help keep our cognitive effort at a minimum. We do not want to think too much; too much thinking may be counterproductive and at times get us into serious cognitive complications. Although the statement looks strange, research evidence suggests that thinking too much about what we are doing can be greatly disruptive and may interfere with our judgments and conclusions.

One important finding of research on social cognition is about a mental structure known as **schema**. As you know schemas are organized patterns of thoughts, beliefs and feelings we acquire through experience about some aspect of the social world. Schemas exert powerful influence on what aspects of the social world we attend to, learn, remember and use in our interactions. They play a key role in understanding others, ourselves and the social world. Individuals in various cultures develop different cultural schemas relating to various activities and relationships. As a result, their schemas for important social roles (familial roles, friendship, religious activities and courtship), may differ greatly.

ATTITUDES: YOUR FEELING AND BEHAVIOR TOWARD SOCIAL OBJECTS

Study of attitudes has long been a central activity in social psychology. Since attitudes determine our social thought and social behavior, a great deal of theorizing and research has been and is in progress in this area. Although psychologists are not agreed upon a comprehensive definition of attitude, for our purpose, it can be defined as a learned predisposition to respond favorably or unfavorably toward persons, objects, events, issues, abstract concepts or ideas. People hold attitudes toward a wide array of objects— democracy, communism, political party, nuclear policy, foreign aid, reservation policy, sex, marriage, divorce, feminism, abortion, music, art, literature, capital punishment and what not. Anything that arouses evaluative feelings qualifies as an object of attitudes.

Social psychologists talk about an **ABC Model of attitude** to suggest that an attitude has three components, namely affect, behavior, and cognition. Affect (A) implies that we hold positive (like) or negative (dislike) feeling toward the attitude object. The behavior (B) component indicates that we have a tendency or intention to act in a particular manner relevant to our attitude. The cognitive (C) component refers to our thoughts, beliefs or opinions about the attitude object. Every attitude has these three dimensions although they vary in terms of which element predominates and the nature of their interrelationship. Suppose you like a particular physician (favorable affect); you know he is efficient, humane and easily accessible (cognition); naturally, you will have an inclination to consult him (behavior tendency). So, we tend to approach, seek out or be associated with things we like; we avoid, shun, or reject things we do not like. Thus, attitudes are simply expressions of how much we like or dislike various things in the social environment. They represent our evaluations (preferences) toward a wide range of attitude objects. The defining characteristic of attitudes is that they express an evaluation of some object. Evaluations may be positive or negative, pro or anti, liking or disliking, favoring or not favoring.

Attitudes are individual expressions representing a summary of evaluations of an attitude object. The expression that one makes publicly may not always be the same as the expressions one does privately to oneself. The relationship between attitudes and behavior is highly controversial.

Attitudes play an important role in how we process information and remember events in our social world. Our attitudes affect how we set our goals and how we interpret the barriers we encounter, while trying to reach the goals. Attitudes guide us as we selectively evaluate information; information that is contrary to our attitudes may be considered unconvincing and we may even try to disprove it. For example, suppose one of your classmates is from the lower socioeconomic strata. If you think that people belonging to that group do not perform well in class, you are prone to think that your classmate will not do well. You look for some evidence of poor performance. You may not notice your friend's well-performed tasks and if notice them, you make up reasons that discount or discredit his/her abilities.

Forming Attitudes

People are not born with well-defined attitudes toward any particular object. Attitudes are acquired or learned. They are learned in the same way as other behaviors are learned. The general theories of learning, such as classical conditioning, operant conditioning and social learning (modeling), explain the acquisition of attitudes as well as they explain acquisition of other forms of behavior.

You have learnt in the chapter on learning that when a neutral stimulus is paired with an unconditioned stimulus several times, the neutral stimulus may begin to elicit a response similar to the one produced by the unconditioned stimulus, a process called classical or Pavlovian conditioning. The same principles hold good in learning of attitudes. Objects, people or events associated with pleasant feelings come to be liked (favorably evaluated), while those associated with unpleasant experiences come to be evaluated unfavorably. Suppose you attended a rally that became violent and you were hurt in the melee; this experience may affect your attitude toward public meetings in general and you may even develop an unfavorable attitude toward high-risk journalism as a profession.

Now, consider how operant learning works in developing attitudes. Suppose you smile at a new comer to your class and she responds with a pleasant smile. Your behavior is positively reinforced. If this happens often, you develop a favorable attitude toward her. On the other hand, if she ignores your greeting, you may think she is a snob and thus develop an unfavorable attitude toward her. When parents reward their children with smiles, agreement or approval when they make a 'right' statement about 'something,' the children develop a liking for that 'something.' This occurs even before the children know much about that 'something.' For example, a child may develop a positive-attitude toward his religion even before he understands what religion means. Thus, parents and elders play an active role in shaping children's attitudes.

A third process through which attitudes are formed can operate even when parents have no desire to transmit specific views to their children. This involves what is called *observational learning* or *modeling*, in which children acquire new forms of social behavior (attitudes) merely through observing the actions of others. For example, a child may learn to go to *pooja* room and prostrate before the idol even before she knows what God or *pooja* is all about. The children do as their parents do. You must have seen young children playing "papa-mama" game. They are simply imitating their parents. In this way, children develop attitudes toward religion, politics, racial discrimination and several other objects by simply modeling their parents.

Often, we develop attitudes through direct personal experience. You may develop liking for classical music just by hearing someone singing. Similarly, you may develop a favorable attitude toward a specific food by eating it once. Research findings indicate that attitudes formed through direct experience are held strongly and they tend to remain stronger than the ones acquired through observing others or other forms of learning. Therefore, if you hold strong attitudes about some aspects of the social world and want someone else to share them, you should arrange for this person to have direct experience with the attitude object.

Is there an inborn tendency to acquire certain attitudes? As you might have guessed, it does not appear so. But some research studies have shown that we may inherit attitudes just as we inherit some of our physical characteristics. The evidence for such a conclusion comes from twin studies. Identical twins exhibit similar attitudes more than fraternal twins. Even identical twins that were reared in different environments exhibit similarity in their attitudes, indicating that there is a genetic influence on attitude formation. But several other researchers doubt the veracity of such findings because of certain defects in the methods used in the study of twins. Until further research supports the genetic theory of attitude formation, we may have to be skeptical about the conclusions.

Influence of Attitudes on Behavior

One of the hotly debated issues in social psychology is the relationship between attitudes and behavior. The basic question here is: Do attitudes guide behavior? Can we predict a person's behavior by knowing his/her attitude? A study of the attitude-behavior relationship by LaPiere in the 1930s showed that the relationship was extremely discrepant; people say one thing and do another. LaPiere (1934) toured the United States with a young Chinese couple and stopped at more than 250 hotels. He and his friends were refused service only once. Several months later, LaPiere asked these hotel-keepers whether they would serve Chinese customers. 92 percent reported that they would not (remember it was in 1934, a time when racial and ethnic prejudice was prevalent in the US). Another study (DeFleur and Westie, 1958) found a consistent relationship between attitudes and behavior. Wicker (1969) reviewed all the available evidence at that time on the attitude-behavior link and came to the conclusion that *attitudes and behavior are at best only weakly related and often there is virtually no relation between them*. In spite of the difficulty in supporting a predictive link between attitudes and behavior, the belief in such a link persists. It appears that the relationship between attitude and behavior is far more complex than common sense would suggest. Several researchers insist that the relationship must be there and we need sophisticated research methods to demonstrate it.

Today, it is widely held that several factors determine the attitude-behavior relationship and unless you take all of them into consideration, the relationship may not be apparent. In general, an attitude is more likely to affect behavior when it is strong, important, relatively stable and directly relevant to the behavior, and when it is remembered easily (Eagly and Chaiken, 1995). Attitudes influence behavior more strongly when situational factors that contradict our attitudes are weak. According to the theory of planned behavior (Ajzen, 1991), our intention to engage in a behavior is the strongest when we have a positive attitude toward that behavior, when subjective norms (our perceptions of what other people think we should do) support our attitudes, and when we believe that the behavior is under our control. White, Hogg and Terry (2002) report that there would be increased attitude-behavior consistency when people consciously think about or are reminded of their attitudes before acting. It is also seen that general attitudes best predict general classes of behavior and specific attitudes best predict specific behaviors.

Influence of Behavior on Attitudes

The attitude-behavior relationship is not a one-way affair. Just as attitudes influence behavior, the behavior can also influence attitudes. Often we develop attitudes that are consistent with how we behave. This phenomenon was demonstrated by Festinger and Carlsmith (1959) in a famous experiment. Since, the study relates to an important theory called **cognitive dissonance** propounded by Festinger (1957), let us examine the theory in some detail.

Theory of Cognitive Dissonance

Cognitive dissonance refers to an uncomfortable state of heightened tension that arises when individuals notice inconsistency between two or more of their attitudes, or between their attitudes and behavior. For example, a smoker who knows that smoking leads to lung cancer holds two contradictory cognitions:

1. I smoke.
2. Smoking leads to lung cancer.

Festinger's **cognitive dissonance theory** predicts that these two thoughts will lead to an uncomfortable state of mind (dissonance). More importantly, the theory predicts that the individual will be motivated to reduce such dissonance in one of the following ways:

1. Modifying one or both cognitions mentioned above.
2. Changing the perceived importance of one of the cognitions.
3. Adding new cognition or information.
4. Denying the relationship between the two cognitions.

Now, the smoker might think that, after all, he does not smoke that much (modifying the cognition); that the evidence linking smoking to lung cancer is weak (changing the importance of a cognition); that the amount of exercise he does compensates for the smoking (adding new cognition); or that there is no strong research evidence linking smoking and cancer (denial). Whatever the technique employed, the result is the same: reduction in dissonance. But what is the preferred technique? Obviously, one that involves least effort (the path of least resistance), changing whatever is easiest to change. Since, it requires effort to change cognitions, to acquire new information, or to minimize the importance of outcomes that are really important, people resort to the easiest course: *changing their attitudes.*

There are several instances in everyday life when you have to say and do things that are inconsistent with your attitudes (counterattitudinal behavior). Let us say that your boss presents an important plan of action in a meeting and asks you for your opinion about its feasibility. The proposal, in your opinion, has serious problems and cannot be implemented. Your boss is a strong and opinionated person and does not tolerate dissent. In fact, he has terminated one of his subordinates for disagreeing with him. Now, what would you do? In all probability, you will praise his proposal because you want to be in good terms with him. Now, your attitude and behavior are inconsistent and you experience dissonance. But still you say your boss's proposal is wonderful. Psychologists call this phenomenon ***forced compliance***. You are forced by circumstances to say or do things contrary to your real views. The effect of forced compliance is a fact of life and you must have experienced the condition on several occasions. When people say or do things they do not believe, they often experience a need to change their attitudes to be in line with the actions. But the important question here is: How strong are the reasons for engaging in counterattitudinal actions? If the reasons are very strong, no dissonance occurs. You have a strong reason to praise your boss's proposal (you do not want to lose your job!). But what if strong and convincing reasons for engaging in such actions are absent? Under such conditions, dissonance will be stronger; you have said something you do not believe even though you had no strong reason for doing so. In this context, dissonance theory makes an unexpected prediction: "the weaker the reasons for engaging in counterattitudinal behavior, the stronger the dissonance-generated and hence greater the pressure to change these views". This paradoxical prediction is called the ***less-leads-to-more effect***. It is to confirm this proposition that Festinger and Carlsmith conducted the experiment referred to above.

In the experiment, participants were offered a small reward (1 dollar) or a large one (20 dollars, a lot of money in those days) for telling another person that some repetitive, boring tasks they had just performed were very interesting (one of the tasks consisted of placing spools on a tray, dumping them out and repeating the process over and over again). After engaging in this attitude-discrepant behavior (telling another person that the tasks were quite interesting when they knew fully well that they were not), participants were asked to indicate their own liking for the tasks. Surprisingly, participants reported greater liking for the boring tasks when they had received a smaller reward than when they had received the large one, thus supporting the "less-leads-to-more" effect. Probably, this is how it happened: the participants who were paid less could not have justified reporting that they enjoyed the task for that amount. To reduce the dissonance between what they did and what they received, they appear to have convinced themselves, unconsciously, that they really did enjoy the task so much that they were willing to say that they enjoyed it even though the reimbursement was very small. The participants who were paid more felt no such compulsion; the money they received, they apparently felt, adequately compensated them for telling someone that they liked the task. For these participants, there was no dissonance to be resolved. (You must have seen eminent film actors in television advertisements making claims that they themselves do not believe. For doing this, they are paid an enormous amount of money; therefore they do not experience any dissonance).

In general, researchers have shown that the less reason there is to engage in a behavior that is counter to an attitude, the stronger the dissonance. Cognitive dissonance does not occur with every inconsistency; it is only experienced by people who believe that they have a choice and that they are responsible for their course of action and thus for any negative-consequence. So, note that less-leads-to-more effect operates only under certain conditions. Also other interpretations have been offered for the occurrence of dissonance. We need not review all of them here. For the time being, we can assume that, generally, dissonance derives from and centers on the effects of inconsistency. That is, when people discover that their various attitudes and behaviors do not fit neatly together, they experience considerable pressure for change. And one of the important things that may give way in such contexts is their attitude. In short, very often, behavior can be said to cause change in attitudes.

Changing Attitudes

As you may have guessed, attitudes are important components of your personality. They determine how you feel about and behave toward people, events and objects in the social world. Some attitudes are desirable, but some of them may be undesirable. Desirable attitudes are to be cultivated and undesirable ones may have to be changed. Whether you know or not, several people around you are attempting to change your attitudes. Then, the question arises: Can attitudes be changed? What factors operate in changing attitudes? A great deal of work has been done in the area of attitude change. Let us see what social psychologists say about attitude change.

Persuasion

Stop for a while, think of the number of people who are trying to change your attitudes. When you are walking in the road, someone gives a leaflet about an event, a new product or a political candidate. He/She is trying to influence you to do something; attend a meeting, purchase a product or vote for the candidate. He is changing your attitude. The newspapers, radio, Television, political speeches and religious discourses are all asking you to do something; all these are attempts to change your attitude. These efforts to change your attitudes are called ***persuasion***. To what extent are such attempts at persuasion successful? What factors determine whether these attempts succeed or not? One of the earliest attempts to study the factors that facilitate persuasion was made by Hovland, Janis and Kelley (1953). They thought that persuasion concerns with *who* says *what* to *whom*. Thus, according to them, persuasion involves three factors:

1. The ***source (who).***
2. The ***message (what).***
3. The ***audience (whom).***

This approach is often called 'Yale model' and the findings of this approach are highly complex and often inconsistent. Let us examine some of their major findings.

Source

The source refers to the origin of the message; it may come from a person (your professor), or a group (your club), or an institution (Supreme court); all these can be grouped together under the general head; communicator. Various characteristics of the source can affect the impact of the message. One important characteristic is the credibility of the source (***communicator credibility***)—how believable is the source of the message. Credibility has two major components: ***expertise*** and ***trustworthiness***. Expertise refers to special knowledge and skills. We judge expertise by whether or not we think the communicator knows what he/she is talking about. Trustworthiness revolves around the truthfulness of the communicator. Trustworthiness is judged by three factors, whether the communicator:

1. Has any special interest in persuading us.
2. The communicator has been consistent in past expressions of attitudes.
3. The communicator has usually been objective.

In general, research has shown that messages attributed to highly credible communicators are more persuasive than are those attributed to communicators with low credibility. We are likely to perceive communicators to be trustworthy when they advocate a point of view that is contrary to their own self-interest. Further it has been found that communicators who are physically attractive, likable and similar to us are more persuasive than others. That is why advertisers spend lots of money to hire attractive, likable celebrities to promote their products.

Message

The message refers to what the communicator is saying—the content of the message. Messages that do not appear to be designed to change our attitudes are often more effective than the ones that seem intended to manipulate us. That is, we usually do not trust the people who are deliberately trying to change our opinion. Generally, people refuse to be influenced by others. It has been found that messages that arouse strong emotions, especially fear, are more effective persuaders. Fear arousal seems to work best when the message evokes moderately strong fear and also provides people with effective, feasible ways to reduce the threat. High fear messages accompanied by inadequate information about "what to do" typically lead to denial. In trying to persuade someone, is it good to present only your side of the issue, or also present the opponent's point of views and then refute them? Research indicates that the two-sided refutational approach is most effective. When the target person initially disagrees with the communicator's point of view or is aware that there are two sides to the issue, a two-sided message will be perceived as less biased. A one-sided approach is most effective when people are either neutral or already favorable to the message; a two-sided message is more likely to win converts from an opposing point of view.

Audience

The audience refers to the receiver of the message. Whether the message influences the receiver depends on certain characteristics of the receiver. One of the factors is the extent to which the receiver's attitude was already in the advocated direction. For example, we have seen earlier that one-sided message was more effective with those who favored the advocated position, while the two-sided message was more effective with those who were initially opposed to the advocated position. People are more susceptible to persuasion when they are distracted by some extraneous event than when they are paying full attention to the message. This may be one of the reasons why political leaders arrange for some spontaneous demonstrations when they are speaking. The distraction often makes the audience accept the speaker's point of view. Janis found that people, who lack self-confidence, and those with low self-esteem, are generally susceptible to persuasion. Messages loaded with logical arguments and facts are highly persuasive with some people, but not with others. There are some who enjoy analyzing the issues and many others do not. This is because people differ with regard to their need for cognition.

Cognitive Approach to Persuasion

The Yale model provides a wealth of information about *when* and *how* persuasion occurs, but not much about why it succeeds. The model does not tell us why people change their attitudes in response to persuasive messages. This issue is being tackled by a modern approach called the **cognitive perspective**, proposed by Petty and Cacioppo (1986). The cognitive perspective does not ask: *Who says what to whom and with what effect?* It asks: *What cognitive processes operate when someone is persuaded?* The focus is on ***cognitive response analysis***, which tries to understand what people think about when they are exposed to persuasive messages and how these thoughts determine whether and to what extent, people experience the need to change their attitude.

Petty and Cacioppo have called their approach **elaboration likelihood model (ELM)** according to which there are two routes to persuasion: central and peripheral. You are taking the **central route** when you pay close attention to the content of the message and carefully examine it; you are influenced by the appeal because you find it to be convincing. The **peripheral route** to persuasion occurs when you do not scrutinize the message, but are influenced by factors such as speaker's attractiveness, the message's emotional appeal, or simply because of the speed with which a person speaks (fast speakers are generally more persuasive than slow speakers). Often, a favorable attitude change can result from simply becoming familiar with something—it is called **mere exposure effect**. Attitude change that results from the central route tends to last longer and predict behavior more successfully than change that results from peripheral route.

People who have a high need for cognition generally follow central route and people with low need for cognition follow the peripheral route. For example, when forming an attitude toward a bank in which you want to open an account, if you think carefully about its customer service in detail, you are following central route. In contrast, if you are influenced by the building or the smart dress of the bank employees, you are taking the peripheral route.

Reciprocity of Persuasion

Attitude change is a two-way process; reciprocity may play a major role in persuasion. That is, we tend to change our attitudes in response to persuasion from others who have previously changed their views in response to our own efforts at persuasion. This is not surprising. In social behavior, reciprocity is the guiding norm. Generally, we like others who like us, help others who help us and fight with others who threaten us. Similarly, the tendency to reciprocate the treatment we have received from others plays a role in persuasion, just as it does in many other forms of social behavior and thought. The greater the extent to which others have yielded to our efforts at persuasion, the greater will be our tendency to yield to others. This may involve shifts in our private attitudes as well as in our publicly stated views.

Resistance to Persuasion

As we said earlier, people are exposed to innumerable number of persuasive messages from various sources every minute in their lives. Suppose they yield to all of them; what would happen? Their views would change from day to day and hour to hour making behavior awfully inconsistent. Fortunately this does not happen, because humans have a capacity to resist persuasions in spite of their charm and charisma. Human behavior remains stable because of several factors. We mention below some of them.

Strength of the attitude: When our attitude is strong about an issue, we are less likely to be persuaded. In fact, it is said that some attitudes, such as the one toward capital punishment (death penalty), are inherited.

Reactance: Reactance is the negative reaction we experience, when we know that someone is bent upon changing our attitude and behavior. Research findings indicate that under such situations we change our attitudes in the opposite direction, a response known as ***negative attitude change***.

Forewarning: When we know in advance that someone is trying to change our attitude, we are less likely to be persuaded. This phenomenon is not universal.

Selective avoidance: This refers to our tendency to direct our attention away from information that challenges our existing attitudes. We may do this by simply bypassing the attempts to persuade us. This is exactly what you do when an advertisement comes on your TV screen—changing channels.

In short, the operation of reactance, forewarning, selective avoidance and of course, the strength of attitude help us in resisting persuasion. It does not mean that attitude change does not occur at all. To say so would mean that all forms of advertisements, propaganda, and political campaign are useless. But it is also true that we are not helpless pawns in the hands of persuaders.

SOCIAL INFLUENCE

Social influence refers to the efforts on the part of one person to change the attitudes or behavior of one or more others. Social influence comes in many forms, some obvious and others subtle. Every day we try to influence others and at the same time we are influenced by others. We have discussed until now one form of social influence, persuasion. There are several other forms of social influence: we go along with others—we behave in the same manner as others in a group or society (conformity); we yield to the request of others (compliance); we obey the orders of some others (obedience). We exhibit all these forms of behavior irrespective of whether we like them or not; we are simply being influenced by others to do something. In this section, we examine these three forms of social influence: **conformity**, **compliance** and **obedience**. We start with conformity.

Conformity

As social beings, we have a strong desire to go along with others—following what others do and fit in with other people around us. This is **conformity** behavior, which can be defined as a change in behavior or attitude brought about by a desire to follow the beliefs or standards of other people. The pressures toward conformity stem from explicit or implicit rules laid by a society called **social norms**—rules that indicate how we should think, feel and behave in specific social situations. For example, we stand up when the teacher enters the classroom and when the national anthem is played. We do not stand very close to strangers; we follow a queue, while purchasing tickets at a movie theater, bus stand or railway station; we leave a tip to the waiter in a restaurant; so on and so forth. Most of us obey social norms most of the time. At first glance, the conformity pressures may appear objectionable to you because they prevent you from doing "what you want to do". But, imagine what would happen when there are no conformity rules and each of us do things in our own way. There would be social chaos.

Asch's Studies of Conformity

Conformity as a social process has been studied extensively by social psychologists for more than fifty years. The research in this field started in the 1950s with an outstanding study conducted by Solomon Asch (1951). In one of his unique researches, Asch asked participants to respond to a series of very simple visual problems. They were shown one card (B) with three lines of varying length and another card (A) that had one line that was equal in length to one of the three lines in the other card (Figs 13.1A and B). The task was seemingly simple and straightforward; the participants had to announce aloud, which of the three lines in the (B) card was identical in length to the standard line in the (A) card. The correct answer was always obvious, the task seemed easy to the participants. All the participants gave correct answers in the first few trials. Now, something odd was introduced in the experiment. Participants, were made to sit along with some others while giving their judgments. These others (6 to 8) were confederates (accomplices) of the experimenter who were coached to give wrong answers most of the time. This was not known to the real participants. The real participant sat in the end by the side of the last confederate (Figs 13.2A to C). The confederates gave the answers aloud before the real participant responded. Remember the confederates gave wrong answers and did so unanimously. For example, they said the standard line was equal to the third line, which was actually shorter than the standard. Now, what would you expect the real participant to say in such a situation? Should he go along with others, or stick to his own judgment? Surprisingly, a large majority of real participants in Asch's study opted for conformity and agreed with the confederates. Strange as it may appear, 76 percent of those tested went along with the confederates' wrong answer at least once. In contrast, only 5 percent of the subjects who were tested in the absence of any confederates made such mistakes.

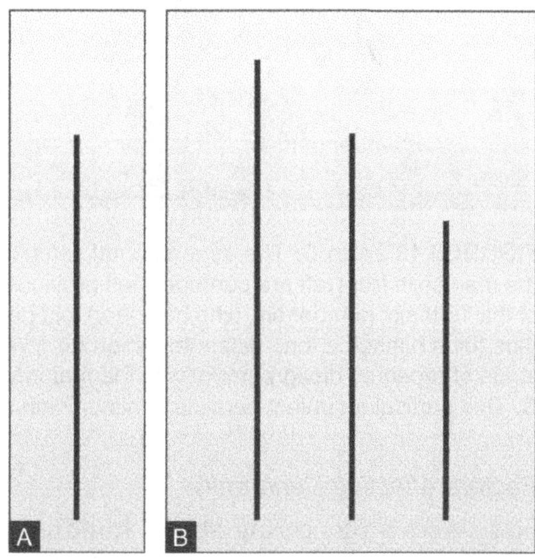

FIGURES 13.1A and B: Asch's conformity experiment. **A.** Standard line; **B.** Comparison lines.

Although most participants conformed at least once, there were a few who resisted such influence on many other occasions. Almost 24 percent never conformed and several others yielded on only a few of the trials on which the confederates gave wrong answers. Yet, a large majority did conform to the confederates' wrong answers at least part of the time. These results and the findings of the later studies point to an unsettling conclusion in social psychology: ***Many people find it easier to publicly contradict the evidence of their own senses than to disagree openly with the unanimous judgments of other persons—even those of total strangers.***

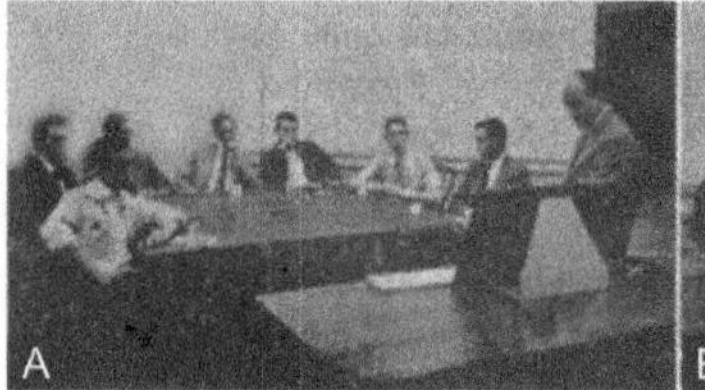

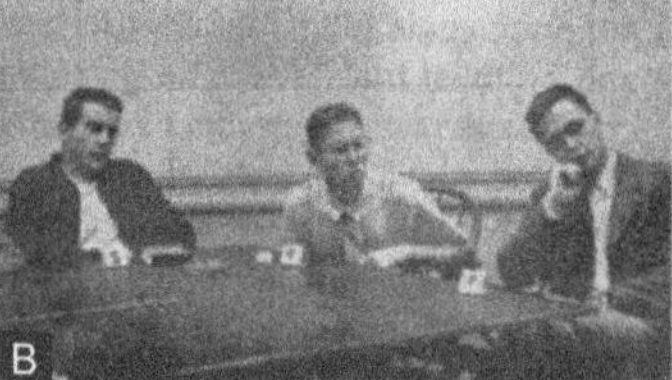

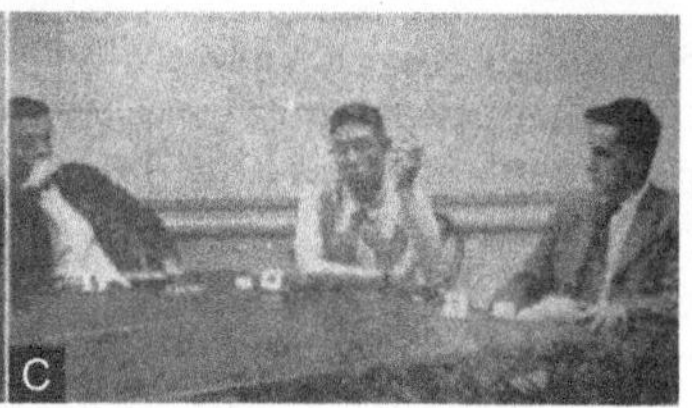

FIGURES 13.2A to C: The experimental setup in Asch's study. **A.** All of the group members except the man sixth from left are confederates previously instructed to give uniformly wrong answers on 12 of the 16 trials; number six, who has been told he is participating in an experiment in visual judgment, thus finds himself a lone dissenter when he gives the correct answers; **B.** The subject showing the strain of repeated disagreement with the majority leans forward anxiously to look at the pair of cards; **C.** This particular subject persists in his opinion saying that "he has to call them as he sees them."

Factors Affecting Conformity

Since Asch's pioneering study, hundreds of researchers have investigated this phenomenon and have come out with several factors that affect conformity. Some of the major factors influencing conformity behavior are given below.

Group cohesiveness: The degree to which individuals like or attracted to other members of the group or to people who attempt to influence them. That is, if the group is more attractive to its members, it produces more conformity.

Group size: Conformity increases as the number of persons exerting conformity increases, but up to a point, about three or four members. Beyond this level, increment in group size has little or no effect on conformity.

Social support: Suppose you discover that someone in the group shares your views, or at least does not go with the majority opinion, then conformity might be reduced.

The way the judgment is given: Conformity is considerably reduced when you are asked to give your judgment privately rather than making a response publicly. Probably, that is the reason why we are given the facility of secret ballot when we vote.

Bases of Conformity

Why do people conform instead of sticking to their own views? Conformity is a basic fact of life. If we do not conform to group standards there would be social chaos. Most of us conform to the norms of our groups or societies most of the time because of two powerful needs possessed by all humans:

1. The desire to be liked or accepted by others.
2. The desire to be right.

How to get others to like us? One of the ways is to appear to be as similar to others as possible. When we demonstrate similarity toward parents, teachers, friends and others, we are accepted, praised, rewarded and approved by them. This source of conformity is known as **normative social influence**. Under its influence, we alter our behavior and attitudes to meet others' expectations.

Secondly, we have a strong desire to be right, to possess accurate knowledge about the world we live in. To achieve this we turn to others. We use their opinions and their actions as guides for our own. This reliance on others for information is an important source of conformity. This source of social influence is known as **informational social influence**. Generally, this type of influence operates when the situation is ambiguous, when there is a crisis or when other people are experts. Together, normative and informational social influences provide a strong basis for human tendency to conform. So, the pervasive and compelling tendency to conform stems directly from our basic need that can be fulfilled only when we decide to "go along" with others.

Resistance to Conformity

But do not go with the impression that conformity pressures cannot be resisted; these pressures are strong and powerful, but definitely not irresistible. Often we stand up and say "no". Where do we get this ability to resist powerful pressures to "go along" with others? Social psychologists point to two factors. One is our desire for *individuation*—the desire to be unique and distinguished in some respects from others. We want to be like others, but not at the cost of losing our individuality or personal identity. So, we choose to disagree with others or to act in unusual ways (sometimes even bizarre ways), even when it is costly to do so. Often the desire to maintain a unique identity overrides the pressures of conformity. The second reason why people resist conformity pressures appears to be the desire to maintain control over the events in their lives. Most people believe that they are the masters of their destiny and they can determine the course of events in their lives. Naturally, yielding to social pressure runs counter to this desire and conformity is interpreted as a restriction of their personal freedom. Hence people resist, at least sometimes, even strong conformity pressures.

Often, some dissenters refuse to be road rolled by conformity pressure. Great thinkers like Socrates, Galileo, Pasteur and Freud stood firm and stuck to their views in the face of severe criticism and widespread opposition. It is reported that dissenting information held by a minority can influence majority views. This happens when the minority is highly committed to a point of view and maintains a highly consistent point of view over time. However, if the minority view appears too unreasonable, deviant or negative, the majority may not yield to minority pressure.

Compliance

Conformity pressures are mostly subtle or indirect. But there are certain situations in which the pressure is direct and explicit. Psychologists call this type of conforming behavior that occurs in response to direct social pressure **compliance**. We may define compliance as a change in behavior brought through a direct request rather than by social norms. Parents, friends, relatives, coworkers and even strangers frequently request you to do something or say something and most often you comply with their requests. When someone asks you for direction to go to a particular address, or asks you "What is the time?" you comply with the request. Compliance is quite straightforward; people state their wishes and hope that these will be granted. But it may also be highly complex; instead of making a direct request, people seeking compliance may use certain techniques to tilt the balance in their favor. We present below some of the procedures that are in use.

Ingratiation

It is a fact of life that when people like us, they are more willing to do things for us, help us, evaluate us favorably and say 'yes' to our requests. Therefore, we engage in some efforts to increase our attractiveness to a target person, so that this person will be more susceptible to yield to our requests. This technique is called **ingratiation**—a procedure for gaining compliance in which requesters first induce target persons to like them and then attempt to change their behavior in some desired manner. When we seek to ingratiate ourselves to others, we employ ***target-directed tactics*** such as flattery, agreeing with their views, showing interest in their manner of speaking, dressing, etc. We may exhibit many positive non-verbal cues such as smiling or leaning in their direction. But remember, when done in excess, these tactics may backfire.

Additional techniques of ingratiation include self-enhancement such as presenting oneself in a positive light through dress and grooming, reporting personal accomplishments, mentioning relationships with eminent persons; self-deprecation such as providing negative information about oneself to create an impression of modesty and self-disclosure, offering personal information even when it is not requested, which fosters the impression that the ingratiator is honest and likes the target person. Research evidence suggests that these techniques succeed if used with skill and care. Using too many ingratiatory tactics too often may backfire and worsen rather than enhance the chances of compliance from target persons.

Foot-in-the-door Technique

This is a strange name given to a technique, which is familiar to you. Here, first you make an insignificant request, if that is complied with, you follow it up with a larger request. For example, in one study (Freedman and Fraser, 1966), a male investigator telephoned housewives and asked what brand of soap they used? The participants complied with the request. Three days later, the same man called "again and made a much larger request". Could he send five or six people to conduct a thorough inventory of everything in the housewife's cupboards, drawers and closets, which may take 2 hours. The results were surprising; around 53 percent of the housewives who had agreed to the simple first request, agreed to this larger second request. In contrast, when housewives did not receive the first request, but were asked to allow the inventory, only about 22 percent complied. Later, studies have confirmed that the **foot-in-the-door technique** is effective in producing enhanced compliance in many settings. Why does agreeing to an initial small request leads to your saying 'yes' to a later and much larger one? Two explanations are given.

First, when you consent to a small request, you develop a favorable attitude toward helping in general. You come to realize that such acts are not costly or risky. As a result, you are willing to comply with later and larger requests. Second, when you agree to a small request, you may experience subtle shifts in your self-perceptions. You may come to view yourself as a helpful person. Therefore, when a second larger request is made, you agree in order to be consistent with your enhanced self-image. Both these explanations have received support from research.

Door-in-the-face Technique

This strategy of gaining compliance is the reverse of the foot-in-the-door technique. Here, you start by asking for a large favor. When it is refused, you make a small request, the favor you really wanted all along. For example, ask for 1,000 rupees; when it is refused, ask for just a 100. You may get it. This procedure, also called '***rejection-then-retreat technique***', appears to be effective in inducing compliance. In one study, Cialdini and colleagues asked college students to serve as unpaid counselors for juvenile delinquents 2 hours a week for the next 2 years, none agreed. Later the request was scaled down. The students were asked to take the delinquents on a 2 hour trip to a zoo. Fully 50 percent agreed. In contrast, less than 17 percent of those in a control group agreed to this smaller request when it was presented alone rather than after the first giant request. Now, why does **door-in-the-face technique** work? There are two possibilities.

When you ask for a huge favor and then scale it down to a small one, the target person views it as a concession. As a consequence, the target person himself feels obliged to make a matching concession and complies with the second, scaled down request. This phenomenon is known as ***reciprocal concessions***. The second explanation relates to our concern over ***self-presentation***—our desire to be seen in a favorable light. When we refuse a large and unreasonable request, our self-image does not suffer. But when we refuse a small one from the same person, we may appear unreasonable or intransigent and hence we yield.

There are several other techniques of obtaining compliance. We shall conclude this section after mentioning two of them. The first one is called ***that-is-not-all technique* (TNA)**, used most often by salespersons. First, you are shown a product with inflated price and immediately after that, you are told that there is a discount, an incentive, or a bonus. You must be familiar with boards that announce: "If you purchase a saree, a blouse piece is free" or "If you purchase a notebook, a pencil is free". The other technique is ***complaining***. You may simply say to your roommate: "Why did you not clean the room today, it is your turn", or your wife may say, "You do not love me anymore". When used sparingly, well-phrased and at least partially justified complaints can succeed in changing others actions and attitude, but chronic complaining may lose its effectiveness if it is repeated frequently.

Obedience

The most direct way of changing the target person's behavior is to order him to do something. This is a less used procedure than conformity pressure or compliance, but it is far from rare. Ordering is common in bureaucracy, business establishments, police departments and military. Even parents and sports coaches seek to influence in the same manner. Obedience to authority figures is far from surprising; they have some means of enforcing their orders; they can punish you when you disobey. But what is surprising is the fact that even persons who do not have such powers can sometimes induce high levels of submission in others. The clearest and most dramatic evidence for such a phenomenon has been reported by Stanley Milgram (1974) in a series of famous and highly controversial experiments.

Milgram's Experiments on Obedience

Milgram, a Harvard psychologist, was interested in finding out whether people would obey orders from a relatively powerless stranger requiring them to inflict a considerable amount of pain on another person—a totally innocent stranger (Figs 13.3A to C). Milgram's interest in this phenomenon derived from several tragic real-life occurrences in which seemingly normal, law-abiding people obeyed such directives. During Second World War, German soldiers obeyed orders to torture and kill millions of unarmed civilians. Similar events occurred in other parts of the world. The My Lai massacre in Vietnam, killing of Kurds in Iraq, and the Tiananmen Square tragedy in China. Milgram expected that Americans would not follow orders to inflict pain on innocent people. To test this hypothesis, Milgram conducted 18 studies between 1960 and 1963; let us examine one of them.

In a crucial experiment, the experimenter told the participants (forty men, ranging in age from 20 to 50 and representing a cross section of occupations and educational backgrounds) that they were participating in an investigation intended to study the effects of punishment on memory, and their task was to administer electric shocks to a "learner" (a middle-aged man who was actually a confederate of the experimenter) whenever he (learner) made an error in a simple learning task. Remember, the real participant was the "teacher" and the confederate was the 'learner.' The teacher presented a series of memory problems to the learner through a two-way intercom system. Each time the learner made an error, the teacher was instructed to administer an electric shock using a machine that had 30 switches, and beginning with 15 volts and increasing step by step to 450 volts (refer Fig. 13.3A). As the 'teacher' watched, the researcher strapped the 'learner' into a chair in an adjoining room and hooked him up to wires from the shock generator (refer Fig. 13.3B). The 'learner' expressed concern about the shocks and mentioned that he had a slight heart problem.

After returning to the main room, the researcher administered the 'teacher' a sample shock (45 volts) to demonstrate the genuineness of the shock generator and ordered the experiment to begin. Notice an important point here; the teacher did not know that the learner intentionally committed many errors and did not actually receive any shock! The learner made verbal protests when shocked, which were standardized on a tape recorder, so that they were the same for all the participants. As the learner's errors increased, the teacher increased the shock. If the teacher hesitated to continue, the researcher issued one or more escalating commands, such as 'Please continue,' "You must continue", and "You have no other choice". At 75 volts, the learner moaned at the shock. At 150 volts, he moaned again and said, "Experimenter! That's all. Get me out of here. I told you that I have a heart trouble. My heart's starting to bother me now. Get me out of here please... I refuse to go on. Let me out". Beyond 200 volts, he emitted agonized screams every time a shock was delivered and yelled "Let me out! Let me out!" At 300 volts, the learner refused to answer and continued screaming to be let out. At 345 volts and beyond, there was only silence. Full obedience was operationally defined as continuing to the maximum shock level of 450 volts.

Participants (teachers) wrestled with a dilemma whether to continue to hurt this innocent person as the researcher commanded or to stop this painful act by openly disobeying the researcher. Most participants became distressed. Some trembled, sweated, laughed nervously or, in a few cases, experienced convulsions. Most participants refused or protested at one time or another and said they would not continue. Before conducting this experiment, Milgram had asked several groups of

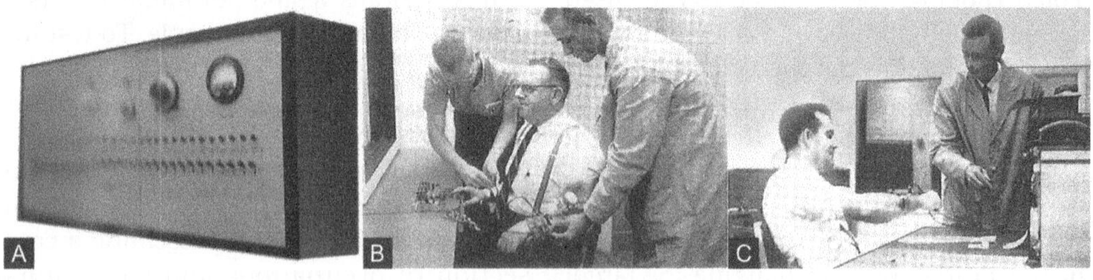

FIGURES 13.3A to C: The 'shock generator' and the 'learner' in Milgram's experiment. **A.** The first picture shows the shock generator used in the experiment; **B.** The second one shows the "learner" being hooked up to the shock-delivery apparatus. The teacher watches it; **C.** The third figure shows the 'teacher' sitting in front of the shock generator and receiving a shock before starting of the experiment. This is to show the teacher the genuineness of the shock generator. The learner and teacher do not sit facing each other. The two are in different rooms and the teacher communicates with the learner through intercom. The teacher does not see the learner; he only hears the taped voice of the 'so called' learner.

people (psychiatrists, university professors, students and middle-class adults) to predict the outcome. They said that virtually no one would obey fully! But in Milgram's study, 26 of the 40 men (65%) obeyed all the way to the end. They continued to give shocks up to 450 volts level, even though they knew they were hurting another innocent person. In contrast, participants in a control group, who were not given such commands, generally administered only very mild shocks during the session.

Later, studies found similar results with women as well as with people in other countries (Jordan, Germany, and Australia) and with children. The results seemed to be alarmingly general in scope. So the question: Why do people obey?

Factors Influencing Obedience

Milgram and others have studied obedience to authority under several different conditions and found that the following factors generally operate in increasing or decreasing such behavior.

Remoteness of the victim: Obedience increased when the learner was in a different room, out of sight. When the "teacher" and "learner" were in the same room, obedience dropped to 40 percent. When the teacher was asked to make physical contact and force the learner's hand onto a shock plate, obedience dropped to 30 percent.

Proximity and legitimacy of the authority figure: Obedience was highest when the authority figure (experimenter or researcher) was close by and perceived as legitimate. When the experimenter left the scene and telephoned his commands to the "teacher" instead of giving face-to-face instructions, obedience dropped to 21 percent. When a college student (a confederate), instead of an older, white-coated experimenter, took over and gave orders to give shock, obedience dropped to about 20 percent. When there were two experimenters (authority figures) who disagreed with each other, no participant administered further shocks.

Diffusion of responsibility: In Milgram's study, the participants psychologically transferred the responsibility for the learner's fate to the experimenter (researcher). They perceived the experimenter as an expert, a legitimate authority figure, who would be responsible for any untoward consequence. Participants openly declared that they "were not responsible" for what happened. When participants asked, "Who is responsible if something happens to the learner?" and the experimenter replied, "I am responsible", the participants felt greater freedom to continue. In real life situations, those who obey harsh or cruel directives from authority figures usually defend their actions by saying, "I was only carrying out orders". Instead of the experimenter, when another "participant" (actually a confederate) flipped the shock switch and the real participant had to perform another aspect of the task, 93 percent obeyed. That is, obedience increases when someone else does the dirty work. When the participants were made to feel fully responsible for the learner's welfare, not a single person obeyed to the end.

Impact of cues from the authority figure: Generally, authority figures wear badges or signs (special uniforms, titles and insignia) that indicate their status and power. The experimenter in Milgram's study wore a white-coat indicating his expertise and authority. These cues remind the participant who is in charge and it is difficult to resist the powerful impact of such cues.

Gradual nature of the punishment: In Milgram's experiment, the participants were first ordered to administer an insignificant amount of shock before going on to give apparently harmful ones. This procedure resembles the "foot-in-the-door technique" of inducing conformity. In fact, when participants were allowed to set the punishment level, no one ever went past 45 volts. In real life situations, you must have noticed police personnel adopting the same procedure: first questioning, then arresting and finally torturing potential victims.

Personality characteristics: Milgram compared the political orientation, religious affiliation, education, occupation, and length of military service of obedient and disobedient participants. The differences were very small or non-existent. Two personality characteristics, **authoritarian submission** and **internal-external locus of control**, appear to be influencing obedience behavior. According to Adorno and coworkers (1950), authoritarian submission refers to the tendency to adopt a submissive, uncritical attitude toward authority figures. Research results suggest that those who are high on this characteristic tend to be more obedient in the Milgram situation than those who are relatively low. The other personality characteristic related to obedience is internal-external locus of control dimension proposed by Julian Rotter (1966). Persons who score high at the *internal* end of this dimension believe that their fate is largely in their own hands. Those who score at the external end believe that they have little control over what happens to them. The results of several studies suggest that externals are more likely to obey commands from authority figures, at least under certain circumstances, than internals. Strangely enough, one study indicated that those who are deeply religious tend to obey more than those who are less religious. These results have to be confirmed by further research.

What lessons shall we learn from Milgram's studies? Does it mean that we are basically apathetic or evil? Of course not. We are not sheep who blindly obey orders whatever the consequence. Remember, the participants of the study were troubled when they were asked to punish the innocent learner. It is the situation in which the person finds himself that determines how he acts. The conclusion therefore is: By arranging the situation appropriately, most people—ordinary, decent citizens—can be induced to follow orders from an authority figure, who is perceived as legitimate, even when doing so harms an innocent person. This research should heighten our responsibility for being aware of the pitfalls of blind obedience and prevent us from being so smug or naïve as to feel that such events "could never happen here". Milgram's research provides yet another example of how social contexts can induce people to behave in ways that they never would have imagined possible.

Can We Resist the Tendency to Obey Blindly?

Social psychologists have made several suggestions that seem to be effective in helping reduce the tendency to obey, especially destructive obedience. Blind obedience can be reduced under the following conditions:

- When individuals who are exposed to commands from authority figures are reminded that 'they'—not the authorities—are responsible for any harm produced
- When individuals are given an indication that beyond a certain point, unquestioning submission to destructive commands is inappropriate
- When people are exposed to *disobedient models*—people who refuse to obey unreasonable commands
- When people question the expertise and the appropriateness of the motives of the authority figure
- When people know about the power of authority figures to command blind obedience.

The power of authority figures to command obedience may be certainly great, but it is not irresistible. Under appropriate conditions, it can be countered. There is always the freedom to choose, which cannot be taken away. But refusing to obey the authority can be dangerous. Those holding power wield tremendous advantages in terms of weapons and technology. Yet, events in recent history have demonstrated that the outcome is by no means certain when committed groups of citizens choose to resist. Ultimately, victory may go to those on the side of freedom and decency rather than to those who possess guns, tanks and planes. The human spirit cannot so easily be extinguished as many dictators would like to believe.

SOCIAL RELATIONSHIPS

When we live in a social set-up, it is but natural that we develop relationships with people around us. We like some of them; we dislike some others. Most others may be placed between these two extremes. Why do we like some people more than others? Probably, we like those with whom our interactions were pleasant and rewarding. Interpersonal relationships play a very important role in our lives. There is nothing more central in your life than your feelings for others. In fact, your success or failure in various walks of life depends on your relationships with people around you, your parents, relatives, teachers, friends and employers, to mention only a few. We have seen that the manner in which we relate to others depends to a large extent on social perception, impression formation and social influence. While these are important, social psychologists have studied several other factors, which contribute to the formation and maintenance of social relationships. We focus on some of these factors in the following paragraphs.

Interpersonal Attraction

When you like someone, you are drawn toward him/her. When the relationship becomes intimate, it may take the form of friendship or even love. A humorist once said, "Friendship is love minus sex and plus reason. Love is friendship plus sex and minus reason". The difference between liking and loving may not be simple, but attraction is indeed the first phase of most friendships and romantic relationships. Therefore, the basic question that social psychologists ask is: Why are we attracted to some people and not others?

Physical Proximity

One basic factor that has been shown to affect the degree of attraction one person feels for another is physical nearness or proximity. We tend to interact mostly with people who are physically closer. Although this may appear obvious, the magnitude of the effect of ***proximity*** or ***propinquity*** on liking or loving is surprising. Residents are most likely to become friends with other residents who live close by and students are more likely to become friends with students seated nearby. A number of studies have shown that propinquity determines who becomes acquainted with whom, who are likely to become friends and even who marries whom. Several explanations are offered for the effect of proximity. One of them is that we simply prefer pleasant interactions with people we meet frequently and make special efforts to ensure smooth interactions with them. The second explanation suggests that repeated exposure to any previously neutral stimulus results in an increasingly positive evaluation of the stimulus. This is often called **mere exposure effect**. Over 200 studies in different parts of the world have shown that repeated exposure to stimuli (classmates, photographs of faces, random geometric shapes and so on), as long as these are not unpleasant and we are not over-saturated, generally enhance liking. The third explanation refers to ***similarity***. Cross-cultural researches overwhelmingly assert that people most often are attracted to others who are similar to themselves. Similarity of attitudes and values seems to matter the most. The old adage, "opposites attract", may occur at times. But more often, opposites repel. When choosing friends and lovers, we rule out those who are dissimilar to us. Relationships among dissimilar people do not last long. The tendency to be attracted toward similar others rests upon several assumptions we make about them. We may perceive the behavior of similar others as more predictable, which leads us to be more confident that interactions with them will be rewarding. We may expect pleasant interactions with them because they are like us.

Physical Attraction

A major factor that determines our liking of others is physical attraction. You may say that "beauty is only skin deep", but it is deep enough to induce in you more proneness to develop liking toward physically attractive (beautiful) people than those who are not. People are drawn to beauty like moths to a flame. Indeed throughout the animal kingdom, species have evolved distinct physical features to attract mates. Among humans, both sexes respond strongly to the physical attractiveness of those they meet, though males are more responsive to female attractiveness than females are to male attractiveness. This tendency is seen even among gay men. The importance of physical attraction can be easily understood when we look at the amount of money spent on cosmetics, exercise, diet products, clothing and even plastic surgery to enhance physical appearance. The desire to appear attractive is so great that some psychologists have developed the concept of ***appearance anxiety***, which is defined as apprehension concerning one's physical appearance, and the evaluation made by others. Using ***Appearance Anxiety Scale***, one researcher found that among college students, women express more appearance anxiety than men and high scores on this scale are associated with experience of social anxiety, feeling unattractiveness in childhood and having had fewer dates in high school. Appearance anxiety has also been found to predict behavior differences in specific social situations.

Research in this area suggests that physically attractive people have many advantages over their unattractive counterparts; they are advantaged with respect to the perceived task performance (perceived as smart workers), their job marketability (they get jobs easily), their expected political success (they may get elected easily) and their perceived persuasiveness. Even mock juries, deciding on the punishment to be given for a crime, give less severe punishment to the physically attractive defendant. Although the important influence of physical attraction cannot be denied, it is felt that the impact of this attribute usually diminishes as a relationship evolves over time. Other rewards associated with social interaction may come to the fore and reduce the dependence on this single superficial determinant of attraction.

CLOSE RELATIONSHIPS

Until now, we have been talking about relationships in general and the factors that contribute to their development. But there are some intimate relationships that play a crucial role in our lives. In spite of the widespread changes around us, we believe that an ideal life includes interactions with parents, cherished relatives, close friends, loving spouses and affectionate children. Given the importance of family, friendship, love and marriage, social psychologists are trying to unravel the dynamics of these close relationships and joys and pains associated with them. This is a vast area and what follows is only a glimpse into it.

Relatives, Friends and Lovers

The common element which runs across all these relationships is interdependence. That is, two people influence one another's lives and regularly engage in joint activities. When college students were asked to identify the one person in the world to whom they are close, they described three types of relationship: family members (14%), friends (36%) and a romantic partner (47%).

Almost all of us grow up in families with parents and siblings. We experience a mixture of love and hate, closeness and rivalry in our relationships with them. No matter how much parents love their children when they were babies, they become anxious when the same young ones approach puberty. Parents are afraid of being rejected and hated by rebellious teenagers. Adolescents report positive feelings about their parents, though they are less close and dependent than they were in childhood. Siblings (brothers and sisters) behave differently at different ages; they are close during childhood, but grow apart in adolescence and young adulthood. Later, they may or may not interact at all. Generally, sister-sister and brother-sister relationships continue to be more closer than brother-brother relationships. It is interesting to note that people continue to maintain cordial relationships with grandparents, especially with grandmother. It is unfortunate that psychologists have not made serious attempts to study these interpersonal relationships in a big way.

We spend more time with close friends, interact with them in varied social situations and we give and receive emotional support. Friendships during adolescence tend to be more intimate than in childhood. When the relationship is intimate, two individuals engage in self-disclosing behavior, express their emotions, provide and receive support, experience trust, and feel relaxed with each other.

Recently, interest in the man-woman relationship is increasing and some social psychologists have initiated research in this form of relationship which is often referred to as romantic relationship. Romance may either endure or fall apart amid emotional turmoil. When the relationship endures, it may be transformed into love and consequently marriage.

Love

Our knowledge of what makes people like one another is extensive, but our understanding of love is limited. In spite of all the poetry, drama, short stories, novels and movies that chronicle, celebrate and eulogize love, its mystery endures. Many early social psychologists thought that love was a phenomenon too difficult to observe and study according to scientific procedures. But since love is such a central theme in human life, social psychologists could not resist the temptation to bring love into the laboratory. As a consequence, nowadays several researchers are examining the components and styles of love and its fate over time. According to modern psychologists, loving is a feeling that is qualitatively different from liking; it is not simply very strong liking, it is a different psychological state. Love is a noble feeling experienced universally, more or less similarly. It is unfortunate that love is often equated with sex.

As we have seen in the chapter on emotion, love manifests in several forms. Erich Fromm (1956) suggested that love flows at least in five directions. Parental love is the love directed toward parents, uncles, aunts, grandparents, all other elders and finally God. Filial love is directed toward children, animals and all helpless ones. Fraternal love moves toward siblings, friends and people in general. Conjugal love is love of spouse. Compared to other forms of love which flow toward many people, conjugal love is directed toward one person. According to Fromm, the fifth and the most important form of love is self-love. Do not mistake it with selfishness. Self-love implies an accurate understanding and evaluating one's self. If you do not love yourself, you cannot love anyone else.

Love is unconditional giving, without anticipating anything in return. It includes understanding, care, respect and responsibility toward the love object. Experience of love elevates your psyche. You do not "fall" in love; you "rise" with love. Love is not 'blind.' It occurs only when you see with open eyes and understand the other person accurately. Fromm was very optimistic about the power of love. He wrote that the one and only sane and sensible solution to all the evils of contemporary (sick) society is love. The focus of contemporary society is to produce more and consume more material goods. How wonderful it would be if we produce more love and consume more love. Fromm's notion of love appears a bit philosophical, but there is a great deal of truth in it.

In modern social psychology, love is studied as an intense form of interpersonal relationship. It is a close relationship involving physiological arousal, an all-encompassing interest in another individual, fantasizing about the other and a passion to be with the loved person. As you can see, the focus here is on the love between a man and a woman. Psychologists have distinguished between romantic love and companionate love. Robert Sternberg (1986) made an even finer differentiation between types of love in his triangular theory of love. Since, we mentioned about Sternberg's views earlier (Chapter 10 on Emotion), they are not repeated here.

STEREOTYPES, PREJUDICE AND DISCRIMINATION

Loving and liking are positive forms of social behavior. But many of us exhibit negative social behaviors. Prominent among them are **prejudice** and **discrimination**. When we interact with people, we often form faulty impressions about them based on their looks, skin color, gender, race, ethnicity, caste and even country. We attribute certain traits to a group as a whole based on experience with one member of the group. This is called stereotyping. **Stereotypes** often lead to prejudice toward people belonging to certain groups. When we think of a group as hostile (stereotype), any member of that group is considered hostile. Prejudices in turn lead to discrimination. These negative attitudes, which are generally mediated by social schemas, create social disharmony and tension. Here, we briefly discuss the origin and development of these negative social behaviors. We start with stereotypes because they are a major cause for the emergence of prejudices and discrimination that are plaguing contemporary society.

Stereotypes

One of the major causes of prejudices is a stereotype, which is primarily a hasty judgment about groups of people based on a single experience with a member of that group. Thus, a stereotype is a belief about people in a particular category. The category may be defined by race, sex, religion, social class, ethnicity, hair color, color of skin, and a myriad of other characteristics. For example, you may have stereotypes such as "Americans are practical," "Britons are conservative," "French are romantic," "Indians are philosophical," "Women are weak," "Men are aggressive," so on and so forth. When you conclude Britons are conservative, it is based on limited experience. You have not examined all Britons. If you do so, you will know your conclusion is wrong. A stereotype may be positive (women are nurturing), negative (business men are cheats), or neutral (Indians eat spicy food). Stereotypes are caricatures, not reasoned formulations, and most often they are incorrect. We interpret incoming information according to the stereotypes we have and do so quickly. We are less likely to attend to and therefore, encode or remember information that is inconsistent with our stereotypes. In fact, we may deny the truth of such information. Once a stereotype is established we respond to a person's membership in the particular group and not to the characteristics of the individual person. Social psychologists believe that stereotyping is a normal cognitive tendency, a kind of cognitive short cut that simplifies the process of making social judgments. Stereotypes allow us to use stored information more effectively about other groups instead of expending all our cognitive resources to evaluate each and every individual member of the group. We develop stereotypes based on race, nationality, gender, age, body weight, disability and sexual orientation, and make inferences about them, which may prove to be unfounded when we get to know them as individuals. The important point therefore to notice is that stereotypes are exaggerated and over-generalized concepts that fail to take into account individual differences. Once stereotypes are formed, they are resistant to change in the face of new information. They damage social relations and justify social inequities.

Stereotypes cause members of the stereotyped groups to behave in ways that reflect the stereotype, through the phenomenon of **self-fulfilling prophecy**. Self-fulfilling prophecies are expectancies about the occurrence of a future event or behavior that act to increase the likelihood that the event or behavior will occur. For example, if a teacher thinks a student is bright, he treats him in ways (gives him more marks) that increase his status. The teacher focuses more attention on the student, asks him questions, gives him interesting assignments and evaluates him more favorably. The most important thing is that the student starts behaving according to the teacher's expectations. He may become a better student; this is self-fulfilling prophecy effect. Similarly, when you think that a person is lazy, you look only at his laziness and ignore instances where he did not behave that way. Over time, the person may become lazy confirming your stereotype. The operation of self-filling prophesies has been well researched by social psychologists. In one study, Rosenthal and Jacobson (1968) administered a test to elementary school students and as though based on the test results, told their teachers that some particular students would do extremely well in the yearend examination. In reality, the particular students were chosen at random. Surprisingly, the students who had been noted to do well in fact did well in the year end examination relative to their classmates who were not so marked. The teachers' impressions and expectations of the students shaped the way they treated the students, which in turn shaped the performance of students in the examination. Often, the self-fulfilling prophesy is called Rosenthal effect after the researcher who studied the phenomenon.

Prejudice

Prejudice refers to a negative attitude toward people based on their membership in specific group. One of the undesirable consequences of stereotyping is prejudice; of course there are other causes of prejudices. Stereotyping and prejudices often lead to **discrimination**, which is treating people unfairly because they belong to a particular group. While prejudice is an attitude, discrimination is behavior. As you can surmise, we live in a social world that has an abundant supply of prejudices and discriminations. Fortunately, some of the blatant forms of these evils are gradually fading. Racial segregation and untouchability that were once highly prevalent in some countries are not condoned nowadays by governmental policies. But many prejudices such as casteism, racism and sexism have gone underground and are difficult to detect and eradicate.

Prejudices can be explicit or implicit. When people express them openly in public, they are called explicit prejudices. When these are hidden from public view, then they are referred to as implicit prejudices. Many people hide their prejudices and express them only when and where it is safe to exhibit them. Prejudices may be conscious and intentional; they may be conscious and unintentional, or even unconscious and unintentional. Whether overt or covert, conscious or unconscious, prejudices originate from a constellation of factors. Then, what are the causes of prejudice? Let us examine some of them.

The origins of prejudices can be traced to historical and cultural norms that legitimize differential treatments of various groups and the socialization processes through which parents and other adults transmit values and beliefs to their children. Social, cognitive, emotional and motivational factors, all contribute to the development and perpetuation of prejudices and discrimination.

Social Origins of Prejudice

None of us are born with prejudices. We learn to hate a particular religious, racial, ethnic or social group just in the same way we learn all other things. Our feelings about these groups are to some extent shaped by the behavior of our parents, friends and other adults. We may simply imitate the behavior of adult models or they may even teach us to dislike certain groups of people. We are instructed not to mix with certain groups of people; not to touch them, not to talk to them and not eat with them. Such social learning processes start at an early age. It is reported that children as young as 3 years show preference for members of their own race and a concomitant dislike of certain other races. Mass media play a crucial role in the development of stereotypes and prejudices. Television shows and movies portray certain groups as Mafia-like mobsters, terrorists, rapists, promiscuous, or lazy. These are imbibed both by children and adults alike. When such inaccurate and unfavorable information concerns minority groups, prejudices toward them is acquired easily and quickly.

Cognitive Roots of Prejudice

For purposes of organizing and simplifying our social world, we have a tendency to categorize people, objects and events. Categorization helps us to understand and predict other people's behavior; but at the same time, it also contributes to the development of prejudices. The first consequence of categorization is the perceptual distinction between **in-group** and **out-group** (us and them). In-group is the group to which we belong and out-group is the one to which we do not belong. People generally think of their own group (in-group) favorably and out-groups unfavorably. The out-group is assumed to possess more undesirable qualities. Our identification with the in-group makes us more inclined to like, trust, help and cooperate with members of the in-group than we like, trust, help and cooperate with members of out-group. The *in-group favoritism* and the *out-group derogation* can lead to prejudice. Although people generally exhibit both these tendencies, the in-group favoritism is usually stronger of the two, especially when we feel threatened.

We also exhibit **out-group homogeneity bias** and **in-group differentiation bias**. We have a tendency to think that members of out-group are more similar to one another than are members of the in-group. We think "they are all alike" and "we are diverse". Therefore, if any member of an out-group exhibits an undesirable trait, we attribute that trait to all the members, because they are all alike. If a member of the in-group displays an undesirable characteristic, we are prone to think that it is an exception, because we have all sorts of people amongst us and we are not all alike. The mere fact that we identify people as Indians, Chinese, Americans, Blacks and Whites reflects out-group homogeneity bias; we do not take note of subgroups among them. Thus, categorization and in-group biases increase the tendency to judge other people based on their perceived group membership rather than on their individual characteristics. So, the "us-them" thinking is a powerful factor in generating stereotypes and prejudices.

What happens when an out-group member exhibits a trait that contradicts our stereotype? That is, suppose we think that members of a particular group are cheats. But we encounter a person in that group who is very honest. Under such circumstances, there is a possibility that we may change our attitude (stereotype) toward that out-group (remember, this is an instance of cognitive dissonance leading to change in attitude). But if our prejudice is very strong, we tend to rationalize the behavior in several ways. We may say it is a rare exception or accidental.

Emotional-Motivational Roots of Prejudice

Our prejudices not only have beliefs and expectations about the group but also an emotional component. Simply thinking about members of a group which we dislike, elicits strong feelings about them. Emotions can influence prejudice in two ways. The *presence of negative feelings* may account for conscious prejudice, whether intentional or unintentional. But even when we do not have negative feelings toward a group, prejudice can arise from the *absence of positive feelings*. In this case, it will be unconscious prejudice. This way, it is possible to have prejudice toward a group with which we never had any contact.

Our ways of perceiving the world—categorizing, forming in-groups and out-groups, often prepare the ground for the development of prejudices. But motivational factors determine how intensely the prejudices are exhibited in life. According to **social identity theory**, prejudices emerge from a need to enhance our self-esteem. Development of self-esteem depends on two factors: a personal identity and a group identity. Self-esteem increases when we acknowledge our strengths and virtues; it also increases when we know we belong to a group that is successful and accomplishing. Experiments have shown that prejudice increases when our self-esteem is threatened and it is restored when there are opportunities to derogate others. When there are threats to our in-group with which we identify and which caters to our self-esteem, naturally self-esteem is also threatened. Derogation of out-group (with prejudices and bias) therefore, restores our self-esteem.

According to **realistic conflict theory**, competition for limited resources is the cause of prejudice. This phenomenon is clearly seen when people fight against minority groups, foreigners and others who are taking away their jobs. Even in advanced countries like the United States of America, when foreign students are employed, the locals develop prejudice against the foreigners who are seen as taking away the jobs. May be the same phenomenon is operating in Australia where foreign students are being treated badly by some locals. Originally, it was thought that threat to personal welfare (fear of losing a job) was the prime cause of prejudice, but now researches have shown that strong prejudices emerge when there is perceived threat to one's in-group. Muzafer Sherif and coworkers (1961) demonstrated experimentally, how competition between groups can lead to intense hostility toward an out-group, in a field study that has come to be known as Robber's Cave experiment.

The researchers divided a set of 11-year-old boys into two groups, Eagles and Rattlers, at a special overnight camp called the Robber's Cave, and made the two groups compete for valued prizes. Intense conflict developed between the competing groups resulting in prejudice. The boys from the competing groups started abusing each other and even destroying each others' belongings. Such behavior was not seen when they were engaged in cooperative activities leading to mutually benefiting goals. It has also been shown that when you are angry and know very well that the out-group is not the cause of your anger, in all probability, you develop prejudice toward the out-group. The emotion of anger is so closely related to competition and conflict between groups that it automatically activates feelings of prejudice toward out-group.

Discrimination

As mentioned earlier, stereotyping and prejudices lead to discrimination. Kosslyn and Rosenberg (2005) quote an interesting instance in the life of a Black student named Bessie, which relates to the operation of discrimination. A White professor failed Bessie on an assignment, which she knew was good. A White girlfriend of Bessie, also a student in the same class, offered to hand in Bessie's work as her own to see what grade the work would be given this time. Surprisingly, Bessie's friend passed with the same work that had earned Bessie a failing grade. Bessie was a victim of prejudice and discrimination. Her professor's behavior was influenced by his prejudice against Bessie because of her race, her membership in a particular social group. Just like prejudice, discrimination may be subtle and sometimes even unconscious. Festinger's concept of cognitive dissonance often helps to reduce discrimination. When we know that discrimination is wrong, if someone points out to our discriminatory behavior, we feel uncomfortable and this may subsequently reduce such behavior. This is an instance cognitive dissonance, a discrepancy between attitude and behavior, which may change either our attitude or behavior.

Techniques of Reducing Prejudice

The effects of prejudice and discrimination are undesirable, harmful and painful. Psychologists have talked a great deal about them. Do they have anything to say about diminishing the effects of prejudice? They have suggested certain techniques, but the task is not easy to accomplish. The following strategies have been found to be effective in reducing prejudice.

Increasing Contact

The contact hypothesis holds that increased contact between the target and the holder of prejudice can reduce the negative attitude. Increasing the amount of interaction between members of different groups under amicable conditions has been found to reduce prejudice (Pettigrew and Tropp, 2000). When two groups interact, the members are likely to become aware of the similarities among them, which can enhance mutual liking. People may become aware of the discrepancies between the stereotypic views and the reality and this fosters a change. Also, increased contact breaks the bubble of out-group homogeneity. Increased contact can reduce prejudice when people are working toward a common goal, have equal status, keep sustained close contact and are supported by broader social norms. When people have a common group identity, such as the one found in a military unit or a cricket team that consists of people from different ethnic groups, there will definitely be a reduction in prejudice.

Recategorization

Another way of reducing prejudice is to remove the boundaries between the in-group and out-group. When the 'us and them' feeling is shattered, the two groups may not feel that they are distinct entities. When the cleaner in a hotel becomes the waiter, the identity of "us and them" changes. When the distinctions between groups are minimized, the groups start thinking that they are a single entity, thus reducing prejudice between them. Working toward a shared goal fosters recategorization. When school children are taught in multiracial learning groups, each child is accorded equal status, and opportunities for sustained close contact are maintained, the reduction of prejudice becomes apparent.

Reducing Stereotype Threat

According to American social psychologist Claude Steele (1997), reducing stereotype is helpful in reducing prejudice. The concept of **stereotype threat** proposes that stereotypes create self-consciousness among stereotyped group members and they start fearing that they will live up to other people's negative stereotypes about their group. For example, African-American students, who receive instructions from teachers who doubt their abilities and who set up special remedial programs to assist them, come to accept society's stereotypes that they are inferior and believe that they are prone to fail. Such beliefs can have devastating effects on their academic performance. Steele suggests that it might be possible to overcome the stereotype threat through certain intervention programs. Minority groups may be trained to see that their vulnerability is inaccurate and they have potential for academic success.

AGGRESSION: HARMING OTHERS

Aggression is a negative social behavior that is in abundant supply all over the world. Everyday, the morning newspapers carry stories of violence both at a societal level (war, invasion, assassination) and at the individual level (street fighting, assault, murder, rape, child abuse, kidnapping and many other cruelties). You are bombarded by such news items the moment you switch on your TV or radio set. The list of inhuman activities by humans seems almost endless. So shall we say humans are inherently aggressive, or is it a form of learned behavior that can be modified by experience? For that matter, what exactly is aggression? Why are people aggressive? What are the roots of aggression? None of these questions can be answered satisfactorily. Even defining aggression is a difficult task (Box 13.1). Tentatively, social psychologists define aggression as any form of behavior that is intended to inflict injury or harm on others. According to Berkowitz (1993), an authority on aggression, the intention or purpose behind the act is important. A physician, who conducts an emergency operation without anesthesia, causing injury and intense pain to his patient, is not aggressive, while rape and murder are aggressive acts.

Aggression takes many forms. Some psychologists distinguish between **hostile aggression** and **instrumental aggression**. The sole aim of hostile aggression is inflicting injury, while instrumental aggression is aimed at obtaining rewards other than the

Box 13.1: What is Aggression?

Read each of the following statements and decide whether it is an act of aggression:
A jailor executes a convicted criminal.
A cat kills a mouse.
A thief is shot when he was trying to escape.
A person kills himself.
A physician gives a painful injection to a crying child.
A sheep is killed for dinner.
A boxer gives a bloody blow on the nose of his opponent.
A tennis player smashes his racket after hitting the ball out.
A lizard eats a fly.
A soldier guns down an enemy.

victim's suffering. The distinction is not clear because what looks like hostile aggression may serve other ends. Most of what is researched in psychology pertains to hostile aggression which may occur in several ways. It can be physical or verbal, active or passive, direct or indirect. These may combine to form different types of aggression (Table 13.1).

Needless to say that aggression is an important and all-too-common form of social behavior and it is hardly surprising that social psychologists have been engaged in the study of the phenomenon for the last several decades and their research has thrown light on the questions raised above—what is aggression? Why does it occur? How to prevent it?

Let us briefly review the work that has been done in the area. We shall start with the theoretical perspectives on aggression.

Theories of Aggression

There are differing views among psychologists, sociologists and ethologists about the nature of aggression, especially human aggression. Some believe that aggression is an inherent tendency among humans. Others assert that people learn to become aggressive. There is some truth in both the views. Let us briefly review some of the major perspectives that throw light on this negative form of social behavior.

Aggression as an Instinct

According *to* ***instinct theory*** of aggression, humans are born with a tendency to fight; their brain is programmed to make them behave aggressively. The earliest supporters of such view were the British psychologist William McDougall, and psychoanalyst Sigmund Freud. McDougall believed that humans have an innate combative instinct. Freud held that aggression is the reflection of death wish or Thanatos possessed by all humans. In recent times, ethologist Konrad Lorenz proposed that we share with our animal ancestors the aggressive drive. It is believed that this instinct developed in the course of evolution because it has some important benefits: one, it has helped to disperse the population over a wide area, thus ensuring maximum use of available natural resources, and secondly, it is related to mating behavior. Fighting ensures that only the strongest will pass their genes to the next generation. Our ancestors evolved as hunters for food. Therefore, their body was anatomically, (physiologically and psychologically) made suitable for hunting, it became strong and fighting fit. The moral was: either attack or starve. Similar views were proposed by sociobiologists and evolutionary psychologists. The implication of these views is that we are by nature

Table 13.1: One Way of Classifying Aggressive Behavior

Type of aggression	*Examples*
Physical-active-direct	Punching, stabbing or shooting.
Physical-active-indirect	Hiring some one to kill another.
Physical-passive-direct	Physically obstructing another from reaching a desired goal.
Physical-passive-indirect	Refusing to perform what is necessary.
Verbal-active-direct	Insulting someone by using abusive language.
Verbal-active-indirect	Gossiping or spreading malicious rumors about others.
Verbal-passive-direct	Refusing to talk to another, to answer questions.
Verbal-passive-indirect	Failing to talk in defense of another when he is being criticized.

aggressive creatures; we have been fighting all along and will continue to do so in the future. War and violence are in our blood. It is reported that approximately there have been 14,600 wars in 5,600 years, and there will be many more in the times to come on the human planet.

Modern psychologists do not completely agree with the view that humans are biologically programmed to fight all the time. There are several cultures where wars are rare. For example, in Norway murder is a rare event; less than one per 100,000 is a victim of homicide; in New Guinea it is almost 800 times higher! In the United States it is more than 8 times higher. Such huge differences indicate that aggression is strongly influenced by sociocultural factors. True, biology plays a role in determining aggressive tendencies, but to say that it is wholly determined by the brain and biochemistry is far from the truth. Today, most psychologists reject the dark, pessimistic, 'human nature' view of aggression and instead emphasize the importance of environmental, social, cultural and psychological factors in the causation of aggressive behavior.

Aggression as a Drive

One of the important alternatives to instinct approach is the **drive theory of aggression**, which proposes that external conditions, such as barriers (obstacles) that thwart motivated behavior (causing frustration), arouse a strong motive to fight. A highly influential drive theory (there are several of them), called '**frustration-aggression hypothesis**', was proposed by John Dollard and coworkers in 1939. This theory asserts that frustration always results in aggression and that all aggressive behavior is caused by frustration. Later, it was shown that this theory is not wholly true. There are several exceptions. First of all, frustration may produce so many other kinds of reactions other than aggression. For example, when people are frustrated, they may withdraw from the situation, give up the task, thinking it is useless to try, take to alcohol or drugs, or positively, they may strive hard to beat the frustration. Secondly, it has also been shown that not all aggression is caused by frustration. Whether frustration causes aggression depends on its intensity.

Intensity of frustration depends on the importance of the goal-directed behavior to the person and the expectations that he/she has about reaching the goal. When the expectations are high, the resulting aggression is high; when low, one may not feel frustrated at all and hence no aggression may result. Suppose you are sure of passing an examination and you are thwarted from taking it for one or the other reason, you will be terribly frustrated, which triggers high level of aggression. Further, when frustration is perceived as due to some arbitrary (unjustified) action, aggression is more likely to occur; when frustration is seen as justified, aggression may not result.

Aggression as Learned Behavior

The **social learning theory** (Bandura, 1973) proposes that aggression, like several other forms of behavior, is largely learned in the social context. We are not born with an aggressive tendency; we acquire it through direct experience or by watching others—social models. This theory stresses the role of imitation (modeling) of others as a cause of aggressive behavior. In both laboratory experiments and everyday life, it was shown that people who have seen others act aggressively are likely to show aggression in a similar situation. In one of his experiments, Bandura (1965) demonstrated how aggression is learned by observing others. In his experiment, children watched a film in which a model acted aggressively toward a doll (Bobo doll, an inflatable plastic clown) punching, kicking and hitting it with a mallet. One group of children saw the model being rewarded for his act, a second group saw the model being punished and a third group saw no consequences for the model. After the film, each child was left in a room with several toys along with the Bobo doll. All children imitated the model by exhibiting aggression, but to different degrees. Children who had seen the model being rewarded exhibited the highest level of aggression. Children who had seen the model punished expressed less aggression than the other two groups. It does not mean that children in this group have not learned to show aggression, they had only inhibited it. Later in the study, when these children were offered attractive rewards to imitate the model, they quickly exhibited aggression.

Bandura's study created interest in the area of the effect of watching filmed or televised aggression on the viewers. Researches strongly suggest that viewing aggressive behavior:

1. Decreases the viewer's sensitivity and concern for the suffering of the victim.
2. May make people become habituated to view films and TV serials that depict aggression.
3. May lead to learning of new ways aggressing.
4. May make one feel that aggression pays.
5. Generally increases the tendency to engage in aggressive acts.

Watching aggression makes people imitate that behavior, agreed. But, what happens when we watch helping (prosocial) behavior? The researchers who tackled this issue suggest that helping behavior is also imitated. We shall discuss about helping behavior in the next section.

In summary, whether we behave aggressively in a given situation depends on our past experience (what happened when we aggressed earlier), the rewards and punishments associated with aggressive behavior, and several other cognitive variables. We learn from past experience whom to attack, whether such behavior is approved or disapproved by others, and the consequences of such behavior (whether it yields rewards or the aggression is retaliated).

Apart from social learning, aggressive behavior can be acquired through Pavlovian and operant conditioning. When aggressive behavior is paired with a neutral stimulus and the combination occurs together often, we develop aggressive tendency toward that neutral stimulus. For example, if your boss insults you in public or behaves violently several times, you may develop a dislike for the person and express aggression toward him/her. Later, the behavior may be generalized and you may show the same behavior toward all authority figures. Operant conditioning occurs when aggressive behavior is reinforced (see the Chapter on Learning). It becomes a habit to express hostility because it is rewarding to do so. Suppose your mother shouts at you asking you to do something and you oblige her; hereafter, she makes it a habit to shout because it is rewarding.

Other Sources of Aggression

Apart from what has been said above, there are several other social, psychological and environmental factors that may elicit aggressive behavior. Probably the most common source of aggression is verbal insult or negative evaluation a person receives from others. The insulting remark may be unintentional. But if it is perceived as intended and if the harmful intent is attributed to the insulter, the insult is perceived as an aggressive act. This act arouses aggression in the person being insulted and this person reacts with counter-aggression. When we are interested in preserving our self-esteem, such insults may end in physical aggression.

Aggression may also result when we have to comply with an authority figure who orders us to aggress against others. This happens when we have to obey an undesirable order. Often, unpleasant or aversive environmental conditions, such as extreme heat, intense noise, provocation, painful stimuli and crowding, may also trigger aggression. It is reported that the presence of weapons in settings where aggression might be expected increases the aggression of people who are already angered. But we do not always exhibit aggression when we encounter these conditions. Most often we inhibit or control aggression and think of non-aggressive ways of dealing with the situation.

Many people use several types of *self-justification* to make it psychologically comfortable to harm others. They may blame the victims for imagined wrongs or convince themselves that they deserve it. Aggressors often dehumanize the victims; the victims may be treated as animals. Freud believed that aggressive impulses build up over time and they have to be released. The discharge of aggressive impulses is called **catharsis**, which reduces the impulse to aggress at least temporarily. But the public expression of aggression is punished by the society. So, Freud thought that these aggressive impulses are channeled into socially approved activities such as sports (hunting, boxing). Or an individual may watch violent sports or identify with people who behave violently, thus discharging his/her own aggressive impulses *vicariously*. For example, you are discharging your aggressive impulses vicariously when you enjoy watching your favorite hero in a movie smashes the villain to pieces.

Gender Differences in Aggression

It is commonly believed that men are more aggressive than women. Is it true? Of course, more men than women are arrested for violent crimes. Does this mean that there is a large and consistent difference between men and women in their tendency to engage in aggressive behavior? Research results are unequivocal in this regard. Several studies show that the incidence of violent acts is more among men than women. Others suggest the differences are not as big as it is believed. It is suggested that feminine violence is often overlooked or condoned by the law-enforcing authorities. Further, men are likely to commit physical aggression (kicking, punching, using weapons) more than other forms of violence, while women are more likely to engage in verbal aggression (abusing, insulting, yelling, and humiliating) than men. Women are found to engage in indirect forms of aggression such as spreading rumors, gossiping about others, ignoring, avoiding or not talking to the target person. A recent study of school children suggests that boys "fight" while the girls "manipulate" when it comes to aggression. Males and females differ to some extent in their attitude toward aggression. Men do not report guilt or anxiety about engaging in aggressive behavior, while women report greater concern over the consequences of aggression (threat to their own safety if the victim retaliates). Remember, there are several factors contributing to inhibition of public show of aggression by women. Contrasting sex-role training practices and socialization processes for boys and girls may be factors contributing to the apparent gender differences. There are some hints that genetic and hormonal factors also play their role in producing gender differences in the expression of aggression.

Prevention and Control of Aggression

By now you have realized that aggression is the result of a complex interplay between a variety of factors—biological, sociological and psychological. External factors (provocation, frustrations), cognitive factors (attributions, memories, perceptions) and biological factors, all contribute to expression of aggressiveness. People may not be programmed to fight and kill. They are taught to do so. As we witness every day, people are trained to kill others as well as themselves (terrorists, and suicide bombers). If so, can we not teach them not to kill? If people can be taught to die, can we not teach them to live and let others live? In short, the question simply is: Can we prevent aggression or at least reduce its incidence. Social psychologists believe that aggression is not an inevitable pattern of behavior and suggest several techniques of controlling its occurrence. While the suggestions offered to limit aggression give us hope, it is difficult to put them into practice. Anyway, we shall review some of the techniques suggested to control aggression.

Punishment

Punishing has been one of the classic approaches to control aggression. We have seen in the chapter on learning that any behavior followed by a punishment suppresses that behavior. Therefore, unpleasant events such as chastisements, fines, embarrassment, arrest, imprisonment and the like may be employed as deterrents to reduce the incidence of aggression. Punishment appears to work when it is strong, when the aggressor is sure of receiving it, when it immediately follows aggressive behavior, when the payoff for aggression is not great, and when the person perceives that the punishment is legitimate and appropriate. But it is evident (as seen in the increasing number of prisoners in our jails) that punishment really is not an effective method of controlling crime and violence. In fact, when punishment is used ineffectively, it may increase aggressive behavior; punishment frustrates the individual and leads to more aggression.

Catharsis

We have seen that catharsis is the name given to the act of discharging pent up aggression. When we are angry, we shout, pound on the table, kick a pet dog or go out and watch a boxing bout; thus we ventilate our anger, we get it out of our mind. Catharsis may temporarily reduce anger, but it does not reduce the likelihood of our becoming angry in the future against the particular person who provoked the anger in us. Cathartic relief comes only when you show aggression against the source of provocation.

Exposure to Non-aggressive Models

If aggressive models can induce aggression in us, can non-aggressive models lessen them? Research says *yes*. When we are exposed to prosocial acts in the media or in real life, the possibility of imitating (modeling) such behavior also increases. Studies have shown that persons exposed to the actions of non-aggressive models, later demonstrated lower levels of aggression than persons not exposed to such models, even under highly provoking situations.

Cognitive Interventions

Often, apologizing sincerely for a wrong doing is likely to reduce the anger. Providing reasonable explanations for provocative actions are found to be highly effective in reducing aggression. Suppose your friend had promised to meet you for an urgent and important work at a known time, but comes an hour late and offers an apology and gives genuine and convincing reasons (traffic jam, car breakdown) for late coming, in all probability, you will not be angry with him/her.

Training in Social Skills

Lack of social skills to handle aggressive encounters is a major handicap in several people. Often people do not know how to respond to provocations from others. Instead of soothing other person's anger, they flame it. Some people do not know how to make their wishes explicit to others and feel frustrated when others do not respond favorably. They have an abrasive style of self-expression and are insensitive to signs of other's emotional states. Because of these inadequacies, such people experience repeated frustrations and say and do things that unnecessarily trigger anger in others around them. Fortunately, psychologists have provided systematic procedures to teach certain social skills. It is reported that those who master these skills show a dramatic decrease in aggressive outbursts. Bienert and Schneider identified among school children deficits in social skills, such as inability in recognizing others' feelings, using self-control, dealing with embarrassment and dealing with teasing. When children with aggressive-disruptive tendencies were trained to acquire effective social skills, their aggressive tendencies decreased.

Incompatible Response

You know one cannot experience two incompatible emotions or make two incompatible responses. This idea can be employed in reducing aggressive episodes. When an angry person is made to experience emotional states such as empathy, mild sexual arousal or humor that are incompatible with aggression, the latter state shows a decline. The positive feelings produced by pleasant emotions will reduce the negative feelings associated with anger and the aggressive tendencies decline.

PROSOCIAL BEHAVIOR: HELPING OTHERS

We see acts of violence all around us very frequently. But we should not lose sight of acts of bravery, kindness and plenty of benevolent deeds performed by humans all over the world. In this section, we shall discuss one of the forms social behaviors known as prosocial behavior. The term **prosocial behavior** refers to acts that are beneficial to others, but that have no obvious benefits to the person who carries them out. Terms such as helping behavior, charitable behavior, and altruistic behavior are also used to refer to good things people do to assist other people who are in need. Often, prosocial behavior may involve an element of risk for the individual who helps. They do it all the same. Why? Why do we help others? Psychologists have tried to determine the variables that predict who does and who does not engage in helping behavior in an emergency.

Early Studies of Helping Behavior

Very little was known about prosocial behavior before 1960. It was a real life incident, which occurred on March 13, 1964, at 3.20 am in New York that kindled research interest in this area. On that fateful night, a 28-year-old lady named Kitty Genovese was returning home after her job as manager of a bar. After parking her car, when she was about to enter her apartment building, a knife wielding assailant tried to rape her. The lady ran, but the assailant chased her and stabbed her. She screamed for help; the lights came on in many apartment windows that overlooked the scene. The attacker retreated, but after a while came back to resume his assault on the screaming young woman. Finally, he raped her and stabbed her repeatedly until she died. The attack lasted about 40 minutes, during which time her screams and pleas were heard by at least 38 neighbors. Many of them came to their windows to see what was happening. Yet nobody came to her rescue; by the time anyone called the police, the lady was dead. The incident created a public furore. Next morning, newspapers and TVs described the barbaric event in detail suggesting that people in general were callous, unresponsive, selfish, apathetic and indifferent to the plight of others. This picture of contemporary humans is not completely true. There are instances when people have lost their lives in a valiant attempt to save others. Consider the heroic efforts of firefighters and police officers who responded to terrorist attacks at the World Trade Center and at Mumbai. Many civilians have lost their lives as they stopped to help others at these sites. Also, think of the people who protested and resisted repressive political regimes at the risk of imprisonment and even death. Therefore, the question is not whether people will help others in need, but under what conditions will they help.

Two psychologists, John Darley and Bib Letané, became interested in finding out why people do or do not help in an emergency. Our indifferent attitude toward people in distress and failure to help others in an emergency has come to be called **bystander apathy**. When people offered help to those who were in difficulty, then that behavior is referred to as **bystander intervention**. Darley and Letané proposed that the inaction of the bystanders in the Genovese case resulted from the fact that there were so many people at the scene, and that no one person felt responsible for taking action. This phenomenon is called **diffusion of responsibility**. The hypothesis that as the number of bystanders increases the diffused responsibility results in a decrease in prosocial behavior has been supported by a number of studies. The finding that as the number of bystanders witnessing an emergency increases, the likelihood of each bystander's responding and the speed of responding decrease has come to be known as **bystander effect**. The bystander effect was demonstrated in one of the ingenious experiments conducted by Darley and Letané (1968). Let us briefly describe the experiment.

Participants in the experiment were college students. They were told that they would discuss with fellow students some of the problems of attending college in high pressure urban setting. The participants were informed that each of them would be assigned to a separate room and could communicate only by an intercom system; they could hear each other, but the experimenter would not be listening. This arrangement was supposed to avoid any embarrassment about discussing personal matters. Some participants were told that they were one of two participants, others that they were part of a group of three, and still others that six students are participating in the discussion. Each student was supposed to talk for 2 minutes after which the listener or listeners would comment on what they heard. In reality, only one participant took part in each session and the other participant or participants were simply tape recordings. Thus, the stage was set for a controlled emergency apparently overheard by varying number of bystanders. In each session, the first person to speak was the tape-recorded individual who was to be the "victim". He said, sounding embarrassed, that he sometimes has seizures, especially when facing a stressful situation such as exams. After the participant (and in two of the conditions, other 'participants') had given a two-minute talk about college problems, the victim spoke. He says that he is having a seizure and needs immediate help without which he may die. Having said this he chokes, and then remains quiet. The experimenters measured bystander intervention in two ways:

1. Whether the participant left the room to look for the imaginary victim.
2. The time taken to initiate action.

As predicted by the researchers, as the number of apparent bystanders increased, the percentage of subjects who attempted to help decreased, and among those who did respond, an increase in the number of bystanders led to increased delay in taking action. Among those who thought that they were the only witness, 85 percent tried to help and did so within one minute (52 seconds). Such responsiveness decreased and slowed down as the number of bystanders increased.

When the subjects thought there were two more participants, 62 percent tried to help and the delay was about 93 seconds; when they thought that there were five more participants, only 31 percent tried to help and the time delay was 166 seconds. So the bystander effect was clearly demonstrated.

The experiment thus nullifies the common belief that *"there is safety in numbers"* when it comes to receiving help. A number of researches conducted by Darley and Letané and several others have added to our understanding of the psychological factors contributing to or interfering with a prosocial response. Now we know that several situational and personal factors, such as not being in a hurry, recently observing a prosocial role model and being in a good mood, increase likelihood of helping someone in need. Based on their work and others' researches, Darley and Letané have proposed a five-step (or choice points) model of prosocial behavior. At each step, various factors, such as the number of bystanders and the characteristics of bystanders, determine the likelihood that someone will or will not help.

Five-step Model of Helping Behavior

Noticing the emergency: Whether a person helps or not depends on whether he notices that there is an emergency situation. If he is preoccupied with other activities and does not attend to the emergency situation, no helping behavior ensues. Only when one notices the emergency, he moves to the next step.

Perceiving that an emergency exists: Helping depends on the correct interpretation of the situation. If the situation is ambiguous and not clear, the likelihood of help declines. If we see that other witnesses are not reacting to the emergency, we keep quiet (effect of **social comparison**). We may suffer from **evaluation apprehension**, a fear that we might be ridiculed if we try to intervene because there may be no emergency at all. Imagine a situation where a husband is beating his wife. If you intervene, the wife may resent your intervention saying: "My husband has every right to beat me. Who are you to come in between?" Therefore, only when we perceive clearly that there is an emergency, we go to the next step.

Assuming responsibility to help: At the third decision point, the bystander asks the question, "Is it my business to help? There are so many others, let them help". If he is alone the tendency to own responsibility increases. If there are others, the diffusion of responsibility comes into operation. If one owns responsibility, he moves on to the next step.

Knowing what to do: Once the responsibility is assumed, the next issue is whether the bystander knows what to do and how to help. Suppose somebody is drowning and you do not know swimming, how can you help? The bystander must be capable and confident, only then can he proceed to the next step.

Deciding to help: The final process is the decision to help or not to help. Among several factors influencing the decision to help is the costs involved. May be you will injure yourself badly or the help is rejected and you look foolish in offering to help. Generally, you help acquaintances rather than strangers.

So, helping behavior is affected by several factors such as the situation (number of bystanders present, the ambiguity of the situation, etc.), temporary influences on the bystander (time pressure), and learned skills (ability to swim, training in first aid). In addition, the personality characteristics of the bystanders and the characteristics of the victim also influence prosocial behavior.

Characteristics of the Helper

Researchers have shown that people with certain characteristics such as a ***need for***

approval, a disposition to feel personal and social responsibility, high agreeableness and an empathic concern for others are more likely to engage in helping behaviors than those who are low on these traits. It is found that helpers tend to have an *internal locus of control* and less concern for their own welfare. Group identity plays a significant role in prosocial behavior; people are more likely to help and cooperate with members of their own group. Children who are exposed to helping models (parents, teachers and significant others) tend to acquire helping behavior. Positive emotional states sometimes increase and sometimes decrease the tendency to engage in helping behavior. Positive emotions lead to prosocial activities if social concerns are involved, the consequences of helping are pleasant rather than unpleasant and the need for help is unambiguous. Positive emotions lead to decrease in helping behavior if the need is ambiguous or if the consequences of helping are unpleasant.

As with positive emotions, negative emotions can increase or decrease the tendency to help depending on the circumstances. Prosocial behaviors increase if there is **empathy** toward the person needing help, if the helpers think that they are responsible for their negative emotions, if the need for help is unambiguous and if the task of helping is interesting. Negative mood inhibits helping behavior if the persons are concerned with themselves and the helpers do not feel responsible for their negative emotions. We help others when we consider it as an opportunity for personal development. The rewards of helping are apparent and the cost of not helping is more as we may feel ashamed and guilty.

Characteristics of the Person Being Helped

We are more likely to help friends, those who are similar to us in age and whom we like. Help is offered more often to an attractive victim than an unattractive one. Variables that increase attraction also increase prosocial behavior. Males tend to help women more than men, whereas women are more likely to help other women than men in need of help. We are likely to help people we believe are not responsible for their plight and those who give a socially acceptable justification for their predicament. A general social norm is that when a person runs into trouble because of his/her own carelessness and irresponsibility, it is up to that person to solve the problem. That is the reason why we do not help a drunkard lying on the footpath. We feel disgusted at the sight of an inebriated person and this negative feeling inhibits our tendency to help. But when we know the person is not responsible for his plight, we respond with empathy, which increases the motivation to help. Thus, we may help an unconscious stranger with injuries lying on the roadside.

One way to get help is to ask for it. But some people find it difficult to ask for help and thus are less likely to get it. For example, shy individuals do not ask for help from members of the opposite sex. Generally, women seek help more often than men, the elderly seek help less often than young adults and people from high socioeconomic strata ask for help more frequently than those from low socioeconomic levels. One reason why people are reluctant to ask for help is the belief that they will be viewed as incompetent when they seek help. One researcher (Nadler, 1993) found that help-seeking could be stigmatizing. He suggests that help seeking activates the basic human dilemma, the conflict between independence and dependence and between personal adequacy and inadequacy; hence people generally tend to refuse help. Also seeking or receiving help reduces a person's self-esteem, especially when seeking help from friends and relatives. Under such circumstances, the victim may respond with negative feelings toward the helper. An American study (Searcy and Eisenberg, 1992) suggests that seeking help from a sibling elicits negative feeling. It was found that receiving help from a sister was less threatening than from a brother. Help from older sisters was less threatening and receiving help from a younger brother was the most threatening.

Why Do People Help? Theories of Prosocial Behavior

A number of explanations have been proposed in answering this question. An exposition of all the theories of prosocial behavior is beyond the scope of this chapter. Because these theories reflect upon important assumptions about human nature (whether humans are basically good or selfish), a brief summary of these theories is given below.

Evolutionary Theory

Evolutionary psychologists and socio-biologists propose that helping behavior is genetically determined and shaped by evolution. Sociobiological concepts are based on the theory of natural selection. It is generally believed that physical attributes are selected for purposes of successful adaptation to the environment. Behaviors that increase an organism's reproductive success are assumed to be represented in subsequent generations more often than behaviors that are irrelevant to reproduction. Prosocial behavior can be seen throughout the animal kingdom. Studies of animals indicate that they tend to help other animals who share their genes, namely, offspring and genetic relatives. This tendency known as the ***"selfish gene"***effect acts to protect and promote survival of those who are genetically similar to yourself. Therefore, organisms tend to help one another, so that they may survive and pass on their genes to the next generation. Each individual is unconsciously motivated to perpetuate his own genes and the species. This process is called **maximizing inclusive fitness**. These concepts are difficult to establish and are subject of controversy.

Empathy-Altruism Theory

Altruism refers to helping another with the sole purpose of enhancing that person's welfare, but without anticipating anything in return. Empathy is the ability to experience and share others' feelings as though it is your own. Daniel Batson (Batson et al, 2004) believes that true altruism exists among humans and it is produced by empathy. We are distressed when we see someone in distress. This behavior appears to be determined by evolutionary processes and it is noticed among monkeys and apes. It is also observed among 12-month-old children. The empathic concern is common among adults, especially those who were raised in families where such behavior is encouraged. Batson's empathy-altruism hypothesis proposes that at least some prosocial behavior is motivated solely by the desire to help the recipient (Batson and Oleson, 1991), and a bystander without empathic concern escapes the scene when it is easy to do so. This observation has also been supported by other researchers.

Social Learning Theory

When we are exposed to prosocial models early in life and taught prosocial norms, the tendency to help others is enhanced. Two social norms contribute to the development of prosocial behavior. One is the **norm of reciprocity**, which states that we should help those who have helped us and the other, **norm of social responsibility**, which states that people should help others and contribute to the welfare of society. We receive positive reinforcements when we adhere to these norms and we are punished when we violate them. According to the principles of social learning, when we observe others being praised for their helping behavior, we try to internalize such behavior.

Egoistic Theory

According to this theory, altruism is based on the individual's selfish desire to feel better. There are two varieties of egoistic theory. One is the **negative-state relief model**, which states that when we are experiencing negative emotions, we are motivated to help others as a way of relieving ourselves from such feelings. The other is the **empathic joy hypothesis**, which proposes that prosocial behavior is motivated by the joy we experience when we observe that somebody's need is satisfied and we are responsible for that. Empathy leads to prosocial behavior only when the helper can observe the consequences of his/her helping. Without this egoistic reward, empathy does not lead to helping behavior.

We shall conclude the section on prosocial behavior with a positive note. Psychologists believe that prosocial behavior among humans can be increased. They have used prosocial modeling (exposing people to helping models), as one method, which is consistent with social learning theory. For example, when you watch people donating blood, you will be tempted to do so. There is research evidence to show that when you develop feelings of empathy and relatedness with others, you are more likely to help. Also, simply learning about factors that hinder or inhibit bystander intervention may increase the tendency to help people in distress.

BEHAVIOR IN GROUPS

We humans are gregarious animals. For that matter, all living beings, except the solitary wasp, and some saints, live in groups. The importance of living in groups can be realized from the fact that one of the severe forms of punishment for crime is solitary confinement. We prefer to live in groups and enjoy it. We belong to a family (primary group), a club (secondary group), a religion, a society, a nation and so many other social institutions (groups). Almost all our behavior occurs in groups. We form groups to share our interests, perform tasks and achieve goals. The impact of groups on us is enormous and it occurs in several ways. We shall examine in this section some of the important ways in which groups influence our behavior. But before that let us know what a group is.

What Constitutes a Group?

The question is simple, but social psychologists have long wrestled with the question and have come with a number of definitions for group. We find some commonalities in their definitions. In any group, there is regular interaction among members, some kind of social and emotional bonding with one another, a common outlook and some degree of interdependence. An acceptable definition of group is that it *consists of two or more interacting persons, who share common goals, have a stable relationship, are somehow interdependent, and perceive that they are in fact part of a group* (Paulus, 1989). The term group does not apply to a collection of people who happen to be in the same place at the same time. Therefore, passengers in a railway coach or people watching a movie do not constitute a group. When we are members of a group, we do not think, feel or act as individuals; we think, feel and act as members of a group. We are not driven by individual goals; we work for group goals.

Why do we join groups? We join groups because it satisfies some of our psychosocial needs. We can achieve certain goals only when we are members of a group. Belonging to a group provides us a sense of security. Group membership enriches our self-image and gives us a sense of identity. Sometimes it is prestigious to be a member of a group such as a reputed club or a political party. There are innumerable other reasons for joining a group; that is why we often try hard to acquire membership of one group or the other.

How do groups influence us? Again, there are several ways in which we are influenced by groups. We are attracted to some groups, we conform to group norms and we are persuaded by group pressures. Specifically, groups affect our behavior in decision making and work efficiency. We shall take up these issues a bit later. Before that let us learn about some general ways in which groups affect us. Psychologists have agreed on four aspects of the group that play a crucial role in this regard; these are roles, status, norms and cohesiveness.

Roles

Behaviors that members in different positions in a group are expected to perform are called **social roles**. Groups create different roles to fulfill different group functions. Every member of a group is assigned a role, which he is expected to play. In a family, father plays his role, mother plays her role and similarly other members are expected to function according to the roles assigned to them. In an organization such as club, association or a political party, there is a president, a secretary, a treasurer and general body members. Each of them fulfills his/her role. A role may be assigned officially by an authority figure of the group like the principal of a college. One may be elected to play a role like the president of the students' union. Sometimes a member may gradually acquire a role, as in the case of an emerging leader. A role may be task-oriented (getting a job done) or relations-oriented (maintaining cordial relationships among members and avoiding friction). Thus, roles clarify the responsibilities and obligations and determine the thoughts and actions of members of the group to which they belong. Sometimes roles come to curtail the freedom of members giving rise to certain negative reactions.

Status

In any group, different roles are associated with different degrees of status. For example, the principal of a college enjoys certain privileges that go with his status. He has a large room, posh furniture and enjoys certain other luxuries. There is a ***status hierarchy*** in which different roles go with varying amounts of power and prestige. You can easily identify a member with high status by his walk, talk and other forms of non-verbal behavior. A high status member can order, criticize and can interrupt the activities of others.

Norms

A set of rules established by a group called '**social norms**' regulate the behavior of each member of that group. Whether implicit or explicit, formal or informal, norms are shared beliefs that are enforced through the group's uses of rewards or punishments. The norms tell the group members how to behave ***(prescriptive norms)*** or how not to behave ***(proscriptive norms)***. Adherence to norms is a basic requirement for membership of a group. Norms may be established by leaders or may result from critical events in the group's evolution or they may be simply carried over from the past. Whatever the way, once formed, norms determine how the individual behaves within the group. Regardless of whether norms are explicit or implicit, one fact is clear: *we obey them most of the time.*

Cohesiveness

All the forces that act on the members causing them to remain a part of the group or belong to the group lead to **cohesiveness** of the group. Generally, the forces are mutual attraction among members, interdependence and shared goals. The degree to which each member likes the other is called ***interpersonal***

cohesiveness and the extent to which group membership helps in the attainment of personal goals is called ***task-based cohesion***. Often cohesiveness is determined by efforts made by the members to get admitted to the group.

Performance in Groups

There are certain tasks that are better performed alone, such as writing a love letter. But most of the tasks are done in the presence of others or with others. Then the question arises: What is the effect of the presence of others on task performance? The issue has been extensively studied by psychologists. There are two aspects to this issue:

1. What is the effect of the mere presence of others on task performance?
2. Is group performance more or less efficient than individual performance?

Performance in the Presence of Others

The term **social facilitation** is used by social psychologists to refer to any effect on performance stemming from the presence of others. The term refers both to increase and decrease in performance. Early researches about the issue yielded conflicting results. Sometimes the performance improved and at other times it suffered when others were present. The first attempt to clarify the issue was made by Zajonc (1965) in his theory, **drive theory of social facilitation**. According to the theory, the presence of others increases the level of arousal. Increased arousal enhances the occurrence of ***dominant responses*** (well-learned, simple responses an individual is most likely to make in a given situation). The dominant responses may be either correct or incorrect in a particular situation. Under conditions of arousal, the theory predicted two possible outcomes:

1. The presence of others will facilitate performance when an individual's dominant responses are the correct ones for the particular situation.
2. The presence of others will impair performance when a person's dominant responses are incorrect for the situation.

Thus, it is implied that the presence of others will facilitate the performance of strong, well-learned responses, but may interfere with the performance of new, complex and as yet unmastered responses. An example will make the points clear. A musician in a concert may perform an old song better than a newly acquired one, whereas he may sing both of them equally well at home. Studies by Zajonc and several others supported the theory. Later, researchers indicated that social facilitation is produced by other factors as well in addition to the presence of others. They have shown that two other factors contribute to social facilitation. One is **evaluation apprehension** (the fear of being judged by others); the other is **self-presentation** (attempts to look good in the presence of others). Finally, a third explanation for social facilitation was provided by RS Baron (1986) and colleagues, which is known as **distraction-conflict theory**. According to this theory, the presence of others produces a conflict between two tendencies:

1. The tendency to pay attention to the task being performed.
2. The tendency to pay attention to an audience.

The conflict produced by these two competing tendencies increases arousal, which in turn enhances the tendency to perform dominant responses. All the three theories have received research support, but still the final answer to the phenomena of social facilitation is awaited.

Group Versus Individual Performance

Earlier we asked the question: Do groups perform better than individuals? The answer is fairly complex. True, working in groups has certain advantages. It permits individuals to pool their resources, knowledge, skill and equipment. It also allows for division of labor. But working in groups has also certain disadvantages. When the group is highly cohesive, members may spend more time in exchanging pleasantries than on task performance. There may be pressure to maintain status quo, which comes in the way of developing more efficient ways of working. There is a possibility that conflicts between members may interfere with efficient performance. With increase in the size of the group, coordination of activities may suffer. But research in the area suggests that whether group performance is better or not depends on the type of tasks. Generally four types of tasks are identified:

1. Additive tasks in which the contributions of each member are combined into a single group product.
2. Compensatory tasks in which the contributions of the various members are averaged together to form a single group product.
3. Disjunctive tasks in which the group's product is determined by the performance of its best or most competent member.
4. Conjunctive tasks in which the group's final product is determined by the poorest performing worker.

Available evidence suggests that on additive and compensatory tasks, groups often perform better than individual members. Groups are about as good as the best member in the case of disjunctive tasks. Finally, groups are less productive than individuals on conjunctive tasks.

Social Loafing

One of the undesirable phenomenon observed when people work in groups is **social loafing**, the tendency among people to expend less individual effort, while working in a group. It is quite common when people are performing additive tasks because it is difficult identify the contribution of each member. Some people work hard, while others pretend as if they are working. The existence of social loafing has been demonstrated both in the laboratory and in real work settings. It occurs in all cultures, in both sexes (although more prevalent among men than in women) and under a wide range of situations. Social loafing can be prevented by instilling a sense of responsibility in each participant, by making the task attractive and by emphasizing the importance of successful performance for the group's well-being. Other members of the group may react to social loafing with anger, resentment, annoyance and even withdrawal. Surprisingly, sometimes it may lead other members to work hard, a phenomenon known as **social compensation**. You must have watched in certain situations some people working very hard, irrespective of whether others work equally well or not.

Decision Making in Groups

Most of the vital decisions that affect our daily life are made by groups. Most of our laws, policies and practices are decided by committees, commissions, boards of directors and such other expert bodies—not by single individuals. Group decision making is common in political parties, military strategists, sport teams and among clinicians engaged in medical treatment. We assume that groups make better decisions than individuals. Is it true? In answering this question, social psychologists have brought into light several interesting phenomena pertaining to group decision making.

Social Decision Making Schemes

When groups make decisions, they generally follow some simple rules known as **social decision schemes**. For example, one such scheme is called ***majority-wins rule***, which suggests that the group will accept the views supported by a majority of members. A second one called ***truth-wins rule*** suggests that ultimately members will make the correct decision (even if it is held by a minority) after they have come to recognize the inherent correctness of the solution. The third one called the ***two-third majority rule*** is self-explanatory. Finally, some groups appear to follow what is called ***first-shift rule***—members tend to adopt a decision consistent with the direction of the first shift in opinion shown by any mèmber. Different rules seem to be effective under different situations. The first one works well when the decision involves judgments or opinions and the second is good for decisions concerning intellectual tasks. The third one is generally followed by the jury in the courts.

Risky Shift or Group Polarization

A student of psychology named James Stoner conducted a small piece of research in 1961 for his masters thesis, which became a talking point for several years. Stoner wanted to know the type of decisions groups make as opposed to individuals. For his study, Stoner asked college students to advise imaginary people to make decisions about two alternatives, one attractive but risky and the other less appealing but safe. For example, in one situation a person had to decide between accepting a low-paid but secure job or a well-paid job with an uncertain future. Which would he prefer? In the first part of the experiment, Stoner asked the participants to make the decision individually and in the second part, after group discussion. Stoner expected that the group decision would be more conservative than individual decisions. But the results showed the opposite trend. The groups appeared to make riskier decisions than individuals. This phenomenon came to be known as **risky shift**.

Early studies about the risky shift appeared to confirm the operation of the phenomenon. Later, the picture became complicated. In some studies, the group discussion tended toward risk taking, but in others the decision making showed a shift toward caution. Eventually, a clear answer appeared. What actually appeared like the risky shift was found to be a shift toward polarization. It was found that group discussion led individual members to become more extreme, not simply more risky or more cautious. That is, if a member initially was mildly opposed to a decision, after group discussion, he/she became more opposed; similarly, if the member was less favorable, he became more favorable after the group discussion. This effect came to be known as **group polarization**. Why does group polarization occur? One reason is that during group discussion a member hears convincing arguments about his initial views and hence his views will be strengthened. Another is that a member realizes that several others are holding similar views and he tries to be better than others, and hence takes an extreme stand. Both explanations are supported by research findings, but some doubts are also raised. Regardless of the precise nature of group polarization, it definitely has important implications. Group polarization may lead many decision making groups to adopt increasingly extreme positions, which may turn out to be dangerous. There are several pitfalls in group decision-making and one that has been studied extensively is groupthink.

Groupthink

Often, smart people make dumb decisions! Several factors emerging out of group discussion can lead groups to take disastrous courses of action. One of the flawed approaches to group-decision making is known as **groupthink**, a phenomenon introduced and studied by social psychologist Irving Janis (1982). Groupthink is a tendency of group members to suspend rational and critical thinking in order to maintain group consensus (Janis called it ***concurrence seeking***). In a group discussion, if the primary concern is to reach a unanimous decision rather than the best decision, then groupthink is in operation. Under such conditions, members are more concerned to agreeing with each other rather than thinking realistically to come to a correct decision.

According to Janis, groupthink is most likely to occur when a group:

1. Is under high pressure to reach a decision.
2. Is insulated from outside information.
3. Has a directive leader.
4. Is highly cohesive.

When groupthink emerges, members come to view their group as invulnerable (one that does not make wrong decisions) and engage in collective rationalization (discrediting or ignoring any information opposed to the group's views). The members start thinking that their group is right, morally superior, and all others are confused. Members who have lingering doubts engage in self-censorship; and if they do not, other members will silence them. Finally, there are some self-appointed "mind guards" who try to shield the members from outside information that is not in agreement with the group's views. All these factors create an illusion of the group's infallibility and an attitude of intolerance toward dissent. Social psychologists have identified several historic decisions that potentially involved groupthink leading to catastrophic consequences. Some of them include the decision by President Kennedy to launch the "Bay of Pigs" military operation in Cuba, the fatal launch of the space shuttle Challenger in 1986 and the fiery disintegration of the space shuttle Columbia in 2003. Probably, the decision to declare emergency in India in 1975 might be considered as a result of groupthink.

Can we prevent the operation of groupthink? Janis believed that we might if the leader remains impartial during discussions, encourages critical thinking, brings in outsiders to offer their opinions and divides the larger group into subgroups—to see if each subgroup independently comes to the same decision. In short, it is accepted that something like groupthink exists and it affects the decisions of important decision-making bodies. The precise nature of groupthink may be somewhat different from what Janis proposed, but the fact remains that he has called our attention to the study of an important aspect of group decision making.

Chapter Summary

You have learnt in this chapter that our thoughts, feelings and behavior occur in a social environment and these are influenced by people around us. Social psychologists have shed light on how we interpret the behavior of others (attribution), how we behave in the presence of others (social influence) and how we relate to others (social relations) among other social phenomena. Society impacts us enormously. We walk, talk, dress and engage in innumerable number of activities in specific ways because of the presence of others. Can you imagine how you would have behaved if you were alone in this world? Difficult, isn't it? But do not think that we are always road-rolled by the society. Often we resist socialization and try to think and behave in the way we want. When the whole world thought that the sun rises in the east and sets in the west, Copernicus thought differently. So, do not think that your behavior is totally under the control of others. You, as a person, have a role in what you think, act and become. Social psychology is the branch of psychology that deals with how our thoughts, emotions and behavior are influenced by our interactions with others. Social thinking is studied under two overlapping processes: social perception and social cognition. Social perception is the process by which we understand people, form impressions, make judgments and develop attitudes about the people and events that constitute our social world. To obtain information about the temporary causes of behavior, we focus on non-verbal cues such as facial expressions, eye contact, body posture, movements and touching. Knowledge about the lasting causes of other's behavior is obtained through attribution.

Contd...

Contd...

Attribution is a personal explanation we form about the causes of our own and other's behavior and events. According to Heider, we tend to explain events by attributing them to either dispositional (internal) causes or situational (external or environmental) causes. There are two important theories of attribution: Jones and Davis's theory of correspondent inference and Kelley's theory of causal attribution. The theory of correspondent inference is concerned with how we decide, on the basis of other's overt actions, that they possess specific traits they carry with them across situations and over time. According to Kelley, three types of information—*consistency*, *distinctiveness* and *consensus*—determine the attributions we make. When consensus and distinctiveness are low, but consistency is high, we attribute behavior to internal causes. In contrast, we are most likely to attribute another's behavior to external causes under conditions in which consensus, consistency and distinctiveness are all high. People make several errors in attributing causes to behavior. The fundamental attribution error refers to our tendency to attribute other's behavior to internal (dispositional) causes and overlook situational (environmental) influences. The tendency to attribute our own behavior to situational (external) causes, but of others to internal (dispositional) causes is called actor-observer effect. The tendency to attribute positive outcomes to internal causes but negative ones to external factors is known as the self-serving bias.

We all think that first impressions are important. We form such impressions by combining available information weighted in terms of its importance. People employ several tactics to make favorable impression on others. These include improved personal appearance and various forms of other enhancement, such as agreeing with others' views and flattery. These are known as impression management techniques and often they succeed.

Social cognition refers to thinking about others and the social world. It consists of processes through which we notice, interpret, remember and later use information about the social world. We use heuristics (mental short-cuts) to minimize the effort in understanding the social world. Two, often used heuristics are representativeness (the extent to which a stimulus is similar to other related stimuli) and availability (the ease with which information can be brought to mind). While engaged in social cognition we pay more attention to information inconsistent with our expectations than to information that is consistent. We tend to notice and emphasize negative social information, a phenomenon called automatic vigilance. We need more information to reach conclusions inconsistent with our initial preference than we do to reach conclusions consistent with these preferences; this phenomenon is called 'motivated skepticism'.

Attitudes are enduring mental representations of features of social or physical stimuli (persons, objects, actions, events) along with evaluations of those features. Attitudes are primarily acquired through experience, and they exert a directive influence on subsequent behavior. They are acquired through classical conditioning, operant conditioning and/or social learning. Attitudes have cognitive, affective and behavioral components. Persuasion is the process of changing attitudes. Early models of persuasion focused on characteristics of communicators, communications and the audience. Newer theories, such as elaboration likelihood model (ELM) and the heuristic model focus on cognitive factors. The principle of reciprocity plays a role in persuasion; that is, the extent to which others yield to our efforts depends on the extent to which we yield to their efforts in changing attitudes. Our ability to resist persuasion is determined by factors such as reactance (efforts to protect personal freedom), forewarning (advance knowledge that someone is trying to change our attitude) and selective avoidance of information inconsistent with our attitude. Contrary to popular belief, people are prone to change their attitudes throughout life. When there is inconsistency between two attitudes we hold, there is cognitive dissonance. Dissonance reduction is often done by changing attitudes.

Social influence refers to the efforts on the part of one person to alter the behavior or attitudes of one or more others. Three types of well-researched social influence (in addition to persuasion) are conformity, compliance and obedience. Conformity occurs when people change their attitudes or behavior in order to adhere to existing social norms. Asch's researches brought to light several startling factors about conformity behavior. Compliance involves direct efforts by individuals to change the behavior of others. Ingratiation, multiple requests, that is not all, foot-in-the-door and door-in-the-face are some of the techniques used to obtain compliance. In obedience direct orders are given by one to change the behavior of another person. It is found that many persons obey commands from authority figure.

Contd...

Contd...

A crucial aspect of human behavior is establishing close relationships. We like and love some people and dislike and hate others. Interpersonal attraction is enhanced by proximity, mere exposure, similarity of attitudes and physical attractiveness. Love is a form of close and intimate relationship.

Prejudices are negative attitudes toward members of specific social groups and discrimination is negative behavior directed toward members of social groups who are the object of prejudice. It may stem from competition between groups for limited resources or due to the tendencies to divide the social world into two camps, "we" (in-group) and "they" (out-group). Prejudices are taught by parents to children. Stereotypes are beliefs that all other members of specific social groups share certain traits. They are cognitive frameworks that strongly influence the processing of incoming social information and a major contributor to the development of prejudice. Prejudice can be reduced by introducing tolerant attitudes in the minds of children, by encouraging direct contact between in-group and out-group and by inducing counter-stereotypic inferences (thinking about people as individuals rather than as members of stereotyped group). Sexism is a prejudice based on gender stereotypes suggesting that all males and all females share certain traits that distinguish them from each other.

Aggression, the intentional infliction of some form of harm on others, is an undesirable social behavior. Freud, McDougall, and Lorenz have thought of aggression as an innate tendency, an instinct. Drive theories suggest that aggression stems from externally generated motive to harm others. Newer theories suggest that aggression stems from negative reactions to aversive experiences, memories and cognitions. Other suggested causes are frustration (interference with goal-directed activities), direct provocation and watching media violence.

Prosocial behavior is a form of positive social behavior. It refers to actions of people that provide benefit to others without anticipating any obvious benefits in return. Latané and Darley have suggested diffusion of responsibility as one of the causes of bystander apathy. They have proposed a five-step decision–making model to predict helping behavior in emergency situations; noticing (attending to) the emergency, perceiving that it is an emergency, assuming responsibility to help, deciding what needs to be done, and deciding to do it (help). People must make the appropriate decisions at each of the five-steps to engage in a prosocial act. Research hints at the presence of an altruistic personality that predisposes people to engage in helpful behavior. Helpful behavior is influenced by the presence of helpful models, helper's emotional state, attraction toward the recipient of help, and the degree to which the recipient is perceived as responsible for the problem. Several theories of prosocial behavior are proposed such as empathy-altruism model, negative state relief model, empathic joy model and genetic determinism model.

A group consists of two or more persons who share common goals, have a stable relationship, are interdependent and recognize the existence of the group's existence. Groups exert influence on members through roles, status, norms and cohesiveness. Social facilitation refers to the effects on task performance (reduction or increase) from the presence of others. Social loafing refers to the tendency of some members to exert less effort when working in a group situation. Decision-making in groups may result in group polarization (a tendency to shift toward more extreme views) and groupthink (a tendency to become more concerned with consensus than with choosing the best alternative).

CHAPTER 14

Health Psychology

PREVIEW

This chapter on health psychology deals with the influence of psychological factors on health, illness, and well-being. For several years in the past, body and mind were considered as different entities. Medical science, until recently, looked upon disease as purely a biological phenomenon. Psychological factors were not taken into account by most healthcare professionals in dealing with physical ailments. Things have changed during the second half of the 20th century. Today, health and disease are found to be determined by the interaction of body, mind and environment.

We are living in a complex and competitive world that is moving very fast and moving in different directions at the same time. The demands made on humans are extremely stressful. Everybody wants something or the other from you, and they want it quickly, here and now. Parents want their children to stand first in the class. Teachers want students to complete the assignments on time. People face stiff competition in all walks of life—to get a seat in school or college, to secure a profitable job or a promotion in the organization, or to get a suitable bride or groom. Your boss is angry that your work is still pending and wants you to stay late in the office and complete it. Your spouse complains that you never took him/her out for a film. In addition, you have a bad headache or increased acidity in the stomach. Adding to all these hazards, there are strikes, traffic jams, accidents, floods, fires, famine, and worse still, a terrorist attack in the neighborhood. Really you are living in the dirtiest world of the, and it is sickening to live in it.

So, several things are driving you toward sickness. The body and the mind interact in keeping you healthy or sick. Very often, you encounter insurmountable difficulties; your expectations go haywire; disappointments increase and frustrations become chronic. As a consequence, your physiological system loses its balance. When the body is sick, you lack energy, become weak, feel dull and depressed. When you encounter an emotional upheaval, you know how your body reacts. Thus, there is a close relationship between thoughts, emotions and the physiological reactions of the body. So, it is very necessary to pay close attention to psychological factors while dealing with physical illnesses and promoting health. In order to deal with the medical consequences of the interaction between body and mind, a movement called **behavior medicine** has emerged and health psychology is a part of this broader movement. Health psychologists in particular are interested in psychological, sociocultural, and environmental factors that produce illness and affect the chances of recovery.

The main focus of health psychology is on the effect of stress on health and illness. The work of Hans Selye, especially his concept of general adaptation syndrome, has influenced the development of health psychology. Health psychologists have studied extensively the varieties of stressors, how stress is perceived by people, how people react to stress, and the strategies people develop to cope with stress. These studies have revealed several interesting insights into the understanding of the dynamics of health and illness. They have also suggested ways of dealing with stress. Therefore, go ahead, read the chapter. You will learn some skills that may help you to ensure that stress will not end in distress. More importantly, you will be dealing with people who are experiencing pain. A few interesting insights about pain are discussed in the chapter. Knowledge about the origins of pain and the ways of coping with pain will be of special interest to you.

Chapter Outline

Health psychology is one of the youngest branches of psychology. American Psychological Association (APA) formed the Division of Health Psychology (Division 38) in the year 1978. According to APA Division 38, health psychology is the aggregate of the specific educational, scientific and professional contributions of the discipline of psychology to the promotion and maintenance of health, the prevention and treatment of illness and the identification of the etiology and diagnostic correlates of health, illness and related dysfunctions. In short, it is engaged in research on the role of psychology in health and illness. Its goal is to understand the role of psychological processes as aids in improving physical health of people.

For centuries, physicians have been following the ***biomedical approach*** to health and illness. This approach assumes that illness can be fully understood and accounted for in terms of deviations of biological variables from the norm. It supposes that any disease process can be understood in terms of invading pathogens, damage to body parts, or a deviant electrical impulse emerging within the organism. Further, it is dualistic in that it assumes that mind and body are independent and do not influence each other. The approach does not take into consideration the role of social and psychological factors in the genesis and progression of disease. The physicians who adhere to the biomedical approach try to find and fix what is wrong in the body. They may prescribe pills or carry out a surgery. Their goal is to repair the machine (body) and put it back on the track and wait until something else goes wrong. In short, the physicians treat the disease and forget the person (patient). On the other hand, health psychologists propose a ***biopsychosocial model***, which is a philosophical point of view that emphasizes the importance and inter-relatedness of biological, psychological, and social factors in determining health and illness. They do not deny the importance of biological factors; they believe that these are not sufficient to understand wellness and disease. The biopsychosocial model does not separate mind and body. It reflects the WHO definition of health as "a state of complete physical, mental, and social well-being, and not merely the absence of disease or infirmity."

Just as disease conditions can influence psychological functions, psychological processes can affect the course of disease or the experience of illness in several ways. For example, a person suffering from terminal cancer will become depressed; a heart attack may affect the lifestyle and self-concept of an individual (influences of disease on behavior). An anxious person exhibits high blood pressure (effect of psychological state on body function). Psychological factors may also contribute to the maintenance of health. An individual with certain personality traits may abstain from alcohol and drugs, not smoke, and exercise regularly. To get well from a disease, pills or surgery may not be sufficient; a person may have to change diet, stop smoking, exercise, relax, and avoid stress.

CONCERNS OF HEALTH PSYCHOLOGY

Health psychology is concerned with, among others, issues such as:

1. Why and how people cultivate certain health-related habits—good habits such as exercising, dieting and relaxing, and bad habits such as smoking, consuming alcohol, and overeating?
2. What are the factors that make a specific intervention effective in changing an individual's health-related behavior?
3. Why people develop an illness, and why all people exposed to the same kind of risky environment do not develop the same illness?
4. Why different people respond differently to the same disease?
5. How do people's coping styles affect the course of disease?

Health psychologists do not simply try to help people to be free of diseases; they are equally interested in helping people to maintain a state of mental and physical health and develop the ability to do things that are meaningful to them in their lives. Contemporary medical care delivery system can benefit greatly from the expertise of psychologists. They can evaluate the psychological aspects of patient care. They can help the patient to evaluate the lifespan changes that are necessary to accommodate the limitations of illness and to adjust to the treatments necessary to maintain optimal functioning. Health psychologists may work with the family members of the patient to assist them to come to terms with the changes in their own lives that result from the patient's conditions. Some health psychologists are engaged in developing health-promoting programs and present them to the community through the media. They have designed many of the health messages—for quitting smoking, avoiding drug abuse, abstaining from unsafe sex, etc.—for educating public and motivating them to lead healthy lives.

During the last two decades of 20th century, health psychology has made tremendous progress in the application of psychological insights to issues concerning health, illness, and medical treatment. They have provided information regarding both effective modes of psychological care for patients, and specific interventions that assist in people's attempts to stay healthy. In the 1990s, **psychoneuroimmunology (PNI)** emerged as an interdisciplinary science guiding theory and research in health psychology. PNI combines behavioral science, immunology, and neuroscience, and attempts to improve our understanding of psychological factors that influence health and disease through the immune system. PNI has helped us to discover that there is a relationship between emotional state and the success of the immune system in fighting the disease. Today, health psychology is emerging as an indispensable accompaniment of public health delivery program. We shall discuss in the following pages some of the important areas (not all of them) with which health psychology is concerned. First, we focus on stress, which plays an important role in the causation of disease and maintenance of wellness.

STRESS AND WELL-BEING

There are not many people in today's world who are not familiar with the word **stress**. Even school children often say that they are under stress. Several adults attend courses on stress management. Stress is a fact of life. But what exactly is stress? Like many other technical terms, it is difficult to define stress precisely. Long ago, stress was conceptualized according to mechanical principles such as load (external force) and strain (damage resulting from load and stress). Gradually, the term has come to be used in the fields of biology, sociology and psychology. Some people view stress as a stimulus (that which produces feelings of tension, discomfort and even threat to the organism's safety); others consider stress as a response (the physiological and psychological responses to events and situations) and still others call it a process (interaction between the person and the environment involving appraisal of the threat and the ways of dealing with it). So, stress is a complicated concept involving physical, psychological, social components or a combination of all the three. For our purpose, stress may be defined as the pressure placed on an organism to adjust or adapt to changing environments.

STRESS AND STRESSORS

Generally, the term stress is used to refer to an organism's physiological and psychological response to stimuli that threaten the organism's state of equilibrium or well-being. The stimuli that threaten the organism's well-being or equilibrium are called **stressors**. A stressor can be anything, a person, an object or event. It may be meeting an estranged friend, a nagging or suspicious spouse, facing an examination, or executing a plan of action for an institution. Sometimes, even good things can be stressing; for instance, getting married, having a child, the first day in office, or even planning a party. Fortunately, these do not cause illness. Only negative events produce results that are detrimental to health.

All of us face stress in life most of the time. In fact, life is continuous process of encountering a series of repeated stress, finding ways of coping with them and finally getting used (adapted) to them. Adaptation to stress may take place without our awareness when it is minor, but adaptation demands major effort when it is severe. Attempts to overcome stress can produce biological and psychological responses that will have implications for health. The most immediate reaction to stress is physiological; there is an increase in heart rate, blood pressure, hormonal output, and changes in electrical conductance of the skin. These responses prepare the body to defend itself from threat (emergency reaction) and cope with stress. But repeated exposure to stress can reduce the efficient functioning of the body and ultimately the organism may become susceptible to disease. On the psychological side, stress can come in the way of adjustment, reduce the ability to deal with emotional problems, and weaken the capacity to face future stress.

Stress affects health in several ways. It can reduce the resistance of the body and increase the susceptibility to disease. It reduces our capacity to recover from illness and face new stress.

The organism's response to stressors is called the **stress response**. Most often it may be **fight or flight response**. This response produces bodily changes that help to cope with the stressor. For example, when you are injured, the body may produce chemicals such as endorphins, enkephalins that work as painkillers and the white blood cells that may congregate at the site of injury to fight against infections. It is body's way of maintaining equilibrium or homeostasis (steady state). A stressor is called *acute stressor* when it is short lived; a long-lasting stressor is called the *chronic stressor*. The daily hassles and annoyances such as traffic jam or quarrelsome coworker are acute stressors, while a serious illness, death of a beloved person, a career failure are chronic stressors. Major catastrophic events such as earthquakes, floods (tsunami) and famine can cause high level of stress. Stressors are classified based on their intensity, duration, predictability, controllability and chronicity. One simple classification with examples is shown in the Table 14.1.

Measuring Stressors

Several attempts have been made to measure stressors. During 1960s, *Social Readjustment Rating Scale (SRRS)* was developed to measure stress in terms of a number of life change events (Holmes & Rahe, 1967). The researchers used 43 positive and negative events each of which was assigned a numerical value from 0 to 100. For example, the death of a spouse was assigned 100, divorce 73, marriage 50, loss of a job 47, change in residence 20, and vocation 13. Depending upon which life changes occurred, the magnitude of stress an individual is facing can be estimated. The SRRS has since been revised and the new version contains 51 major life events (Hobson et al, 1998). Research using revised SRRS has shown that people agreed amazingly well about which events were more stressful. The stressful events fell generally into five major categories: death and dying, health and illness, crime, finances and family problems. In 1990, Smith and coworkers developed a *self-report measure of positive and negative life events for adolescents*, which also measures stress in terms life event changes. Kanner and coworkers (1981) developed the *'hassles scale'*, which quantifies stress in terms of 117 disruptive minor hassles of everyday life, such as breaking a glass full of milk, misplacing keys, getting caught by police while transgressing traffic rules and so on. Daily hassles may appear as minor inconveniences but in the long run have been shown to have negative cumulative effects on health. Several researches have indicated that minor hassles are as important (if not more) as major stresses in the genesis of pathology both at physical and psychological levels. Renner & Mackin (1998) have developed the *'college life stress inventory'* to measure the amount of life stress experienced by college students.

Table 14.1: Examples of Stressors

Types of stressor	*Acute*	*Chronic*
Physiological	Injury caused by a fall or an accident	Suffering from cancer or tuberculosis
Psychological	Preparing for a job interview or an important test	Working under an authoritarian boss
Social	Insulted by a close friend; rejection by a lover	Nagging spouse; solitary confinement; overcrowding

SOURCES OF STRESS

Life is full of stress. Taking an examination, appearing for a job interview, having a relationship, getting married, having a baby, working for difficult boss, and several other activities in contemporary world can be stressful. It all depends on how you view the situation. Cognitive appraisal (the way you look at it) determines whether a stimulus is a stressor or not. The amount of control (perceived control, not actual control) you think you have over the situation determines the emotions you experience. Remember, it is the perception of the stimulus that determines the response, not the stimulus as such. Psychologists have found that certain types of stimuli are more likely to be appraised as stressful. We shall examine a few of them.

Hassles of Everyday Life

Most people think it is only the major events in life—death, serious illness, divorce, or job loss—that produce stress. Recent research has shown that a number of small problems predict stress related illnesses better than major changes in life. The "little things"—daily hassles such as fear of losing a job, concern over the health of someone in the family, suspicious spouse, troublesome kids, having too many things to do, trying to lose weight—add up to create more stress. According to Kanner et al, (1981), the 10 most troublesome hassles reported by American college students were:

1. Troubling thoughts about the future.
2. Not getting enough sleep.
3. Wasting time.
4. Inconsiderate smokers.
5. Physical appearance.
6. Too many things to do.
7. Misplacing or losing things.
8. Not enough time to do the things you need to do.
9. Concern about meeting high standards.
10. Being lonely.

Several researches have shown that those who report more daily hassles also report more psychological problems and physical symptoms, and are more likely to have problems with the immune system as well as higher cholesterol levels. Providing long-term care for an ailing patient at home can be a source of stress for the caregiver. Constant interruptions (unsolicited phone calls, door-tapping by sales persons) when one is engaged in an important task can be stressful. Interruptions during a mentally challenging task have been found to increase cortisol level. When you have control over the interruptions, it would not be stressful. For example, you can switch off your mobile phone when you do not want to receive any calls. This means you have control over the stressful situation. Suppose you have to attend to four tasks every day; you are under stress. If the number of tasks can be reduced to two a day, that is less stressful. On the other hand, suppose you are attending to one task only per day and it is increased to two, then it becomes stressful. So, it is all in your perception, how you think of it. If you perceive a situation as an improvement, you will experience the stimulus as less stressful than if you perceive things as getting worse.

Conflicts and Frustrations

Often conflicts produce stress. People are said to experience a conflict when it is difficult to make a choice between two alternative goals. When you are in conflict, you vacillate or shift back and forth between competing goals. The more you remain in conflict, the more stressed or frustrated you feel. Neal Miller (1944) categorized three kinds of conflicts: **approach-approach conflict**, **approach-avoidance conflict** and **avoidance-avoidance conflict**. When two goals are both positive and equally desirable, the individual experiences approach-approach conflict. For example, when you have to choose between two equally attractive jobs, you experience approach-approach conflict. Although there is an element of stress in this situation, it will not produce any unpleasantness because both options are equally good. Avoidance-avoidance conflict results when both courses of action are unpleasant. For instance, you are offered a job which you do not like or you remain unemployed. Both choices are unpleasant. Approach-avoidance conflict occurs when a goal or course of action has both positive and negative implications. Sex is a classic example of this type of conflict; you desire to have a sexual experience, but at the same time you are afraid of the consequences (refer Chapter 9).

Frustration is a state of negative arousal brought about by obstacles to goal directed behavior. You feel frustrated when obstacles placed in your path prevent you from achieving your goals or when you set very high goals that are beyond your reach. Students desiring to go for higher education may be frustrated when they do not have the necessary financial support.

Work-related Stress

A satisfying job is a great source of happiness. But work can be a source of stress also. Unpleasant working conditions—bad light, noise, crowding, and demands of shift work can make life of the worker miserable. Social atmosphere—dictatorial boss, inconsiderate supervisor, uncooperative coworkers and lack of social support—may produce stress. The job itself may be a source of stress when there is a demanding work-load. Commutation to the workplace can be stressful. Chronic stressors on the job, physical and mental exhaustion, lack of job satisfaction, absence of a sense of achievement and a sense of cynicism often add up to produce a condition called **burnout**. Strikes, lockout and workplace violence add to the workers stress load. Those whose jobs have low social status, and those who are paid less tend to live in poor neighborhoods that lack recreational facilities, healthcare facilities and absence of good schooling for children. Naturally, people living under these conditions suffer from ill health. Stressful living conditions that are related to a lack of financial resources can outstrip available coping resources and create a chronic stress response.

STRESS RESPONSE

The pattern of cognitive, physiological and behavioral reactions to demands that exceed a person's resource is called the **stress response**. Generally, response to stress has two components: cognitive and physiological. One of the well-known principles in psychology is that "perception determines response." We do not simply respond to a stimulus; we respond to stimulus as perceived by us. This has led to the cognitive appraisal theory of stress.

Cognitive Appraisal of Stress

The starting point for the stress response is the cognitive appraisal of the situation and its implication to the organism. According to Richard Lazarus (1991), there are two phases in the appraisal of potential stressors. The first is ***primary appraisal***, which involves the person's assessment of the nature and demands of the situation—relevance and the potential negative implication of the event. The person may think in ways such as: Is the event dangerous to me? Is it a threat to my future? Is it likely to thwart my goal-directed behavior? The second phase is the ***secondary appraisal***, which involves the person's realization whether he/she has the resource and the ability to deal with the threat posed by the situation. In making a cognitive appraisal, people will also take into account the consequences of failing to cope successfully with the stressor, including both the seriousness of the consequences and the likelihood they will occur. When they appraise consequences of failing as costly, the perceived stressfulness may increase. Often there will be distortions and mistaken appraisals; people may overestimate the seriousness of the situation, underestimate their own resources, exaggerate the seriousness of the consequences and the likelihood they will occur. These will cause inappropriate stress responses. According to cognitive appraisal theories, it is only after appraisals have been made that the individual reacts. The assumption is that human beings think before they act; they interpret what they encounter and then respond.

Physiological Changes in Stress

In the early part of the 20th century, Walter B Cannon described stress as response to a threatening stimulus and named the behavior pattern **fight** or **flight response** in which the organism either fights the stimulus or runs away from the situation. The response is characterized by increase in blood pressure, heart rate, blood sugar level, sweating and rate of respiration. Cannon proposed that repeated stress impairs homeostasis and the organism will be vulnerable to disease. Following the footsteps of Cannon, an Austrian-born Canadian physiologist (endocrinologist) Hans Selye (1907–1982) made the word stress a household name through his research and theorizing on the concept.

General adaptation syndrome (GAS) is the name given by Selye (1976) to the predictable pattern of responses made by the body when under stress and suggested that it has three distinct phases: alarm, resistance and exhaustion. The **alarm stage** is triggered by the perception of a stressor followed by the flight or fight response. Perception of stress activates the sympathetic nervous system and inhibits the parasympathetic division. Neurotransmitters such as epinephrine and norepinephrine are released; these in turn cause increase in breathing, heart rate and blood pressure. The functioning of the immune system is altered. These changes bring in more oxygen to the muscles; the pupils dilate so that one can see better, and palms sweat helping a better grip. Cortisol (a glucocorticoid) is released to provide extra energy (cortisol also has an anti-inflammatory effect and can cure injuries). In short, all these activities prepare an organism either to fight the threat or flee from it. During the **resistance stage**, the organism makes efforts to take action to overcome the stress or learn to adapt to the stressor (resistance phase is often called the adaptation phase). The body's resources are mobilized by the continued release of stress hormones (epinephrine, norepinephrine and cortisol). If the resistance continues for a relatively long time, the body's resources are depleted and functioning of the immune system is partially suppressed by the stress hormones. If the stressor is very strong and persists for too long a period, the body becomes exhausted because of its limited resources to deal with stress. Now, it reaches the **exhaustion stage** in which there is increased vulnerability to disease (in several cases collapse and death). According to Selye, whatever body system is weak (e.g. cardiovascular, respiratory, gastrointestinal) it will be the one, most affected.

Selye found that all stress produce the same pattern of reaction. For GAS to be activated the organism does not have to be chased by a tiger; the daily hassles such as a traffic jam, an unreasonable boss, a quarrelsome spouse or a midterm examination can produce the same reaction. Historically, Selye's GAS is an important model because it depicts the mechanism by which stress leads to physiological damage. Most importantly, his work led to the emergence of an exciting area of study called psychoneuroimmunology.

PSYCHONEUROIMMUNOLOGY

Psychoneuroimmunology (PNI) is a field of study that investigates the interrelationships between psychosocial processes, nervous, endocrine, and the immune system functioning. Most of the researches in PNI have focused on the impact of stress on immune functioning. Research has shown that stressors can affect the immune system in various ways. Nerve fibers from the brain stimulate the lymph tissues to release a wide variety of chemicals that bind to receptors on white blood cells, thus influencing immune functions. Although it is known that stress affects immune functions, how it happens is highly complicated (Box 14.1).

Researches have shown that psychological stress can alter susceptibility to infectious agents influencing the onset, course and outcome of certain infectious pathologies (Biondi & Zannino, 1997). When demands imposed by events exceed the individual's ability to cope, a psychological stress response composed of negative cognitive and emotional states is elicited. It is these responses that are thought to influence immune function through their effects on behavioral coping and neuroendocrine response (Cohen & Herbert, 1996). If the immune system is functioning well, people probably will live longer. But stress can harm the immune system. Stress can impair the functioning of white blood cells and hence it takes a long time to heal wounds. Major stressors such as floods, earthquakes and victimization (being raped or robbed) can affect the immune system. But not all people who are exposed to stress respond in the same way.

Box 14.1: Immune System

The immune system guards the body from infection. The function is believed to be done by two types of white blood cells: B cells and T cells. The B cells are formed in the bone marrow and T cells in the thymus (an organ located in the chest). B cells produce antibodies to fight foreign invaders. T cells secret chemicals that aid in a process by which attacking microorganisms are ingested and destroyed. There are several other cells and blood components—(mast cells, monocytes, macrophages, natural killer cells)—involved in immune responses. Natural killer cells (NK cells) are reported to detect and destroy damaged or altered cells such as precancerous cells before they become tumors. Glucocorticoids, which are released when one is under stress, hinder the formation of some white blood cells (including NK cells) or kill other white blood cells making the body more vulnerable to infection and tumor growth. People who exhibit higher sympathetic nervous system responses to stress show the most changes in immune system functioning, indicating that changes in the immune system are moderated by changes in the sympathetic nervous system. Exposure to some chronic psychological stressors can increase inflammation and the risk for autoimmune disorders.

STRESS AND DISEASE

By now we know stress can contribute to the development of diseases. Let us examine how stress operates in some selected diseases.

Cancer

Stress does not cause cancer, but it is found to affect the growth of cancerous tumors. This happens when the immune system is suppressed and NK cells (natural killer cells) are not working optimally to prevent the spread of tumor cells. It is also found that stress can facilitate the growth of capillaries feeding the tumor. Therefore, there will be an increase in blood flow to the tumor site and thus nourishing the tumor to grow. However, it must be emphasized that stress does not cause a tumor to develop; it only assists the growth if one is already there. Several psychological factors are implicated in the development of cancer. It is believed that perception of inadequate social support, feelings of distress, lack of control over the happenings, fatigue and lack of joy in life can all weaken the immune system and thus help cancerous growth. In fact, there is talk of a type of personality called *cancer personality (Type C)*—a name given to a constellation of traits, such as the tendency to deny or suppress emotions, to avoid conflicts and to be overly agreeable, which facilitates the onset of cancer. But there is not enough research evidence to support the existence of such a personality type. It is found, however, that people who adopt a fighting spirit are more likely to recover from cancer than those who meekly submit and suffer.

Coronary Heart Disease

Most people believe that stress can lead to heart disease. We all know that stress increases blood pressure, which in association with hormonal conditions can lead to narrowing or blocking of the coronary arteries (arteriosclerosis), which in turn may promote atherosclerosis (the buildup of fatty deposits called plaques, on the inside wall of the arteries). The plaques, formed in the coronary arteries obstruct blood flow hampering oxygen supply to heart muscles, which produces chest pain (angina pectoris). When there is severe or prolonged blockage of blood to the heart, it may lead to heart attack (myocardial infarction). Coronary heart diseases (cardiovascular diseases) are the major killers in the USA and Europe. Coronary heart diseases (CHD) have many risk factors such as tobacco smoking, obesity, sedentary lifestyle, diabetes, hypertension, high serum cholesterol and family history. Hypertension is a major risk factor for CHD and several other conditions such as stroke and kidney diseases. Obesity, sedentary lifestyle, diet, alcohol and familial problems contribute to the development and maintenance of hypertension. People suffering from hypertension are more likely to express hostility and suspiciousness than those with normal blood pressure. Hypertension seems to be more common among individuals working in high-stress jobs such as air traffic controllers. It may also be the result of overcrowding.

While discussing the role of psychological stress in the genesis of CHD, it is customary to talk about the **Type A behavior pattern (TABP)** introduced by cardiologists Meyer Friedman & Rosenman. The TABP is characterized by competitiveness, hostility and incessant struggle to achieve more and more in less and less time. Most of the type A people are ambitious and workaholics. In contrast, persons with **Type B behavior pattern** are cooperative, not aggressive, less competitive, not working in a strictly time-bound programs, generally calm and collected, taking life as it comes. Because of his/her hostile, competitive, and achievement orientation, the Type A person is highly aroused (mobilized) most of the time. Earlier researches found a strong relationship between CHD and TABP, but later researches have reported a limited relationship between the two. These researches have suggested that people who are energetic, expressive and animated may not develop heart complaints. Only those who exhibit chronic hostility, anger, aggression and distrust of others are the ones who are prone to CHD. One study found that medical students who scored in the top 20 percent on a hostility scale were more than four times as likely to develop heart diseases 25 years later as were their low-hostility peers. Among lawyers increased mortality was found to be associated with an untrusting and cynical view of people, repeated negative emotions in personal interactions and recurrent expression of overt anger and aggression in the face of difficulties or frustrations. People high in hostility are more likely to have a higher heart rate and blood pressure throughout the day, no matter what their mood. In contrast, people low in hostility showed cardiac changes only when they were in a negative mood.

Stress generally elicits negative emotions such as fear, anger, sadness and helplessness. These emotions elicit a long lasting increase in heart rate. Chronic stress has been found to produce helplessness, depression and despair. Anxiety is also associated with heart disease. Healthy changes in lifestyle—changing diet, regular exercise, adopting effective stress management techniques and availability of social support—are found to reduce the incidence of heart complaints.

Post-traumatic Stress Disorder

Sometimes, people undergo highly harrowing and extremely stressful experiences such as fire, floods and other natural calamities, sexual abuse, rape and painful war experiences, which will have serious effects on them even after months or years after the events have occurred. These individuals may experience exaggerated startle reactions, sleep disturbances, extreme guilt, flattened affect, intense watchfulness and even relieving of some of the traumatic experiences. Such people are diagnosed as suffering from **post-traumatic stress disorder (PTSD)**. This condition has been linked to weakening of the immune system and the usual hormonal changes associated with stress. People suffering from PTSD generally take to alcohol, drug abuse and smoking. Often they may attempt suicide.

Psychophysiological Disorders

Physiological disorders that are influenced by psychological factors are called **psychophysiological disorders**. Psychological and physiological factors are so very closely interacting in these conditions that it is difficult to separate them. Among the most prominent psychophysiological disorders are blood pressure, migraine headache, backache, ulcers, asthma, dermatological and gastrointestinal problems. Each of these diseases is chronic and widespread, but their precise causes are not known. However, it is known that both have a physical and a psychological component. The two factors occur together, but which is the cause and which is the effect is not clear. Chronic stress or negative emotions do not cause diseases. There is a correlational relationship between negative psychological factors and illness. Whether psychological factors cause physical illnesses is not established. However, there is some evidence to say that negative psychological factors precipitate illness, facilitate its development and hinder the curative process.

COPING WITH STRESS

There is sufficient evidence to say that stress can affect the immune system and can reduce the organism's ability to defend itself from microbial invaders. Death of a loved one, for example, can lead to reduced production of lymphocytes, which are necessary to fight infection. Facing a tough examination can lead to immunosuppression, which in turn can cause respiratory disorders and other infections. But an intriguing phenomenon about stress is that not all people who are stressed respond to it in the same way. One may be overwhelmed by stress and break down, while the other may barely notice it. Several people when under stress engage in health-impairing behaviors such as smoking, alcohol or drug abuse, risk taking, poor nutrition, unsafe sex and not exercising. Such people damage their health. Several of them do not appraise the risk and ignore the risk factors. Some of them think that they are invulnerable and do not take necessary precautions. These are negative coping strategies. Different people tend to use different coping strategies depending upon the situation and the emotions aroused. People may engage in reactive coping, which involves responding to present or past stressors, or proactive coping, which involves responding to potential stressors such as an expected job loss. Proactive coping refers to taking action before an event has occurred, not in response to the event. Coping strategies are categorized in two ways: problem-focused coping and emotion-focused coping.

Problem-focused Coping

Problem-focused coping involves taking direct action to change a stressful situation or to prevent or reduce its effects. It includes strategies to alter the environment or the way in which the person and the environment interact. An individual may anticipate a stressful event and be prepared to face it. He may learn the methods of coping with the situation. This is proactive coping. This mode of coping is adopted by people who believe that there is something they can do about the stressful situation and they have the resources to do it. It is found that people who score high on conscientiousness, one of the Big Five personality factors, engage in problem-focused coping.

Emotion-focused Coping

Emotion-focused coping involves attempts to regulate or reduce the emotional consequences of the stressful event. One, who adopts emotion-focused coping, uses strategies to change his/her emotional responses to the stressors. For example, when your boyfriend deserts you, you may cope with the distress by taking active part in sports or studying well for securing a good grade in the examination. Or you may think in the following lines: "After all, the relationship was really not that good; fortunately it is over now, sooner than later." As you might have guessed, this is reactive coping, which is used after the stressful event has occurred. This type of coping brings down the level of arousal. People who think that they cannot alter the stressor try to change their perception of, or response to, the stressor. Studies have shown that people who perceive that they have less control over the stressful events are less likely to use problem-focused strategies and more likely to employ emotion-focused strategies.

People use more than one strategy in dealing with a stressful event. The effectiveness of the strategy used depends in part on a person's ability to estimate whether the environment can be altered. Suppose you do not have enough money to pay the next term fee; you may think of various ways of raising the money. Here you are using the problem-focused coping strategy. You may start giving tuition to raise the required money. If so, you are using two problem-focused strategies: active coping and suppression of competing activities. That is, you try to work hard and avoid all other distracting activities (going to films, attending parties, making purchases).

The specific coping strategy a person uses depends on the intensity and frequency of the stressor. If the stress occurs very frequently, people may use avoidant coping strategies such as behavioral disengagement or mental disengagement. In ***behavioral disengagement***, people reduce their efforts to deal actively with the stressor. In its extreme form, disengagement can lead to helplessness. In ***mental disengagement***, people try to divert their attention from the stressor. Avoidant coping strategies are used when the individual realizes that nothing can be done to change a stressor. These coping strategies are summarized in Table 14.2.

Cohen & Lazarus (1979) suggested the following five coping strategies, which of course, overlap with the list presented in the Table 14.2:

1. ***Taking direct action:*** Dealing directly with the stressor whenever it is possible.
2. ***Inhibiting action:*** Suppressing the desire to take action; keeping quiet instead of yelling at your boss.
3. ***Engaging in intrapsychic efforts:*** Ignoring upsetting thoughts or reframing them into positive ideas.
4. ***Seeking information:*** Learning about the successful ways of dealing with stressors.
5. ***Calling on others:*** Seeking help from others for maintaining both physical and emotional safety.

Table 14.2: Coping Strategies

Strategy	*Activity*
Problem-focused Strategies	
Active coping	Removing the stressor or reducing its effects
Planning	Thinking about the ways of managing stressors
Instrumental social support	Seeking advice, assistance, and information
Suppression of competing activities	Putting all other activities aside and concentrating only on coping strategies
Restraint coping	Waiting to act at the appropriate time
Emotion-focused Strategies	
Emotional social support	Seeking encouragement, moral support, sympathy, and understanding from others
Venting emotions	Focusing on and talking about distress
Positive reinterpretation	Reinterpreting events in positive ways
Behavioral disengagement	Reducing efforts to deal with stressors
Mental disengagement	Turning to other activities to divert attention

Evidence from researches on coping suggests that no specific coping strategy is equally effective in all situations. The effectiveness of a technique depends on the characteristics of the stressor, the appropriateness of the technique and the skill with which it is applied. People are likely to adapt to stress well when they have multiple techniques and are aware how and when to apply them. In this connection, it is good to remember the prayer: "God, give me the courage to change those things that can be changed, the forbearance to accept those that cannot be changed and the wisdom to discern the difference."

Emotional Disclosure

There is some truth in the saying that "sorrow shared is sorrow lessened." Researches have demonstrated that hidden traumatic feelings might prove to be harmful to both body and mind. When people hide their feelings, their bodies respond with increased heart rate, blood pressure and sweating. Therefore, you are advised to "talk to somebody". **Emotional disclosure** refers to the act of revealing your inner feelings to other people. The disclosure may take the form of talking or writing. Disclosing the event helps the release of the stress to some extent. The release may help people to forget the event or learn to live with it. Talking provides an opportunity for social comparison. The person to whom you are talking might have had similar experience and he/she might tell you how it was handled. This will provide you with some amount of emotional-social support and give some hint to deal with your problems. James Pennebaker (1997) asked college students to talk about their past traumatic experiences to an experimenter seated in an adjoining room or to tape record or write about their experiences. Many of them recounted incidents involving personal disappointments, familial catastrophes, frustrated love affairs, sexual abuse and traumatic accidents. Participants of a control group were asked to talk or write about mundane trivial events of their life. Blood samples were taken from the students before and after the sessions and examined. The results indicated an enhanced immune system functioning in those who had purged themselves of negative emotions.

But in those who had not ventilated their traumatic experience such an improvement was not seen. Further, it was found that among the students who made emotional disclosure, there were 50 percent fewer visits to the campus health center over the next six months compared with the control group. In another study, Denise Sloan & Brian Marx (2004) found that writing or talking about traumatic events produce similar improvement. One problem here is that not many people among your friends or relatives are prepared to hear your problems; they may not have either the patience or time to listen to your woes. Only when you have a compassionate listener, emotional disclosure will be effective. Probably a trained listener such as a counselor may be useful during emotional disclosure.

Social Support

Social support is an important factor that helps in the alleviation of stressful experience and its consequences. The knowledge that we can rely on others for help and support in times of crisis can reduce the impact of stress and increase the capacity to cope with it. ***Social support*** refers to the support or help offered by friends, coworkers, relatives, family members and professionals (such as counselors) when you are under stress. These people may provide ***tangible support***—financial or medical help; taking care of your home or children when you are under duress. They may offer you ***informational support*** by suggesting ways of dealing with your problems. They may also give you ***emotional support*** by reassuring you that there are people who love you, care for you and value you. These forms of social support have been found to go a long way when one is recovering from a serious illness. Generally, it is found that highly sociable people are more resistant to infectious diseases and other forms of illnesses.

In one of the studies done on 37,000 people for over 12 years, researchers found that those with weak social ties were twice as likely to die during the period of study as those with strong ties to others (House et al, 1988). Social support is found to protect against stress by enhancing immune system functioning. Several other studies have shown that social support decreases psychological distress in people who are tackling stress of all kinds. Apart from enhancing immune system functioning and reducing psychological distress, social support has some other benefits. People who feel that they belong to a social system experience a greater sense of identity and meaning in their lives, which in turn results in greater psychological well-being. Having the backing of others can increase control over stressors. Social support helps both the recipient as well as the help giver. Stephanie Brown and coworkers (2003) found those who help and support others had lower mortality rate than those who did not. In a study of over 4,000 men and women in California, the death rate among socially isolated people was twice that for people with strong social ties. Even holding hands or touching was found to be a beneficial form of social support. For those undergoing surgery, talking with their doctor the night before surgery was found to be effective during recovery. Among people suffering from CHD, half of the people without social support died within 5 years; it was three times the rate for those who had a close friend or spouse. College students under stress developed depression when they had no social support.

Receiving social support may have certain disadvantages. Help given may carry with it an implicit requirement to reciprocate. There is also a possibility that those who try to help will intrude into the private life of the one being helped. Sometimes, the help-giver may thrust a solution so vehemently, which in itself may become a burden and a source of further stress. For example, you must have come across people who ask you to change the physician or the drugs; both of which may not be to your advantage.

PERSONALITY AND COPING

How a person copes with stress also depends on certain personality characteristics. In fact, coping style itself can be thought of as a personality trait. Let us examine a few of the personality traits that have been studied in the context of coping with stress.

Hardiness

You must have come across some people who, despite highly stressful conditions, maintain or even improve their health. How is it possible? Salvatore Maddi & Suzanne Kobasa proposed the concept of hardiness to explain this intriguing phenomenon. **Hardiness** is a psychological construct that refers to an individual's characteristic way of responding to stressors. It is composed of three components namely, ***commitment, control*** and ***challenge*** (sometimes called the three Cs). Hardy individuals are committed to their work, social relations and family; they are extremely involved in what they do and believe that what they are doing is important. They believe that they are having control over the outcomes and can influence events rather than feeling helpless and powerless in the face of external forces (this is similar to internal locus of control proposed by Rotter). They place considerable emphasis on their own responsibility for their lives, feel that they are capable of acting on their own, without being directed by others. Finally, hardy people accept events in life as challenges and are not threatened by them. They anticipate and even welcome changes in life as opportunities for growth. They are optimistic, open, and flexible in thought and action; they have a high tolerance for ambiguity. Individuals who exhibit hardiness have generally been found to be less susceptible to develop illness when under stress (Kobasa, 1979; Kobasa, Maddi, and Kahn, 1982; Maddi and Khoshaba, 1994).

Optimism and Pessimism

Optimism is a good buffer to stress. Optimism is a key concept in the developing movement in psychology known as ***positive psychology***; it refers to the way an individual perceives the world. An optimist views the future positively and expects things to work out well. Optimism has been found to be a relatively stable trait. Optimists report facing a less number of stressful situations in their college life; students scoring high on this trait report better moods, coping skills and immune system functioning during examination. Optimists report higher levels of psychological health during stressful periods than those who were non-optimists. The incidence of depression is found to be low among the optimists. Edward Chang (1998) found that optimists felt less hopeless in the face of stress and adjusted to negative life events better than pessimists. Optimistic women exhibited lower level distress during high-risk pregnancies and recovered better from breast cancer than pessimists (Lobel et al, 2000). Optimists were found to recover more quickly after surgery than non-optimists. They were less likely to be rehospitalized following heart bypass surgery (Scheier et al, 1999). For that matter, optimists are less likely to die of heart ailments.

Pessimism is associated with anxiety, depression, poor health and stress-proneness. There are two types of pessimism: ***true pessimism*** in which negative expectations are anchored in past experience of failure and ***defensive pessimism***, in which more negative outcomes are expected than warranted by facts. Defensive pessimism may be considered as a type of proactive coping strategy in which negative or lowered expectations of performing in a task, motivates coping behavior. An individual may expect that he would not do well in tackling the forthcoming task and may try to avoid doing anything to ward off the anxiety associated with failure. Optimists employ problem-oriented coping strategies involving direct action. They are prepared to accept the reality of the stressful situation and generally learn from their experience. On the other hand, pessimists deny or avoid the stressful situation and give up when they cannot manage the situation.

Coping Self-efficacy

Related to hardiness and optimism is Bandura's concept of **self-efficacy**, which refers to the belief that we have the necessary skills and sufficient resource to perform well in the face of adversity. Self-efficacy depends on previous experience; if an individual was successful in dealing with similar tasks, it increases and if not, decreases. Self-efficacy expectations increase when you observe others coping successfully and you receive encouragement from others. Feelings of efficacy strengthen both body and mind to deal with stress. The immune system appears to function well when you have a feeling that you can get things to go alright.

Avoiders and Non-avoiders of Stress

Another personality factor associated with health and illness is the extent to which people avoid or face (think of) stress. Avoiders are often referred to as ***repressors*** and non-avoiders as ***sensitizers***. Avoiders may use thought suppression strategy—not thinking about stress-arousing and distressing ideas (see below under mental control) whereas non-avoiders habitually think about them. Although they report fewer stress-related problems, sensitizers are more likely to have high blood pressure, lowered immune system functions and other such negative effects on health. However, the research evidence is not unequivocal in this regard. Some studies have shown that sensitizers exhibit more anxiety and high physiological stress response than repressors.

RELIGIOUS BELIEF AND COPING WITH STRESS

Humanistic theorists emphasize the role of religious and spiritual beliefs in dealing with stressors. They propose that people with a religious orientation try to find a higher meaning for their adversity and misfortune in life. For example, it is found that parents who lost their children coped better with their grief when they had a religious belief. It is reported that people who found some higher meaning in the death of a family member experienced less distress. Religious orientation may yield both positive and negative results when under stress. In one study, it was reported that elderly people suffering from physical and psychological problems started thinking that God was punishing them and that they were under the influence of demonic forces; as a result they started expressing anger toward God and questioning their faith. So, religious belief may yield positive results in dealing with some types of stress, but not with others. It is found that religious beliefs help in coping with losses, diseases, and personal failures, but not in facing marital conflicts and abuse; in the latter cases they may have a negative impact by inducing guilt feelings or introduce internal pressures on the individual to remain in the stressful relationship. This area is still in the formative period. We hear often about faith healing, holistic therapy and such other procedures. The major emphasis in the area has been the effect of mind over matter or the mind as a healer or a slayer.

TRAINING FOR STRESS MANAGEMENT

Stress occurs universally; it impairs physical and mental health. Can we teach people to manage stress? One of the main jobs of clinical health psychology has been designing interventions that help to reduce stress in everyday life. Much effort has gone into developing methods of reducing stress and to enable people to live healthier and productive lives. Numerous interventions have been suggested to serve specific functions such as improving the efficacy of the immune system, calming down the nervous system and eliciting effective cognitive coping strategies. Coping strategies can be grouped under three heads such as behavioral, cognitive and physiological. Behavioral interventions focus on altering the individual's activities such as engaging in active exercises. Cognitive interventions focus on altering the thought processes (cognitive restructuring). Physiological techniques include somatic relaxation training, meditation and biofeedback.

Behavioral Interventions

The best known behavioral intervention technique is exercise. Several researches have shown that exercise could be an effective method of coping with stress. Exercise helps to reduce physical and emotional strain, bring down blood pressure and heart rate. Exercise appears to be a good outlet for physiological arousal. People who exercise regularly are found to be physically fit and experience lower levels of anxiety. Regular exercise can help to keep you healthy in the face of stress. It is reported that regular exercise could enhance the efficiency of heart and reduce the risk of heart attack. The frequency of premature death has been found to be low among people who exercise regularly. A study of college students has shown lower level of test anxiety among those who exercise. In a study of executives under stress, exercise was found to be associated with lower overall illness reports.

Cognitive Interventions

By now you must have realized that the intensity of stress depends upon how you interpret the situation (cognitive appraisal). If you think that the stress is too much for you to handle and you do not have the resources to handle the situation, the stress response will be too severe. On the other hand, if you look at stress as a challenge, not as a problem (like hardy people) and think that you are in control of the situation, the chances are that the stress response will be less severe. Having this view in mind, several cognitive therapists have proposed certain cognitive stress management strategies. According to Albert Ellis (1962), who developed rational emotive behavior therapy, several irrational beliefs are at the root of negative maladaptive feelings, e.g. thoughts like:" I must succeed in all that I attempt," "All people should appreciate my work," and "It will be awful if I do not get a first class in the examination." Such illogical and unrealistic beliefs are referred to by Ellis as *musterbating, awfulizing* and *catastrophizing*. Such thoughts generate unnecessary anxiety, anger and despair; they can be replaced by more realistic rational thoughts such as: "If I do poorly in this examination, I shall work hard and get good grades in the next one." The technique used to replace negative beliefs by positive ones is called **cognitive restructuring**, in which attempts are made to detect, challenge and replace irrational thoughts by rational thoughts.

Another stress management strategy suggested by Donald Meichenbaum (1985) is **stress inoculation training**. It is a way of cognitively preparing persons to face the threat just like immunizing an individual against an illness. Stress inoculation is done in three steps: conceptualization, skill acquisition and rehearsal, and application and follow up. During the ***conceptualization*** stage, the client and the therapist sit together to analyze and understand the problem. The second is the ***skill acquisition and rehearsal*** stage in which the individual is trained in relaxation and desensitization techniques.

The client is taught to redefine the problem and provided with certain practical aids to overcome stress-producing situations. Finally, during the ***application and follow-up*** phase, cognitive and behavioral techniques are used to bring about change in behavior. The therapist and client may engage in "role playing" the stress-producing situation to enable the client to practice the skills that have been acquired by him.

Mental Control

In recent times, a technique called ***mental control*** has been proposed by some researchers (Wegner & Pennebaker, 1993). It is a technique in which people suppress a thought, concentrate on a sensation, inhibit an emotion, maintain a mood, stir up a desire, soften a craving or otherwise exert influence on their own mental states. During mental control, an individual generally makes a self-statement to alter his/her mental state. It may take forms such as ***thought stopping***, ***cognitive distraction***, or ***thought avoidance***. In thought stopping, the individual tells himself "stop" when a thought occurs in his mind. In cognitive distraction, the individual starts thinking about something else to distract the occurrence of an undesirable thought. In thought avoidance, the individual simply tries not to think about something that is troubling. It is found that maintaining thought control over time is difficult. These techniques must be well practiced to be effective and they require hard work on the part of the individual.

Thought suppression sometimes may produce a phenomenon called ***rebound effect***; that is, trying not to think about something can have the paradoxical effect of causing the suppressed thought to pop up into consciousness more than it does when you are not trying to suppress it. Some people use thought suppression more often than others. Such people have less success in suppressing stress-related thoughts. Because of the rebound effect, the subsequent increase in thoughts about the stressor may lead to excessive focus on it and to depression. Attempts to suppress thoughts that are emotionally charged have also been found to be associated with changes in the sympathetic nervous system.

Physiological Interventions

Behavior therapists have developed a number of physiological interventions to cope with stress. The well-known technique of **systematic desensitization** developed by Joseph Wolpe involves progressive muscle relaxation and related procedures in reducing stress.

Relaxation Techniques

Relaxation techniques are popularly used in behavior therapy. These are also used in stress management. They are found to be effective methods of reducing somatic tension, heart rate and blood pressure. There are two forms of relaxation techniques: ***somatic relaxation*** and ***cognitive relaxation***. In somatic relaxation (also called systematic desensitization or ***progressive muscle relaxation***) the client is trained to focus on specific muscle groups and alternately to tense and relax the muscles. The individual might start with the hands and arm muscles and work up through head, neck, abdomen, thorax and legs. With each muscle group, the individual may tense the muscles for ten seconds and then relax them for the same amount of time. During the relaxation phase, the individual is asked to notice how pleasant the experience is compared to tense state. He may also be asked to imagine some pleasant instances. With some training the individual learns to relax the whole body and experiences the pleasant feelings associated with it. Relaxation training is based upon the technique developed by Jacobson (1938) and described by Wolpe (1990) in detail. Many individuals learn to relax the entire body with about a week's practice. Because relaxation is incompatible with arousal, relaxation training provides a means of voluntarily reducing and preventing arousal associated with stress. Relaxation training has become the cornerstone of most stress management programs.

The extensively used form of cognitive relaxation is meditation. Meditation relaxes both body and mind. It produces cognitive relaxation, a peaceful clear state of mind. During meditation, the individual sits quietly in a comfortable position with eyes closed and concentrates on an idea, a word, or an image (or even a body function such as respiration) for about 20 minutes. This produces a state of relaxation. Meditation has been found to reduce anxiety, hypertension and such other components of the stress response. Cardiologist Herbert Benson has developed a meditation-based method of relaxation for stress management, which is popularly known as the **relaxation response** (Benson et al, 1974). The method has been used extensively with corporate and business executives. Several people all over the world practice meditation to counter the effects stressors in their day-to-day life.

Biofeedback is another effective technique used to help people relax. It involves an electronic device that emits a signal (a light or buzzer sound) to inform the client about the body state. The information may be about the tension in a muscle or general state of arousal of sympathetic or parasympathetic nervous system. Based on the information, the individual may try to maintain an optimal body state. This is in fact a kind of operant conditioning procedure of retaining bodily or mental comfort with the help of reinforcement. Biofeedback appears to have the same level of effectiveness as progressive somatic relaxation.

GENDER, CULTURE, AND COPING

Research reports suggest that women in Western cultures experience more stress than men. This is supposed to be because of multiple roles modern women play, especially working women. Modern urban woman plays the role of house wife, mother, daughter and employee and she has do cooking, cleaning and shopping. The multiple roles have both positive as well as negative effects. Often women may feel hassled, depressed, anxious and hostile because of the pressure of a number of things she is expected to do. On the other hand, multiple roles may also confer advantages such as increased feelings of self-esteem, financial gain, control over family affairs and social support from colleagues. Marital stresses differ for husbands and wives. Women experience more stress and negative health effects from marital conflicts, but they also experience more happiness from their marital relationships and motherhood. Men and women also differ in the ways they cope with the stressors. When under stress, women seek out social support whereas men tend to be more action oriented; men try to fight the causes of stress.

Culture also determines how people perceive stress, how they cope with it and the extent of control they have on the stressful situations. For example, in Western cultures people perceive crowding as a serious problem, while in Asian societies, population density, crowding and living conditions are viewed as less serious problems. It is reported that Asians can create a sense of privacy even under crowded conditions. In one study, Indian students were found to prefer emotion-focused coping strategies more than to the Canadian students. It is found that social cohesiveness found in Japanese culture protects its members from heart ailments. It is also observed that people in collectivist cultures seek lesser social support than those in individualistic cultures; they know it is available and there is no need to ask for it.

PAIN AND PAIN MANAGEMENT

Pain is a universal human experience and definitely one of the most unpleasant realities of life. It is an unpleasant sensory and emotional experience associated with actual or potential tissue damage. Pain is a psychological experience that includes a personal, private sensation of hurt. One third of all humans experience pain that requires medication at some time in their lives. A large number of people suffer from either backache or headache or both. In spite of its discomfort, pain has important survival functions. It serves as a danger signal that something is wrong somewhere in the body. It warns that the body is being threatened or damaged and triggers a variety of behaviors to cope with the threat. It is pain that brings people to a physician.

Generally, people think of pain as sensory phenomenon, but it is more than that. It is a complex perceptual phenomenon involving a number of psychological processes. Pain depends heavily on our thoughts and emotions. There are people who experience excruciating pain even in the absence of tissue damage. There are others who suffer severe physical damage, but experience no pain. For example, people with cardiac complications and cancerous growth, which are life threatening, do not seek help because often these conditions are not associated with pain. Women report that the pain experienced during childbirth is moderated by the joyful nature of the incident.

Several people do not seek medical help because of the fear of pain associated with treatment such as surgery or extraction of a tooth. However, people do consult physicians and take medicines for pain more often than any other symptom or disease. Often, reduction of pain is more important than satisfying hunger or thirst. Several people commit suicide when pain becomes intolerable. People fear intractable pain (pain that cannot be relieved) more than death. For these and several other reasons, health psychologists are immensely interested in the study of pain. Thankfully, several pain control techniques and medications to reduce pain are available nowadays. But, what is pain? What causes it? How to control pain? In the past three to four decades, medical and psychological researchers have struggled to find answers to these questions. A brief summary of what is known today about pain is given in the following pages.

Pain generally is understood as a sensory and emotional discomfort, that is usually (but not necessarily) related to tissue damage. In certain respects it is a sensation and in others it is an emotional-motivational phenomenon that leads to escape and avoidance behavior. According to Sternbach (1968) pain is a psychological experience which includes:

1. A personal, private sensation of hurt.
2. A harmful stimulus which signals current or impending tissue damage.
3. A pattern of responses which operate to protect the organism from harm.

Pain may be acute or chronic. Acute pain is temporary and lasts less than 6 months. Acute pain may cause considerable distress, but it subsides soon. When pain lasts longer than 6 months, it becomes chronic. Chronic pain can be intermittent or continuous, may be dull and mild, or sharp and unbearable, and generalized or local. Three varieties of chronic pain are recognized. *Chronic recurrent pain* (such as neuralgia) is not life threatening, but produces intense episodes of pain followed by periods of relief. *Chronic intractable benign pain* (such as low back pain) is always present, but unrelated to a progressive condition. *Chronic progressive pain* (for example, advancing arthritis) involves continuous discomfort that becomes progressively more intense as the condition worsens. Whatever its status, the discomfort caused by pain motivates the individual to avoid, escape, or fight the causative factors and their consequences. People suffering from chronic pain may become preoccupied with somatic concerns and experience a heightened sense of dependency; they may develop a sense of helplessness and even depression.

Perception of Pain

When an individual's body is injured, signals of the tissue damage flow from different neurons of the peripheral nervous system to the dorsal horn of the spinal cord and then to various areas of the brain, including the thalamus, hypothalamus and the cerebral cortex. The pain receptors (free nerve endings) are found in all body tissues except the brain, bones, and certain non-living parts of the body organs. When activated, these nerve endings generate impulses that travel to the brain. The sensory information about the intensity of pain and its location is relayed by the thalamus to the somatosensory and frontal areas of the cerebral cortex. Messages from the thalamus also go to the limbic system, which is involved in motivation and emotion. Thus, pain has both a sensory and an emotional component. When there is painful sensation and negative emotional response, the individual suffers from pain.

Pain sensations arise primarily when two different kinds of nerves are stimulated. These nerves have fibers that differ in size and the speed with which they carry impulses. As a consequence, we experience what is called ***double pain***: first a sharp pain at the time of injury, which is followed by dull and diffuse pain. Perception of pain is not always straightforward. Sometimes, pain originating in one part of the body is perceived as though it is coming from another part. This is called **referred pain**. Pain may also be experienced in the absence of apparent tissue damage. **Neuralgia** is one such condition. Another condition, called **causalgia**, involves severe burning sensation after the injury has healed. One of the strangest experiences is **phantom-limb pain** in which an individual experiences pain in a part of the body that has been amputated.

Brain Mechanisms in Pain

In the early 1980s, an important explanation of the neurological mechanisms in pain was presented by Canadian psychologist Ronald Melzack and physiologist Patrick Wall (1965) that has come to be known as **gate control theory**. The theory acknowledges specificity in pain transmission, the importance of patterning and summation of impulses and the role of psychological processes in the pain experience. The gate control theory proposes that pain impulses on their way to the brain are modulated by an opening and closing of the gating mechanism in the nervous system and the degree of pain experience depends on these processes. Events in the spinal cord can open a system of spinal cord gates and allow the nerve impulses to travel toward the brain. Certain other events can block the sensory inputs on their way to brain by closing the gates partially or fully and thus blunt the experience of pain. For example, scratching an itch can produce relief. Gate control theory suggests that acupuncture relieves pain because the needles used stimulate mostly receptors that close the pain gates. A psychologically important feature of the gate control theory is that it suggests that nerve impulses descending from the brain can also influence the spinal gates, thereby increasing or decreasing the flow of pain stimulation to the brain. This ***central control mechanism*** allows thoughts, beliefs and emotions to influence the experience of pain, thus emphasizing the role of psychological (cognitive) factors in pain, in addition to the physical ones. Gate control theory has been valuable in suggesting ways for pain control and in stimulating research on the psychological factors in pain.

Melzack and his associates have contributed a great deal to our understanding of pain all of which cannot be discussed in a chapter. Recently, Melzack (1999) has proposed a modified theory of pain known as the neuromatrix theory of pain, which suggests that every individual has an innate, genetically prescribed neural network called neuromatrix. The neural network consists of feedback loops between the thalamus and the cortex and between the cortex and the limbic system. These loops are modified through experience with pain. When sensory inputs are received, they cycle through this matrix and are synthesized creating a unique pattern called neurosignature. Thus, all sensory inputs become imprinted in the neuromatrix and these neurosignatures are projected to specific brain centers known as the sentient neural hub where they are converted to conscious.

Recent research has shown that in addition to neural mechanisms, the immune system plays a role in the management of pain. It is found that glial cells (the cells, which support and service neurons within the spinal cord) are involved in the production and maintenance of pain. Glial cells are activated by immune challenges (viral or bacterial infection) and by substances released by neurons within the pain pathways. They can amplify pain by releasing cytokines (messenger molecules) that promote inflammation. This may help explain why we experience "ache all over" sensation when we are ill.

Neurochemical Basis of Pain

It is well known that opiates (such as opium, morphine and heroin) have been used for centuries to relieve pain. These substances produce their effects by locking into specific receptor sites in brain regions associated with pain. But why would the brain have these receptors for opiates unless there was some natural chemical in the brain for the receptors to receive? The answer is that the brain has its own built-in painkillers (analgesics) with opiate-like properties. These natural opiates are called **endorphins** (endogenous or internally produced morphines). Endorphins are found to inhibit the release of neurotransmitters involved in the synaptic transmission of pain impulses from the spinal cord to the brain and thus control pain experience. Some endorphins are extremely powerful; one of the recently isolated endorphin has been found to be 200 times more potent than morphine. Researchers have identified three main groups of endogenous opiates: beta-endorphins, proenkephalin and prodynorphins. Recent researches have shown that various regions of the brain including thalamus, amygdala and certain sensory areas of cortex release endorphins when experimental subjects were administered painful stimuli. It was also found that people differed in their pain experience despite identical pain stimulation. The differences were linked to variations in the number of opioid receptors the participants had for the endorphins to bind to and their own ability to release endorphins. The studies clearly indicate that both biological as well as psychological factors underlie differences in people's ability to tolerate pain.

Psychological Factors in Pain

Pain experience is the result of innumerable factors apart from the physiological ones. Pain is influenced by personality, gender, age, beliefs, expectations, social support and cultural factors.

Personality Factors

The personality trait that influences perception of pain is **neuroticism**, the tendency to experience negative emotional states such as depression, anxiety, insecurity and reactivity. People who score high on neuroticism are found to experience more pain than others both in relation to medical conditions and in controlled laboratory administrations of painful stimuli such as electric shock. In contrast, those who are optimistic and have a sense of personal control over their life report lower levels of pain experience. Patients with chronic pain accept the pain rather than blame their fate, respond emotionally to it, have less disability, better adjustment and higher work efficiency. Another factor associated with pain is ***private body consciousness*** (PBC), which refers to the tendency to pay close attention to physical sensations. Researches showed that both college students and patients who were high in PBC report more pain.

Some researchers have classified people into two groups: augmenters and reducers. ***Augmenters***, also called *sensitizers*, perceive stimulation as greater than average; they respond to external stimuli directly and try to do something to deal with it. ***Reducers***, also called *avoiders*, on the other hand, play down external stimulation and even deny it; they see pain stimuli around them as part of the larger field in which other stimuli are embedded. Reducers tend to have a body image with definite boundaries; they are extroverted, have low levels of anxiety and minimize stimulation.

Some people may use pain to attain certain goals. For them, pain can be a way of dramatizing their unhappiness, eliciting care and sympathy from others. Pain can also be a way of avoiding and escaping from threatening and difficult situations. Generally, readiness to use pain as a symptom occurs among people who are old, anxious, neurotic and self-punishing. People with hypochondriasis, reactive depression, psychosomatic conditions and those who use pain to manipulate others suffer more pain than others.

Age Differences

Until recently, it was believed that older people had a higher threshold for pain. This was thought to be due to their lowered sensitivity to stimuli and their reluctance to label noxious stimuli as painful. Recent researches have disputed these claims; some of them have reported an actual decrease in pain threshold as people grow old.

There were some mistaken notions about the experience of pain among infants and young children. There was a belief in the medical community that infants do not experience pain since it was a subjective and psychological phenomenon. For this reason, circumcision was conducted during infancy. Just because infants cannot communicate pain in words, it does not mean that they do not experience pain. They do experience pain and it can be seen in their facial expressions, which are very much similar to those of adults. You must have seen young children making a hell of a scene when a nurse or doctor tries to give them a prick. Are children more sensitive to pain than adults? Although there is not enough research evidence to support age-related difference to pain, there are some indications that children are more sensitive to pain than adults.

Gender Differences

Boys and girls, men and women, appear to differ somewhat in their perception of and reaction to pain, but the evidence is not enough to come to a definite conclusion. Laboratory studies have indicated that women have a lower pain threshold, lower pain tolerance and greater ability to make fine discriminations among pain stimuli. But these differences appear to be small, apply to certain kinds of stimulation and the differences are influenced by a multitude of situational factors. Males and females seem to have different attitudes toward pain because of their early upbringing and socialization process. The tentative conclusion is that generally women tend to report more pain than men, have different modes of coping with pain and exhibit different responses to treatment. Attempts are afoot to see whether hormonal differences between the sexes have anything to do with pain experience. Other researchers are searching for differences in brain structure to explain gender differences in pain.

Sociocultural Factors

How we interpret pain experience depends partly on the culture in which we are brought up. Culture refers to the set of shared beliefs, customs, values, traditions and expectations about the appropriate ways to behave in certain situations in a society. The beliefs we hold about pain and the meanings we attach to painful stimuli often determine the extent of suffering from pain. For example, childbirth is considered as a painful ordeal in Western cultures and many women express considerable anxiety about going through it. But in some cultures, it is the most glorious event and women show virtually no distress about childbirth. In one culture studied by anthropologists, it is the husband who gets into bed and groans as if he were in great pain, while the woman calmly gives birth to the child. The husband stays in bed with the baby to recover from his terrible ordeal, while the mother goes to work in the field almost immediately. In several other cultures, childbearing mothers do not attach strong negative emotions to the associated sensations and as a consequence suffer far less pain.

In India, people engage in some terribly painful rituals during religious festivals. They break coconuts on their heads, pierce sharp needles through various parts of the body and walk on burning cinder. The most painful of these rituals is hook hanging in which a person hangs from a pole with hooks embedded in his back. He hangs from the hooks with his entire body weight with no evidence of pain. When the hooks are removed the wounds heal rapidly and are scarcely visible within a couple of weeks. The religious meaning attached to the hook hanging and other painful ceremonies probably transform the perception of sensory input coming from these acts.

The role of cultural factors in pain perception has been studied among modern Western subcultures. Cultural and social differences in pain tolerance appear to be caused by the anxiety stemming from pain related attitudes, especially the willingness to deny or avoid dealing with pain and the desire to avoid or eliminate pain. In one study, 372 medical patients representing six different ethnic groups (Old Americans, Hispanic Americans, Italian Americans, Irish Americans, French Canadians and Polish Americans) were examined. All of them suffered from chronic pain that was beyond the point of healing. The patients completed self-report measures about their pain experiences. The groups did not differ overall in the type of physical affliction, the duration of illness and the treatment they received. But they differed in the pain levels reported by them and these differences were associated with different attitudes and beliefs they held about their pain. The Hispanic and Italian Americans believed that they had no control over their pain; they were worried and angry about it and reported that they would be unhappy as long as they experienced it. They also believed that it was appropriate to express their pain openly. These two groups experienced intense pain and suffering. In contrast, Old Americans (US-born Caucasians) and Polish Americans felt it best to suppress the outward expression of pain; they were less upset by pain and reported having control over their lives. They reported less suffering from their pain. Researchers have studied Italians, Irish Jews, New Englanders, Eskimos and Native Americans and several other racial and ethnic groups around the world and found intriguing diversity in pain perception. Overall, it was found that different meanings attributed to the pain stimuli and the belief system held about it resulted in very different levels of suffering.

The effect of belief on pain has been vividly demonstrated in studies using **placebos** (inert substances that have no medical value, but are thought by the patients to be helpful). In one study, 122 surgical patients who were suffering from postoperative pain were administered either a *placebo* or morphine. Among those who received morphine, 67 percent found relief, but 42 percent of those who were given a *placebo* also reported similar relief. In some other studies, *placebo* effects have yielded even higher rates of pain relief, as large as 100 percent. So, pain depends on how we interpret it.

Treatment of Pain

The phenomenon of pain has tremendous economic consequences. It is estimated that $170 billion is spent annually in the US (the figure may be an underestimate because several people do not report about their pain-related injuries and illnesses). About 31 million Americans suffer from back pain and the productivity loss because of back pain is estimated to be $28 billion. Therefore, the need for developing new methods of treatment for pain is of paramount importance. During the last few decades, several methods of treating both acute and chronic pain have been developed. Some of them are medical treatments and others are psychological interventions. Whatever the procedure, the aim is the same: to eliminate or reduce pain, or to help the individual to tolerate and if necessary, to live with it.

Medical Treatment

The most common and preferred form of treatment of pain is the use of drugs. Plenty of drugs called analgesics (pain killers) are available today in the market. Several types of drugs such as local anesthetics, sedatives and barbiturates are used to obtain relief from pain. Local anesthetics prevent affected nerve cells from generating pain impulses; these drugs block impulses in pain fibers as well as in motor neurons. Sedatives and barbiturates help to depress pain responses by decreasing the transmission of nerve impulses throughout the central nervous system. These drugs do not really affect pain, but rather reduce the patient's anxiety and help patient to sleep, thereby avoid the pain experience temporarily. Antidepressants work directly by affecting pain-related neurotransmitters and also by reducing the feeling of depression often associated with pain. Peripherally-acting analgesics are the best known of all the forms of pain treatment drugs; these include Aspirin and other non-steroidal anti-inflammatory drugs (NSAID). These drugs reduce inflammation at the site of tissue damage and inhibit the synthesis of neurochemicals that facilitate the transmission of pain impulses. Centrally-acting analgesics (narcotics such as morphine, codeine, methadone and heroin) are pain killers that work by binding to opiate receptors in the central nervous system. Narcotics are very effective in pain reduction. The difficulty with narcotics is their side effects—tolerance and addiction. Clinicians generally do not advocate the use of narcotics for nonmalignant pains.

Psychological Approaches

The most commonly used psychological interventions in the management of pain include cognitive strategies, behavior therapy, progressive relaxation, meditation, biofeedback and hypnosis. Cognitive errors, faulty logic and emotional distress often distort pain experience and interfere with an individual's ability to deal with pain. A meta-analysis (a statistical technique that combines results from several studies to draw relevant conclusions) of 47 studies revealed 85 percent of investigations reporting a positive impact of cognitive strategies on pain reduction or pain tolerance. Generally, the cognitive errors that interfere with an individual's ability to deal with pain are:

1. Catastrophizing—exaggerating the adverse consequences of injury.
2. Overgeneralizing—believing that painful experience will continue forever.
3. Low frustration tolerance—avoiding present discomfort at the cost of long-term gains.
4. External locus of control—believing that external factors determine one's life.
5. Mislabeling somatic sensations—interpreting all bodily sensations as pain.
6. Feelings of worthlessness—reduction in personal usefulness because of pain.
7. Feelings of unjust treatment—believing that one has been treated unfairly by fate.
8. Cognitive rehearsal—continuously brooding over pain.

What we think about pain can significantly influence our perception of pain and its consequences. When cognitive appraisal is characterized by hopelessness, lack of personal control over the events, and a sense of inability to deal with the situation, it generally results in anxiety and depression. Both anxiety and a lack of control over pain can heighten the severity of pain experience. Substituting positive cognitions (hopeful thoughts) in the place of negative ones will go a long way in helping an individual to deal with pain effectively. Diverting attention from pain towards other stimuli can often reduce pain experience. For example, hearing the melodious music when you are having a splitting headache may reduce the intensity of the pain experience. Non-pain imagery (imagining a beautiful valley or waterfalls) has been found to be a good aid in tolerating pain. Often, coping self-statements such as "I am all right," "I can manage the pain," have been found to do a lot of good in helping an individual to put up with pain.

Progressive Relaxation Technique

The progressive relaxation technique has been used successfully in the treatment of back pain, arthritis and headache. Researchers have shown that muscle tension causes the buildup of lactic acid in muscles and decreases blood flow, which in turn aggravates the experience of pain. Psychologists have developed several techniques of progressive relaxation of muscles during their work with behavior therapy. A simple technique is to consciously tense and then relaxing certain muscles experiencing the comfort associated with the relaxed state. Simultaneously, the person might empty the mind of all thoughts and focus on pleasant images. An important aspect of relaxation is deep breathing and keeping the body and mind in peace. Any of these methods can be used to relieve pain. Progressive relaxation has been found to be more effective than drugs in the treatment of pain.

Meditation

Meditation is one type of relaxation. It incorporates an additional element of focus, especially on current sensory experience. A technique called mindfulness meditation involving deep breathing and relaxation has been used successfully to reduce pain and negative emotions. Here the individual is required to concentrate on the pain, but with a "detached observation". The procedure has been found to reduce the emotional distress that accompanies pain. Mindfulness meditation not only reduces negative feelings but also enhances positive affect, activity level and self-esteem. These effects are long lasting and reported to be effective even after 15 months.

Biofeedback

Biofeedback is a technique in which an electronic gadget signals to the individual by means of light or sound to bring about some particular change in body functions.

For example, tension in the forehead muscle, amount of blood flow to the extremities, or skin temperature might be measured using electrodes attached to these specific parts of the body. Muscle tension may be measured using an electromyogram (EMG) biofeedback; temperature and blood flow may be assessed by thermal biofeedback. Biofeedback works on the principle of classical conditioning and teaches people to be aware of their bodily processes and to alter them consciously. This method is extensively used in controlling migraine and tension headaches. Using biofeedback, people have been taught to activate their parasympathetic system, which brings about relaxation during stress or anxiety.

Hypnosis

Hypnosis is often used to alleviate pain. Hypnosis is an altered state of consciousness (artificially produced sleep-like state) brought about by suggestion. It may involve several components such as relaxation, distraction (directing attention away from pain) and suggestion (telling that the pain is getting reduced, and replacing, pain experience by a pleasant sensation). But whether hypnosis really blocks pain or it simply interferes with the reporting of pain by the patient is an issue that is being debated. Hypnosis does not work for everyone; there are significant individual differences in the susceptibility to hypnosis and a complete understanding of the dynamics of hypnosis has not yet been achieved. But there is strong evidence that hypnosis can be used successfully to control certain types of pain among certain groups of people.

There are several other techniques of pain management such as behavior modification based on operant conditioning procedures, physical therapies based on the principle of counterirritation, transcutaneous electrical nerve stimulation and acupuncture. Interested students may consult advanced books on health psychology.

BEHAVIORAL FACTORS IN HEALTH AND ILLNESS

In the beginning of the 20th century, the leading killers were diseases like influenza, pneumonia, tuberculosis, gastroenteritis and heart problems. Today, thanks to the advances in the field of medicine, some of these have been largely controlled. The major killers in modern times are heart diseases, cancer and stroke. These are attributed to health-impairing behaviors. Health experts are of the opinion that the major causes of early mortality can be traced to risky behaviors such as cigarette smoking, excessive alcohol consumption, use of illicit drugs, insufficient exercise, poor food habits, unsafe sex, automobile accidents and failure to adhere to the physician's instructions. It is believed that improvement in the health of modern man is more likely to be the result of efforts to prevent disease and promote health than from new drugs and medical technologies. In this context, the crucial role of behavior in the maintenance of health has been recognized and health psychologists have helped in the identification of psychological and social causes for risky health behavior. They have emphasized the need for lifestyle interventions to promote health and suggested procedures to bring about positive changes in behavior that can contribute toward healthy living. It has been found that modifying people's health behavior as a form of illness prevention can considerably reduce medical cost and avert physical as well as psychological discomfort that diseases produce. Health-related behaviors fall into two categories: health-impairing behaviors and health-enhancing behaviors; we shall briefly examine these two.

Health-impairing Behaviors

Many people, when under stress, engage in self-destructive behaviors such as overeating fatty foods, using tobacco in one form or the other, drug abuse, excessive alcohol consumption, unprotected sex, poor nutrition and lack of exercise. These are referred to as ***health-impairing behaviors*** and they can damage health. People know that these activities definitely endanger their health but still engage in these risky behaviors. Why? Researches have shown that there are several factors that prompt people to engage in such behavior. One of them is ***perceived risk***—how much, we think, a behavior will endanger our health. Another is ***perceived severity***—how much severe, we perceive, the health problem to be. Mostly, our assessment of long-term risks is inaccurate. We may see ourselves as invulnerable and thereby underestimate the risk of health-impairing activities. Despite the evidence regarding health problems that can develop as a result of a variety of undesirable behaviors, we think that these problems do not affect "us."

In fact, one of the major obstacles to the prevention of many diseases is our reluctance to believe that some aspect of our lifestyle requires change. Every day we are bombarded by health-relevant information and have to decide whether or not to accept what we are told by the media about the newly identified threat. Generally, we do not accept such information. We defend ourselves against the threat in ways that are maladaptive. In one study, Liberman & Chaiken (1992) found support to the hypothesis that the more relevant the health threat to the individual, the less likely that person is to accept the truth of the message. The researchers gave their subjects (women), bogus information (supposedly from the *New England Journal of Medicine*) about a medical research that purportedly found a link between caffeine and a breast disorder. The information was either highly threatening (follow-up studies supported the finding) or low in threat (follow-up studies were inconsistent). Personal relevance was defined in terms of the coffee-drinking habits of the participants. The researchers assumed low relevance for those who did not drink coffee, and high relevance for those who drank two to seven cups a day. Surprisingly, women to whom the threat was most relevant (regular coffee drinkers) were less likely to believe either the high threat or the low threat message than women who did not drink coffee. Because information about possible health threats arouses fear and anxiety, the more relevant such messages are to one, the less one believes in them. It appears that when a health threat is relevant to oneself, one processes the information in a biased way, which defuses the threat, reduces anxiety and therefore makes it unnecessary to change one's present behavior. As you can see, the rejection of relevant, threatening information is extremely maladaptive.

Changing Health-impairing Behavior

Changing people's unhealthy behaviors such as smoking, drinking and overeating is not easy. Programs that attempt to change people's problematic behavior suggest that they may either change their behavior or they continue it. But researches by Prochaska and his colleagues have proposed a different conception of change, which has come to be known as the ***transtheoretical model*** (Prochaska et al, 1998). The model identifies six major steps in the change process.

Precontemplation: The person has no intention to change unhealthy behavior; does not perceive the problem; denies the existence of problem itself or feels powerless to change. He/She may change under pressure from outside, but the problem will relapse once the pressure is removed.

Contemplation: The person acknowledges the existence of a problem and starts thinking of the desirability of a behavior change or doing something about it, but has not yet decided about the action. The real action, though, is seen as far in the future, not now.

People generally get stuck at this phase. It is like a smoker who knows the hazards of smoking, but still cannot decide to quit the habit. Unless he realizes that the benefits of quitting outweigh the cost of his efforts, he will not take action.

Preparation: The person is aware of the problem and its causes and wants to change his behavior. He develops tentative plans to change and is committed to change as early as possible. The smoker takes preliminary steps and cuts down the number of cigarettes per day. But still he has mixed feelings about change and starts vacillating whether to take action or not. The intended plan may not be put into practice.

Action: The person has decided to act and starts changing his behavior. The smoker throws away his cigarette pack and stops smoking. This stage requires the greatest amount of behavior-control skills to stick to his decision. External social support helps the person to stick to his/her decision.

Maintenance: The person has not smoked for the last six months and controlled the temptation to smoke. Still he is afraid of the relapse, but in view of the benefits of not smoking—the food tastes better, the cough is under control, the family appreciates his behavior, etc., he maintains his changed pattern of behavior. The struggle is not completely over; the temptation to smoke may still be there. He may in fact start smoking again but he reinstates the change efforts. It may take three to five cycles of "starting and quitting" the habit because it is strongly entrenched.

Termination: If the decision to change is very strong and there are personal control and social support, the chances of relapse are minimal; the problem may not recur.

The model outlined above is based upon observation that, most people go through stages of change, each stage having its own tasks that must be completed in order to go on to the next stage. People may not go through these stages smoothly; they may move forward and backward through the stages as they try to change their behavior over time. Many people may make repeated attempts to change before they completely succeed. Failure at a given stage is likely to occur if the previous stage has not been completely mastered.

The transtheoretical model has important applied implications. When we know that people go through different stages in changing their problem behavior and they need different types of interventions, we can develop suitable strategies for this purpose. In fact psychologists have designed some stage-matched interventions that help in moving from contemplation to action and maintenance stage. Some such interventions are mentioned below.

Strategies that Help Change

During the earlier stages in the model suggested above, consciousness raising and social liberation can be of help in changing undesirable behavior. *Consciousness-raising* involves becoming aware of the problem and the way the person avoids facing it. Precontemplators need consciousness-raising information that convinces them that there is a problem and there are ways to deal with it. A smoker may feel that smoking will take care of itself when his other problems are solved, and does not bother to do anything about it. Such person may have to be convinced about the health hazards of smoking and the ways of quitting it. *Social liberation* refers to external forces that may help in providing information about the problem and the alternatives to it. Social forces work in several ways. For example, you cannot smoke when you are in your work place and when you are at home. You may have to go out to smoke and look out whether someone is watching you. This makes smoking a cumbersome process, less comfortable and less pleasurable. Similarly, social forces warn about drunken driving or over-speeding. During the latter stages of the model, emotional arousal and self-re-evaluation may help in changing the problem behavior. *Emotional arousal* refers to becoming intensely concerned about the consequences of problem behavior. For example, a smoker may become anxious about his developing lung cancer or heart complaints. A car driver may think about serious accidents when he is driving speedily or when he is drunk. *Self-reevaluation* involves thinking about the pros and cons of continuing or changing the health-impairing behavior. The person may take stock, both intellectually and emotionally, whether this is what (sticking to problem behavior) he/she wants to be.

Health-enhancing Behaviors

Researches during the last three decades in health psychology have clearly shown that by adhering to certain behavior patterns people can remain healthy and live longer. One longitudinal study of 7,000 adults revealed that there is a significant relationship between seven good health practices and life expectancy. These include sleeping 7 to 8 hours a day, eating a good breakfast, not eating between meals, maintaining an optimum body weight, not smoking and consuming a minimum of alcohol. For both men and women, these practices predict a longer life. Let us examine some of these health-enhancing behaviors and how people can be encouraged to cultivate them.

Exercise

An American medical expert once remarked that if exercise could be prescribed as a capsule, that would be the most sold drug in the world. True, everybody asserts that exercise is associated with health and longevity. Activities such as jogging, cycling, swimming and aerobic exercises have been found to produce many physical benefits. In a body that is well conditioned by regular aerobic exercise, the heart beats more efficiently, the oxygen is better utilized, cholesterol level is reduced, slow-wave sleep is increased, the body can cope with stressors and more calories are burned. Despite the known benefits, it is unfortunate that people do not realize the importance of exercise and prefer to lead couch potato lives. Many people nowadays do not engage in active manual work and remain lazy most of the time. Sedentary lifestyle can give rise to several health problems including heart diseases, obesity and diabetes. A study that followed 17,000 Harvard students into their middle age revealed that death rates were one quarter to one third lower among moderate exercisers than among those who were leading a less active life. Surprisingly, extremely high levels of exercise were not associated with enhanced health; moderate regular exercise produced the best health benefits. Such exercise has a positive impact on mental health also; the incidence of anxiety and depression was low among moderate exercisers.

Why do people not engage in exercise? Research has shown that factors like low self-efficacy for success in exercising regularly ("I can't do this"), type A personality ("I have no time to exercise"), inflated opinion about one's good health ("I am perfectly fit, there is no need to exercise"), and inactive leisure time activities (watching TV most of the time) contribute toward people's lack of interest in exercise. Psychologists have suggested that improved methods of educating people to engage in exercise must be introduced early in life.

Weight Control

Nowadays there is an increasing tendency among people to eat more and grow fat, especially in developed societies. Even children and adolescents tend to be overweight. As a consequence, death rate due to obesity is increasing. It is reported that if this trend continues, 500,000 people will die every year in the United States of America alone. Obesity predisposes people to a variety of chronic diseases such as cardiac complaints, kidney disorders and diabetes. Abdominal fat deposit is a far greater risk factor for cardiovascular disease, diabetes and cancer than fat deposits in the hips, thighs or buttocks.

Weight reducing programs involve behavior interventions. The program may begin with a period of self-monitoring, during which you would keep careful records of what, when and how much you eat. This will give you an idea of your food habits and the situational factors (antecedents) that induce you to eat. Then you would learn to have control over the antecedents. For example, you may increase the intake of raw vegetable and reduce eating high calorie foods. You are advised to confine your eating to one particular place and time. You learn to eat slowly, with pauses between mouthfuls. You bite, chew, and swallow slowly. This way you eat less. But eat items with high nutritional value. You try to enjoy every mouthful. The goal is to enjoy more and eat less. These behavioral interventions reduce your food intake. You arrange to positively reward yourself for eating less and enjoying it more. Add to this a program of regular exercise. You are sure to reduce your weight considerably, and you know, you will enjoy the weight loss more than the food.

Self-regulation

Researches have shown that mere medical treatment is not enough for speedy recovery from illness. If treatment is associated with lifestyle changes, recovery is quicker and better. In one study, William Haskell and coworkers (1994) divided people suffering from coronary artery disease into two groups. Group-A was given the best of the available medical treatment. Group-B was put under a behavioral self-regulation program, which included active exercise, control of smoking, weight reduction, nutritive food habits and meditation. A 4 years follow-up study revealed that the group-A (which received the medical treatment only) showed either no improvement or worsening of the disease condition. On the other hand, those who received behavior self-regulation training (group-B) showed significant improvement. They reduced their fatty food intake, showed reduction in the level of bad cholesterol (LDL) and increase in the level of good cholesterol (HDL), engaged in active exercise and improved the efficiency of their cardiovascular functions. Group-B members had 47 percent less buildup of blockage material in their artery walls. During the 4 years follow-up period, 45 percent of the group-A patients either died or had non-fatal heart attacks or other cardiac complications compared with only 24 percent deaths in group-B. The study demonstrates the value of psychologically-based interventions in the promotion of health. In this context, I am reminded of the advice given by a cardiologist to a person who has undergone cardiac bypass surgery: "If you don't change your lifestyle, I may have to bypass the bypass."

MAINTAINING POSITIVE BEHAVIOR CHANGE

Several people, after a change for the better, unfortunately fail to maintain the positive behaviors. The biggest problem facing an individual who strives to adopt healthy practices and eliminate unhealthy ones is relapse. *Relapse* can be defined as the recurrence of bad habits (behaviors or symptoms) after a period of improvement. The ex-smoker, who did not touch cigarettes for several months, begins to smoke regularly. The person who was dieting to control weight starts eating fatty food. This is a major problem in behavior change. The dropout rate is high. Why do people relapse into their problem behaviors? What can we do to prevent this tendency? After investigating this issue, the researchers have proposed an intervention program known as ***relapse prevention***. The purpose of the intervention was to reduce the risk of relapse. Observations on drug abusers have shown that most relapses (return to undesirable habits) tend to occur after the person has suffered one or more lapses (occasional slips) in the face high-risk situations such as interpersonal conflicts, pressure from peers to engage in undesirable behaviors, stressful situations and negative emotions. Relapse occurs among people who have not developed coping skills to deal with high-risk situations. Such people have low self-efficacy and believe that they do not have enough strength to resist the temptations or for them, the pleasures of bad habits (such as smoking, unprotected sex, drug abuse, etc.) are more important than their ill effects. Under such circumstances, relapse occurs and it is followed by a reaction called **abstinence violation effect**, which is characterized by blaming oneself for the inability to control the undesirable behavior. The person starts thinking that he is weak-willed and will never be able to resist the temptation. This sense of helplessness puts the person in such a situation that he/she will abandon all attempts to change. Only those who have effective coping skills associated with a sense of self-confidence to handle the situation can avoid relapse even when there is a lapse. Psychologists have developed relapse-prevention training programs, which include:

1. Studying the lapse carefully to identify the causes that have led to it.
2. Identifying the specific cognitive, emotional and social antecedents.
3. Learning to handle the antecedents effectively.
4. Practicing the skills to improve self-efficacy.
5. Focusing on "progress, not perfection."
6. Enhancing the level of motivation to continue healthy habits by suitable rewards.

With effort, cultivation of positive health behavior and the avoidance of negative ones can be maintained indefinitely. With knowledge, skill and social support, people really can change their lives and improve their health. Relapse prevention training has been found to be effective in changing many problematic behaviors such as smoking, drug addiction, overeating and sexual offenses. In short, relapse is caused by a combination of factors such as negative emotional states, inadequate initial motivation, lack of skill to cope with the pressures to relapse, physiological factors (craving for smoking), lack of social support and environmental stimuli that favor the unhealthy behavior.

PHYSICIAN-PATIENT INTERACTION

In the interaction between physician and the patient, what happens to the patient is what matters most. It is better to have a patient get well and never know precisely what was the illness than make a distinguished diagnosis and have the patient die. In the light of this observation, it is assumed that the interaction between the doctor and the patient is an important determiner of health and illness. The relationship that develops and the type of communication between the two are the essential features of medical treatment. It is unfortunate that many physicians do not have either the time or the patience to talk to their patients. Doctors today treat the disease and forget the patient. The spoken words are extremely powerful tools in medical care;

they establish the reality of suffering. Let us briefly discuss some of these issues.

Physician-patient Relationship

The patient-physician relationship depends upon the circumstances that surround their association and upon their beliefs about the appropriate locus of responsibility and power in the relationship. Generally, the relationship takes one of three basic forms: the active-passive model, the guidance-cooperation model and the mutual participation model (Szasz and Hollender, 1956). The ***active-passive model*** exists when the patient is unable, because of his/her medical condition, to participate in care and to make decisions regarding personal welfare. The physician takes over the responsibility of the patient's welfare and the patient has no say in what is being done. In the ***guidance-cooperative model***, the physician is largely responsible for diagnosis and treatment. The patient simply answers questions and provides information. The doctor makes the decision. In the ***mutual participation model***, the doctor and the patient make joint decisions about all aspects of diagnosis, treatment and medical care. Questions and discussions take place freely and there is an exchange of information. The responsibility is shared. Some researchers have modified the basic models, but the total picture more or less remains the same. Also, the styles may vary depending on various aspects of the medical care. ***Mutuality*** is an important element in the medical relationship because it balances the power and responsibility between the doctor and the patient. The achievement of mutuality requires dedication and open-mindedness on the part of both parties and it is better than other models because it combines the expertise of the physician and the patient.

Physician and Patient Communication

It is through the process of communication the practitioner and the patient attempt to gain a common understanding of the illness and the course of treatment. Long ago, Sir William Osler, an eminent Canadian physician who practiced and taught in Canada, Great Britain and the USA, observed that "if physicians would only listen to their patients, the latter would tell them the diagnosis." Even today, it is held that talking is the main ingredient of medical care and that communication is the most important means of achieving therapeutic goals. But, unfortunately there are many hurdles to communication between the doctor and the patient. Many patients are reluctant to talk or they talk too much. The reasons for the reluctance to talk are many and varied. The patient may think that the doctor is an "all knowing" person and he/she will be able to find out the source of the problem by a thorough physical examination. This is an impossible proposition; diagnosing a medical problem is more an art than a science, and the doctor may not be always successful in this regard. Secondly, the physicians enjoy a relatively high degree of social prestige and power; this may inhibit the patient from talking out of fear of being misunderstood or committing a social blunder. Patients may not volunteer information thinking that it would cast them in a bad light or they may feel embarrassed to talk about the illness. Finally, many patients are unable to report accurately the nature of their problem.

Physicians generally dominate the interview; they may not have the patience or time to hear the patient. Some of them may not be skilled at encouraging the patient to provide necessary information or talk in such technical language that the patient does not understand. Often the physician does not give an opportunity to the patient to participate in the treatment because he/she believes that the patient's participation is not valuable and not worth the trouble. More than all, the physician may be very busy; there may be many patients waiting in the queue to be seen, and he/she may not have time to talk to the patients in detail (as it happens in many underdeveloped countries). Some patients talk too much, explaining every bit of their problem in such detail; the doctor may consider listening to it as simply waste of time. Whatever the source of difficulty, insufficient or inefficient communication is a major handicap in medical practice. As modern medicine becomes more and more dominated by technology, many medical professionals tend to give reduced attention to patient-doctor communication.

Listening to patients is an important component of medical care. Practitioners who listen carefully to what patients say are more likely to make a much better diagnosis and chalk out an effective form of treatment. The most often heard complaint of the patients is; "The doctor did not listen to anything; I tried to say". Listening requires "no talking." Several studies have shown that patients do not have much of a chance to talk because physicians talk so much. Listening with empathy goes a long way in understanding the patient's problem and facilitating the cure. Remember, words too are therapeutic tools.

Adherence to Medical Regimens

One of the major consequences of insufficient patient-physician communication is the lack of compliance with medical advice. Compliance with or adherence to medical regimens is an important factor, which has been studied by medical men, psychologists and sociologists. The terms refer to the degree of success a patient has in carrying out the medical treatment recommendations given to him/her by a health professional. On the other hand, non-compliance or non-adherence refers to patients' ignoring, forgetting or misunderstanding the regimen as prescribed by the health professional and thus carrying it out wrong or not carrying it out at all. Surveys show that perhaps 85 percent of patients do not fully comply with their physician's advice. One comprehensive survey of over 500 studies found high rates of non-compliance. Patients kept only 50 to 75 percent of their scheduled appointments and failed to take medicines as directed by their doctors 23 to 50 of the time. Non-adherence appeared to be more frequent when the medications had to be taken over a long period of time. Patients do not follow the advice regarding diet, alcohol consumption and smoking. Non-compliance is a real threat to successful health maintenance and a major problem in the delivery of effective medical service. The development of certain types of drug-resistant pathogens is traced directly to the problems of non-compliance of patients with drug regimens.

Why do patients not comply with the physician's advice? The answer is not simple. Many patients stop taking the drugs the moment there is some relief; they think that they no longer need them. Some people keep the drugs in safe custody, so that they may take them when there is a relapse. Some other patients practice ***creative non-adherence***, in which they modify a treatment advised by their doctor based on their own judgment or experience. Non-compliance may be a result of psychological **reactance**, a negative cognitive and emotional reaction toward attempted control of one's freedom. People often become hostile when someone tries to restrict their freedom and in this case, they do so in a self-destructive manner by refusing to accept medical advice. A patient will not carry out a health behavior if significant barriers stand in the way or if the steps to carry out the behavior actually interfere with favorite activities. Often the high cost of drugs may become an impediment for poor people.

Can compliance be increased? Although compliance does not guarantee that the disease will disappear, it does optimize the possibility that the patient's condition will improve. Several suggestions have been made to increase patient compliance. For one thing, the person must somehow be committed to comply with the regimen. True and internally motivated commitment comes when the patient believes that adhering to medical advice is going to be beneficial and it will bring about valued outcomes. Real commitment emerges when the pros and cons of following the physician's advice are carefully evaluated from several angles (wishes of the family, friends and the social circle). Social support enhances adherence to the medical regimen. When the physician maintains good, warm relationship with the patient, compliance will be better. The instructions he/she offers must be clear. Physicians who provide clear, accurate, honest information produce greater compliance. Patients want to be informed about the drug, its side effects if any, and the number of days it may take for the symptoms to subside. This will create in the patient greater confidence toward the doctor. Patients will be less anxious and more confident about the outcome of the medical treatment. In short, a positive interaction with the physician brings with it the potential for substantial health benefits.

Most people under a doctor's care are able to achieve and maintain control over their diseases if they carefully follow the treatment recommendations made by their doctors. Patients who strictly follow antihypertensive regimens are more likely to have lower blood pressure than are those who fail to comply with prescribed medications and health behaviors. People with heart diseases who regularly take the prescribed medicines are less likely to die than are those who do not. If a prescribed treatment is the correct one, it is not surprising that the patient becomes well by following it. What is surprising is the fact that people benefit from sheer adhering to treatment even when it has no direct effect on the disease. This is the well-known ***placebo effect***. A placebo is an inert object (such as a sugar pill) that has no direct effect on the body. A practitioner administers a placebo instead of a drug to the patient (who does not know it is a placebo) and assures that it will work. Often, it works, the patient becomes well, which is an instance of mind over body. Sometimes, in what is called the '**double blind situation**', both patient and the doctor are unaware of the fact that the administered drug is placebo. Even then cure has occurred. Researches have shown that pure and strict adherence to regimen in itself can bring about improvement in health. It is observations such as these that projected health psychology to the forefront in recent times.

CONCLUDING WORDS

Stress is a fact of life. Pain is a universal phenomenon. Diseases are widespread. Fortunately, stress can be managed, pain reduced and diseases prevented if certain elementary principles of living are cultivated. Life is a continuous process of adjusting to environmental demands. When these demands go beyond the individual's capacity to cope with, he/she experiences stress. People try to cope with stress by changing the environment or their behavior. Certain amount of stress is necessary to keep people active, alert and energized. Only when stress goes beyond a limit, we experience *distress*. Whether stress energizes or drains you physically and psychologically depends on your life style. Health psychologists have made significant contributions to help people reduce health-impairing behaviors and healthy lifestyle. So, what can we do to keep the stress within manageable limits and see that it does not become distress? What principles should we follow to stay healthy? Health psychologists suggest the following tips to maintain stress within a manageable level and lead healthy life:

1. Know your limits; you cannot do everything; avoid attempting more than what you can accomplish. Wherever possible, delegate responsibilities to

others. Unrealistic expectations are a major source of stress. Set realistic goals.
2. Have a time table for things you want to do. Arrange them according to their importance; attend to the most urgent tasks. You can attend to less essential ones later.
3. Learn to live with hassles, especially when you do not have control over them. If there is a traffic jam, do not grumble; instead spend the time reading a newspaper or a book.
4. Learn to relax; listen to music; read something interesting—not a textbook.
5. Take care of your body. Have a balanced diet. Avoid rushing through your meals. Get enough sleep. Exercise regularly.
6. Avoid drug abuse; control smoking, reduce alcohol consumption. Get regular medical checkup.
7. Expand your social network. Social support reduces the effect of stress and vulnerability to illness.
8. Prevent burnout.
9. Learn to say "No" when people make unreasonable demands on you.
10. Avoid stress-inducing thoughts, disappointments, setbacks, disasters. Do not keep upsetting feelings bottled up. Express your feelings.
11. Control type A behavior pattern. Avoid unhealthy competition. Take things easy. Rome was not built in a day. Remember, the world can go on without you; you are not indispensable.
12. Prevention is better than cure. Try to follow elementary principles of hygiene. Undergo immunization and get vaccinated for some of the dreadful diseases.

Chapter Summary

Health psychology is concerned with the study of psychological factors that affect the origin, development, prevention and treatment of physical illness. An important phenomenon that, contributes to ill health or well-being is stress. But, what is stress? Some researchers think of stress as stimulus, some others as a response and still others look at it as a process. Although there is no agreement on the exact meaning of stress, it can be defined as people's reaction to demanding situations; it is the pressure placed on an organism while adjusting or adapting to the environment. The threatening situation or object that produces stress is called stressor. For example, daily hassles, financial problems, job-related problems, significant life changes, conflicts, frustrations, persistent pain and a medical disorder are stressors. Both major negative life events and minor everyday hassles can produce undesirable psychological consequences such as anxiety and depression. Stress can increase vulnerability to physical illness by impairing the functioning of the body's immune system, Psychoneuroimmunology (PNI), an interdisciplinary area studies the relationship among psychological factors, the immune system, and the brain. Stressors can bring about negative health changes; increase the risk of illness, worsen the pre-existing diseases or even increase the chances of death.

Hans Selye made significant contribution to our understanding of stress. He described the physiological response to stress as the general adaptation syndrome, which involves the stages of alarm, resistance and exhaustion. Alarm reaction involves mobilization of the body's resources to cope with immediate stress. Resistance stage is characterized by body's attempt to adjust or adapt to persistent stress. The third stage, exhaustion is characterized by the depletion of bodily resources to stress-related conditions. The autonomic nervous system (ANS) and the endocrine system play a key role in the body's response to stress. Cognitive appraisal plays an important role in determining people's responses to stressors. People appraise the nature of the demands, the resources available to deal with them, the possible consequences of the situation, and the personal meaning of these consequences. Distortions in any of these processes can lead to an inappropriate stress response.

Contd...

Contd...

Several ways of managing stress are available. Three major ways of coping with stress are problem-focused coping, emotion-focused coping, and seeking social support. Emotional disclosure can bring about positive changes in the state of body and mind. Emotional constraint may be a risk factor in the development of physical disorders. Stress-management teaches people adaptive coping skills for handling stress. Cognitive restructuring and self-instructional training can be used to develop coping skills. Behavioral interventions, biofeedback, relaxation techniques and meditation are helpful to control physiological arousal associated with stress. Personality factors such as hardiness, coping self-efficacy, optimistic outlook and positive attitudes to life and living can fortify body and mind against stressful events.

Pain is a universal phenomenon and it can be a major source of stress. The experience of pain is influenced by physiological, psychological, and sociocultural factors. At the level of physiology, the major receptors of pain appear to be free nerve endings. Gate control theory attributes pain to the opening and closing of gates in the spinal cord and certain other influences emanating from the brain. Endorphins in the nervous system are believed to play a role in pain reduction. Glial cells are also implicated in pain. Expectations of relief produced by *placebos* can markedly reduce the experience of pain. Cultural and religious factors influence the appraisal of pain. Negative emotional states are found to increase the suffering and decrease tolerance for pain. Psychological techniques such as dissociative and associative cognitive strategies (dissociating oneself from painful stimuli; associating with the stimuli by studying it objectively), providing sensory and procedural information to increase cognitive control and increasing activity level are used to counter chronic pain.

A transtheoretical model consisting of six stages has been proposed to change health-impairing behavior and increase health-enhancing behavior. The stages are: pre-contemplation, contemplation, preparation, action, maintenance, termination. The model has inspired stage-specific interventions to help people move toward action, maintenance, and termination stages. Researchers have identified seven good health-improving practices such as exercise, sleeping 7 to 8 hours, eating a good breakfast, rarely eating between meals, avoiding alcohol, maintaining a prescribed body weight and engaging in regular physical activity. Exercise had been found to be an effective health-enhancing behavior, but people fail to adhere to exercise programs. Social support influences adherence. If people can stick to an effective exercise program for three to six months, further adherence is easy. Inability to control the weight increase has been a severe problem and this has prompted researchers to development of several behavioral weight-control measures, such as stimulus control (not being tempted by the sight or smell of food), self-monitoring (what have I eaten, what I should not eat) and training people to eat less and less. A good exercise program can contribute to weight loss. Combating health-impairing behaviors include avoiding unprotected and high-risk sexual activities, homosexual practices and drug abuse. Drug abuse is associated with other disorders and is part of a larger pattern of maladjustment. Multimodal treatments including aversion training, stress management, coping-skill training, and positive reinforcement procedures have been found useful in bringing about a change in self-defeating behavior. Relapse prevention is designed to keep lapses from becoming relapses by building effective coping skills to deal with high risk situations and countering the abstinence violence effect when lapses occur.

In recent times, health psychologists are concentrating on the study of physician-patient interaction as an important determiner of speedy recovery and health maintenance. Communication pattern between the doctor and patient play a significant role in diagnosis, treatment and prevention of illnesses. Unfortunately, modern doctors talk too much and have no time to listen to the client. One of the major complaints of people who go to a doctor is—"The doctor did not listen to me." The physician should not forget that empathic listening is a potent therapeutic tool.

A serious problem impeding recovery is the bad habit of not adhering to the medical regimen, the non-compliance of medical advice by the patients. They do not take medicines regularly, do not keep the appointment with the doctor and do not obey the instructions such as not smoking, avoiding certain foods, engaging in physical activities or taking bed rest. It is reported that the non-compliance is as high as 85 percent. The importance of compliance has been shown in placebo studies. Patients who follow the medical regimen get cured soon even when the drug administered is a placebo. Unfortunately, many people who do not comply do so for a number of reasons. One important reason is lack of proper supervision or inadequate communication between the doctor and the patient. The other is patient reactance (a negative emotional state produced by curtailment of personal freedom). Sometimes the patients stop taking a drug when there is slight improvement in their condition. Some patients preserve the drug for later treatment. This is a psychological problem and a fit subject for investigation by psychologists.

15

CHAPTER

Abnormal Psychology

Study of Psychological Disorders

PREVIEW

All along we have been discussing normal adaptive behavior. But there are some individuals who engage in maladaptive behavior for reasons unknown to them. Even some normal people at times exhibit maladaptive, deviant or abnormal behavior. The terms abnormal and abnormal behavior are often used as roughly equivalent to psychological disorder or mental disorder. This chapter deals with abnormal behavior, its meaning, conceptualization, classification, causes and course. The treatment of these disorders will be discussed in the next chapter.

Although the term appears simple, psychologists have struggled over the years to provide a precise definition to the term abnormality. A person who exhibits behavior that tends to be distressing, unusual or dysfunctional may generally be considered abnormal. But this one criterion is not enough, abnormalities rely on multiple criteria. Psychologists, while defining abnormality, take into account several characteristics of behavior such as its unusualness, social deviance, maladaptiveness, dangerousness, faulty perceptions and interpretation of reality, and emotional distress caused by such behaviors.

In ancient times, mental patients were viewed as possessed by demons. Treatment consisted of drilling holes in their skull to drive away the evil spirits. Abnormality was linked to witchcraft, and patients were tortured and burned at stakes as witches. Patients were whipped, starved, immersed in hot water. The treatment was worse than the illness. It took several years to develop a humanitarian view of mental patients. Fortunately, today, we have an enlightened view of these unfortunate people and this awakening parallels the developments in medicine and psychology.

The first breakthrough in understanding abnormality came in the form of the medical model of mental illness, which considered abnormality as a product of changes in the neurophysiological factors in the body. The second view looked at these disorders from the psychological angle. The most famous of these psychological perspectives was that of Sigmund Freud, who proposed that abnormality stems from unconscious conflicts that have their roots in the early childhood. Today, differing explanations are given to abnormal behavior by different groups of psychologists, psychiatrists and psychoanalysts. Among them, behaviorists think of abnormality as a form of learned maladaptive behavior. Cognitive psychologists believe that most of the abnormalities result from the irrational beliefs, perfectionist expectations and faulty thinking. Humanists view abnormality as resulting from barriers to growth and self-actualization. According to them, if human beings are allowed to become what they can, everything would be perfectly all right. Each of these viewpoints suggests not only different causes of abnormal behavior but also different forms of treatment. Some of these approaches are found to be more successful with particular disorders than others.

The knowledge you acquire by reading this and the next chapter will go a long way in understanding your patients. It is said that about 70 percent of the people who visit a outpatient medical clinic are suffering more from psychological disturbances than the physical diseases. The information given in this chapter may raise your awareness about the psychological problems of people you deal with and perhaps even some of the problems you encounter in your own life. But this is only an introduction; it is not intended to make you a diagnostician. If it stimulates a desire in you to study further, the purpose of the chapter is served.

Chapter Outline

WHAT IS ABNORMALITY?

As the name suggests, abnormal psychology deals with behaviors that are unusual, deviant, undesirable, dysfunctional, maladaptive, impaired, dangerous, distressing or simply abnormal. Sarason and Sarason (1996) defined abnormal psychology as the area within psychology that focuses on maladaptive behavior—its causes, consequences and treatment. Although it is easy to describe abnormal behavior, it is difficult to distinguish between normal and abnormal, and to give a crisp non-controversial definition to the term abnormality. Not that there are no definitions, there are, but they are not universally accepted. Although there is no consensus on any single definition, there is some agreement as to what constitutes abnormality and what conditions do not.

There are some very clear elements that suggest abnormality, but no one element of abnormality is sufficient to define the term. All that we can do is to select the major components of abnormality and determine the extent to which an individual exhibits these tendencies. Based on some major components we can define (describe) abnormality as follows.

Abnormality as impairment: The extent to which an individual's behavior is impaired and disorganized, causing disability to the individual. For example, an officer who is anxious cannot make accurate decisions; to that extent his/her behavior is abnormal.

Abnormality as discomfort: The degree of distress or suffering the person is experiencing because of the behavior he/she is exhibiting. For example, a lady who bursts into tears and expresses hopelessness about future for no apparent reason is exhibiting distress.

Abnormality as inability to function effectively: The extent to which the behavior is maladaptive, useless and dysfunctional. A person is exhibiting abnormality when he withdraws from family and friends, and is unable to work for months.

Abnormality as deviation from the average or the ideal: The extent to which the behavior deviates from the normal standards, and violates sociocultural norms. Often, statistically infrequent conditions such as mental retardation are taken as abnormal.

Abnormality as social discomfort: The extent to which an individual's behavior causes discomfort to people around him/her. Suppose somebody sitting beside you in a railway compartment blurts out that he/she is going to jump out of the running train, how do you feel? Is it not terribly discomforting?

Abnormality as irrationality and unpredictability: The Unorthodox, unconventional and unexpected forms of behavior are often considered abnormal. Suppose your copassenger in a bus, suddenly starts screaming and yelling obscenities at you for no reason; the behavior is disorganized, unexpected and does not make sense to you.

Abnormality as dangerous behavior: Any behavior that is harmful to the individual and others can be called abnormal. For example, a person who is depressed may attempt suicide and a paranoid may attack indiscriminately people around him/her.

Abnormality as insanity: The term **insanity** is a legal concept, not a psychological construct. The legal system makes a distinction between normal and abnormal based on the concept of insanity. When a court tries a person for an offense, he may not be held responsible for the crime he has committed if the person is found to be suffering from insanity. But the definition of insanity varies from country to country and one state to another. In one country, a person who cannot understand the difference between right and wrong is considered insane. In another country, a person who lacks impulse control or is incapable of understanding the criminality of his behavior is dubbed as insane. In some other states, courts do not allow any plea of insanity.

None of the above definitions is broad enough to cover all instances of abnormal behavior. None of them help us to judge whether a behavior is normal or abnormal. For example, a death in the family causes immense suffering, but it cannot be considered abnormal. A contract (supari) killer kills for money; that is the way he makes his living. Is his behavior abnormal? When a student is talking to himself when he is alone in his room, we may call the behavior crazy. But suppose, in fact, he is practicing "Mark Antony's Speech" from Hamlet for a public performance on the college day, what would you say? Of course, it is easy to distinguish between normal and abnormal in the case of severe mental disorders such as schizophrenia. People with psychotic disorders exhibit certain bizarre symptoms such as **hallucinations** (having sensory experiences in the absence of appropriate stimulation) and **delusions** (entertaining certain absurd false beliefs). But even these symptoms do not help us to define abnormality because in some societies, these symptoms are not at all regarded as unusual or abnormal. There are some societies in which hearing voices, or being possessed by a spirit is considered as divine intervention rather than psychological disturbance. For example, in some North African and Middle Eastern cultures people experience a condition called 'zar,' or spirit possession. Those affected may shout, laugh, hit their head against a wall and show other bizarre behaviors. This condition does not bother anybody in that culture, although it appears abnormal to you. In some countries, homosexuality is not considered abnormal, marriage between same sexed partners is tolerated; such behavior is considered crazy in several cultures. Therefore, be warned; it is not as easy as it appears to distinguish normal from the abnormal.

Probably one way to solve the problem is to view normality and abnormality as two ends of a continuum rather than as two qualitatively distinct conditions. Behavior then can be evaluated in degrees ranging from completely normal to extremely abnormal. Most people's behavior falls somewhere between the two extremes. You may say that a normal person is less abnormal and an abnormal person is less normal. Abnormal behavior or a psychological disorder involves a constellation of cognitive, affective and behavioral components that produce significant distress to the person; it impairs his/her performance in educational institutions, occupational settings and social relations; it interferes in daily living and may lead to significant risk of harm. Therefore, no single criterion is sufficient to capture the meaning of abnormality; most conceptualizations of abnormality rely on multiple criteria.

CLASSIFICATION OF ABNORMAL BEHAVIOR

The number of abnormal behaviors is so large that it becomes impossible to comprehend them without some sort of classification. Most sciences rely on classification; biologists classify living organisms into kingdom, phyla and classes, chemists classify elements according to the periodic table. With an agreed classification system, we can be confident that we are communicating clearly. When your friend tells you "I purchased a car," you have a mental image that approximates to that of a car. There are of course a variety of cars varying in size shape and color and yet, you have no difficulty in recognizing the essential features of "carness." This "carness" is what psychologists refer to as a "cognitive prototype" or "pattern." In abnormal psychology, classification involves the attempt to delineate meaningful subvarieties of maladaptive behavior. Classification of some sort is the necessary first step toward introducing order into our discussion of the nature, causes and treatment of abnormal behavior. Classification makes it possible to communicate about particular clusters of abnormal behavior in agreed upon and relatively precise ways.

Mental health professionals classify abnormal behaviors into several categories called psychological disorders or mental disorders. They designate a single indicator of abnormality a symptom. Symptom may involve emotion (e.g. anxiousness), cognition (e.g. thought disturbances) or behavior (e.g. eating disorders). A group or pattern of symptoms that occur together consistently in a disorder is called syndrome. A syndrome represents the typical picture of a disorder and can be taken as indicative of a particular disorder.

Although there have been several attempts to classify mental disorders down the ages, it was Emil Kraepelin, a German psychiatrist, who developed an early synthesis and classification system of the hundreds of mental disorders by grouping them together based on common pattern of symptoms. He demonstrated that mental disorders showed specific patterns in their genesis, course and outcome. The current systems of classification, to some extent, are based on the work of Kraepelin. At present, there are two systems of classification that are popular. One is the Classification of Mental and Behavioral Disorders (CMBD), which is a section of the World Health Organization's International Classification of Diseases (ICD-10) and the other, is the Diagnostic and Statistical Manual of Mental Disorders, popularly known as **DSM**, published by the American Psychiatric Association. Both the systems are currently in use. The ICD-10 is widely used in Europe and many other countries whereas DSM is the standard guide in the United States. Since, DSM is an important tool, let us see how it was developed.

Development of Diagnostic and Statistical Manual of Mental Disorders

Diagnostic and statistical manual of mental disorders is the official system of classification of psychological and psychiatric disorders, prepared and published by the American Psychiatric Association. It is the major guide to diagnosis, classification, treatment and prognosis of psychological disorders. The first version, DSM-I, was published in 1952 and subsequent revisions (II, III, III-R, and IV) appeared in 1968, 1980, 1987 and 1994 respectively. DSM-IV was revised slightly in 2000 and it is known as DSM-IV-TR (TR stands for Text Revision). The latest revision includes more up-to-date information on incidence rates and cultural factors, but without changing the diagnostic categories or the criteria. The fact that DSM has undergone so many revisions is proof that diagnosis of psychological disorders is hardly a science. During the several revisions the number of mental disorders has increased from 100 to about 350. Social, cultural and even political factors have played their role in determining maladaptive behaviors. A noteworthy feature of DSM is that disorders are specifically defined and the emphasis is on thoughts, feelings and behaviors. Another important feature of the recent manual is that it does not rely on any specific theory of the causes of disorders; it is theoretically neutral and bases the identification of disorders on a growing body of empirical research.

Taking into consideration the interaction between the individual and the environment, the DSM includes diagnostic information from five axes. Axis I includes major clinical disorders and axis II includes personality disorders and mental retardation. Axis III describes general medical conditions, such as blood pressure that might be relevant to a diagnosis on axis I or II. Axis IV notes the psychosocial and environmental issues and Axis V mentions the coping resources of the person. An appendix to the manual outlines aspects of the patient's cultural context that a clinician should take into account when making a diagnosis. The most important diagnostic categories included in DSM-IV-TR are mentioned below.

Anxiety disorders: High levels of anxiety, tension, worry; phobic disorders; panic disorders; stress disorders; anxiety due to medication; drug abuse and others.

Mood disorders: Depressive disorders; bipolar disorders; mood disorders due to use of medicines and substance abuse.

Somatoform disorders: Physical symptoms with no apparent medical cause; somatization disorders; conversion disorders; pain disorders; hypochondriasis, body dysmorphic disorders, etc.

Factitious disorders: Self-induced physical symptoms apparently to play the role of a patient; Munchausen syndromes.

Dissociative disorders: Include amnesia, fugue, depersonalization and identity disorders.

Schizophrenia and other psychotic disorders: Various types of schizophrenia, schizophreniform disorders, schizoaffective disorders, delusional disorder, brief psychotic disorders and psychotic disorders due to medication and substance abuse.

Substance-abuse disorders: Alcohol, amphetamine, caffeine nicotine, opioid, hallucinogen, cocaine, cannabis, inhalant, sedative-related disorders and other polysubstance related disorders.

Sexual and gender identity disorders: Difficulty in the expression of normal sexuality; sexual desire disorders, arousal disorders, orgasmic disorders, sexual pain disorders and sexual dysfunction due to medication; paraphilias such as exhibitionism, fetishism, sadism, masochism, voyeurism, transvestic fetishism; confusion about gender identity.

Eating disorders: Significant disturbances in eating such as anorexia nervosa and bulimia nervosa.

Sleep disorders: Dyssomnia (insomnia, hypersomnia and sleep-wake schedule disorders); parasomnia (somnambulism, dream-anxiety disorder and sleep-terror disorder); disturbances in sleep-wake cycle; excessive daytime sleepiness and sleep disorders related to other mental disorders.

Impulse-control disorders: Kleptomania; pyromania; intermittent explosive disorder; pathological gambling; trichotillomania (compulsive pulling of one's hair to the point of pulling it out).

Adjustment disorders: Persistent emotional or behavioral reactions in response to identifiable stressors confronted in life (such as negative life events). The reactions may take the form of anxiety, depression or withdrawal.

Disorders first diagnosed in infancy, childhood or adolescence: Learning disorders; motor skills disorder; communication disorders; pervasive developmental disorders; attention deficit and disruptive disorders; feeding and eating disorders; tic disorders; elimination disorders; others such as autism, stereotypic movement, separation anxiety and reactive attachment.

Delirium, dementia and amnesic and other cognitive disorders: Delirium due to substance intoxication or substance withdrawal; dementia due to HIV disease; head injury; Parkinson's disease; Huntington's disease; Pick's disease and general medical condition.

Personality disorders: Schizoid, schizotypal, paranoid, antisocial, borderline, histrionic, narcissistic, avoidant, dependent-personality disorder and obsessive-compulsive personality disorders.

Mental retardation: Impairment of intellectual functioning and learning, classified as mild, moderate, severe, or profound mental retardation.

Limitations of DSM Classification

Several authorities are critical about DSM for various reasons. Some researchers do not agree with the attempts of defining medical problems as psychological, which is a way of pathologizing mental health. DSM does not provide a discrete boundary separating normality from abnormal; it is left to the clinician's judgment to determine whether the degree of impairment is clinically significant. Often the real problems of real patients do not fit into the precise lists of signs and symptoms used in the manual. The clinical reality is that the disorders people actually suffer are often not finely differentiated as indicated in the DSM. In certain cases, there is no clear distinction between one disorder and another. For example, among personality disorders and some of the axis I disorders, there is an extensive overlap. The reliability and validity of diagnosis in these categories are difficult to establish because of overlap. DSM provides little information about the causes of abnormal behavior. Finally, the major criticism of DSM is the sheer number of disorders included, which is too unwieldy.

Despite the criticisms, DSM is the most often used tool in diagnosing mental disorders. Its multiaxial approach has some unique value because it emphasizes the value of integrating information about the severity of stress and previous life adjustment, as well as long-lasting personality patterns of people. DSM is better than all other diagnostic systems and the good thing about it is that it is being continuously revised and improved.

Advantages and Disadvantages of Classification

A widely recognized classification system is an asset in clinical diagnosis and treatment of psychological disorders. If every clinician creates his own system, communication becomes difficult. For example, when one clinician reports that a patient is suffering from schizophrenia, the other clinician understands what the first one is talking about. The first clinician's diagnosis may or may not be correct. In fact, both of them may not be sure of what schizophrenia is, but both of them understand what they are talking about. Labeling a pattern of symptoms as a disorder helps to determine the incidence of that disorder. That is one advantage of diagnosis. But unfortunately, labeling (diagnosis) has certain disadvantages. Diagnostic labels can have personal, social and legal consequences for people who are labeled. For example, when a person is labeled as a schizophrenic, a dehumanizing stigma is attached to that person. People view that person differently. People accept the label as an accurate description of the individual, rather than his/her behavior. Labeling might make it difficult for a former patient to get a job, get admission to a professional course, get married and claim custody of a child. Diagnostic categorization not only influences social perception but also self-perception. When people come to know that a psychiatric label has been attached to them, it becomes a **self-fulfilling prophesy** and they may start developing the expected symptoms. Further, the diagnosis often is unreliable. There are two major sources of unreliability. One is the clinician's training or theoretical orientation, which influences diagnosis. The other is that diagnostic labels are attached to individuals and not to their behaviors. No two individuals are alike; the same patient may describe his symptoms differently on two different occasions depending upon how he/she is feeling at that time. Two patients with similar problems might describe their conditions differently and therefore be classified differently.

Psychiatrist Thomas Szasz (1961) has long been an outspoken critic of psychiatric diagnosis. He asserts that mental illness is a myth; it is a carryover from medical model of physical illness. There are no physical criteria for mental disorders as there are for bodily diseases. According to Szasz, mental disorders are problems of living, rather than some inner illnesses. Szasz is of the opinion that society invented the idea of mental disorder to make it easier to control or change people whose behavior upsets or threatens the existing social order. Of course, some people do not agree with Szasz's point of view (which is often called antipsychiatry) about mental illness, but many agree that there is some arbitrariness in psychiatric diagnosis.

There are several legal implications of psychiatric diagnosis. When an individual is judged to be dangerous to himself and/or others because of his mental condition, he can be involuntarily committed to a mental hospital. Then the person loses some of the civil rights and may be detained indefinitely in the institution until his/her condition improves. Courts also take into consideration the mental status of a criminal in passing judgment. Two important legal concepts that are talked about in this context are competency and insanity. Competency refers to an accused person's state of mind at the time of judicial hearing (not at the time of committing an offense). Insanity refers to the presumed state of mind of the criminal at the time the crime was committed. Criminals may be declared not guilty because of insanity. If it is proved that the accused was severely mentally impaired when the crime was committed, the law takes a lenient view and the accused may be given a lesser punishment. The person may be sent to mental hospital instead of jail. Of course, the insanity plea is a hotly debated issue and several countries do not accept the plea.

The errors committed in psychiatric diagnosis were dramatically demonstrated in a famous study by an American clinical psychologist, David Rosenhan (1973). He along with eight of his colleagues went to mental hospitals in five different states in the US and reported to mental health professionals that they were hearing strange voices (unclear voices that were empty, hollow and thud). In truth, they were perfectly normal and none of them was hearing 'voices.' Surprisingly, each of them was immediately admitted to the hospital and received the diagnosis of schizophrenia. Once admitted, they behaved normally in the hospital; answered questions during the interview normally performed normally on several psychological tests and reported that they no more heard the voices. Despite their normal behavior, the 'pseudo-patients' were kept in the mental hospitals from 3 to 52 days with the average stay being 19 days. When they were discharged, most of the 'patients' left the hospital with the label ***schizophrenia in remission***, which implied that the cure was temporary and the illness could recur any time in future. Interestingly, none of the pseudo-patients were identified as imposters by the staff of the institutions. The study clearly indicates that diagnosis of mental disorders is not always accurate and that labeling individuals influences how their behaviors are perceived and interpreted.

MAJOR PSYCHOLOGICAL DISORDERS

Now that we have familiarized ourselves with the basic issues concerning psychological disorders, let us move on to the study of some of the major psychological disorders, especially those mentioned in the Axis I and Axis II of DSM. We shall start with one of the most prevalent conditions, anxiety disorders.

Anxiety Disorders

Anxiety is a condition that most of you are familiar with. All of you must have experienced anxiety at some time or the other. Remember what happened when you were asked to make a public speech for the first time in your life. In all probability, you experienced dryness in the mouth, thumping of the heart, profuse sweating and blankness in the head. It means you have experienced anxiety. Generally, anxiety is considered as a vague, unpleasant emotional state with qualities of apprehension, dread, distress and uneasiness. Anxiety is mostly distinguished from fear by its being often (some say usually, others say always) objectless, whereas fear assumes a specific feared object, event or person. When you are afraid of something (say a snake), you are experiencing fear. When you experience intense fear in the absence of a specific stimulus (and you do not know why), you are experiencing anxiety. But the meaning of anxiety is more complex than what is said here and you will come to know its complexity as you read through the chapter.

When anxiety becomes severe, uncontrollable, worrisome and is associated with a persistent sense of dread and not associated with any known cause, it becomes an anxiety disorder. In **anxiety disorders**, the frequency and intensity of anxiety responses are out of proportion to the situation that arouses them and the conditions interfere with day-to-day living. Generally, anxiety responses have four components:

1. A subjective emotional component including feelings apprehension and tension.
2. A cognitive component, which includes worrisome thoughts, and a feeling of inability to deal with them.
3. Physiological responses, such as heavy breathing, increased heart rate, blood pressure, muscle tension, dryness in the mouth and often frequent micturition.
4. Behavioral responses, such as impaired task performance and avoidance of certain situations.

Large scale population studies indicate that anxiety disorders are the most prevalent disorders in the United States affecting about 23 million Americans at some point in their lifetime. According to American Psychiatric Association, approximately three percent of people suffer from anxiety at any given point in time. The incidence of anxiety disorders is not different in other parts of the world. Fear and anxiety are part of life, but people who suffer from anxiety disorders experience intense or pervasive anxiety and engage in extreme attempts to avoid these feelings.

Types of Anxiety Disorder

Anxiety disorders occur in several forms, and DSM-IV-TR recognizes seven primary types of anxiety disorder. These are phobic disorders (specific or social type), generalized anxiety disorders, panic disorders (with or without agoraphobia), obsessive-compulsive disorders and post-traumatic stress disorders.

Phobic Disorders

Phobic disorders are the most common type of anxiety disorders. A **Phobia** is strong, persistent, irrational fear of certain objects or events that are not generally fear producing. There is a strong need to avoid the phobic object or situation, although there is no actual danger. The word phobia is derived from *Phobos*, the Greek God of fear. Psychologists and psychiatrists have identified innumerable number of phobias, some of which are given in the Box 15.1.

DSM identifies three main types of phobia: specific phobia (refer Box 15.1), social phobia and agoraphobia.

Box 15.1: Some Specific Phobias

Acrophobia: fear of height
Agoraphobia: fear of being alone in public places
Algophobia: fear of pain
Androphobia: fear of man
Anemophobia: fear of wind
Acquaphobia: fear of water
Astraphobia: fear of lightning
Bathophobia: fear of depth
Bibliophobia: fear of books
Claustrophobia: fear of closed places
Cyberphobia: fear of computers
Cynophobia: fear of dogs
Demophobia: fear of crowd
Epistemophobia: fear of knowledge
Ergophobia: fear of work
Erotophobia: fear of sex
Gamophobia: fear of marriage
Hemophobia: fear of blood
Hypnophobia: fear of falling asleep
Iophobia: fear of being poisoned
Kainophobia: fear of new things
Kenophobia: fear of empty spaces
Lalophobia: fear of speaking
Macrophobia: fear of large objects
Microphobia: fear of small objects
Monophobia: fear of being left alone
Mysophobia: fear of dirt
Nyctophobia: fear of night and darkness
Ophidiophobia: fear of snakes
Parturiphobia: fear of childbirth
Pyrophobia: fear of fire
Scopophobia: fear of being seen by others
Tapophobia: fear of graves
Thanatophobia: fear of death
Theophobia: fear of god
Toxophobia: fear of poison
Tricopathophobia: in women, fear of facial hair
Triskaidekaphobia: fear of number 13
Xenophobia: fear of foreigners
Zoophobia: fear of animals

In specific phobia a person shows strong, excessive and persistent fear of some specific object or situation such as animals (snakes, dogs, spiders, etc.), water, storm, heights and sight of blood or injury, tunnels, bridges, elevators, flying or driving and enclosed spaces. People with these phobias go to any length to avoid encounters with such objects or situations. Avoidance is the cardinal symptom of phobias. Animal fears are common among women; men exhibit fear of heights. Phobias may develop at any time of life, but many of them emerge during childhood, adolescence and early adulthood. Once developed they seldom go away; they may broaden and intensify over time. One kind of specific phobia known as ***blood-injection-injury phobia*** is characterized by a unique pattern of physiological responses. When some people see blood or injury, they show an initial acceleration followed by a dramatic drop in both heart rate and blood pressure along with nausea, dizziness, and/or fainting, which do not occur with other specific phobias. Specific phobias are quite common, especially in women. About 90 to 95 percent of people with animal phobia are women. Among people with one specific phobia, over 75 percent have at least one other specific phobia.

Social phobia is characterized by disabling fear of one or more specific social situations such as public speaking, eating or writing in public places, or urinating in a public toilet. In these situations, some people fear that they may be exposed to the scrutiny and potential negative evaluation by others. Therefore, as far as possible, they avoid such situations. The most common social phobia is public speaking. There are some who avoid almost all social situations and these people are said to be suffering from ***generalized social phobia***. It is estimated that some 10 to 12 percent of the population suffer from social phobia at some point of time in their lives and about 60 percent of them are women. More than half of people with social phobia also suffer from one or more anxiety disorders; some of them suffer from depressive disorders. Many of them abuse alcohol to avoid anxiety.

Agoraphobia is fear of open or public places from which escape would be difficult (*agora* is a Greek word for public places). It includes fear of busy streets, shopping malls, movie theaters and other crowded places. Agoraphobics also avoid standing in a queue, busy restaurants, sport meets, elevators, escalators, trains, buses, airplanes, bridges and tunnels. Some people with agoraphobia are frightened by their own bodily sensations and therefore avoid activities that will arouse those—activities such as watching scary films, drinking coffee, aerobic exercise and sexual activities. The condition is so disabling that some people do not go out of their homes or even enter a particular part of the home.

Agoraphobia is a frequent complication of panic disorder. But it can occur without full-blown panic attacks. When this is the case, fearfulness gradually spreads to more aspects of the environment outside the home. Cases of agoraphobia without panic are extremely rare. The lifetime prevalence of agoraphobia without panic is estimated to be about 1.4 percent. Approximately about 4 to 5 percent of adults are found to suffer from panic disorders with or without agoraphobia.

Generalized Anxiety Disorders

Generalized anxiety disorder (GAD) is characterized by chronic, excessive and baseless anxiety and worry about many aspects of life. It was earlier called ***free-floating anxiety***. People suffering from anxiety generally complain that they have no control over it. The condition is diagnosed as GAD if it continues for more than 6 months. People suffering from GAD show marked vigilance for possible threats from the environment and engage in subtle avoidance behavior such as constant checking, procrastination and constantly enquiring about the safety of near and dear ones. Patients complain about restlessness, irritability, loss of sleep, muscle tension and fatigue. They experience a state of apprehension, chronic tension and diffuse worry about the future. It is reported that about five percent of people between the ages 15 and 45 suffer from GAD and about six percent of the population suffer from the condition at some point in life. It is twice as common in women as in men. The onset tends to occur during childhood and adolescence, but it can occur among people of all ages. The condition, as can be expected, creates distress and markedly interferes with day-to-day activities even when the symptoms are not continually present.

Panic Disorder

In contrast to GAD, which is marked by chronic anxiety, **panic disorder** is characterized by intense, unexpected and terrifying bouts of anxiety attacks. The unpredictable nature of panic attack makes it mysterious and horrifying to the victims. The attack comes as a bolt from the blue and in the absence of any known cause. The attack may occur either during daytime or during sleep. When the attack occurs during sleep (***nocturnal attack***), the victim is awakened with cold sweat and along with the fear that he/she is dying. According to DSM-IV-TR, a diagnosis of panic disorder is made when a person exhibits four or more of the following symptoms: palpitation and pounding of heart, sweating, trembling, shortness of breath, feeling of choking, chest pain, nausea, dizziness, derealization (a feeling that the external world is strange or unreal) or depersonalization (a feeling of being detached from oneself), fear of death, going crazy or losing control, chill or hot flashes. Note that most of the symptoms are physical. Many people who suffer from panic attacks also develop agoraphobia. In fact, DSM identifies two types of panic disorders: panic attack with and without agoraphobia.

The first panic attack generally occurs following feelings of distress or stressful events, such as the death of a loved one, loss of job or criminal victimization. Once the disorder develops, it tends to have a chronic and disabling course. But not all people develop panic attacks after stressful events. It is reported that 7 to 30 percent of people experience at least one panic attack in their lifetime, but most do not develop full-blown panic disorders. Panic disorder is about twice as prevalent in women as in men. Among people with severe agoraphobia, roughly 80 to 90 percent are women.

Obsessive-compulsive Disorders

Obsessive-compulsive disorder (OCD) consists of two components: cognitive and behavioral. The cognitive component called **obsession** is characterized by the occurrence of certain unwanted and intrusive thoughts, impulses or distressing images over which the individual has no control. The behavioral component, called **compulsion**, is some uncontrollable act, which the person is compelled to perform. These behaviors are performed to neutralize the unwanted thoughts, impulses and images emerging from within. Note that obsessions specifically refer to recurrent unwanted thoughts, images or impulses and compulsions to acts that are undertaken to neutralize the anxiety associated with unpleasant obsessive thoughts. The disorder may be characterized by the presence of obsession, either alone or in combination with compulsive acts. Commonly, obsessions may involve thoughts of contamination ("I may develop an illness if I closely move with him"), repeated doubts ("Have I put off the stove?"), or a thought to hit someone who is urinating in public. Compulsions are repetitive tasks such as handwashing, counting steps when climbing a staircase, praying regularly, or uttering certain words silently a known number of times. The patient is actually driven to engage in these ritualistic behaviors and he/she feels miserable if these acts are not performed. The OCD patients know that what they are doing is absurd, and in fact, do not want to engage in them, but they cannot help; it is beyond their control to stop acting that way.

Most of us experience obsessive thoughts and may engage in repetitive tasks, but in OCD these stereotyped or repetitive behaviors are excessive, much more persistent, highly distressing and uncontrollable. Compulsions are strengthened through a process of negative reinforcement, because they help the person to avoid the anxiety associated with the unpleasant obsessions. The disorder generally begins during late adolescence or early adulthood (during 20s). It may also develop among others including children. Among children, it is more common in boys than girls. It is reported that 2.5 percent of people suffer from OCD. The disorder creates difficulties in establishing and retaining interpersonal relation in social circles and occupational settings. The prevalence of OCD has been found to be more frequent among divorcees and unemployed people.

Post-traumatic Stress Disorders

Post-traumatic stress disorders (PTSD) are severe anxiety attacks that occur when people are exposed to extremely stressful (traumatic) events in life. Sudden, unexpected crises such as divorce, separation and death of intimate people, earthquakes, hurricanes or the horrors of war are the major causes of PTSD. Generally, PTSD patients experience severe anxiety, arousal and distress that were not there before the traumatic event. The victims relive the traumatic event in fantasy or dreams. They meticulously avoid everything that reminds them of the trauma and several of them experience ***survivor guilt*** (a feeling that others were killed and somehow the patient survived), as it happens during war, floods or devastating fire. In fact, the studies of PTSD came into force after examining war returnees. Recent studies have shown that civilian war victims were even more vulnerable than soldiers to this type of anxiety disorder. Inhuman activities such as war, torture or rape tend to precipitate PTSD more often than natural calamities such as earthquakes and floods. When exposed to traumatic events, women exhibit twice the rate of PTSD symptoms compared to men. One of the recent events that are threatening to cause PTSD is terrorism. It is reported that among the residents around the World Trade Center that was attacked on September 11, 2001, the incidence of PTSD was as high as 20 percent. Women who experienced PTSD have double the risk of developing depressive disorders and three times the risk of developing alcohol-related disorders. These findings emphasize the need for providing prompt post-trauma interventions to prevent the development of PTSD.

Causes of Anxiety Disorders

Anxiety is a highly complex mental state experienced by most humans all over the world. One textbook of abnormal psychology described 20th century as an age of anxiety. But what exactly causes anxiety? A straight answer to this question cannot be given. Psychologists have written a great deal about anxiety. Psychoanalysts, behaviorists, and humanists have offered different interpretations to anxiety. Each of the anxiety disorders mentioned above has different cause and course. It is not possible to discuss all of these within a chapter. A brief outline of the general causes of anxiety disorders is given below.

Contemporary psychologists use a schema called **vulnerability-stress model** to explain psychological disorders and the same can be adopted to understand anxiety disorders also. According to this model, all of us have a degree of **vulnerability** for developing a psychological disorder, given sufficient stress. Vulnerability refers to the likelihood with which people respond maladaptively to stressful situations; it is a disposition ranging from very low to very high. Vulnerability can have biological, psychological, environmental bases and any of these factors can dispose people to respond to stressors in certain ways that facilitate the development of anxiety disorders. We shall discuss these factors briefly.

Biological Factors

Available research evidence indicates that there are modest genetic causes for each of the anxiety disorders and that at least part of the genetic vulnerability may be non-specific or common across the disorders. One of the evidences for the belief that there is a biological basis for anxiety attacks comes from studies of twins. Among identical twins, the **concordance** rate for anxiety disorders is reported to be about 40 percent. That is, if one of the identical twins is having anxiety disorder, the chance that the other also has the disorder 40 percent. On the contrary, the concordance rate for fraternal twins is 4 percent. The genetic vulnerability may take several forms. One of them is over-activity of the autonomous nervous system to perceived threat causing increased physiological arousal. Some researchers report that there is the involvement of the neurotransmitter GABA (**gamma-aminobutyric acid**) in the production of anxiety states. GABA is an inhibitory neurotransmitter that reduces neural activity in the **amygdala** (a brain structure that is significantly involved in the emotion of fear) and other brain structures that elicit emotional arousal. It is believed that low levels of inhibitory GABA activity in those arousal areas may cause some people to have highly reactive nervous system, which quickly produces anxiety responses when they are under stress. Support for this belief has come from brain scan studies, which have shown that people with a history of panic attacks have a 22 percent lower concentration of GABA in the occipital cortex than those without panic disorder. Other neurotransmitter systems may also be involved in the production of anxiety disorders. For example, it is proposed that serotonin plays a role in OCD, based on the observation that serotonin-based drugs (such as Prozac) reduce OCD symptoms.

Amygdala, which is believed to be the central area involved in what is called ***fear network,*** has connections with several minor and major areas of the brain including ***locus coeruleus*** (a small group of cells deep in the brain stem) and prefrontal cortex. Animal studies suggest that locus coeruleus is the seat of "alarm system" that triggers an increase in heart rate, faster breathing, sweating and other components of the "flight or fight" response and these bodily responses lead to the experience of panic. In simple words, it is said that an over-sensitive locus coeruleus gives rise to panic attacks. The electroencephalographic (EEG) studies have also found an unusually strong activation in the right frontal lobe (compared with left) when people suffering from panic attacks encounter panic-inducing stimuli. This suggests that the brain system involved in withdrawal emotions is relatively easily activated in people with panic disorders.

It has been generally observed that more women suffer from anxiety disorders than men. Such gender difference exists even among children as young as 7 years. This observation has prompted some researchers to think that there is a sex-linked biological predisposition for anxiety disorders. Although there is always some biological factor in the causation of anxiety disorders, the role of psychological and sociocultural factors cannot be overlooked. For instance, in the studies of identical twins, as we have seen earlier, the concordance rate is only 40 percent; if biological factors alone were responsible, the concordance rate should have been 100 percent. This indicates the importance of psychological and environmental factors in the causation of anxiety disorders.

Psychological Factors

Psychologists have researched and written extensively about anxiety and anxiety disorders. Psychoanalysts, behaviorists and cognitive psychologists have proposed slightly differing views about anxiety. According to Sigmund Freud, there are three types of anxiety: ***reality anxiety, neurotic anxiety*** and ***moral anxiety***. Reality anxiety is what we generally refer to as fear. We are afraid of several things around us—snakes, floods, earthquakes, fires and so on. The important point here is that we know what we are afraid of. But in the other two varieties, we are afraid, but we do not know the cause of the fear. The causes are in the unconscious. Neurotic anxiety occurs when repressed, undesirable and unacceptable impulses threaten to enter the conscious. These may be forbidden sexual or aggressive impulses. Moral anxiety is experienced when there is a wish to engage in a forbidden, unethical, sinful act. Neurotic anxiety is the central construct in psychoanalytic theories of abnormal behavior. According to psychoanalysts, neurotic anxiety results when the repressed, unconscious, unacceptable impulses try to overrun ego's defenses. How the ego deals with neurotic anxiety determines the form of anxiety disorder. When neurotic anxiety is displaced onto some external object, the result is phobic disorder. When the anxiety is unattached to any specific external object and is free floating, then the result is generalized anxiety disorder. Psychoanalysts believe that obsessions and compulsions are mechanisms developed to deal with anxiety. An obsession is symbolically related to, but less threatening than, an underlying anxiety. A compulsion is a way of dealing with neurotic anxiety resulting from an impulse to engage in a dirty act, such as "sex" or aggression. Panic attacks occur when the ego's defenses are not strong enough to counter the dangerous impulses, but are strong enough to hide the underlying conflict.

According to behaviorists, anxiety is a learned response. Behaviorists assert that conditioning (both classical and operant) and/or observational learning contributes to the development of anxiety disorders. For example, a boy who was confronted by a ferocious dog in a narrow lane may develop ***claustrophobia***. A man who watched a terrible airplane accident on TV may develop fear of flying; this is the product of observational learning. Often, when you hear a vivid description of a dangerous event, you may develop anxiety for similar events. The role of operant conditioning in the development of anxiety disorders is as follows: We are motivated to avoid or escape anxiety because it is unpleasant. Then, any behavior (such as a compulsion) that reduces anxiety is acquired through **negative reinforcement**. For example, compulsive handwashing wards off the fear of contamination and hence, we develop a compulsion to wash. An individual, who is suffering from agoraphobia, prefers to stay at home where he feels safe; thus avoids a panic attack that may occur when he goes out into the open. Once the anxiety is learned, either by conditioning or vicarious learning, it will be elicited later either by internal cues (thoughts and images of the threatening stimuli) or by environmental cues.

Cognitive psychologists emphasize the role of maladaptive thoughts and beliefs in the development of anxiety disorders. People with anxiety disorders magnify threats and expect the worst to happen. They think that they have no powers to cope with the events effectively. In PTSD, the thoughts about a previous trauma intrude forcibly into the mind and the presence of such thoughts predicts the later development of the illness. According to cognitive theorists, panic attacks are triggered by exaggerated misinterpretations of normal anxiety symptoms. For example, heart palpitation or dizziness may be taken as an indication of an impending heart attack. Such catastrophic appraisals may create even more anxiety until the processes go out of control resulting in a full blown panic attack.

Sociocultural Factors

In a cross-national study of over 60,000 people from 14 countries, conducted by the World Health Organization (WHO) in 2004, it was found that anxiety disorders were the most common forms of psychological disorders reported in all but one country (Ukraine). Although cross-cultural studies indicate that anxiety is a universal phenomenon, there are some differences in the prevalence and the forms in which anxiety is expressed in different cultures. The occurrence and the course of anxiety disorders depend upon the sociocultural milieu in which the person is living. The presence of a close relative or friend—often referred to as a "safe person"—goes a long way in decreasing panicky thinking. Social support from family and friends immediately after a trauma may help decrease the likelihood that PTSD will develop. In the case of those exposed to trauma in the battle field, social support after coming back home can reduce the risk of PTSD. Cultural factors play a major role in the development of obsessive-compulsive disorders. In societies, which are highly religious, compulsive praying is common. The role of culture can be clearly seen in culture-bound disorders that occur in certain cultures only. For example, a specific type of social phobia called *'Taijin Kyofusho'* is found in Japan. People suffering from this disorder are pathologically afraid of offending others by emitting foul smell, blushing, staring, or improper facial expression. This is supposed to be the result of the high value Japanese people attach to interpersonal sensitivity and social prohibition toward expressing negative emotions or causing discomfort to others. Anorexia nervosa has an obsessive component. In developed countries, being thin or slim is a cultural obsession. Among Khmer refugees, panic attacks are associated with symptoms of ***Kyol Goeu*** (wind overload)—a fainting syndrome that occurs when one stands up from a lying or sitting position. Those who are suffering from this condition are more likely to be sensitive to signs of autonomic arousal in their bodies and to have negative beliefs about what the arousal means; this increased anxiety makes panic attacks more likely. In China, a disorder called *'**Koro**'* is exhibited. Men, who suffer from Koro, fear that their penis is shrinking into their body, and when this process is complete, they will die. Women fear that their nipples are retracting and their breasts shrinking. In many societies, women are generally shy—they are expected to be so and valued for being so—and as a consequence suffer from social phobia. Under such circumstances, they do not suffer from social phobia; they live with it.

Therefore, take note that there is no single cause for anxiety disorders. The individual's brain, the psychological makeup and the social environment; all combine to contribute toward the development and maintenance of anxiety states. People's personality traits and their world view influence the level of anxiety experience. Also, underscore the fact that anxiety is a common symptom in several psychological disorders. Basically this is an emotion-based disorder. Now we shall examine another group of emotion-based disorders called somatoform disorders.

Somatoform Disorders

Somatoform disorders are a group of disorders that exhibit physical symptoms and complaints, which look like medical problems, but do not have any demonstrable physiological basis, and are not produced by the individual. These disorders appear like ways of avoiding anxiety, stress and managing the problems of life that threaten to overwhelm people's coping capacity. Some of the major forms of somatoform disorders are hypochondriasis, somatization disorders, pain disorders, conversion disorders and body dysmorphic disorders.

Hypochondriasis

In **hypochondriasis**, the patients are extremely worried about any physical symptom they notice, and convinced that they have, or are about to have, a serious physical disorder. They diagnose themselves as suffering from cancer, tuberculosis, AIDS, and numerous other ailments and immediately run to a doctor. When the doctor says that there is nothing wrong, they doubt the doctor's conclusion; go to another doctor, and so on. Often these people are called "clinic shoppers". They are sincere in their conviction that the symptoms they notice represent real illness. They are not malingering.

Somatization Disorder

Somatization disorder is characterized by many different physical complaints that start before age 30 years and continue for many years leading to medical treatment. The condition is diagnosed as somatization disorder when patients complain of at least two gastrointestinal symptoms, one sexual symptom, one pseudoneurological symptom and four pain symptoms. The condition cannot be adequately explained medically. The symptoms are not intentionally produced or feigned. The illness appears similar to hypochondriasis, but there are certain features that distinguish somatization disorder from hypochondriasis. For example, with hypochondriasis the patient has one or two symptoms, but in somatization disorders exhibit multiple symptoms. Somatization disorder was formerly called Briquet's syndrome after the French physician who first described it.

Pain Disorder

In pain disorder, the patients experience persistent and severe pain in one or more areas of body for which there is no physiological basis. The pain causes significant distress and impairs effective functioning. The pain is genuine and not feigned. Pain may be associated only with psychological factors or both psychological and medical conditions, but the role of psychological factor is judged to be more important. In either case, pain may be acute (lasting for less than 6 months) or chronic (lasting for more than 6 months). The patients go from one doctor to another seeking treatment or confirmation of the symptom. The prevalence of pain disorder is more among women than men. The condition is comorbid with anxiety and mood disorders.

Conversion Disorders

Conversion disorders are marked by sensory or motor dysfunctions for which no neurophysiological basis can be demonstrated. Typical symptoms are blindness, deafness, paralysis and pseudoseizures. The symptoms are precipitated by emotional or interpersonal conflicts and severe stress. But it should be noted that the person is not faking the symptoms. Early observers, dating back to Sigmund Freud, suggested that in the conversion disorder, the patients are not worried, anxious or afraid of their condition. This seeming lack of concern for the deficit was called ***'la belle indifference'*** (the French for the "beautiful indifference"). In fact, this point was considered important in diagnosing conversion disorder. But, in recent times, it is observed that patients are really anxious about their symptoms and as a consequence, la belle indifference is not included as a criterion for diagnosing conversion disorders.

The term conversion disorder is relatively new. Historically this disorder was one of several disorders grouped under the term *hysteria*. Freud called this disorder ***conversion hysteria*** and thought that the symptoms were an expression of repressed sexual desires. According to him, the anxiety associated with repressed, unconscious, sexual conflicts gets converted into bodily ailments; this was one way of avoiding the sexual conflict. For example, one who wants to masturbate may develop paralysis of the hand. Of course, the person is not aware of the origin and meaning of his ailment because the whole process occurs unconsciously. Also the person gets the sympathy of others when he develops a defect; this, Freud called **secondary gain**. The **primary gain** is the escape from the stressful situation.

Body Dysmorphic Disorders

The DSM-IV-TR includes **body dysmorphic disorder (BDD)** as another type of somatoform disorder. Patients of BDD are preoccupied with certain aspects of the body; they are obsessed with some imagined or perceived flaw in their appearance. The preoccupation is so intense that it creates enormous amount of distress and disrupts social and occupational functions. People with BDD are so scared about their imagined body defect that they go on checking repeatedly for hours together in front of mirror to ascertain whether everything is alright with their appearance. Because of the fear that others may notice the (imagined) flaw, they avoid all kinds of activities. Often they lock themselves up in their room and never go out even for work. They imagine that they are too thin (or fat), have blemishes on the skin, their breasts are very small (or big), so on and so forth. One recent study found the following locations where flaws were noticed by patients suffering from BDD (percentage of people noticing the flaw given in the brackets): skin (73), hair (56), nose (37), eyes (20), legs (18), breasts/nipples (21), stomach (22), lips (12), body build (16), and face size/shape (12). These people spend a lot of time in front of the mirror trying to set right the defect and engage in excessive makeup to camouflage the imagined flaw. They frequently seek reassurance from others about their appearance, but are not satisfied with the reassurance given. The age of onset is usually during adolescence, and the condition is equally prevalent in both the sexes.

Causes of Somatoform Disorders

Somatoform disorders appear to run in families. But the evidence is not enough to conclude that they are hereditary. May be the children imitate their parents in expressing the symptoms. This argument is supported by the fact that somatoform patients are highly suggestible; their hypnotic suggestibility has been found to be more than average. It is believed that learning and social facilitation play a role in the manifestation of the bodily symptoms. Biological and environmental factors may predispose people to develop the illness. It is reported that somatoform disorder is more prevalent among cultural groups that discourage open display of emotions. When people cannot express their feelings or talk about them, they tend to express them in the form of bodily symptoms. Among police and military personnel, open discussion of emotions and self-disclosure of psychological issues are frowned upon. Therefore, somatic symptoms may be the only option left for them to express their psychological distress.

Dissociative Disorders

Dissociative disorders exhibit disturbances or alterations in consciousness, memory and personal identity. Normally, we experience a sense of unity and coherence in our personality; we know who we are, where we are, and what we are doing. There is consistency in the ways we think, feel and act. Memory plays an important role in providing this integrity. It connects the past and present and provides us with a sense of personal identity over time. In dissociative disorders, there is a breakdown in the normal integration of personality resulting in alterations in memory and self-identity. The identity may be forgotten temporarily; the person may assume a different identity and start thinking that he is a different person. Stress plays a significant role in bringing about the dissociation. Like somatoform disorders, dissociative disorders are employed as a means of avoiding anxiety and stress that are overwhelming, which the person cannot handle. The DSM-IV-TR mentions several varieties of dissociative disorders, such as dissociative amnesia, dissociative fugue, dissociative identity disorder and depersonalization disorder.

Dissociative Amnesia

In **dissociative amnesia** (also known as *psychogenic amnesia*), there is extensive or selective memory loss. A person may forget everything about the past or forget certain selected items such as names of places, persons or events, but the memory for other functions, such as cognitive activities, language and motor skills, are intact. The gaps in memory occur generally after an intolerable stressful event and the memory loss cannot be attributed to any brain damage. The amnesic episode may last between a few days to a few years. Some people experience only one such episode, while others have many of them during their lifetime. Some people may recall the lost memories, while others may never remember them.

Dissociative Fugue

In **dissociative fugue**, people experience memory loss for some or all of the past. They may run away from home or work and live in a different place with a different name and identity (the term fugue is derived from Greek word *fugere*, which means "to flee"). They do not remember anything about their past and live a normal life with their changed identity. Fugue can be considered as a more profound form of dissociative disorder, which is triggered by a stressful event or trauma. It may last from a few hours or days to several months or even years. It is reported that married fugue patients may marry someone else and lead a new life. Generally, the fugue ends 1 day and the person recovers his original identity. The person wakes up mystified and distressed at being in a strange place and strange circumstances.

Dissociative Identity Disorder

Dissociative identity disorder (DID), which was formerly known as *multiple personality disorder*, is a dramatic dissociative disorder in which an individual exhibits two or more distinct personalities that alternate in taking control of behavior. It has been a popular theme based on which several movies were made (*The three faces of eve*, *Sybil*, and *Psycho*) and books written (*Dr Jekyll and Mr Hyde*). Each personality may have a different personal history, self-image and name. The one identity that is most frequently exhibited, called ***host identity***, carries the real name of the individual, but it may not be the best adjusted one. The ***alter identities*** may differ in striking ways. They may assume different gender and age; exhibit different handedness, handwriting, language, voice, general knowledge, religious affiliation and sexual orientation. The female patients frequently have different menstrual cycle for each identity. Some have dissimilar EEG patterns. Epileptic patients with DID have seizures in one personality, but not in another. The alter identities take control at different points of time and the switch over occur very quickly. The alter identities have amnesia for each other. But in some cases, there is one-way amnesia; that is, A is aware of B, but B is not aware of A.

In a majority of cases, DID begin in early childhood, mostly in response to physical or sexual abuse. It is said that due to trauma and their helplessness to resist it, children engage in something like self-hypnosis and dissociate from reality. This is the ***trauma-dissociation theory*** of dissociative identity disorder proposed by Frank Putnam (1989) after studying 100 diagnosed cases. The DID is a controversial disorder. Some critics doubt its prevalence and others its very existence.

The DID is unknown in some cultures. Whether DID is real, imagined or imitated is being hotly debated even today. Only about 100 to 200 cases were reported before 1979. But after the publicity it received through films and stories, the incidence appears to have increased. By 1919, over 30,000 cases had been reported in North America alone. Several researchers believe that this increase in the prevalence of DID is simply artifactual.

Mood Disorders

Mood disorders are psychological disorders characterized by persistent or episodic emotional disturbances that interfere with the normal functioning of individuals. These include depression and/or mania and together with anxiety disorders, mood disorders are the most prevalent psychological disorders. The common mood disorders, among others, include **major depressive disorders** and **bipolar disorders**.

Major Depressive Disorders

A large number of people report that they have felt sad or were in the "blue" at some time or the other during their lifetime. Most people experience some type of disappointment, pain or loss in life and as a consequence, feel sad, apathetic, passive and discouraged. For them, the future looks bleak; they often say they are depressed. Such reactions are normal and the feelings fade away after the distressing event has passed or the person gets used to the event. But these people cannot be branded as suffering from a psychological disorder. In major depressive disorder (MDD), the individual's affect (A), behavior (B), and cognition (C) are disturbed; it is an intense depressed state that leaves the person incapable of functioning normally and effectively in life. The negative mood state is the central feature of depression. It is reported that at least 20 percent of people suffer from depression and it is the most common psychological disorder in the US. It is found among all cultures and the prevalence is about the same for men and women. According to DSM, a person is diagnosed as suffering from MDD when he/she has been experiencing depressive mood for at least 2 weeks and exhibits at least five of the following symptoms:

- Remain depressed most of the day, almost every day
- Exhibits loss of interest in nearly all daily activities
- Loss of appetite and significant loss of weight
- Suffers from loss of sleep (insomnia) or sleeps a lot (hypersomnia)
- General psychomotor retardation or intense restlessness
- Fatigue or loss of energy
- Feelings of guilt and sense of worthlessness
- Inability to think and concentrate
- Recurrent thoughts of death or suicide.

Some people suffer from a less intense form of depression called **dysthymia**, which is more chronic and long lasting. The condition may continue for years with some intervals of normal mood that never lasts more than a few weeks or months.

Bipolar Disorders

When a person suffers from only depression, the condition is called **unipolar depression**. When depression alternates with **mania** (excessive excitement), the condition is called bipolar disorder. During a manic episode, the person experiences euphoria and a sense of grandiosity and feels that anything under the sun can be achieved. Manic people engage in frenetic activity, be it in work, in sexual relationship or in other areas of life and are not worried about failure. Generally, manic people are hyperactive; their speech is rapid or pressured as if they must say as many words as possible in the allotted time. They may become irritable and aggressive when their activities are frustrated. The psychomotor overactivity associated with the manic state may cause exhaustion and sleeplessness. The person may go for several days without sleep.

Some patients exhibit cyclical mood changes less severe than bipolar disorder; this condition is called **cyclothymic disorder**. When the manic symptoms are less severe, the condition is called **hypomania**. Bipolar disorders were earlier called ***manic-depressive insanity***. Kraepelin in 1899 introduced that term and described the condition as a series of attacks of mania and depression, with periods of relative normality in between. The DSM-IV-TR has named this illness bipolar disorder and has distinguished between two kinds of disorders known as **bipolar I disorder** and **bipolar II disorder**. Bipolar I disorder is distinguished from major depressive disorder by at least one episode of mania or a mixed episode. A **mixed episode** is characterized by symptoms of both full-blown manic and major depressive episodes for at least 1 week. In bipolar II disorder, the person does not experience full-blown manic episodes, but has experienced clear-cut hypomanic episodes as well as major depressive episodes.

Prevalence of Mood Disorders

Epidemiological studies in the US have shown that about 5 percent of Americans suffer from severe depression and the chances are that at least one in five of them will have a depressive episode in their lifetime. Depression occurs at all ages. Infants as young as 6 months, who have been separated from their mothers for prolonged periods, were found to have suffered from depressive episodes. Depressive symptoms among children and adolescents are as high as the adult rate. Data also suggest that the rate of depression is increasing among 15- to 19-year olds dramatically in the US. The illness occurs equally among various socioeconomic and ethnic groups. The number of women suffering from unipolar depression is twice as that for men, but there are no sex differences regarding bipolar disorders. Women are likely to have their first episode of depression in their 20s and men in their 40s.

Once a depressive episode has occurred, it follows one of the following three courses:

1. In about 40 percent of the cases, depression will not recur after recovery.
2. In a number of cases there is recurrence after recovery.
3. In about 10 percent of cases there will be no recovery and the people will remain chronically depressed.

Manic episodes are less common than depression. According to one report issued by the American Psychiatric Association, one percent of Americans suffer from manic attacks and the recurrence rate is more than 90 percent.

Causal Factors in Mood Disorders

As in anxiety disorders, biological, psychological and sociocultural factors interact with each other in the production of mood disorders. The person, the brain, and the society, all the three contribute to the development of mood disorders. But we see more emphasis on neurobiological factors than on psychological and environmental factors.

Biological Factors

Several researchers have implicated the role of genetic and neurochemical factors in the causation of depression. Depression tends to run in families. The evidence for genetic factors comes from the study of twins. The concordance rate for identical twins is about 67 percent in comparison with 15 percent among fraternal twins for experiencing depression. But remember, what is inherited is not the illness, but a disposition to develop a depressive disorder, given certain kinds of environmental conditions such as loss of social support.

In recent times, there have been an increasing number of studies searching for the biological bases for mood disorders. One influential theory suggests that depression is a disorder of motivation caused by underactivity of certain neurotransmitters such as norepinephrine, dopamine and serotonin. These transmitters are believed to play significant roles in several parts of the brain involved in experiencing pleasure from reward. When neural transmission is decreased in these areas, individuals feel lack of drive and loss of pleasure, which are the essential features of depression. Further support for such belief comes from studies of the action of antidepressants. Powerful antidepressant drugs increase the activity of the neurotransmitters, which in turn stimulates the neural systems that underlie positive emotions and goal-directed behavior. Unfortunately, the results of these studies are sketchy and the exact mechanisms of how the neurotransmitters influence the brain structures are not yet understood.

Bipolar disorder in which the depressive episode alternates with less frequent manic attack appears to have a strong genetic base compared with unipolar depression. The risk of developing bipolar disorder is just below one percent in both men and women. About 50 percent of patients with bipolar disorders have a parent, grandparent or child with the same disorder in the family. The concordance rate for bipolar disorder is five times higher in identical twins than in fraternal twins suggesting a genetic basis. Manic disorder may be produced by the overactivity of the same neurotransmitters that were underactive in depression. For instance, lithium chloride that is often used to calm down manic patients works by decreasing the activity of these transmitters in the brain's motivational and pleasure-activating systems.

Psychological Factors

Stressful events in life are important factors in the causation of mood disorders. Although it is not clear how stress operates in the production of unipolar and bipolar disorders, researchers believe that it is a promising hypothesis and it should be investigated further. Psychoanalysts (Freud and his followers) believed that traumatic events during childhood create a personal vulnerability for later depression by triggering a grieving and rage process that becomes part of the individual's personality. Subsequent losses reactivate the original loss and cause a reaction not only to current event but also to the unresolved loss from the past. Loss of one or both parents during childhood has been found to be a risk factor in the causation of depression both among men and women, especially among women.

American psychiatrist Aaron Beck is an important researcher in the area of depression. He emphasized the role of cognitive factors in causing depression. According to Beck, depressives victimize themselves through their own faulty assumption that they are defective, worthless and inadequate. They have a totally negative view of the future and believe that only bad things will occur to them because of their personal defects. Generally, the negative thoughts concern three areas: the world, oneself and the future. This thought pattern is called the **depressive cognitive triad**. The depressive people report that these negative thoughts automatically enter into their consciousness and they do not have the power either to control or suppress them. They are prone to remember only sad faces and unfortunate events around them indicating their perceptual sensitivity to the negative. Beck suggests that depressive people exhibit what he calls the ***depressive attributional pattern***, which is a tendency to attribute success or other positive outcomes to environmental factors failure and negative outcomes to personal factors. They think that they have failed even when they have won. Since, they do not take credit for personal achievements and always blame themselves for failures, they suffer from lower self-esteem. It is argued that people with unstable self-esteem, coupled with unrealistic standards for what constitutes success generally develop bipolar disorders.

Another cognitive thought pattern exhibited by depressive people is what Seligman calls **learned helplessness**, which is a general expectancy that bad things will definitely occur and that there is nothing that one can do to prevent or cope with them. Learned helplessness theorists suggest that depression occurs as a result of negative attributions for failure that are personal ("It is entirely my fault"), stable ("It will always be like this way for me") and global ("I am a total loser"). Thus people, who attribute negative events in their lives to factors such as intellectual inadequacy, physical repulsiveness or an unlovable personality, tend to believe that their personal defects will render them helpless to avoid negative events in the future, and this sense of helplessness places them at significantly greater risk for depression.

Learning theorists believe that depression is triggered by a loss, by some other punishing event, or by a decrease of positive reinforcement that people receive from their environment. As depression develops, people stop performing things that previously provided positive reinforcement. Depressive people, by the way they behave, also make other people feel anxious, depressed and often hostile. These other people fail to understand why the depressed ones cannot come out of their depression, feel fed up with them, and gradually try to avoid them. Thus, the depressed people lose the social support from the near and dear ones. Research shows that loss of social support is an important predictor of subsequent depression. Behavior theorists thus assert that depression is the result of a vicious circle in which depression-induced inactivity and aversive behavior reduce positive reinforcement from the environment and thereby increase the depression still further. They suggest that in order to feel better, depressed people must break this vicious circle by initially forcing themselves to engage in behaviors that are rewarding and pleasure producing. Positive reinforcement generated by this process of behavior activation will begin to counteract depressive affect and undermine the sense of hopelessness, which is the hallmark of depression, and increase the feeling of personal control over the environment.

Sociocultural Factors

Although depression occurs in all cultures, the form it takes and its prevalence differ widely. For example, in China and Japan, the rate of depression is relatively low. Chinese and Japanese people do not exhibit symptoms of depression, such as feelings of guilt and self-accusation (common among Western cultures), but show somatic symptoms, such as disturbed sleep, loss of appetite, weight loss and reduction in sexual interest. This is said to be due to the philosophy of life in the Eastern cultures. In Western cultures, people view themselves as independent and autonomous. When failure occurs, they attribute it to themselves and feel guilty and entertain negative thoughts. The lifetime prevalence rate for depression in Taiwan is estimated to be about 1.5 percent, while in the US it is estimated to be around 17 to 19 percent. But with increasing industrialization, adolescents in the East are also succumbing to mood disorders.

Several researchers propose that social environment such as family plays an important role in the development of mood disorders. For example, Constance

Hammen (1991) studied the family histories of depressed people and concluded that children of depressed parents often experience poor parenting and face many stressful experiences as they grow up. As a result, they may fail to develop good coping skills and a positive self-concept, making them more vulnerable to stressful events later in life, which can trigger depressive reactions. This conclusion is supported by findings that children of depressed parents exhibit a significantly higher incidence of depression and other psychological disorders as adolescents and young adults.

Depression and Suicide

According to the WHO, nearly 500,000 people commit suicide every year—almost one per minute. The number of people who engage in non-fatal suicide attempts is ten times that number. In the US, suicide is the most frequent cause of death (after accidents) among school and college students. Women attempt suicide three times more than men, but men are three times more likely to actually kill themselves. The suicide rate for both men and women is high among those who have troubles in the family (divorce, separation, widowhood). In women, suicide is generally triggered by failure in love relationships, whereas in men career failure is the main cause. The important thing to notice here is that depression is the strongest predictor of suicide. According to Beck, suicidal attempts are associated with depression and the feeling of hopelessness. It is reported that about 15 percent of the depressed people kill themselves. It is estimated that 80 percent of suicidal people are depressed. A strange feature is that suicides do not occur when depression is intense; instead they occur when people are recovering from the condition. The lifting of depression may provide the energy needed to complete the suicidal act, but not reduce the feelings of hopelessness and helplessness in the person.

What are the motives for suicide? Researchers have found two:

1. Some people use suicide as a solution to their problems; they want to put a full stop to their emotional distress by killing themselves; some others attempt suicide thinking that they are a burden to people around them.
2. Some others use the threat of suicide to manipulate and coerce people around them into doing what the former wants; for example, attempted suicide may be used to prevent a lover from ending a love relationship or to induce guilt in others.

   The attempts that do not end in death are often referred to as ***parasuicides***. In these attempts, people use less lethal methods (small doses of sleeping pills) and attempts are made when they are sure that there are people to stop them from committing suicide. There are instances when people die to save others; these are called ***altruistic suicides***. For example, a soldier may dive on a hand grenade to save his buddy; a pregnant mother may prefer to die and save her baby instead of aborting, which would have saved her.

We can do several things to prevent suicide. People have several misconceptions about suicide. For example, when someone talks about suicide, we generally think that he/she does not mean it. This is a wrong assumption. Verbal or behavioral threats to commit suicide are the best predictors of suicidal attempts and such threats must be taken seriously. People with suicidal tendency are lonely; it is important that they be given social support and empathy. When you show genuine concern toward them and help them to ventilate their problems, it will go a long way to prevent their suicidal thoughts. If a person has suicidal tendencies, do not leave him alone. When a person realizes that there are people who care and help the intensity of suicidal tendencies will subside. In several cities there are centers to provide professional help to suicide-prone people.

Schizophrenia

Schizophrenia is the most highly talked about and researched condition among the mental disorders. This is the disorder, which mostly corresponds to what common people call lunacy, madness or insanity (these terms are not used in scientific writing). In spite of its popularity, not much is known about schizophrenia. It still remains an enigma, a highly puzzling and bizarre state of mind. The cause and cure of this illness are baffling and a complete understanding of the disorder continues to elude mental health professionals. The majority of patients in any psychiatric hospital are people suffering from schizophrenia. It is estimated that the disorder affects about one in a hundred. It is more common in men than in women. Treatment of schizophrenia accounts for about 75 percent of all mental health expenditure.

It was the German psychiatrist Emil Kraepelin who first described the illness in detail. He called it ***dementia praecox*** to emphasize its early onset and irreversibility of the condition. Later, the Swiss psychiatrist, Eugen Bleuler coined the term **schizophrenia** to refer to the disorder. The term is derived from two Greek roots, *schizo* (or German term *schizien*), meaning "to split" and *phrenia*, meaning "mind" or "reason." Because of its origin, the term has been misconceived by the general public as split personality (as seen in the classical "Jekyll and Hyde" type). However, this is not what Bleuler intended the word 'schizophrenia' to mean. Rather, he was referring to the splitting of the thought pattern—split between words, between thoughts, emotion behavior and in general a split from reality. There is a breakdown in the logical structure of thinking and speech characterized by looseness between expressed ideas. In fact, many specialists consider schizophrenia basically as a thought disorder.

Today, the term schizophrenia is used to refer to a group of disorders exhibiting severe impairment in attention, perception, speech, thought, emotion and behavior. The person suffering from schizophrenia misinterprets reality, cuts off social relations and as time passes, starts exhibiting general deterioration. Several types of schizophrenia have been identified, but the distinctions between them are not always clear.

Symptoms of Schizophrenia

Schizophrenic patients exhibit a variety of bizarre symptoms. The DSM-IV has identified two groups of symptoms:

1. Positive symptoms.
2. Negative symptoms.

1. The **positive symptoms** include **hallucinations**, **delusions**, disorganized speech and bizarre behavior. These are called positive symptoms not because they are desirable, but because they reflect the presence of excessive distortions in normal behavior.
2. The important **negative symptoms** are blunted emotional expressions (apathy, anhedonia), poverty of speech, especially alogia (very little speech) and avolition (lack of will to initiate and continue goal-directed activities). The patients may sit and stare at things without any feeling.

Schizophrenic patients may exhibit both positive and negative symptoms but excessive negative symptoms indicate that the prospect of recovery is poor. Let us examine some of these symptoms.

Hallucinations: A hallucination refers to a sensory experience in the absence of any eliciting external stimuli. That is, the person hears where there is nothing to be heard, sees where there is nothing to be seen, or feels where there is nothing to be felt. Hallucinations may occur in any sense modality, but in schizophrenia auditory hallucinations are the most common; 75 percent of the patients report that they hear "voices." Visual hallucinations are reported less frequently. The voices may come from familiar or strange people and sometimes from God or devil. The voices may be pleasant and encouraging or rude and abusive. The patients become so involved in the auditory hallucinations that they may actually act on them; that is, they may do what the voices ask them to do. Are the patients really hearing the voices? The brain mapping studies show that there is increased activity in the speech centers indicating that they are really hearing voices. Researchers have concluded that auditory hallucinations are really a form of misperceived subvocal speech.

Delusions: The delusions are erroneous and/or false beliefs that are firmly held despite clear contradictory evidence. People with delusions believe things that others around them do not believe. A delusion is a thought disorder; the thinking is logical, but the content of thought is wrong. All schizophrenics may not have delusions, but almost 90 percent have them. The contents of delusions are characteristic of schizophrenia. The patients believe that their thoughts, feelings and actions are controlled (***delusions of control***) by external agents or that their private thoughts are being broadcast indiscriminately or thoughts are being inserted into their mind by external agents or some external agency is robbing their thoughts (***delusions of persecution***). There are some ***delusions of reference*** in which the patients think that some external events (such as TV program, a story, a conversation between two persons, or a person looking at the patient) have personal meaning intended only to them. There may also be ***delusions of grandeur*** (belief that one is an important person), and of bodily changes, such as believing that some body part has changed or not working properly.

Speech disorders: The schizophrenic speech does not make sense although it is grammatically correct. The speech appears to be an external manifestation of schizophrenic thought. Poor speech cannot be attributed to either intellectual deficit or lack of education. Several researchers refer to this condition as a form associative disruption. Terms such as "cognitive slippage", "thought derailment" and "incoherent talk" have been used to describe schizophrenic speech. Often new words that have meaning only to the person are constructed; the process is called ***neologism***.

DSM-IV suggests the following criteria for the diagnosis of schizophrenia:

1. Delusions.
2. Hallucinations.
3. Disorganized speech.
4. Grossly disorganized behavior.
5. Negative symptoms.

If two or more of the above symptoms are present for a significant portion of time during one-month period, the condition is diagnosed as schizophrenia. Only one symptom is enough if the delusions are bizarre or if the hallucinations consist of a voice keeping up a running commentary on the person's behavior or thoughts, or two or more voices conversing with each other. The other indications are lack of interpersonal relations and self-care as well as, impaired work performance.

The average age of onset of schizophrenia is 20 years, but in some cases it may occur later in life. The onset is gradual, with the prodromal phase (the period between the occurrence of the first symptom and the actual onset of the illness) marked by slow deterioration in functioning, such as withdrawal from social relations, poor hygiene, and outbursts of anger. Finally, the disorder enters an active phase in which positive and negative symptoms emerge. Approximately 1 percent of people worldwide are estimated to develop schizophrenia sometime in their life. 25 percent of the cases have only one episode and recover completely, 25 percent improve enough to live independent life, 25 percent improve but not enough to lead an independent life, 15 percent do not improve and remain in a chronic state, and 10 percent commit suicide.

Subtypes of Schizophrenia

We said in the beginning that schizophrenia is a group of disorders having different causes, course and outcome. Questions have been raised about subtyping, but still clinicians prefer to do so. The DSM-IV-TR mentions five major types and several minor kinds of schizophrenia. A brief review of the same is given below.

Paranoid schizophrenia: **Paranoid schizophrenia** is characterized typically by delusions, especially delusions of persecution. Patients generally think that others are trying to harm them. Some of them suffer from delusions of grandeur in which they believe they are very important persons born to achieve something great. The patients suffering from paranoid schizophrenia are generally suspicious, anxious, and often aggressive. When these people are not talking about their delusions, they appear normal; their intellectual and emotional functions are not deviant. They sometimes experience auditory hallucinations. The suicide rate among them is more than average. The recovery rate is relatively high.

Disorganized schizophrenia: **Disorganized schizophrenia** is characterized by grossly disorganized speech, bizarre behavior and flat or inappropriate affect (emotions). It occurs early in life and the onset is gradual. The condition was earlier called ***hebephrenic schizophrenia***. As the illness progresses, the patient starts exhibiting silly, infantile behavior. A silly smile and inappropriate shallow laughter with little or no provocation are common features. The thought is so disorganized that it is difficult to communicate with them. Speech is un-understandable and may include baby talk, silly giggling and repetition of similar-sounding words. Delusions, if present, are not as organized as in the case of paranoid type. Patients suffering from disorganized schizophrenia cannot manage their day-to-day life. No treatment is effective in the case of these patients and the prognosis is very poor.

Catatonic schizophrenia: The clinical picture of **catatonic schizophrenia** is dominated by ***catatonic stupor*** (exhibition of an immobile body posture) or ***catatonic excitement*** (excessive motor activity). The two states may alternate. During stuporous state, the patients assume bizarre, immobile body postures, exhibit stereotyped behaviors or peculiar mannerisms. They may exhibit a condition called ***waxy flexibility*** in which their limbs can be molded to any position that is maintained for any length of time. Catatonic patients exhibit extreme negativism: they refuse to change from the position they have assumed, may remain mute, refuse to eat and may not comply with any request. During the excitement state, they are oblivious to reality, appear agitated, talk incessantly, pace rapidly back and forth and may indulge in sexual activities in the open. They may attack someone impulsively or even commit suicide. Some of these patients are highly suggestible and will automatically obey any command or imitate the actions of others (***echopraxia***) or mimic whatever is said (***echolalia***).

Undifferentiated schizophrenia: As the name itself suggests, schizophrenic types that do not show the specific symptoms of paranoid, disorganized or catatonic categories are diagnosed as belonging to undifferentiated type. Although the patients suffer from hallucinations, delusions, thought disturbances and emotional disorders in varying combinations, on the whole, the condition does not clearly fit into any of the major types because of mixed symptom picture.

Residual schizophrenia: The fifth type mentioned by DSM-IV-TR is **residual schizophrenia**. This diagnosis is made for people who have suffered at least one episode of schizophrenia, but now do not show any prominent positive symptoms such as hallucinations, delusions, disorganized speech and grossly disorganized or catatonic behavior. However, there are negative symptoms such as flat affect and social withdrawal along with some mild psychotic symptoms (odd beliefs, eccentric behavior and unusual perceptual experiences).

Other Schizophrenia-like Disorders

The DSM-IV-TR mentions certain other psychotic disorders that resemble schizophrenia. One of them is ***schizoaffective disorder*** in which the symptoms of schizophrenia coexist with symptoms of mood disorders. The second one is ***schizophreniform disorder***. A person is diagnosed as suffering from this type if he exhibits schizophrenic symptoms that last for at least a month but not lasts for six months. The third type is called ***delusional disorder***. This diagnosis is made when the person suffers from well systematized delusions, is absorbed in them, and sometimes takes action on the basis of the delusions. But the patient does not exhibit gross disorganization. The performance deficiency as found in schizophrenia and behavioral deterioration is rare even when it proves chronic. A major delusion observed among patients, especially women, is ***erotomania***—a belief that a great person is in love with her or him. The fourth type is called ***brief psychotic disorder***, which exactly implies what the name suggests—the sudden onset of schizophrenic symptoms, which last for a short period, too short to diagnose as schizophrenia. The final type is named ***shared psychotic disorder***, which is well-known in its French name, ***folie á deux***. This is a strange type in which schizophrenia operates as a contagious disorder. Suppose a person X is closely related to Y, who is suffering from schizophrenic delusions. Over time, X comes to acquire and believe in the delusions of Y. Thus, X comes to share the disorder of Y. Sometimes, the disorder may spread even further and the whole family may adopt the same delusional thinking.

Etiology of Schizophrenia

What causes schizophrenia? This is a billion dollar question. In spite of innumerable research efforts for the past several years, the etiology (causal pattern) of schizophrenia remains an enigma. Schizophrenia really is a puzzling, and indeed a mystifying disorder. It is difficult to implicate any one single factor as the cause of schizophrenia. As is in the case of other psychological disorders, schizophrenia is believed to be a result of an interplay of various complex factors—biological (genetic, neurological and hormonal), psychological (cognitive, affective) and environmental (familial and sociocultural). Let us briefly review the role of these factors in the causation of schizophrenia.

Genetic Factors

A number of twin and family studies indicate that there is a genetic basis for schizophrenia. It has long been believed that schizophrenia "runs in families." The prevalence of schizophrenia has been found to be higher than expected rates among the biological relatives of "index" case ("***proband***", the individual, diagnosed as suffering from a disorder, who provides the starting point for the investigation of that specific disorder). For example, the prevalence of schizophrenia in the first-degree relatives (parents, offspring and siblings) of a proband with schizophrenia is about 10 percent. For second degree relatives (aunts, uncles, half-siblings, nephews, nieces and grandchildren), who share only 25 percent of their genes, the lifetime prevalence is only 3 percent. Twin studies have shown that identical twins have higher concordance rates than fraternal twins or ordinary siblings. According to one exhaustive review of studies (Torrey et al, 1994), the concordance rate for identical twins varies between 48 and 65 percent and for fraternal twins, three and nine percent. The overall pairwise concordance rate is 28 percent for identical twins and 6 percent for fraternal twins. The results are not unequivocal. However, one thing is clear. The prevalence of schizophrenia is more among identical twins than among fraternal twins and siblings. If schizophrenia were entirely a genetic disorder, the concordance should be 100 percent; it is not the case. Among the fraternal twins the concordance rate is only 6 percent. Although small, it is greater than the expected rate in the general population, which is one percent. From these observations, we can draw two conclusions. First, genes undoubtedly play a role in the causation of schizophrenia. Second, genes themselves do not tell the whole story. No specific gene that might cause the disorder has been identified. Therefore, it has to be inferred that along with genetics other factors—psychological, sociocultural and environmental—play a significant part in the development of schizophrenia. Researchers aver that schizophrenia is a genetically influenced, not genetically determined disorder.

Brain in Schizophrenia

Studies of the brains of schizophrenic patients have shown certain structural abnormalities. One view called ***neurodegenerative hypothesis*** proposes that destruction of certain brain tissues can cause schizophrenia. Neuroimaging studies have shown mild to moderate brain atrophy (deterioration of neural tissues) in the cerebral cortex and the limbic system (especially in the thalamus and amygdala). Also, there are enlarged ventricles (fluid-filled spaces that lie deep in the brain), suggesting a decrease in the quantity of brain cells. Note that the atrophy is centered in the areas of brain that are involved in cognitive and emotional functions. This information is used as a basis to explain the thought disorders and inappropriate emotions among schizophrenic patients. Certain abnormalities in the thalamus (the organ that collects and relays sensory information to other parts of the brain) are used to explain the disorders of attention and perception in the schizophrenic cases. Studies have also shown a decline in the brain size as the disorder progresses. But it has to be emphasized that most schizophrenic patients have brains that are basically normal and that many of the differences reported are not specific to schizophrenia.

Neurotransmitters

Abnormalities in the functioning of the neurotransmitter **dopamine** are implicated in the causation of schizophrenia. Once it was thought that an overproduction of dopamine was responsible for schizophrenia, a view known as **dopamine hypothesis**. This hypothesis was supported by researches. For example, when the amount of dopamine was reduced through medication, there was a decrease in the number of positive symptoms among schizophrenic patients. Also, when people without schizophrenia were given drugs to increase the amount of dopamine, they exhibited symptoms of schizophrenia. But now it is believed that dopamine hypothesis is too simplistic an explanation for a complex condition such as schizophrenia. But the fact that dopamine has an influence in the development of schizophrenia cannot be denied. Other neurotransmitters such as glutamate, (an excitatory neurotransmitter), are probably involved in the disorder as well.

No doubt abnormalities in the brain structures and the biochemical variations are found among the patients suffering from schizophrenia, but whether these are the causes or the result of schizophrenia has yet to be established. Future research may shed light on the role of other biological and biochemical factors in the etiology of schizophrenia.

Psychological Factors

Sigmund Freud thought that schizophrenia was the result of regression (retreat to an earlier level of safety) to an infantile level of development in the face of severe stress or conflict. This idea has been used to explain the general social withdrawal, which is a predominant symptom of schizophrenia. Although Freud's regression point of view has not found any research support, it is generally believed that life stress has a significant influence in the development of schizophrenia.

Cognitive psychologists believe that schizophrenic patients have difficulty in processing and responding to sensory stimuli. According to them, the patients have a defect in the process of attending. As we know, attention filters out irrelevant information and helps us to focus on relevant stimuli emanating from the environment. When attention is impaired, irrelevant stimuli and images flood the consciousness causing distractibility and thought disorganization. People start experiencing disconnected ideas and are overwhelmed by stimulus overload. As a result, they may see inanimate objects moving around them, may not be able to determine the importance of new information, and may have difficulty in understanding the social cues. Ultimately, they may not realize that they have problems (lack of insight). As mentioned earlier, the thalamic abnormality may be behind such sensory and perceptual disturbances.

Environmental Factors

Several environmental factors, such as intrauterine conditions, familial and sociocultural environment have been implicated in the etiology of schizophrenia. Maternal stress, illness and birth-related medications are found to produce certain structural changes in the fetal brain, which in turn, creates a vulnerability to develop schizophrenia. Stressful events seem to interact with biological and/or personality vulnerability factors. A highly vulnerable person breaks down under stress. Some 50 years ago, family was considered as an important culprit in the causation of schizophrenia. Mothers were singled out for criticism. A mother, who was cold and aloof toward the children, was called ***schizophrenic mother***. Another influential concept, **double bind hypothesis**, was popular in clinical circles, while talking about schizophrenia. A double bind occurs when parents present the child with ideas, feelings, and demands that are mutually incompatible. For example, a mother may complain that the child has no love for her and when the child expresses affectionate feelings, she freezes or punishes the child. But no solid evidence has ever been found to support the idea of a schizophrenogenic mother or double bind communication. However, the role of familial environment in the genesis of schizophrenia cannot be completely ruled out.

Research has shown that having a sick person at home may cause conflicts and disturbances in the family. George Brown and colleagues have observed that when a schizophrenic patient returned home to live with parents or spouse after treatment, the risk of relapse was more than when they lived alone. These researchers have developed a construct known as **expressed emotion (EE)**, a measure of the family environment that is based on how a family member speaks about the patient during a private interview with a researcher. The EE has three major elements: *criticism* "All you do is read the newspaper", *hostility* "We are fed up with your crazy behavior" and *emotional overinvolvement* "Do not go out anywhere unless I accompany you". Later studies have shown that high EE home environment predicts relapse in patients with schizophrenia (Vaughan and Leff, 1976). Well, even here, the results are not conclusive.

There is some evidence to show that there is a higher rate of schizophrenia in urban areas and in lower socioeconomic classes. Two factors, social selection and social causation, are put forward to explain this finding. ***Social selection*** refers to the drifting (social drift) to lower socioeconomic classes of those who become psychologically disabled. This occurs among those who cannot work effectively and those who have no family support. ***Social causation*** refers to the chronic psychological and social stressors in the urban environment, especially for the poor. These stresses trigger schizophrenia in people who are biologically vulnerable. It is also reported that schizophrenia is more prevalent and its recovery rate is lower in industrialized nations than in developing countries. The explanations given for these findings are not convincing.

Many researchers today believe that psychological disorders can best be explained by a **diathesis-stress model** (the word diathesis means vulnerability or predisposition). This conceptualization states that for a given disorder, there is both a predisposition to the disorder (diathesis) and specific factors (stress) that combine with the diathesis to trigger the onset of the disorder. Although usually genetic in nature, the diathesis may include other biological factors, such as complications during pregnancy and childbirth, psychological factors such as maladaptive personality characteristics or dysfunctional thinking patterns. According to this model, only people who have some genetic predisposition will develop schizophrenia and only if they are exposed to so much stress that they are unable to cope with. Joseph Zubin assumes that schizophrenia is not a permanent disorder, but rather a permanent vulnerability to a disorder. Each person has a level of vulnerability (which may be high or low) to schizophrenia determined by genetic, prenatal and postnatal physical factors. When a high level of vulnerability interacts with stress, it produces schizophrenia. Researchers have shown that the heightened susceptibility to stress comes about because of the effect of cortisol on dopamine activity (which is to produce an overactivity of dopamine systems), which, in turn, can worsen symptoms of schizophrenia.

These findings prompt us to fall back on to the often repeated conclusion that schizophrenia, like several other psychological disorders, is the result of interaction of biological, psychological and environmental factors. A biological vulnerability in combination with psychosocial and environmental factors determines whether an individual develops the disorder or not.

Personality Disorders

We have learnt in chapter 11, that each of us has a personality that determines the characteristic way in which we respond to life events. All of us do not respond to all situations in similar ways. Personality styles can be maladaptive, if an individual is unable to change his/her behavior in appropriate ways with changing environmental conditions. If personality traits are not flexible enough to allow an individual to respond adaptively to day-to-day situations, he/she is said to have a personality disorder. Therefore, **personality disorders** can be defined as a set of relatively longstanding, maladaptive and inflexible ways of responding to environmental stimuli. These disorders limit an individual's approach to stress-producing situations because his/her style of thinking, feeling and acting permit only a narrow and rigid range of responses. The dysfunctional traits of personality can cause distress or difficulty with functioning in school, work, family and social relationships. Personality disorders can usually be noticed in childhood or at least by early adolescence and may continue through adult life. These may occur alone or accompany other psychological disorders. The DSM-IV-TR has identified a number of personality disorders and grouped them under three clusters based on common symptoms. The clusters and the personality disorders under each cluster are summarized below.

Cluster-A: Includes paranoid, schizotypal and schizoid personality disorders and these are characterized by odd or eccentric behaviors. The major symptoms exhibited by people suffering from cluster-A disorders are distrust, suspicion and social detachment.

Paranoid personality disorder is characterized by the following behaviors: pervasive suspiciousness and distrust of others to the extent that other people's motives are interpreted as harmful and ill-intentioned; unjustified doubting of the trustworthiness of spouse, friends and other close associates; reading hidden or threatening meaning into benign remarks of others; unforgiving of insults; expression of anger to perceived attacks on his/her integrity or reputation. The paranoid personality disorder is to be distinguished from paranoid schizophrenia. The former does not exhibit delusions and hallucinations like the latter.

The person suffering from ***schizoid personality disorder*** neither desires nor enjoys close social relationships including members of the family; he/she has no friends or confidants and engages in solitary activities; emotional expressions are narrow, cold and detached; does not show interest in members of the opposite sex and exhibits indifference toward praise or criticism.

The people with ***schizotypal personality disorder*** exhibit ideas of reference (believing that the conversation, smiling or other gestures of people have reference to oneself), social anxiety (fear of mixing with others), odd beliefs (believing that one has magical powers), unusual perceptual experiences, bizarre speech and thinking, suspicion, strange or eccentric behavior and inappropriate emotions. The person does not have close friends or confidants except family members).

Cluster-B: Includes histrionic, narcissistic, borderline and antisocial personality disorders. People suffering from these disorders exhibit behaviors that are dramatic, emotional or erratic.

People with ***histrionic personality disorder*** experience discomfort in situations where they are not the center of attraction, exhibit sexually seductive or provocative behavior that is inappropriate, display rapidly shifting shallow emotions, and use physical appearance to draw attention to themselves. Their speech is impressionistic and they exhibit relationships as more intimate, which is not true. These people are highly suggestible.

Individuals with ***narcissistic personality disorder*** show grandiose (exaggerated) sense of self-importance and are preoccupied with fantasies of unlimited power, success, brilliance and beauty. They believe that they are special and unique, and exhibit excessive need for admiration. The other characteristics are: exploitative tendency; lack of empathy; being envious of others or believing that others are envious of self; arrogant and haughty behavior and a sense of entitlement (claim that they are great and deserve better things).

The clinical features of b***orderline personality disorder*** include frantic efforts to avoid real or imagined abandonment, unstable and intense interpersonal relationships, unstable sense of self, impulsivity (in spending, sexual encounters, reckless driving and drug abuse), suicidal and self-mutilating thoughts and behavior, emotional instability (frequent mood change), feelings of emptiness, inappropriate anger and transient stress-related paranoid ideation or dissociative symptoms.

People suffering from ***antisocial personality disorder*** fail to conform to social norms (violating laws); they are deceitful, manipulative, impulsive (fail to plan ahead), irritable and aggressive, reckless and have disregard for the safety of self and others. They are irresponsible, lack empathy, do not care for how others feel, and do not experience remorse after having hurt, mistreated or stolen from others. They exhibit superficial charm and blame others for any adversity that comes their way.

Cluster-C: Includes avoidant, dependent and obsessive-compulsive personality disorders; the major symptoms shared by these disorders are anxiety and fearfulness.

People suffering from ***avoidant personality disorder*** are introverted and avoid social contacts. They are unwilling to involve in any social relationship unless they are sure of being liked. They do not prefer to work in an environment where interpersonal relationships are involved. They avoid intimate relationship because of the fear of being ridiculed and rejected. They are hypersensitive and suffer from a sense of personal inadequacy. They generally feel inferior to others and are preoccupied with the thought of being criticized or rejected. They are reluctant to take risk and do not engage in any new activity for fear of embarrassment. They feel bored and lonely, desire the affection and company of others, but are afraid of failing to establish a comfortable relationship. As a consequence, they experience acute anxiety. Ineptitude and a sense of social inadequacy are the two most stable and glaring features of the avoidant personality disorder.

As the name indicates, people with ***dependent personality disorder*** express an intense desire to be looked after by others and want others to take all responsibilities for most of the major decisions of life. They are submissive and cling to people around them, are scared of disagreeing with others because of the fear of loss of support or approval. They exhibit acute fear of the possibility of being separated from others and being alone. Because they build their lives around others, they subordinate their own needs and views to keep these people involved with them. They have difficulty in making even simple decisions and initiating projects without the advice and assurance from others. Several features of dependent personality disorder overlap with those of borderline, histrionic and avoidant personality disorders.

People suffering from ***obsessive-compulsive personality disorder*** exhibit extreme perfectionism, inflexibility, preoccupation with control and excessive concern for maintaining order. They are so preoccupied with details, schedules, order and rules that they will forget the central theme of an activity, the concern with perfection is so great that it interferes with the completion of the task on hand. These people are rigid, stubborn, over-conscious, miserly and excessively concerned with morality, ethics, or values. They are so devoted to work that they deny themselves leisure. They are reluctant to delegate work to others unless they are sure that others do the same thing in the same way. Research indicates that rigidity and stubbornness, as well as reluctance to delegate, are the most stable traits of people having obsessive-compulsive personality disorder.

In addition to the ones mentioned above, clinicians have come across several other personality deviations such as affective (depressive, cyclothymic and anxiety-ridden) personality disorder, explosive personality disorder and passive-aggressive personality disorder. The list is not complete. Note that there is a good deal of overlap of symptoms among the various disorders.

Causation and Prevalence of Personality Disorders

Not much is known about the causal factors of personality disorders. One major problem in studying the etiology stems from the high level of **comorbidity** (occurrence of one or two of these disorders along with other psychological disorders). Researchers have found that 85 percent of patients who qualified for the diagnosis of one personality disorder also qualify for several more. It is estimated that about three quarters of people diagnosed with a personality disorder also have an Axis-I disorder of DSM-IV. Several of the so-called "normal" people suffer from personality disorders and society tolerates them. People with personality disorder do not think they are sick and do not come for treatment; and as a consequence, doing research on them is a problem. Not many *prospective studies* (observing cases before the onset of a disorder and following them over a period of time to see who develops problems and what the causal factors are) have been conducted in this area. The majority of researches are conducted on people who already have the disorders and these have relied on retrospective recall of prior events. Some of them have relied on observing current biological, psychological and social factors. Therefore, any conclusion about the causes of personality disorders may have to be considered tentative. It is also difficult to diagnose personality disorders because these are not sharply defined; the disorders are not mutually exclusive. People often exhibit more than one personality disorder.

These disorders do not stem from debilitating reactions to stress in the recent past; rather, they stem largely from the gradual development of inflexible and distorted personality and behavior patterns that result in persistently maladaptive ways of perceiving, thinking about and relating to the world. It is estimated that about 13 percent of people in the general population suffer from personality disorders and these people often cause at least as much difficulty in the lives of others as in their own lives. Therefore, it is necessary that serious attempts are made to study the etiology, diagnosis and treatment of personality disorders.

OTHER PSYCHOLOGICAL DISORDERS

There are a number of other psychological disorders such as eating disorders, drug abuse and dependence, disorders pertaining to sexual behavior, cognitive disorders and childhood disorders. All these cannot be discussed in a chapter. Interested students can study them in one of the standard textbooks of abnormal psychology (Sarason & Sarason 1996, Carson, Butcher, Mineka & Hooley, 2007). A brief review of these is given in the following pages.

Eating Disorders

In contemporary society, several people, especially people in developed countries, suffer from eating disorders due to their preoccupation with their weight and body image. People are crazy about maintaining their figure like those who walk on the ramp. Being thin and lean has become the standard. More than 90 percent of those diagnosed as suffering from eating disorders are women; but in recent times, the incidence among men is also increasing. Anorexia nervosa and bulimia nervosa are the two eating disorders frequently encountered in clinical practice.

Anorexia Nervosa

Anorexia nervosa is characterized by the refusal to maintain even a low normal body weight, and intense fear of gaining weight. The term anorexia nervosa literally means lack of appetite induced by nervousness. It is a fatal disorder in which the person pursues thinness regardless of physical consequences. Among those hospitalized with anorexia nervosa, 10 percent will eventually die. General symptoms necessary to diagnose the condition are: distorted body image (distorted perception of body shape and size), fear of becoming fat, refusal to maintain a healthy weight, and amenorrhea among females (absence of at least three consecutive menstrual periods). Patients know that they are underweight; yet, when they stand in front of a mirror, see fat in the body that is not there. Generally, they overestimate their body size. They are obsessed by thoughts of food as bad or good that are generally illogical and irrational. Although they are thin or even emaciated, patients deny having any problem. In fact, some of them are proud of their appearance and body size.

There are two types of anorexia nervosa: The ***restricting type*** in which every effort is made to restrict food intake, and the ***binge eating/purging type*** in which the patients binge, purge, or binge and purge. A binge involves eating excessively. The binge may be followed by efforts to purge or removing the food by vomiting or misuse of laxatives. In professions where slender body is emphasized (film stars, fashion models, ballet dancers), anorexia is more prevalent.

Bulimia Nervosa

Bulimia nervosa is characterized by binge eating and preventing weight gain by purging using self-induced vomiting or excessive exercise. The word bulimia roughly means "eating like an ox," and was first used by the British psychiatrist GSM Russell in 1979 and was included in the DSM in 1979. The binge-eating/purging type of anorexia nervosa and bulimia nervosa appear to have several symptoms in common and some writers argue that there is no need for two terms. But there is a difference between the two. Anorexic patients are generally underweight and it is not so with bulimia nervosa; bulimia patients typically have normal weight.

Anorexia nervosa and bulimia nervosa are considered "modern disorders." and it is only during the 1970s and 1980s, the two have come to attract the attention of clinicians. The disorders generally occur during late teens and early adulthood. The age group of highest risk is women aged 20 to 24. Although eating disorders occur in males, these are far more common among women. The conditions occur with depression, obsessive-compulsive disorders and drug addiction. No single cause has been proposed for eating disorders. In all probability, the disorders develop from the combined effect of biological, psychological and sociocultural variables.

Addiction Disorders

Behavior characterized by a pathological craving for or abuse of **psychoactive substances** is referred to as addictive behavior or substance abuse disorders. The psychoactive substances include alcohol, nicotine, cocaine, barbiturates, tranquilizers, amphetamines, heroin and marijuana among others. These are chemicals that produce alterations in consciousness and affect behavior. Continued consumption of addictive substances creates serious mental health problems. Several problems of alcohol or other substance abuse stem from their intoxicating effects and ***toxicity*** (the poisonous nature of the substance). The DSM-IV-TR and ICD-10 have identified two major categories of addiction disorders: substance abuse disorders and substance dependence disorders.

Substance abuse refers to the use of one or the other of the psychoactive substances to the degree that a severe and long-lasting impairment in function occurs; the addicted person may engage in potentially hazardous behavior, such as reckless driving, while intoxicated. He/She may continue to use the substance in spite of it producing persistent social, psychological and occupational problems. **Substance dependence** is a more severe form of maladaptive substance-related disorder involving tolerance for the substance and withdrawal symptoms. **Tolerance** refers to a condition resulting from repeated use of a substance in which the same amount of substance produces a diminished effect and more of the substance is required to achieve the same effect. Tolerance results from biochemical changes in the body affecting the rate of metabolism and elimination of the substance from the body. **Withdrawal symptoms** are uncomfortable (or even life-threatening) effects such as profuse sweating, tremors and tension that may be experienced during withdrawal or the cessation of the use of the substance. Tolerance and withdrawal symptoms typically occur with the use of alcohol, barbiturates, amphetamines, cocaine, lysergic acid diethylamide (LSD), marijuana, morphine and heroin. The term ***psychological dependence*** is often used to describe situations in which the individual develops an intense craving for a drug because of its pleasurable effects. Many factors influence substance dependence including genetic predisposition, personality traits, religious beliefs, cultural norms, familial environment and the type of friends.

Alcohol Abuse and Alcohol Dependence

Alcohol is the most widely used (and abused) recreational drug all over the world. It is a depressant (not a stimulant as is believed by the general public), which decreases the activity of the nervous system by increasing the activity of gamma-aminobutyric acid (GABA), the brain's major inhibitory transmitter, and by decreasing the activity of glutamate, a major excitatory neurotransmitter. The subjective feeling of pleasure or euphoria is due to the action of several neurotransmitters such as dopamine. At higher doses, alcohol disrupts brain's control centers. Thinking is disorganized, physical coordination impaired and fatigue may set in. The blood alcohol level (BAL) is a measure of alcohol concentration in the blood. High BAL impairs reaction time, muscular coordination and decision making. It also increases the tendency to engage in risky behavior. A substantial number of traffic-accident deaths involve alcohol abuse. Alcohol also produces a condition called ***'alcohol myopia'***—shortsighted thinking caused by the inability to pay attention to as much information as when one is sober. The psychological effects of alcohol include impairment in the ability to think abstractly, conceptualize information, notice situational cues and interpret ambiguous social situations. More complex effects include a phenomenon called inhibitory conflict (difficulty of inhibiting a behavior that would normally not be expressed when sober) and increased aggression, especially sexual aggression. Alcohol abuse increases sexual desire, but lowers sexual performance. Organic impairment, including brain shrinkage, occurs in proportion with high alcohol dependence, especially among binge drinkers (people who abuse alcohol following periods of sobriety). For pregnant mothers, even a moderate amount of alcohol is believed to be dangerous. It is reported that the children born to them suffer from a condition called **fetal alcohol syndrome (FAS)**, which may cause birth defects and mental retardation. Alcoholism is associated with several psychotic states such as *idiosyncratic intoxication, withdrawal delirium (formerly called delirium tremens), alcoholic amnestic disorder (formerly known as Korsakoff's syndrome), chronic alcoholic hallucinosis* and *dementia.*

Alcohol abuse and dependence are major problems in advanced countries and are among the most destructive psychological disorders. Heavy drinking is associated with vulnerability to injury and involvement in intimate partner violence. The lifespan of an alcoholic is about 12 years shorter than the average person. More than 35 percent of alcohol abusers suffer from at least one coexisting psychological disorder. Alcohol disorders are associated with over half of deaths and injuries suffered in automobile accidents each year, and over 40 to 50 percent of murders. It is reported that one in every three arrests in the United States is related to alcohol abuse. Alcoholism is more prevalent among men than women. Marriage, higher level of education and being older are associated with lower incidence of alcoholic disorders.

Psychoactive Drugs

Depressants, such as barbiturates (Nembutal, Seconal, Veronal and Tuinal) and tranquilizers (anti-anxiety drugs such as Valium), mimic the effects of alcohol by depressing the nervous system activity. **Barbiturates** are prescribed by physicians to aid sleep and reduce anxiety, but they can become lethal when combined with alcohol. In higher doses, barbiturates cause slurred speech, dizziness, poor judgment and irritability. People may also develop tolerance and withdrawal symptoms. Withdrawal may be accompanied by agitation and restlessness, hallucinations, and delirium tremens. Anti-anxiety drugs—***benzodiazepines*** such as Valium (diazepam), Librium (chlordiazepoxide) and Miltown (meprobamate)—are also used as sedatives (sleeping pills), but these are less habit forming than barbiturates.

The other psychoactive drugs, most commonly associated with abuse and dependence are stimulants, such as cocaine and amphetamines (which increase feelings of alertness and confidence); narcotics such as opium and its derivatives, including heroin (which alleviate pain); psychedelics and hallucinogens such as LSD, mescaline, and PCP (phencyclidine), which produce hallucinations. The LSD, an odorless, colorless and tasteless drug is the most potent of the hallucinogens. An amount of LSD smaller than a grain of salt can cause intoxication. Mescaline, which is derived from the small disc-like growths at the top of the peyote cactus and psilocybin, which is derived from a Mexican mushroom (*Psilocybe mexicana*), both have mind altering and hallucinogenic properties. They distort experience—enabling the user to see, hear or otherwise experience events in unaccustomed ways. The user may be transported into a realm of "non-ordinary reality." The varieties and effects of psychoactive drugs are summarized in Table 15.1.

Another dangerous substance Ecstasy, or MDMA (3, 4-methylenedioxy-methamphetamine), a popular party drug, is both a hallucinogen and a stimulant. Marijuana, which is derived from the leaves and the flowering tops of the hemp plant Cannabis sativa, is a mild hallucinogen. The drug, colloquially called "grass," is smoked in the form of cigarettes (variously referred as weed, stash, joints, reefers, etc.), or in pipes. Hashish, another stimulant related to marijuana, but stronger than the latter, is also smoked. Both the drugs produce a sense of well-being and a state of relaxation.

The causes of drug abuse include biological predisposition, personality factors, and sociocultural influence. The influence of peer groups, the existence of 'drug culture,' and availability of drugs has all been found to play a role in drug abuse.

Sexual Variations, Abuse and Dysfunctions

It is not easy to distinguish between 'normal or acceptable' and 'deviant' forms of sexual behavior. Time and place are important factors that shape sexual behavior and attitudes. Sex and sex-related behaviors

Table 15.1: Psychoactive Drugs and their Effects

Classification	*Drug*	*Effect*
Sedatives	Alcohol	Reduce tension, facilitate social interaction produce pleasurable feelings
	Barbiturates	Reduce tension
	Nembutal	
	Seconal	
	Veronal	
	Tuinal	
Stimulants	Amphetamines	Boost arousal and increase feelings of alertness and confidence
	Benzedrine	Decrease feelings of fatigue
	Dexedrine	Stay awake for long periods
	Methedrine	Increase a sense of physical strength and endurance
	Cocaine	Produce a sense of euphoria stimulate sex drive
Narcotics	Opium and its derivatives	Alleviate physical pain
	Opium	Induce relaxation and pleasant reverie
	Morphine	Alleviate anxiety and tension
	Codeine	
	Heroin	
	Methadone	Treatment of heroin dependence
Psychedelics and hallucinogens	Cannabis	Induce changes in mood thought and behavior
	Marijuana	
	Hashish	
	Mescaline	Expand one's mind
	Psilocybin	Induce stupor
	Lysergic acid diethylamide (LSD)	
	Phencyclidine (PCP)	
Anti-anxiety drugs	Librium	Alleviate tension and anxiety
	Miltown	Induce relaxation and sleep
	Valium	
	Xanax	

Courtesy: Carson RC et al, 2007.

are influenced by social expectations, attitudes, beliefs and the state of biological and medical knowledge of a given period. What is normal sexual behavior has been changing dramatically over time and differs from culture to culture. During early 1900s, masturbation (sexual self-stimulation) was believed to cause a number of physical and mental disorders such as dyspepsia, headache, epilepsy, spinal diseases, impaired eyesight, palpitation of the heart and bleeding in the lungs. Such a view appears bizarre today. It is reported that over 90 percent of all males and over 60 percent of all females have masturbated at least once. Until recently, homosexuality (sexual activity with same-sexed partner) was viewed either as criminal behavior or as a form of mental illness. Modern mental health professionals view masturbation and homosexuality as normal sexual variants. It is estimated that around 20 to 25 percent of males and about 15 percent of females have had at least one homosexual experience during adulthood. Today, it is accepted that sexual behavior can be expressed in a variety of ways and we view as normal what was once considered as unnatural or abnormal. But, the fact remains that there are several deviations and dysfunctions in the realm of sexual behavior and these are grouped by DSM-IV-TR under three heads: sexual dysfunctions, paraphilias and gender identity disorders. We shall learn some elementary facts about these problems in the following pages.

SEXUAL DYSFUNCTIONS

The term **sexual dysfunction** refers to impairment either in the desire for sexual gratification or in the ability to achieve it. Dysfunction can occur in the first three of the four phases of the human sexual response: the desire phase, the excitement phase and orgasm (Master and Johnson. 1966). The major problems included under sexual dysfunctions, are sexual desire disorders, sexual arousal disorders, orgasmic disorders, and sexual pain disorders. These are summarized below.

Sexual Desire Disorders

1. **Hypoactive sexual desire disorder:** Either a man or woman shows little or no sexual drive or interest.
2. **Sexual aversion disorder:** The person shows extreme aversion to and avoidance of, all genital contact with a partner.

These disorders typically occur in the absence of obvious physical pathology, but physical factors may at times play a role. Hypoactive sexual desire problems are found to increase with age; these problems are more prevalent among women.

Sexual Arousal Disorders

1. **Male erectile disorder:** Persistent or recurrent inability to attain or maintain erection until completion of sexual activity.
2. **Female sexual arousal disorder:** Persistent or recurrent inability to attain or maintain arousal until completion of sexual activity.

Masters and Johnson have hypothesized that male erectile dysfunction is primarily due to anxiety about sexual performance. Erectile problems occur in as many as 90 percent of men who are on antidepressant medication. Others have hypothesized that cognitive distraction associated with anxiety interferes with arousal.

Orgasmic Disorders

1. **Male orgasmic disorder:** Persistent or recurrent delay in, or absence of, orgasm following a normal sexual excitement phase during sexual activity.
2. **Female orgasmic disorder:** Persistent or recurrent delay in, or absence of, orgasm following a normal sexual excitement phase.
3. **Premature ejaculation:** Persistent or recurrent ejaculation with minimal sexual stimulation before or shortly after penetration, and before the person wishes it.

Men who are completely unable to ejaculate and experience orgasm are rare. In women, orgasmic disorder is reported to be more prevalent. In most cases, this is supposed to be due to absence of sufficient stimulation. However, several cases of lifelong orgasmic dysfunction among women are reported. What causes female orgasmic disorder is not well understood. Explanations for premature ejaculation have ranged from psychological factors such as anxiety to physiological factors such as increased penile sensitivity. But neither of them has received empirical evidence.

Sexual Pain Disorders

1. **Dyspareunia:** Recurrent or persistent pain associated with sexual intercourse in either male or female. It is common among women, especially young women. The most obvious cause of dyspareunia among women is physical, such as chronic infections or inflammation of the vagina or internal reproductive organs, vaginal atrophy occurring with aging or insufficiency of sexual arousal. This condition is generally associated with vaginismus. Women who suffer from vaginismus also have sexual arousal disorder. Dyspareunia may be a result of conditioned fears associated with earlier traumatic sexual experiences.
2. **Vaginismus:** Recurrent or persistent involuntary spasm of the musculature of the outer third of the vagina that interferes with sexual intercourse.

PARAPHILIAS

Paraphilias are persistent sexual behavior patterns in which unusual objects, rituals or situations are required to obtain full sexual satisfaction (paraphilia means attraction to the deviant). People with paraphilias have recurrent, intense sexually-arousing fantasies, sexual urges, or behaviors that generally involve:

1. Non-human objects.
2. The suffering or humiliation of oneself or one's partner.
3. Children or other non-consenting persons.

DSM-IV mentions eight specific paraphilias:

1. Fetishism.
2. Transvestic fetishism.
3. Voyeurism.
4. Exhibitionism.
5. Sexual sadism.
6. Sexual masochism.
7. Pedophilia.
8. Frotteurism.

There are some rarer disorders such as telephone scatologia (making obscene phone calls), necrophilia (sexual desire for corpses), zoophilia (sexual interest in animals), apotemnophilia (sexual excitement and desire about having a limb amputated) and coprophilia (sexual arousal to feces). Although mild forms of paraphilias probably occur among normal people, a paraphilic person is diagnosed as suffering from these conditions depending on the insistence and relative exclusivity with which his/her sexuality focuses on the acts or objects in question—without which orgasm is often impossible. Paraphilic persons are obsessed with the objects, which they choose for sexual gratification. Nearly all paraphilic persons are males and the reported cases of female paraphilics are extremely rare. A summary of the major paraphilias is given below.

Fetishism is characterized by recurrent, intense sexually arousing fantasies, urges or behaviors involving the use of non-living objects, such as female undergarments, shoes, perfume, hair, and similar objects associated with opposite sex. Sexual excitation and gratification is commonly obtained by masturbating, while kissing, fondling, tasting or smelling the objects. The objects may be obtained through burglary, theft or even assault.

Transvestic fetishism refers to recurrent, intense sexually arousing fantasies, urges or behaviors involving cross-dressing in a heterosexual male. Transvestism generally starts during adolescence and involves masturbation, while wearing female dress or undergarments. Studies indicate that a majority of cross-dressing men are heterosexual and married. They keep their cross-dressing a secret. When wives find out, they feel disturbed. It is said that cross-dressing men are aroused by the image of themselves as women and not by women outside them.

Voyeurism is marked by recurrent intense, sexually arousing fantasies, urges or behaviors involving the act of observing an unsuspecting person who is naked in the process of disrobing or engaging in sexual activity. These "Peeping Toms" masturbate, while watching their favorite acts. These offences are generally committed by young men who are curious about sexual activity, but feel shy and uncomfortable in their relationship with women. Voyeurism satisfies their curiosity and to some extent sexual needs.

Exhibitionism refers to recurrent, intense, sexually arousing fantasies, urges or behaviors involving the indecent exposure of one's genitals to an unsuspecting stranger. The exposure may take place in secluded places such as an escalator or public places like department stores. Men who engage in exhibitionism often cause emotional distress to the viewers because of the impulsive quality of the act, along with its explicit violation of propriety norms. Society considers exhibitionism as a criminal offense. Women are the targets of voyeurism and exhibitionism.

Sexual sadism is marked by recurrent, intense, sexually arousing fantasies, urges, or behaviors involving real acts in which the psychological or physical suffering of the victim is sexually exciting to the person. The term is derived from the name of Marquis de Sade (1740–1814), who inflicted cruelty on his victims for sexual pleasures; he was eventually committed as insane. A sadist may slash a woman with a razor; prick her with a needle, bite, whip or burn the victim. Sadists may mentally replay their torture scenes later, while masturbating. Unfortunately, nobody knows why people become sadists.

Sexual masochism refers to recurrent, intense, sexually arousing fantasies, urges, or behaviors involving real acts of being humiliated, beaten, bound or otherwise made to suffer. The term is derived from the name of the Austrian novelist Leopold V Sacher-Masoch (1836–1895), whose fictional characters dwelt lovingly on the sexual pleasures of pain. In sexual masochism, a person experiences sexual stimulation and gratification from the experience of pain and degradation in relating to a lover. Masochism appears to be much more common than sadism and occurs in both sexes.

Pedophilia is characterized by recurrent, intense, sexually arousing fantasies, urges, or behaviors involving sexual activity with a pubescent child or children (generally age 13 years or younger). Pedophilia frequently involves fondling or manipulating a child's genitals and occasionally penetration. Nearly all pedophiles are male and about two thirds of their victims are girls typically between the ages of eight and eleven years. They may be homosexuals or heterosexuals; homosexual pedophiles tend to have more victims than heterosexual pedophiles. Pedophilia usually begins in adolescence and persists over a person's life.

Frotteurism refers to sexual gratification derived by touching or rubbing against a non-consenting person. The act itself (frottage) is usually carried out in crowded places such as buses and trains. Frotteurism is a relatively new category of paraphilia and has not been satisfactorily researched.

Several general facts about paraphilia have to be remembered. First, nearly all persons with paraphilia are male. Females with paraphilia are so rare that they are found in the literature (novels and short stories) only as case reports. Second, paraphilias usually begin around the time of puberty or early adolescence. Third, people with paraphilia have more than one of them. Why paraphilias are more prevalent among men? It is suggested that male vulnerability to paraphilias is closely related to their greater dependence on visual sexual imagery. Sexual arousal in men depends on physical stimulus features to a greater degree than in women. In women, arousal depends more on emotional context such as being in love with a partner. Men form sexual associations to non-sexual stimuli after puberty when the sexual drive is high. These associations may develop as a result of classical conditioning, operant conditioning or observational learning. When people watch paraphilic stimuli (for example, photographs of scantily dressed women} or fantasy about them, they masturbate, which is reinforcing and as a consequence, the attraction to paraphilic stimuli are strengthened.

Gender Identity Disorders

There are some rare individuals who feel uncomfortable and unhappy with their biological sex and strongly desire to change to the opposite sex. These are having problems with their gender identity. **Gender identity disorder** is characterized by two essential elements:

1. Strong and persistent **cross-gender identification**—i.e. the desire to be or the insistence that one is of the opposite sex.
2. **Gender dysphoria**—persistent discomfort about one's biological sex or the sense that the gender role of that sex is inappropriate.

The disorder may occur in children or adults and both among males or females. Boys with gender identity disorder show a preference to engage in feminine activities. They prefer feminine dress and play with feminine dolls. They avoid rough and tough games and often express the desire to be a girl. Girls with this disorder refuse to be dressed in feminine attire. They cut their hair short. They identify with super heroes such as Phantom or Spiderman. They are not interested in dolls and want to be in big sports. Cross-gender behavior in girls is better tolerated than in boys. That may be the reason why more boys with gender disorder come to clinics than girls. Parents do not mind when girls behave like boys, while they are concerned about the femininity in their sons. The most common outcome of boys with gender identity disorder is homosexuality during adulthood.

Transsexualism

Transsexuals are adults with gender identity disorder who desire to change their sex. Modern surgical advances have made this goal partially feasible although expensive. **Transsexualism** is a very rare disorder. Studies in Europe suggest that approximately 1 per 30,000 adult males and 1 per 100,000 adult females seek sex reassignment surgery. Some researchers think that transsexualism is the adult version of childhood gender identity disorder and indeed it is often the case. But most children with gender identity disorder do not become transsexuals. Most female-to-male transsexuals are sexually attracted to women. There are two types of male-to-female transsexuals: homosexual and autogynephilic transsexuals. Homosexual transsexual men are generally very feminine and are sexually attracted to biological males. Autogynephilic (heterosexual) transsexuals may report sexual attraction to women, to both men and women or to neither.

Sexual Abuse

Sexual abuse refers to sexual contact involving psychological or physiological coercion with at least one individual who cannot reasonably consent to the contact (for example a child). In these instances, the sexual target is unwilling, uninformed, vulnerable, or too young to give consent. Among the clearest examples of such sexual abuses are pedophilia, rape and incest. Some cases of child abuse (pedophilia) and rape are examples of paraphilias; others are examples of sexual gratification through aggression or in the case of child abuse, desire for an easily obtainable and easily coerced sexual partner. These three are social problems and society views the perpetrators as sex offenders and they are subject to a variety of treatments, including imprisonment. Research on sexual abuse has moved in two directions, one dealing with the effects of these acts on the victims, and the other with the characteristics of the perpetrators and the settings in which these acts occur.

Child Sexual Abuse: We have already mentioned about pedophiles who engage in child sexual abuse. But not all child sexual abusers are pedophiles. Pedophiles have a special attraction toward children, but there are other sexual abusers who seek sexual gratification from children because they are easily available. Unlike pedophiles, these people are not drawn exclusively to children as sexual objects; they may be attracted to a variety of other sexual targets available to them. It is reported that in the United States 100,000 to 500,000 children suffer from sexual abuse. Probably many more are abused, but these are not reported because of fear of retaliation or embarrassment. When these acts are carried out by a family member, definitely they are not reported. In the majority of reported cases, children are abused by people they knew. Children in foster and adoptive families appear to be the ones that are mostly abused. Sexual abuse in childhood may produce several problems such as depression and low self-esteem during adulthood. Adults who suffered sexual abuse during childhood may avoid sex altogether or engage in promiscuity or prostitution.

Rape: One of the most under-reported sexual crimes in modern society is rape, the forced sexual intercourse with a non-consenting partner. Only about 15 to 20 percent of such cases are reported, probably because of the emotional trauma experienced by the victim. While both male and female rapes occur, it is the women who are the victims in the majority of cases. Many cases of male rape—by other males—have been reported in prisons. Rapes are classified into three categories:

1. Power rape.
2. Anger rape.
3. Aadistic rape.

In ***power rape***, the victim is intimidated and threatened by (a person) who generally feels inadequate and awkward in interpersonal relationships. In ***anger rape***, the person seems to be taking revenge on women in general and ventilating his rage through physical and verbal abuse; he seems to be not very much interested in sexual pleasure as such. In ***sadistic rape***, sexuality and aggression are combined and the focus is on the suffering of the victim. It is believed that in rape there is more aggression than sex. Across history, rape is traditionally most frequent during and following wars. This may be because the perpetrators perceive that they will not be punished or look at it as a way of expressing their antagonism and contempt toward the enemy.

Most rapes are planned and committed by people in the neighborhood and not by strangers. About a third or more of all rapes involve more than one offender (gang rape). The after effects of rape on the victim are highly damaging both physically and psychologically. The psychological trauma in women is more severe leading to a condition called ***rape trauma syndrome***, which is being recognized as a post-traumatic stress disorder. The condition is associated with severe sex problems. The other unfortunate factors in rape are the possibility of pregnancy or contracting sexually transmitted disease. A rape may have a negative impact on the victim's marriage prospects or other intimate relationships. Rape is a bullying, intrusive violation of another person's integrity, selfhood and personal boundaries. Rape deserves to be viewed with more gravity than often been the case. The victim has to be viewed with more compassion and sensitivity.

Rape is usually a young man's crime committed by people who are around 25 years old. About 30 to 50 percent are married. As a group, they come from lower socioeconomic strata and commonly have a prior criminal record. They are likely to have experienced sexual abuse, a violent home environment, and inconsistent caregiving in childhood. There is evidence that some rapists are afflicted by paraphilias such as exhibitionism or voyeurism. In terms of personality, rapists are characterized by impulsivity, short temper, lack of interpersonal sensitivity and intimate relationships. Many of them show some deficits in social communication skills as well as in their ability to understand a woman's feelings and intentions. They lack conversation skill that is necessary for developing relationship with women. They cannot decode women's negative cues during social interaction and interpret friendly behavior as sexually provocative.

Incest: A culturally prohibited sexual relationship between family members, such as brother and sister, or a parent and child, is called incest. Incest is a universal taboo among human societies. Even animals tend to avoid mating between close relatives. Incest produces children with mental and physical problems because of shared genes. Among humans, incest avoidance appears to stem from lack of interest in people to whom they are continuously exposed from an early age. Because incest is rarely reported, its prevalence cannot be ascertained accurately. Brother-sister incest appears to be more common than other varieties. Father-daughter incest is also reported, although infrequently. Girls living with stepfathers are at higher risk for incest because they are not blood relatives. Frequently, incest offenders do not stop with one victim in a family. Some incestuous fathers involve all of their daughters serially as they mature. Mother-son incest is relatively rare. Incestuous child molesters tend to have some pedophilic arousal patterns.

Childhood Psychological Disorders

Psychological disorders can occur at any time in life including childhood. The number of children afflicted by psychological disturbances is considerable. One review of 49 studies involving over 240,000 children across many countries found the average prevalence rate to be 12.3 percent. In most studies, maladjustment was found to be more prevalent among boys than girl (a ratio of 1.7 boys to 1 girl). It is reported that boys suffer mostly from emotional disorders and girls from eating disorders. Although children may suffer from any type of psychological disorder including schizophrenia and depression, DSM-IV-TR mentions some specific disorders, such as attention-deficit/hyperactivity disorder (ADHD), autism, separation anxiety disorders, oppositional defiant disorder, feeding, eating, elimination disorders, learning, reading and communication disorders. Three among these disorders are mentioned below.

Attention-deficit Hyperactivity Disorder

Attention-deficit hyperactivity disorder (ADHD) is the most often mentioned of the childhood disorders, which is characterized by difficulties that interfere with task-oriented behavior in children. The most important features are impulsivity, inattention and exaggerated motor activity. Hyperactive children are highly distractible and fail to follow directions. They exhibit restlessness and often are found to be low in intelligence. They talk incessantly, are socially intrusive and appear immature; they do not get along with their parents because of their disobedience, and are viewed negatively by their peers. Their performance in school is poor and they often exhibit learning and reading difficulties. They pose problems to their teachers in classrooms. ADHD occurs most frequently among preadolescent boys, and is 6 to 9 times more prevalent among boys than girls. It occurs most frequently before the age of 8 years and tends to become less frequent thereafter. Often, the residues of ADHD are seen among 50 to 80 percent of adolescents and 30 to 50 percent of adults. Adults with ADHD have adjustment problems at home, work and in interpersonal relationships. It may occur along with other childhood disorders such as oppositional defiant disorder. The disorder is thought to occur in about 3 to 5 percent of school-going children. Although several researchers implicate environmental, psychological and genetic factors, the exact causes of ADHD remain unclear. One study suggests that family pathology (especially personality disorders in parents) contributes to the development of ADHD, but in many cases the results are inconclusive.

Autism

Autism is one of the most baffling and pervasive of the childhood disorders, first reported by the American child psychiatrist, Leo Kanner (1943) and for that reason it is called Kanner disease (it is also called infantile autism). It is a developmental disorder involving a wide range of problems, such as deficits in language, perceptual and motor development. Autism is noticed during early childhood (before 3 years). Autistic children exhibit lack of empathy, inattention to others and the inability to imitate. They do not show any need for affection or contact with anyone and may not even recognize their parents. They are believed to have "social deficit." There is marked impairment in cognitive abilities. Many of the autistic children form strong attachments with unusual objects such as rocks, keys, electric switches and film negatives. When attempts are made to separate them from these objects, they become disturbed and may show violent temper tantrums. Mostly, they are emotionally flat and are thought to have mind blindness. Autistic disorders afflict thousands of children all over the world, from all socioeconomic levels, and its incidence is believed to be increasing. The precise causes of autism are not known. They are supposed to be born with defective cognitive-perceptual functioning. The concordance rate observed in twin studies is high (80 to 90 percent). Therefore, several researchers believe that autism is a heritable form of psychopathology. But nothing is known about the exact nature of genetic transmission.

Oppositional Defiant Disorder and Conduct Disorder

The essential feature of **oppositional defiant disorder** is a recurrent pattern of negativistic, defiant, disobedient and hostile behavior shown by children toward authority figures. It is believed to be an important precursor for the antisocial behavior seen in children who develop conduct disorder. Oppositional disorder begins by the age of 8, whereas conduct disorders typically emerge during middle childhood through adolescence. The important symptoms of **conduct disorder** are persistent, repetitive violation of social rules and disregard for the rights of others. Children with conduct disorder exhibit overt or covert hostility, disobedience, both physical and verbal, aggressiveness, quarrelsomeness, vengefulness, cruelty toward animals, and destructiveness. They engage in stealing and lying, are sexually uninhibited and may show sexual aggression. They often stay out at night despite parental prohibitions.

There is impairment in social, academic and occupational functioning. Temper tantrums, bullying, vandalism, robbery and homicidal acts are common. Conduct disorders often comorbid with substance abuse disorders. Children with conduct disorders are prone to develop antisocial personality disorder later in life. The link between conduct disorder and antisocial personality is stronger among children belonging to lower socioeconomic class. Severe problems of conduct can lead to other psychological problems such as depression. A genetic predisposition is believed to cause low verbal intelligence, mild neuropsychological problems and bad temperament, all of which set the stage for early development of conduct disorder. Ineffective parenting, parental neglect or rejections, harsh and inconsistent discipline at home are other causative factors in the genesis of conduct disorders.

The other common psychological disorders of childhood are ***enuresis*** (bedwetting), ***encopresis*** (lack of proper bowel control), ***somnambulism*** (sleep walking), ***tics*** (intermittent and persistent muscle movements), ***mental retardation*** (lack of intellectual abilities), ***learning disabilities***, anxiety and depression. (These are interesting problems. Interested students should consult a standard textbook on abnormal psychology and familiarize with these problems).

PREVALENCE OF PSYCHOLOGICAL DISORDERS

Do not be surprised! The number of people suffering from psychological disturbances is huge. At least, it is so all over the world. It is estimated that every second person you meet on the road in the USA is likely to suffer from some psychological disturbance at some point of time in his/her life. In a massive study of the prevalence of psychological disorders in the USA, 8,000 men and women between the ages 15 to 54 years were interviewed. According to the results of the study, 48 percent of the people interviewed had experienced a psychological disorder at some point of time during their lives (Kessler et al, 1994). The common problem was depression (17%), followed by alcohol dependence disorder (14%). The others were drug dependence and panic disorders. Another study indicated that the number of people who experienced psychological disorders increased from 19 percent in 1957 to 26 percent in the mid 1990s (Swindle et al, 2000). These figures apply to the US. The results in other cultures may differ significantly. It is estimated that the probability of people suffering from at least one episode of depression is only 1.5 percent in Taiwan, 2.9 percent in Korea, 11.6 percent in New Zealand, and 16.4 percent in France (Weissman et al, 1996). The figures clearly indicate the impact of sociocultural factors in the genesis of psychological disorders.

ARE PEOPLE WITH PSYCHOLOGICAL DISORDERS DANGEROUS?

There is a popular misconception that people suffering from psychological disorders are dangerous and are more prone to engage in violence. The violence committed by mental patients is often exaggerated in the media. Fiction, films, TV and newspapers depict such people as dangerous. In fact, the way people in mental health institutions are depicted in films is far from the truth. A study of TV portrayal of mentally ill characters revealed that 73 percent of them committed violence compared with 40 percent of normal characters. Part of the stigma attached to psychological disorders is the popular belief that such people are prone to commit violent acts. Of course, people suffering from antisocial personality are prone to violence. Paranoid and catatonic schizophrenics, who have stopped medication, may also engage in violent acts. But people with anxiety disorders and depression are no more dangerous than average people. In fact, severely depressed people are more dangerous to themselves than to others. Severe disorders, such as schizophrenia are more prevalent among lower socioeconomic groups, where violence is also more common. Also, such severe illnesses are very rare. Therefore, it should be remembered that the danger from mental patients is not as much as it has been portrayed.

SOME CAUTIONARY NOTES ON PSYCHOLOGICAL DISORDERS

We have learnt in this chapter symptoms of some of the psychological disorders that people generally suffer from. When you peruse the range and variety of these symptoms, it would not be surprising if you start thinking whether you are also suffering from one or the other of these problems. This is a common perception among both medical and psychology/psychiatry students—a feeling that you suffer from the symptoms you are studying among your patients. A beginning medical student, after examining a patient, may begin to imagine that he also has some of the symptoms the patient is having. This is often called the "medical student's disease." Similarly, there is also the "psychology student's disease."

We face severe problems in life at various points—excessive stress, emotional upheaval, conflicts and frustrations. Under such circumstances, we may react in ways that bear some resemblance to the symptoms of disorders discussed in this chapter. But it does not mean that it we are suffering from these problems at a clinically significant level to be considered as psychological disorders. In addition to the three D's (***distress***, ***dysfunction***, and ***deviance***), associated with abnormal behavior, the frequency with which the behavior occurs, its intensity and persistence are to be taken into consideration in deciding whether the behavior is indicative of severe maladjustment. We have seen how difficult it is to differentiate normal and abnormal behavior. A statement made by Thomas Szasz is pertinent in this context. He says that "***When we talk to God, we are praying, but when God talks to us we are schizophrenic!***" Therefore, do not be tempted to use the knowledge you acquired in this chapter to diagnose your friends, family members or yourself. The ability to diagnose psychological disorders accurately requires detailed knowledge and extensive training. However, when psychological problems interfere with your happiness or personal effectiveness, you should not hesitate to seek the help of a mental health professional. It is unfortunate that significant prejudice and discrimination are directed toward people with psychological disorders. When you are physically sick, you do not hesitate to go to a doctor. Then, why hesitate to consult a mental health professional when you are mentally disturbed? Mental illness is like any other illness; it can be cured when proper treatment is given. (Information about the mental health professionals and the treatments available for psychological disorders is discussed in the next chapter).

Chapter Summary

Distinguishing abnormality from normality is not easy. Several criteria have been suggested to define abnormality. Ultimately abnormality turns out to be a social judgment. However, the following factors may be kept in mind in calling a behavior abnormal:

1. The behavior must be distressing to the person and/or to the people around him/her.
2. The behavior must be unusual, dysfunctional, maladaptive and self-defeating and/or.
3. The behavior must be socially deviant and uncomfortable to others and it must not be caused by environmental factors.

Contd...

Contd...

These criteria may not be enough to capture the concept of abnormality; most conceptualizations rely on multiple criteria—statistical, emotional, sociocultural and dysfunctional.

One of the major attempts to classify psychological disorders has been made by the American Psychiatric Association through a publication known as the *Diagnostic and Statistical Manual of Mental Disorders (DSM)*, which is now in its fourth edition (DSM-IV-TR). Diagnosing, in spite of its scientific utility, has important personal, social and legal consequences for the people who are being diagnosed. Once a diagnostic label has been attached to a person, the person may have to suffer several disadvantages such as in getting a job, being socially accepted, getting a spouse, etc. Legally, the person may be denied certain civil rights. Diagnostic labels may worsen a psychological disorder or a label may actually increase the likelihood that a person will act in an abnormal way. Some thinkers like Thomas Szasz assert that there is nothing like a 'mental disorder,' and there are only 'problems of living.' According to Szasz, 'mental illness is a myth;' it is a poor analogy to physical illness. Szasz is often referred to as a leader of antipsychiatry movement. Despite the drawbacks of labeling, DSM-IV has had an important influence on how professionals approach psychological disorders and it provides a logical way of describing abnormal behavior under several heads.

The most prevalent of the psychological disturbances are the anxiety disorders. These are marked by excessive physiological arousal, psychological fear and worry that may disrupt normal functioning. Anxiety disorders include phobic disorders (irrational fear of a specific object or event), generalized anxiety disorders (free-floating anxiety), panic disorder (recurrent episodes of extreme fear), obsessive-compulsive disorder (persistent and uncontrollable thoughts or compelling need to perform repetitive acts) and post-traumatic stress disorder (severe anxiety associated with some traumatic event). Anxiety disorders may be caused by biological (genetic, biochemical), psychological (unconscious conflicts, cognitive distortions) and sociocultural factors.

Somatoform disorders involve bodily complaints that have no biological basis. These include hypochondriasis, somatization disorders, pain disorders, conversion disorders and body dysmorphic disorders. People suffering from hypochondriasis are unduly worried with the idea that they are suffering from a serious illness, which may actually be a result of misinterpretation of normal bodily functions. Somatization disorders are long-lasting preoccupations with body symptoms that have no identifiable physical cause. Those suffering from pain disorders experience intense pain that is disproportionate to whatever medical condition they have or for which there is no physical basis. In conversion disorders, people suffer from physical problems, such as blindness or paralysis that have no identifiable basis. It is said that the underlying anxiety expresses (converts) itself as a physical symptom. People with body dysmorphic disorder imagine that they have some flaw in one or the other part of the body or in their appearance. Somatoform disorders are considered as one of the ways of dealing with anxiety. While in anxiety disorders anxiety is manifest, in somatoform disorders the presence of anxiety is inferred.

Another group of disorders that may also be regarded as ways of avoiding anxiety are dissociative disorders in which there is breakdown of personality integration, resulting in significant alterations in memory and personal identity. Major dissociative disorders include dissociative amnesia, dissociative fugue and dissociative identity disorder (DID). Dissociative amnesia is characterized by an inability to remember one or more important personal informational details. The person, for example, may forget his/her personal identity or family history. The memory loss may last for a few hours or even years. In dissociative fugue the individual forgets his identity and runs away from home and lives in some other place with a different identity. Sometime later, he/she wakes up and returns to the first residence. In dissociative identity disorder, which was earlier called multiple personality disorder, an individual may alternate between two or more distinct identities or personalities. The incidence of DID is rare and some even doubt the very existence of such states. Somatoform disorder runs in families, but it is unclear whether it is due to genetic factors or product of social learning.

Mood disorders are characterized by prolonged, disabling emotional disruptions such as depression or excessive excitement (mania). Depressive disorders exhibit a variety of symptoms that include cognitive, emotional, motivational and somatic components. In a manic state, there are psychomotor overactivity, a sense of euphoria, and flight of thought. A major depressive episode is characterized by an intense depressed mood that leaves the person unable to function effectively. In bipolar disorders, depression alternates with periods of mania. Both genetic and neurochemical factors may be involved in the causation of both depression and bipolar disorders. One theory links neurotransmitters such as norepinephrine, dopamine and serotonin to depression.

Schizophrenia is the name given to a group of severe psychotic conditions characterized by disorders of thought and speech, poor contact with reality, inappropriate emotional expressions, cognitive impairments such as delusions and hallucinations. There are several subtypes of schizophrenia including paranoid, catatonic, disorganized and undifferentiated schizophrenia.

Contd...

Contd...

Sufficient evidence is available to suggest that there is a genetic basis for schizophrenia. Studies of identical twins reveal that the concordance rate is more than 60 percent. One theory states that schizophrenia is caused by overactivity of dopamine. The prevalence of schizophrenia is the same across cultures. Despite the enormous amount of research on schizophrenia, not much is known about the cause, course and cure of schizophrenia. Large proportions of inmates in psychiatric hospitals all over the world are chronic schizophrenics indicating the seriousness of the problem.

Personality disorders show stable, maladaptive way of thinking, feeling and behaving, which impair social relations and normal living. People with personality disorders adopt inappropriate coping strategies when they encounter problems of life and their emotional controls break down. The DSM-IV-TR describes ten personality disorders under three clusters. Anyone suffering from personality disorder has an increased likelihood of developing disorders described in Axis I of DSM. The presence of personality disorders along with major Axis I disorders makes the recovery from the latter difficult.

Apart from the major psychological disorders, there are a number of other impairments that create problems to the people who suffer from them and others around them. Included among them are eating disorders, addictive disorders, sexual disorders and childhood disorders. Among eating disorders, anorexia nervosa is characterized by intense fear of gaining weight coupled with refusal to eat the necessary food. Bulimia nervosa is marked by heavy eating and purging the food because of the fear of gaining weight. Addictive disorders such as alcohol or drug abuse are the most widespread and intransigent psychological problems facing contemporary society. Alcohol abuse produces alcohol myopia, changes in brain structure, fetal alcohol syndrome (in children of alcoholic mothers) and increased number of automobile accidents. Several psychotic states such as withdrawal, delirium, chronic alcoholic hallucinosis and dementia are associated with alcoholism. Drug abuse disorders may involve physiological dependence on substances such as opiates or barbiturates, as well as psychological dependence on substances like marijuana. Biological, psychological and sociocultural factors are all implicated in making a person an addict.

It is difficult to draw a line between normal and deviant sexual behavior. The distinction depends on the person, place, time and society. However, certain forms of psychological problems associated with sex are identified. These include sexual dysfunctions, paraphilias, sexual identity disorder and sexual abuse. Sexual dysfunction involves impairment either in the desire for sexual gratification or in the ability to achieve it. There may be a lack of desire or arousal (erectile disorders), absence of orgasm and pain during intercourse (vaginismus and dyspareunia). Paraphilias involve patterns of persistent sexual gratification obtained through unusual ways. These include fetishism, voyeurism, exhibitionism, sadism, masochism and pedophilia. Sexual abuse includes pedophilia, incest and rape. Gender identity disorder is characterized by strong cross-gender identification and gender dysphoria (discomfort about one's biological sex). The disorder may occur in children or adults, among males or females. Transsexualism is a gender identity disorder in which people try to change their sex through sex-reassignment surgery; it is a rare disorder.

Psychological disorders can occur at any point of time in life. Children are found to suffer from variety of disturbances that may become the precursors of psychological disorders in adulthood. Attention deficit/hyperactivity disorder (ADHD) and autistic disorder originate in childhood and often persist into adulthood. ADHD is one of the more common behavior problems of childhood. In this condition, the children are impulsive, overactive and inattentive to such an extent that the symptoms interfere with normal functioning. Autism is a pervasive developmental disorder beginning in infancy involving a wide range of problematic behaviors including deficits in language, perception, motility and communication. Some children may develop conduct disorders, which are marked by negativistic, defiant, disobedient and hostile behavior.

The prevalence of psychological disorders varies from country to country suggesting the impact of sociocultural factors in their genesis. The differences may be indicative of the tolerant attitude shown toward psychological disorders, non-reporting of their incidence or due to life styles prevalent in certain cultures. The misconception that mental patients are dangerous is gradually disappearing; most of them are not dangerous. All of us are maladjusted to some extent, but that does not mean we need psychiatric treatment.

16 CHAPTER

Treatment of Psychological Disorders

PREVIEW

In this chapter, we discuss the ways of helping people who suffer from psychological disorders. The history of treatment of mental disorders does not make a pleasant reading. Although there were some rare attempts to treat mental illnesses scientifically, throughout the major part of history, society's treatment of these people was characterized by utter neglect and horrific remedies. Mental patients were considered as possessed by demons, and holes were drilled in their skull to drive away the evil spirits. For several years, mental patients were thought of as dangerous and were imprisoned, tied or chained to poles. Sometimes, they were branded as witches and tortured or burnt at stakes. The belief that mental patients are possessed by demons still persists in some societies. Even today, mental patients are being treated in monasteries and temples using exorcism (symbolic acts performed to drive away the evil spirits).The humane treatment of these unfortunate people started toward the end of the 18th century when Philippe Pinel, a medical director of the psychiatric ward at La Bicêtre in Paris, unchained the mental patients in 1793. Later, the humanitarian trend spread to other parts of the world. Today, fortunately a scientific view of psychological disorders is developing and people suffering from emotional and behavioral problems are treated compassionately with science-based techniques.

Today, various forms of treatment are available to persons who are suffering from psychological disturbances. Despite diversity, contemporary approaches to treatment fall into two main categories: psychological and biological therapies. Psychological approaches therapies are called psychotherapies. Psychotherapy is a form of treatment offered by a trained professional whose aim is to help people overcome psychological problems, resolve conflicts and bring about personal growth. There are different forms of psychotherapy that are derived from different theoretical perspectives to psychological disorders. There are psychodynamic, behavioristic, cognitive and humanistic therapies. It has been estimated that hundreds of therapeutic procedures, ranging from Freudian psychoanalysis to Zen meditation, exist today. Although diverse in many respects, the goal of psychotherapies is to bring about a change in behavioral patterns of people and help them in dealing with problems of living. This goal is achieved through discussions and interaction between the therapist and the client (psychotherapists call the psychologically disturbed persons "clients", not patients).

Biomedical therapies rely on drugs and other physical-chemical and surgical procedures. Biomedical therapies are administered by psychiatrists, who are medical persons trained in the treatment of psychological disorders. Today, it is recognized that mental disorders may have their origins in the body, mind and/or the environment. The type of treatment offered depends on what one considers is the cause. Psychiatrists, who are medical men, treat the body. They use drugs to bring about changes in the central nervous system. Drug treatment gives immediate relief to patients, but there may be a number of side effects.

Among psychologists, especially clinical psychologists and counseling psychologists, insight therapists (psychodynamic, cognitive and humanistic psychologists) attempt to treat the mind (mental functioning) and behaviorists try to change the environment. In fact, today the trend is to combine the good features of all approaches and follow an eclectic approach. This chapter does not attempt to make you therapists. But an understanding of the dynamics of therapy, both psychological and biological, will go a long way in helping you to appreciate the psychological problems of people and how they are being handled by specialists.

Chapter Outline

Psychological disorders have been in existence ever since humans were born on earth and there have been concerted attempts to identify the causes and cures for these afflictions. Religious leaders such as Moses, Mohammad and Buddha, and philosophers such as Lao Tzu, Socrates, Plato and Aristotle have all tried to heal human mental suffering through educational and spiritual procedures. There have been pragmatic practitioners such as Hippocrates who offered many insights into the functioning of the human mind, the insights we take for granted today. Hippocrates (460–377 BC) believed that mental illnesses are diseases just like physical diseases and suggested that mental illnesses are caused by disturbances in the brain. He attempted a classification of mental illnesses and personality disorders. Unfortunately, there were not many improvements on Hippocrates' ideas until the last two centuries. During the medieval period, the preferred form of treatment for emotional disturbances was burning of patients at the stakes. Demonology propagated the view that mentally disturbed people were possessed by demons, and trephining (drilling a hole in the skull to allow the devil to get out) was the popular form of treatment. In other cases, exorcism was used. Exorcism consisted of symbolic acts, such as magic, prayer, incantation, sound-making and the use of holy water or obnoxious concoctions, for casting the evil spirit out of an afflicted person. During the 16th and 17th centuries, more than 100,000 people with psychological disorders were identified as witches and they were hunted down and executed. It is surprising that even today such superstitious rituals are prevalent in some cultures including advanced countries.

It was during 1800s, Western medicine returned to viewing mental ailments as based on physiological factors. The emphasis on the importance of biological factors on the genesis of psychological disorders (the **medical model**) received a fillip with the discovery that **general paresis**, a disorder characterized by psychological deterioration and bizarre behavior, was caused by massive brain pathology due to sexually transmitted disease called syphilis. This was taken as evidence to assume that psychological disorders have a biological base; this discovery is often considered as the ***first mental health revolution***. In the early 1900s, Sigmund Freud proposed the importance of psychological factors in the causation of behavioral disorders, which came to be recognized as the ***second mental health revolution***. In the 20th century, the importance of sociocultural and other environmental factors in the causation of psychological disturbances were recognized, and as a result, community based treatment modalities of these disorders became a new trend. This view called ***community mental health program*** is often referred to as the ***third mental health revolution***. Although several issues remain unanswered, today we are told that biological, psychological and environmental factors interact in causing psychological disorders. Based on the assumptions about the causes of psychological disorders, researchers have developed several approaches to the treatment of these disorders. Contemporary approaches to treatment fall into two broad categories: psychological therapies and or biomedical therapies. Psychological therapy (or **psychotherapy**) is a form of treatment in which several psychological techniques are used to help people recover from behavior pathologies. Psychotherapy is offered by a trained professional, called a ***psychotherapist***, whose goal is to bring about a positive personality change and growth in the patient. The biomedical approaches rely on drugs and other medical procedures to treat psychological disorders and to improve psychological functioning. Generally, **psychiatrists** (medical men trained in the treatment of psychological disorders) administer drugs and employ other medical procedures in the treatment of mental disorders. In this chapter, we briefly examine some of the major forms of treatment used by psychotherapists and psychiatrists, how the treatment works and what research says about the effectiveness of the treatment procedures.

PSYCHOLOGICAL APPROACHES TO TREATMENT

It is estimated that there are some 400 different types of psychotherapies. Although there are differences in these approaches, all of them aim at solving problems of living, changing maladaptive thoughts, feelings, behavior patterns, and helping people gain a better understanding of themselves, their past, present and future. In short, the goal is to help people live happier and productive lives. In psychotherapy, therapists generally are engaged in three activities: *listening*, *understanding* and *responding*. The therapist listens to the client in order to learn about the client's problems. Listening provides a basis for the therapist to understand the client's self-concept and his/her view of the world. Listening and understanding enable the therapist to respond to the client. The response may be a question to elicit more information or simply a comment. The comment may be an interpretation of what has been going on during the therapy session or in the client's interpersonal relationships. In most of the therapeutic procedures, it has been found that the relationship between the client and the therapist is the prime determinant of therapeutic success. Within the helping relationship, therapists employ a variety of techniques to promote positive changes in the client. These techniques differ widely depending on the therapist's theoretical orientation and training.

A number of professional groups are engaged in providing psychotherapy, the chief among them being clinical psychologists, counseling psychologists and psychiatrists. In addition to these, other professionals who engage in psychological treatment are psychiatric social workers (who work in community agencies), marriage and family counselors (who specialize in problems arising from family relationships), pastoral counselors (who tend to work with spiritual problems) and substance-abuse counselors (who work with substance and sexual abusers). Although there are a number of approaches to psychotherapy, most of these fall into one or the other of the four major categories: psychodynamic, behavioral, humanistic and cognitive therapy. Each of these is based on a characteristic personality theory. A brief summary of each of these is given below.

Psychodynamic Therapy

Psychodynamic therapy is a form of treatment that focuses on the client's individual personality dynamics. It has its root in the classical psychoanalytic theories developed by Sigmund Freud. He was a genius. Single-handedly, he propounded a theory of personality and a theory of psychotherapy that have had tremendous influence on psychology. Freud's theories have been modified by some of his followers and others who deviated from his theories. Still, psychoanalytic principles are at the core of all psychodynamic approaches. The main focus of all psychodynamic therapies is on the individual's internal conflicts and unconscious dynamics that are believed to underlie psychological disorders. Since it is the first and the most famous form of psychological treatment, let us examine the fundamental tenets of psychoanalysis in some detail.

Psychoanalysis is the oldest form of psychological treatment. The aim of psychoanalysis is to unearth the unconscious conflicts, fears, thoughts and repressed memories (most of which have their origin in childhood experiences) and bring them into the client's awareness. When this is done, the psychic energy used by the people to keep the unconscious conflicts under control will be available to them to lead a more productive conscious life. According to Freud, most of the psychological problems emerge because of the conflicts between the three components of personality, the id, the ego and the superego. The id strives for the immediate gratifications of biological urges (mostly sex and aggression). The superego imposes severe moral restrictions on the satisfaction of these instinctual desires. The ego tries to balance the demands of these two warring components and the external reality. Most of these processes occur at an unconscious level. When the ego fails to satisfy the harsh masters, its integrity is threatened. Then, the ego tries to develop certain defense mechanisms as temporary measures to retain personal integrity. When these processes also fail, ego breakdown occurs resulting in psychopathology. The goal of psychoanalytic therapy, therefore, is to make the person understand the origin of these unconscious conflicts. When an individual realizes the source of his problems, that is, when he gets "insight," Freud believed that the individual can change his maladaptive behavior patterns and thus the symptoms generally disappear. Because of its emphasis on gaining insight, psychoanalysis is often referred to as an "insight-oriented therapy."

To achieve this goal, Freud used the method of **free association**, in which the person is asked to talk aloud, freely, without any inhibition whatever comes to mind, regardless of its apparent irrelevance. During the therapy session, the client lies on a couch (the well-known 'Freudian Couch') and the analyst sits out of the client's line of sight in order to avoid distracting the client from the process of free association. This way, Freud thought he could reach the unconscious world of repressed memories, desires and conflicts that are at the root of abnormality. Freud believed that most of the conflicts stem from early psychosexual development. In order to unearth the unconscious conflicts, Freud also used **dream analysis** because he thought of dream as "the royal road to unconscious." The client was asked to free associate to each element of the dream. Based on the associations, the meaning of dreams was determined. Freud believed that the contents of the unconscious can be found in the client's stream of thoughts, memories, images and feelings expressed during free association.

Often, free association did not directly lead to unconscious material. During analysis, Freud encountered certain hurdles; for example, after a few sessions, the patients were found to stop talking freely and refuse to discuss certain memories, thoughts, fears and feelings. This behavior was called **resistance**, and it might be expressed in several ways such as a sudden change of subject matter, forgetting what was being discussed, stop coming to therapy and so on. It was an unwillingness or inability to talk about repressed memories, thoughts and experiences. Freud considered resistance as an important event in therapy. It was the sign that anxiety-arousing materials were being approached. An important task of analysis was to explain to the client the reasons for resistance, which would both promote insight and guard against further resistance—the stopping of coming to therapy.

As the therapy progressed, the patients started developing intense affectionate relationship with the therapist. The client takes the therapist as a blank screen to project his/her important perceptions and emotions. Suddenly the therapist becomes an important person, the loved one or even the hated one to the client. This behavior called **transference** was another highly significant event during therapy. Transference is a form of displacement of affect, once shown toward significant persons (father, mother or some other) by the client, toward the therapist. Transference might be positive or negative. In positive transference, the client develops an intense liking (even love) for the therapist and in the negative transference, hatred. If the therapist starts reciprocating these emotions, it was called **countertransference**. It was essential that the therapist guard against countertransference for the success of therapy. For this reason, Freud insisted that all therapists themselves be analyzed before engaging in therapeutic practice. Freud called these irrational events during therapy, *transference neurosis*. An important and final step in therapy was the **interpretation** of the meaning of resistance, transference and dreams to the client. The aim of interpretation was providing insight into the client's behavior. The interpretative statements help the clients to admit into their consciousness, materials that they have avoided all along. Interpretation is a highly rated skill. It is a general rule that interpretation must start with contents that are near the surface, the ones the client can digest. Interpretations of deep contents should be held back even if they are correct until an appropriate time. This is one reason why psychoanalytic therapy takes a long time.

Freud's therapeutic procedure declined in its popularity over time for a number of reasons. For one thing, it was lengthy and costly. Therapy was held four to five times a week, over several months and even years in certain cases. It is reported that the patients attend, on the average 835 sessions before completing psychoanalysis. Thus, it becomes very expensive and time consuming and not all people can afford this form of treatment. The most important reason is that it is not effective with all people, and with all psychological disorders. It is found that psychoanalysis is useful with people who are "young, adaptable, verbal, intelligent and successful (YAVIS)."

Because of the limitations, alternative procedures with certain modifications to classical psychoanalysis were developed and these are called psychodynamic therapies. **Psychodynamic therapy** tends to be shorter, usually taking not more than 3 to 4 months or about 20 sessions. The therapist takes a more active part than what Freud did in controlling the course of therapy through advice and direction. The therapist and the client sit facing each other and discuss the problems confronting the client. Instead of free association, there is direct conversation between the therapist and the client. There is less emphasis on childhood experience, sex and aggression. The goal is the same, to bring unconscious wishes and conflicts into awareness. Doing so leads to the development of intellectual and emotional insights, which are supposed to give the client more control over his/her unfulfilled, repressed, unconscious impulses. With this control, the client can now act on consciously chosen desires rather than acting under unconscious forces. However, both psychoanalysis and psychodynamic therapies try to relate the present problems of the client with his/her past experiences, and both consider the client's relationship with the therapist an integral part of treatment. The therapist interprets the client's words and behavior in the light of unconscious motivations. Slips of the tongue (Freudian slips) are given their actual unconscious meanings. Through analytic interpretations, the client understands the real meaning of his defense mechanisms. In short, the client becomes reality-oriented instead of being defensive.

Recently, a brief therapy known as **interpersonal therapy (IPT)** has come into existence. IPT arose from American neo-Freudian, Harry Stack Sullivan's theory of interpersonal relations and today, it is a well-researched, manual-based treatment. This form of treatment concentrates on clients current relationships with significant people in their lives and how the relationships affect their mood. The procedure is highly structured and does not take more than 15 to 20 sessions. The goal of therapy is to resolve marital conflicts, adjusting to changed conditions (such as death of loved ones and loss of relationships), identifying and correcting social deficits in social skills that come in the way of developing effective social relationships and improving client's interpersonal communication. The therapist works actively in finding solutions to these problems. He invites the client to review the present problems and compare them with those in the past, reassuring the client that what happened in the past need not be carried into the present. The outcome studies of interpersonal therapy have shown that this form of treatment is effective with several psychological disorders, especially depression. The IPT for depression rests on the assumption that if interpersonal relationships work well, there will be relief from depression. The brevity and its cost effectiveness have made this therapy very popular among contemporary practitioners.

Critics are not happy with psychoanalysis or its modified version, psychodynamic therapy. They question its theoretical basis, maintaining that there is no proof that constructs such as 'unconscious' exist. The overemphasis on infantile sexuality and aggressive impulses in the genesis of psychopathology, the emphasis on the remote past and the neglect of the client's immediate problems and several such themes do not go well with contemporary thought. More importantly, modern critics question the effectiveness of psychodynamic therapy in comparison with contemporary psychotherapeutic techniques. They assert that there are no objective ways of knowing whether the patient has improved except through the patient's or therapist's words. Despite criticisms, brief psychodynamic therapy has been found to be effective in the treatment of depression and bulimia nervosa.

Behavior Therapy

Behavior therapy is based on the assumption that abnormal behavior, like all other behaviors, is learned, and if it is learned, it can be unlearned. People who exhibit maladaptive behavior have either acquired faulty forms of behavior or failed to acquire useful skills necessary for effective living. The dysfunctional behaviors are maintained through some type of reinforcement. Therefore, to modify these maladaptive behavior patterns, they must be unlearned using appropriate techniques based on the principle of learning. Behavior therapists do not look into the past history of the client or his inner mental states. They consider the present abnormal behavior itself as a problem and think of methods of modifying it. Behavior therapists do not believe in the importance of inner conflicts or unconscious dynamics in the causation of behavior disorders. They are not concerned with what has caused the problem. Their goal is changing the maladaptive behavior. Just change the abnormal behavior using appropriate technology, the problem is solved and the illness is cured. The therapeutic techniques are derived from research on classical conditioning, operant conditioning and observational learning. Behavior therapists believe that learning principles can be effectively applied to change the behavior patterns seen in schizophrenia, anxiety disorders and problems of children and adults that seemed resistant to traditional therapies.

Historically it was Joseph Wolpe, a South African psychiatrist, who initiated the work on behavior therapy with the publication of his book *Psychotherapy by reciprocal inhibition* (1958). While Wolpe focused on treatment methods derived from Pavlov's classical conditioning procedure, Skinner developed behavior modification techniques based on operant conditioning. A third type of behavior therapy evolved from Albert Bandura's social learning theory. Whatever the theoretical orientation, the behavior therapist concentrates on the following three aspects called the *ABC of behavior*:

1. The ***antecedents A:*** The stimuli that are eliciting the problem behavior.
2. The problematic ***behavior B.***
3. The ***consequence C:*** factors that are maintaining the problem behavior.

As indicated earlier, the behavior therapist is not interested in the "unconscious" roots of problematic behavior. His interest is in the distressing symptoms, which the client has "learnt" and how to "eliminate" them. The emphasis is on behavior and performance. The therapist takes an active and directive role in eliminating the maladaptive behaviors. He is interested in the results of treatment that can be directly observed and measured. Several techniques of treatment have evolved from the three models of learning—classical conditioning, operant conditioning and social learning.

Techniques Based on Classical Conditioning

Exposure Therapy

The most preferred form of treatment used in the elimination of phobias and other forms of fear is the extinction technique called **exposure therapy**, in which the clients are asked to expose themselves to feared stimulus in a planned and gradual manner. It is a technique based on classical conditioning that rests on the principle of habituation or extinction. People may be exposed to real life events (***in vivo exposure***) or asked to imagine scenes involving the feared stimuli (***imaginal exposure***). The stimuli will, of course, elicit considerable anxiety in the beginning, but the anxiety will extinguish in time if the client remains in the presence of the phobic stimulus and in the absence of original aversive stimulus that was associated with the phobia. Another type of exposure is computer based ***virtual reality exposure*** in which highly realistic virtual environments are created to simulate the original experience. Exposure technique is being used extensively in the treatment of anxiety disorders, especially phobias.

Flooding

Flooding is a form of exposure therapy in which the client encounters anxiety-producing situation for a prolonged time either ***in vivo*** or imaginal form. In flooding, the clients are prevented from engaging in their usual maladaptive responses to anxiety-producing stimuli. Although the client experiences anxiety during the exposure, the feared consequences do not occur. Remaining exposed to a feared stimulus for a prolonged period without engaging in any fear-reducing behaviors allows for anxiety reduction.

Systematic Desensitization

The most popular form of behavior therapy is **systematic desensitization**, which was first used by Mary Cover Jones and later refined by Joseph Wolpe (1958, 1982) as a method of eliminating anxiety and fear. This is also a form of exposure therapy in which the client is exposed gradually to imagined anxiety-producing situations, when the client is in a relaxed state. Wolpe viewed anxiety as a classically conditioned emotional response and asserted that it could be eliminated by a procedure called **counterconditioning**. Counterconditioning involves establishing (by conditioning) a new response that is incompatible with the experience of anxiety such as being relaxed or having a pleasant emotional experience when one is about to experience anxiety. While exposure technique involves extinction and habituation, Wolpe's technique uses a substitute response to counter the anxiety response.

There are three steps in systematic desensitization: The first step is teaching the client the skill of *progressive muscle relaxation* (Box 16.1) using a technique similar to the one developed by Jacobson (1938). The second step is the construction of an anxiety hierarchy, which is an ordered list of situations that lead to fear reactions. The client is asked to imagine a series of anxiety-provoking situations beginning with the least anxiety-producing and ending with the one the client is afraid of (Box 16.2). Finally, the desensitization proper begins after the client has learned the skill of muscle relaxation and the anxiety hierarchy is ready. In the relaxed state, the client is asked to imagine the least anxiety-provoking scene in the hierarchy. If the client experiences anxiety, he is asked to resume the relaxed state. A state of deep relaxation is incompatible with the experience of anxiety; one cannot be afraid and relaxed at the same time. Hence, the client learns to be comfortable with the imagined anxiety-producing scene. In this

Box 16.1: Progressive Muscle Relaxation

Jacobson is credited with developing a progressive relaxation procedure, which has since been modified, refined and used with systematic desensitization, and several other behavior therapy techniques. The relaxation training involves several components that require some 4 to 8 hours of instruction. Generally, the therapist instructs the client how to relax the muscles (often a recorded version of the instructions is used). Clients are instructed to contract and relax alternatively their muscles one by one from head to toe focusing on the pleasantness associated with the state of relaxation. Generally, the arm muscles are relaxed first followed by the head, the neck and shoulders, the back, abdomen, and thorax. The clients are encouraged to experience tension under the condition of contracting the muscles, and to enjoy the pleasant feelings under the state of relaxation. Gradually, the client develops the habit of relaxing and enjoying the pleasantness that comes with relaxation, and experiencing the difference between the two conditions. The relaxation training was used primarily with systematic desensitization till recently. But nowadays it is applied to a variety of clinical problems, either separately or in conjunction with related methods. The most common use has been with problems related to stress and anxiety, which are often observed with psychosomatic symptoms. The technique is also used to bring relief to patients having high blood pressure, cardiovascular complaints, migraine headache, asthma, and insomnia.

Box 16.2: Anxiety Hierarchy and its Use

1. The word dog on paper.
2. Hearing the word dog uttered by somebody.
3. Oneself-uttering the word dog aloud.
4. A picture of a chained dog on paper.
5. A picture of a free dog on paper.
6. A chained live dog with the owner on the road.
7. A free dog with the owner on the road.
8. A free dog with nobody around.
9. A dog in the client's compound.
10. Clint going near the dog.
11. Touching the dog.
12. Hugging and playing with the dog.

Assume that a child with a phobia for dogs is being treated. While using systematic desensitization, the child learns to relax first and then asked to *imagine* the first item at the top of the hierarchy (imagining the word dog written on paper). If he becomes anxious, he is asked to stop imagining that scene and try to enter into a state of relaxation. The same procedure is repeated with the second item. Similarly, he is asked to proceed with other items. Whenever he experiences anxiety, he is asked to stop to engage in relaxation procedure. The procedure is continued in the same way until the child can imagine the final scene in the hierarchy without experiencing anxiety.

way, the therapist moves progressively down the hierarchy. Whenever the client reports experience of anxiety, the scene is terminated and relaxation is induced again. In the same way, the client continues down the hierarchy. The treatment ends when the client is able to remain in a relaxed state, while imagining the scene that was formerly the most anxiety-evoking. The purpose of systematic desensitization is repeated exposure to anxiety-producing situations until the client learns to imagine the situation without experiencing any anxiety.

Systematic desensitization is the widely used treatment procedure all over the world. Wolpe treated 100 phobic patients successfully using this procedure. In many controlled studies, the success rate has been found to be 80 percent or more in the treatment of several types of phobic disorders (Rachman, 1998; Spiegler and Guevremont, 2003).

Aversion Therapy

A time-tested treatment based on classical conditioning is **aversion therapy**, which involves creating unpleasant reactions to stimuli that an individual previously enjoyed. The procedure is simple and is used in the treatment of pedophilia, alcoholism, drug abuse and smoking. For example, a person who habitually consumes alcohol is injected a drug (Antabuse) that causes severe nausea and vomiting. When the two are paired a number of times, the alcohol becomes associated with the vomiting and the individual starts disliking alcohol. Highly impressive results are reported in treating alcoholics using aversion therapy (Wiens and Menustik, 1983). Sometimes an electric shock may be used when one is engaged in an undesirable behavior (pedophilia). Although aversion therapy works reasonably well to inhibit several bad habits, its long-term effectiveness is questionable. For instance, a recovering alcoholic or a drug addict, who watches friends consuming alcohol or drug in a party, is likely to have difficulty in resisting the temptation.

Techniques Based on Operant Conditioning

Behavior therapists, who make use of the principles of operant conditioning, call their technique **behavior modification**. These procedures may make use of positive reinforcement, negative reinforcement, positive punishment or negative punishment. The focus of the therapist here is observable behavior that is targeted for change. Behavior changes are objectively measured and suitable modification in the technique is made if the change is not taking place in the desired direction. Behavior modification is used in the treatment of patients such as of hospitalized schizophrenics, mentally challenges individuals and profoundly disturbed children, where other forms of therapy were ineffective. For example, a procedure called **token economy** is used in the treatment of chronic schizophrenic patients who have deteriorated due to an extended stay in psychiatric hospitals. These patients receive plastic tokens for the performance of desirable behaviors such as personal grooming, housekeeping, completing assigned jobs, helping other patients, participating in vocational training and exhibiting appropriate social responses. These tokens can be exchanged for a wide range of tangible reinforcers such as a dinner, some recreational activities (watching a TV or a movie), having a private room with good furniture, spend time talking to a friend and walking freely around the hospital. Using this technique, researchers have found a remarkable increase in adaptive behavior among the clients (Ayllon and Azrin, 1968). Token economy has been used extensively in schools, prisons, business organizations and homes to increase desirable behavior. Operant reinforcement techniques are found to be used in teaching social skills. In rare cases, punishment is used to eliminate undesirable behavior among children, of course, with the permission of their parents. Generally, punishment is avoided because of its side effects.

Techniques Based on Social Learning

Social learning or modeling is an effective procedure used in behavior therapy, especially to treat children having problem behaviors and persons with phobias. Clients observe people (models) interacting with the feared stimuli in a relaxed state and learn to imitate the same. Modeling is extensively used in teaching social skills to people who lack them. In ***social skills training,*** the clients learn new skills by observing and then imitating a model that performs a socially skilled behavior. It is often used in conjunction with other forms of treatments to jump-start new adaptive behaviors that can then be strengthened by natural reinforcers in the client's everyday environment. Social skills training has been used with many groups including delinquents, hospitalized patients and individuals who have minor deficits in social skills. Observing successful models also increases self-efficacy by encouraging the thought "if he can do that, so can I." Increased self-efficacy makes social skill training easy. There are various types of modeling. Live modeling involves direct observation of the model. In participant modeling, the client practices a behavior by interacting with the model. Symbolic modeling refers to the observation of a model that is shown in a film. An extension of symbolic modeling is covert modeling, in which the individual is asked to imagine that he is observing a model.

Humanistic Approaches to Treatment

Humanistic therapists view psychological disturbances as the direct result of contemporary social environment that impedes positive personality development. We live in a society dominated by self-interest, industrialization, mechanization, computerization and mass deception. We experience alienation, loneliness, depersonalization, dehumanization and fail to find meaning in life. Problems like these cannot be solved by the analysis of unconscious forces or behavior manipulation. Humanistic therapists aver that these types of problems need altogether different approaches. They emphasize the clients' self-responsibility in developing their own personality. They believe that clients have control over their behavior, freedom to choose the kind of life they would like to lead, can take responsibility for their choices and behaviors and can solve their problems by themselves under suitable therapeutic conditions. They view therapy as a meeting between equals. The therapist's goal is to create an environment in which clients can engage in self-exploration to remove the barriers that block their personal growth. You have seen how humanistic psychology is referred to as the "third force" in contrast to two other major forces, psychoanalysis (which looks upon humans as domesticated animals) and behaviorism (which considers humans as machines). Similarly, humanistic therapy can be regarded as a third force in psychotherapy, an alternative to psychodynamic therapy and behavior therapy. There are several humanistic approaches to therapy. The best known and widely used ones are Carl Rogers' client-centered or person-centered therapy and Gestalt therapy developed by Fritz Perls.

Person-centered Therapy

Person-centered therapy was propounded by the American psychologist and psychotherapist Carl Rogers (review the section on Rogers in Chapter 11 on Personality). During the 1940s, Rogers called his procedure *non-directive counseling*; during 1950s he renamed it as **client-centered therapy** and still later during the 1970s and 1980s he called his approach **person-centered therapy**. The changes in nomenclature, in a way, reflect the gradual evolution in Rogers views about human personality and psychotherapy. In the early years, Rogers named his counseling procedure "non-directive" as a reaction against the directive approaches to therapy adopted by psychoanalysts and behavior therapists. He challenged the validity of commonly accepted therapeutic procedures such as advice, suggestion, direction, persuasion, teaching, diagnosis and interpretation. He proposed that clients have an intrinsic capacity to grow, and if a proper therapeutic atmosphere is provided, they can solve their problems. Rogers' emphasis was on the creation of a permissive and non-directive climate during therapy. Therefore, he called his procedure non-directive. Later, he named it client-centered therapy to emphasize the fact that the focus of therapy was the client and not the non-directive methodology. Rogers believed that the best vantage point to understand the client was from his/her internal frame of reference and hence it should be client-centered. Toward the latter part of his life, Rogers extended his counseling to family, education, industry, conflict resolution, and the search for world peace. Now, his focus was on the entire humanity, which is implied in the name person-centered therapy. But many practitioners recognize Rogers' procedure as client-centered therapy only.

For Rogers, psychotherapy is a process of removing obstacles for personal growth. He believed that humans have a natural capacity to grow called ***actualizing tendency***. According to Rogers, many of the human problems arise because of a lack of coherent, unified sense of **self (or self-concept)**. There is a mismatch (**incongruence**) between what a person actually is (his/her ***real self***) and what he/she would like to be (***ideal self***); the individual does not accept all his basic (organismic) experiences as his own. In short, the clients do not accept themselves as they are. The aim of therapy, therefore, is to lessen the incongruence, to help the clients to accept themselves, their inner experiences and to bridge the gap between the real self and the ideal self. To achieve this goal, the therapist creates a psychological atmosphere in which clients feel that they are accepted unconditionally, understood and valued as persons (**unconditional positive regard**). The therapist also makes an empathic reflection of the client's inner world (a reinstatement of the client's description of his problems). Under these conditions of therapeutic warmth, the client begin to feel free to explore their real feelings and thoughts and to explore their assets and liabilities, likes and dislikes, loves and hates, and the ugly and the beautiful parts of themselves. In an atmosphere marked by therapeutic warmth, the clients learn to accept themselves as they are. Their self-concept becomes more congruent with their actual experience, the self-ideal self-discrepancy is reduced, they become more self-accepting and more open to new experiences and new perspectives. In short, the client becomes what Rogers called "**fully functioning person**." Being such a person includes characteristics such as openness to experience, the absence of defensiveness, accurate awareness, ***unconditional self-regard***, and harmonious relations with others.

Person-centered therapists do not ask questions, do not answer queries, nor do they interpret what the clients say. They do not probe the unconscious conflicts. They simply listen attentively and acceptingly what the clients are telling, interrupting only to restate in an empathic manner what the clients are saying. Such non-judgmental, non-interpretative and non-directive reflection of clients' statements by the therapist helps clients to examine and clarify their feelings and thoughts—a process of self-examination leading to restructuring of self-concept. Rogers believed that as clients experience a constructive therapeutic relationship, they exhibit increased self-acceptance, greater self-awareness, enhanced self-reliance and increased comfort in social relationships and improved functioning in life. The therapist's personality plays an important role in the effectiveness of person-centered therapy. A significant element in therapy is the genuineness of the therapist. He expresses his true feelings in an open and honest way. Researches have indicated that therapy will be successful when the therapist is perceived as genuine, warm and empathic. The therapist's attitudes are more important than his knowledge, theoretical orientation and the techniques he uses.

In spite of significant contributions to psychotherapy, Rogers' theory did not go without critics. Some of the criticisms leveled against Rogers' therapy are:

1. It is too simple.
2. It is only concerned with listening and reflecting.
3. There is no proof to say that clients have within them a potentiality to grow—the actualizing tendency.
4. It gives too much responsibility to the client and reduces the role of counselor as an expert.
5. All counselors cannot give "unconditional positive regard," because everything ultimately is conditional.
6. Clients often do not know what is happening to them and you cannot accept all they say as true.

One of Rogers' significant contributions to the field of counseling is his presenting the propositions and concepts in the form of testable hypotheses for purposes of conducting research. In fact, it was Rogers who opened the field of psychotherapy to research. He and his associates undertook ingenious researches in the area of personality change as a result of psychotherapy (Rogers and Dymond, 1954). He insisted on subjecting the transcripts of therapy sessions to critical examination and applying research methods to counselor-client dialogues. Even the strongest critics of Rogers give credit to his research orientation, which has inspired many others to conduct extensive studies of the counseling process and outcome.

Gestalt Therapy

Frederick S (Fritz) Perls, a Berlin-born psychiatrist, was the founder (along with his wife Laura Perls) of **Gestalt therapy**. Perls was a psychoanalyst (analyzed by a psychoanalyst Wilhelm Reich and supervised by Karen Horney) during his early years. His association with Kurt Goldstein, a Gestalt theory-oriented neuropsychologist, changed his outlook and made him the founder of Gestalt therapy. Perls migrated to the United

States in 1946, where he became a popular theorist and therapist within the humanistic perspective. Gestalt therapy makes use of several basic principles of Gestalt psychology. An important assumption of Gestalt therapy is the idea that people tend to perceive only a part of their whole experience—the figure and ignore the background against which the figure appears. The background includes important thoughts, feelings and desires that are blocked from awareness because they are anxiety-producing. The Gestalt therapist encourages the clients to examine their earlier experiences (that are in the background) and complete any "unfinished business" from their past that are still affecting present-day behavior and relationships. The therapist helps the client to reintegrate the disowned parts into his/her self-system so that the individual may function like a unified whole. The therapy includes reenactments of specific problems the clients experienced in the past, and bring them to awareness so that they may be faced realistically.

Gestalt therapy, like other humanistic therapies, has an existential, experiential and a phenomenological flavor. It is phenomenological because it focuses on the client's perception of reality (immediate experience), existential because it is grounded on the notion that people always are in the process of becoming, remaking, rediscovering themselves, and experiential in that clients come to grips with *what* and *how* they are thinking, feeling and doing as they interact with the therapist. Gestalt therapists emphasize the value of being fully present during the therapeutic encounter. They believe that growth occurs out of the genuine contact between client and therapist.

To achieve their therapeutic goals, Gestalt therapists employ a variety of imaginative techniques (called ***experiments*** and ***exercises***). These are active, dramatic procedures designed to help the clients to get in touch with certain aspects of their inner self that have all along been avoided. For example, let us examine the popular **empty-chair technique** (also called ***double chairing***), which employs a kind of internal dialogue and role play. Perls believed that most people have two opposing poles in their personality such as the ***top dog*** that is righteous, bossy, demanding, manipulative, and moralistic, and the ***underdog*** that is apologetic, helpless and weak, playing the role of a passive victim. Using two chairs, the therapist asks the client to play the role of the top dog, and then shift to the other chair, and become the underdog. The dialogue continues between both sides of the client. In doing so, the client experiences the conflict between the two sides more fully. The conflict can be resolved by the client's understanding, acceptance and integration of both sides of their personality. While this exercise helps clients to get in touch with a side of themselves that they may be denying, it does not aim to rid oneself of certain traits; it only helps to learn to accept and live with the polarities. Perls has developed a number of such exercises (literally hundreds of them) to challenge and confront the client's attitudes and behaviors. These exercises help the client to gain full awareness, experience internal conflicts, resolve inconsistencies, and work through an impasse that is preventing completion of unfinished business.

Recently, attempts have been made to combine person-centered therapy and gestalt therapy resulting in what has come to be called ***process-experiential therapy***. This form of treatment emphasizes the experiencing of emotions during therapy. Clients are asked to reflect on their emotions and are encouraged to create meaning from them. Just like all other forms of humanistic therapy, the therapeutic relationship is considered very important. But the therapist in Gestalt therapy plays a more active role in guiding the client to experience the emotions more vividly, than in Roger's approach.

Gestalt therapy is rich in strategies to help the clients, but it lacks a clearly articulated theory. Its empirical base is also limited. One important criticism of this approach is that it is often manipulative and controlling. Further, there is no emphasis on teaching the clients useful life skills. It is viewed as gimmicky having a high potential for abuse. It is considered as anti-intellectual because of its stress on experiential aspects and neglect of cognitive factors.

Cognitive Therapies

Cognitive psychologists believe that the way people perceive, think and interpret the world around them determines their behavior. They have demonstrated that people's thoughts (cognitions), not just their learning histories, influence their feelings and behaviors, both normal and abnormal, in various ways. For example, just thinking about a positive love relationship of last year can put you in a good mood and thinking about an unhappy love affair can have the opposite effect. Therefore, cognitive therapy aims to help clients to cultivate thinking rationally in order to reinterpret events that otherwise produce distressing feelings and behaviors. Cognitive therapists assert that it is the interpretation of the stimulus, not the stimulus, which determines the response to that stimulus. They try to identify maladaptive ideas, irrational thoughts, beliefs and self-statements, challenge their rationale and help the clients to correct them. Among several cognitive approaches to therapy, one developed by Albert Ellis and the other by Aaron Beck need special mention.

Ellis's Rational Emotive Behavior Therapy

Albert Ellis (Fig. 16.1), who was earlier trained in psychodynamic therapy, became convinced that it is the individual's irrational thoughts and not the unconscious dynamics that were at the root of behavioral disorders and developed a method to treat such disorders. Ellis (1962) called his technique rational emotive therapy (RET), but later changed the name as **rational emotive behavior therapy (REBT)**, because it made use of several principles of behavior therapy. The aim of REBT is to change a client's maladaptive thought processes and emotional responses and thus behavior. Ellis asserts that healthy people behave rationally and in tune with experienced reality. But many people engage in unrealistic thoughts and develop perfectionist attitudes. They expect too much from themselves and when they fail, acquire irrational beliefs that they are worthless and thorough failures. For example, they may think that they *should* succeed in all they attempt, *must* be liked by everyone, and *ought* to be right always. Such irrational and unrealistic expectations and self-demands inevitably spell disaster in their lives (Box 16.3).

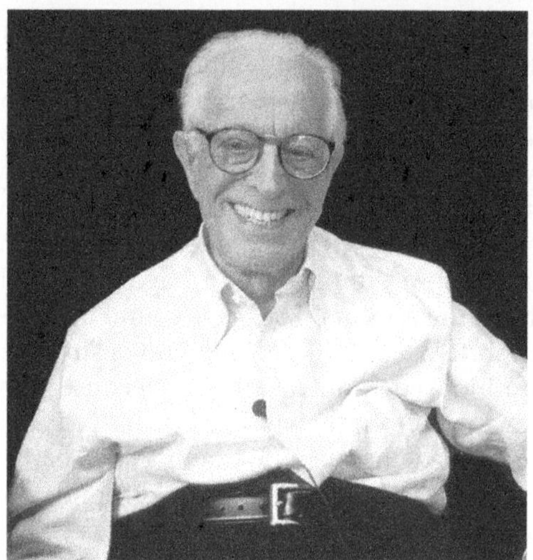

FIGURE 16.1: Albert Ellis

Thoughts and behaviors are viewed as irrational if they create significant emotional conflicts with others, block goal-directed behavior, are not in line with objective reality or unnecessarily threaten life. In the beginning, Ellis proposed eleven irrational beliefs, which were later reduced to the following four:

1. *Awfulizing:* Characterized by habitual exaggeration of reality by "disasterizing"

Box 16.3: Examples of Irrational Beliefs

- I must be loved and approved by virtually all the people around me
- I must succeed in all the ventures I undertake
- It is awful and catastrophic if things do not go the way I expect them to
- People should love each other and must treat all others nicely
- It is terrible if I cannot solve my problems successfully and quickly
- I should have got the job; I deserved it; it is unfair that I was not given

about the future, focusing on the worst possible outcome, and experiencing a major emotional upheaval even out of a minor disappointment. Example: "I have failed in this examination again, I will probably never pass it."

2. *"I can't stand it":* In reality, we can stand everything except death. But there are people with low frustration-tolerance who cannot tolerate even minor irritants. Life's normal setbacks become elephantine in size; they distort the relative significance of things when they do not go their way.
3. *Musterbating:* The constant use of words such as "must" "should" and "ought" and the underlying thoughts they represent indicates that the person expects special treatment and expects everyone to cooperate to provide what is demanded. It is irrational to do so for the world around rarely cooperates.
4. *Self-judgments:* Evaluating things in absolute terms as good, bad, right or wrong, and condemning all below a standard performance represent this type of irrational belief. It is irrational to expect perfection from anyone, because it is impossible. Example: "She is an idiot; she can't do anything right any time."

Ellis proposed a theory, called the ***A-B-C theory of emotion/personality*** as the guiding model for the practice of REBT. Here *A* refers to the activating event, *B* the belief and *C* the emotional and behavioral consequence or reaction of the individual. The reaction can be healthy or unhealthy. According to Ellis, *A* (the activating event) does not cause *C* (the emotional consequence). Instead, *B* (the person's belief about *A*) causes *C* (the emotional reaction). For example, if a person experiences depression after a divorce, it is not the divorce that causes depression, but the belief about being a failure in married life or being rejected. Thus, people are largely responsible for creating their own emotional reactions (Box 16.4).

Showing clients how they can change the irrational beliefs that directly cause their emotional disturbance is the central point in REBT. Therefore, the therapist attempts to restructure the individual's belief system, especially the irrational ***shoulds, musts*** and ***oughts*** that are preventing the person from developing positive sense of self-worth and an emotionally satisfying life. Toward this

Box 16.4: ABC Theory of Emotions

A	B	C
Activating Event *Being divorced*	**Belief or Interpretation of Event** *I am a bad wife; failed in life*	**Emotional or Behavioral Consequence** *Frustration and anxiety*
D	**E**	**F**
Disputing Irrational Beliefs *Being divorced does not mean I am bad. It is not such a terrible situation. It is difficult, alright, but I can manage it.*	**Emotional Effect** *Relief*	**End Result** *New feeling*

end, the therapist uses several methods, such as disputing irrational beliefs (D), changing his/her language, employing humor, role playing rational emotive imagery, shame-attacking exercises and doing cognitive homework. The REBT practitioners regularly make use of behavior therapy procedures such as operant reinforcement, relaxation, systematic desensitization and modeling. They combine cognitive, emotive and behavioral methods in a single session with a given client. If a particular technique is not working well, they switch on to others. In fact, their technical eclecticism and therapeutic flexibility make controlled research on the effectiveness of REBT difficult.

The REBT has been widely used in the treatment of anxiety disorders, personality disorders, problems of love, sex and marriage, in addition to mood disorders and other psychotic disorders. It is used to cultivate effective child rearing practices and managing adolescents in the family. Often, the technique is used in social skill training and self-management. The REBT is well suited as a brief form of therapy for individuals, families, couples and groups. However, Ellis does not assert that all clients can be helped through logical analysis and philosophical reconstruction. Those who cannot reason logically (children, schizophrenics, mentally retarded and some with character disorders) cannot benefit from REBT. Because role of the counselor in REBT is so verbal, active and directive, the client often may feel overpowered and not responsible for the therapeutic outcome. Also, it is difficult for some counselors to practice REBT if they are not outgoing, confrontational, combative and do not enjoy vigorous debate.

Beck's Cognitive Therapy

Aaron Temkin Beck (Fig. 16.2) (1921), an American psychiatrist, developed a form of cognitive therapy (CT) that has several similarities to REBT. Both are active, directive, present-centered and brief. Beck developed his therapy independently of Ellis, but the two exchanged their views frequently. The CT, like REBT, is based on the rationale that how people think, feel and behave is determined by the way they perceive and interpret their experience. Beck's cognitive therapy (Beck, 1976) emphasizes recognizing and changing negative thoughts and maladaptive beliefs in clients. The theoretical bases of Beck's therapy are:

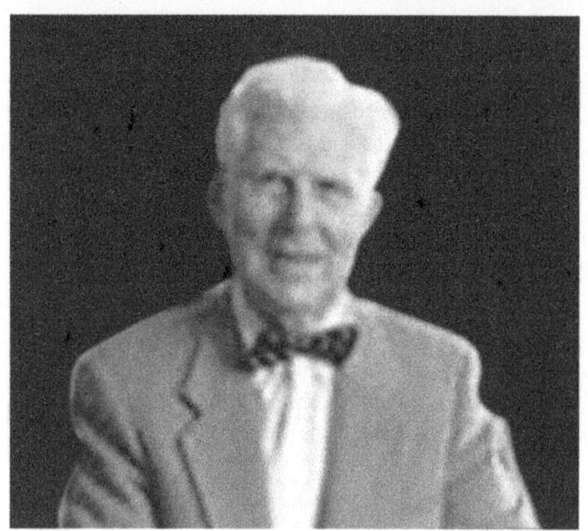

FIGURE 16.2: Aaron Beck

1. That people's internal communication is accessible to introspection.
2. That client's beliefs have highly personal meanings.
3. That these meanings can be discovered by the client rather than being taught by the therapist.

The theory holds that to understand the nature of emotional disturbances, it is necessary to focus on the cognitive content of the client's reaction to the upsetting event or stream of thoughts. The goal is to change the way the clients think by using their automatic thoughts to reach the core schemata and begin to introduce the idea of restructuring the schema. This is achieved by encouraging the clients to gather and weigh the evidence in support of their beliefs. The clients are taught to identify their own automatic thoughts (such as, "I am a total failure") and to keep records of their thought contents and their emotional reactions. With the help of the therapist, the clients then identify the logical errors in their thinking (called ***cognitive distortions***) and learn to challenge the validity of these automatic thoughts. For example, the clients realize that they perceive the world selectively as harmful, while ignoring the evidence to the contrary, are overgeneralizing based on limited experiences, are magnifying the significance of undesirable events; are emphasizing the negative aspects of things, while filtering out the positive and engaging in absolutistic thinking. The process of helping clients shift their thinking away from automatic, dysfunctional thoughts to more realistic ones is called **cognitive restructuring.**

In Beck's therapy, clients do not change their beliefs by debate as is common in REBT. Rather they are encouraged to gather information about themselves and test the cognitive errors that interfere with their effective living. They are encouraged to discover the faulty assumptions or dysfunctional schemas that are making them vulnerable to psychological disorders. Cognitive therapy also makes use of ***psychoeducation*** in which the clients are educated about therapy and research findings pertaining to their problems. This knowledge is then used to help the clients develop more realistic, rational, undistorted view of their problems. Beck's therapy has been successfully used in the treatment of depression and anxiety disorders. It is also used in treating phobias, hostility, psychosomatic disorders, panic disorders, personality disorders and substance abuse. The therapy has been found to be most useful in helping basically healthy people to cope better with everyday stress and in preventing them from developing full-blown anxiety or depressive disorders.

It is difficult to distinguish between cognitive therapy and behavior therapy. The two are not really distinct; the difference is only a matter of emphasis. Behavior therapy aims at behavior change and cognitive therapy involves change in cognitions. Feelings are the affective accompaniments of behavior and you cannot think of behavior that is devoid of feeling. In recent times, therapists have been using cognitive and behavioral techniques in treating the same client with the realization that cognitions and behavior affect each other and both affect feelings. Today, altering cognitions, feelings and behavior is considered the essential part of all psychological treatment techniques. Cognitive techniques change thought, which then affect both behavior and feelings. Behavioral techniques change behaviors, which in turn lead to new experiences, feelings and ways of relating, which then change both how people think about themselves and the world around. In fact, the terms cognitive therapy and cognitive behavior therapy have come to be used interchangeably in recent times. Cognitive behavior therapy can be used in the treatment of several psychological disturbances, especially the stress-related problems by providing clients new coping strategies and new ways of mastering skills. Other variants of cognitive behavior therapy have been proposed by Meichenbaum (1977) and Lazarus (1989).

Group Therapy

Group approaches to psychotherapy have become popular for several reasons. These are less costly and are found to be as effective as individual therapies. An important feature of group therapy is that clients learn both by observing other group members' adaptive and maladaptive attempts to solve personal problems and by comparing their own relationship with the therapist, and with those of other members. Some proponents of group therapy believes that it produces better results than individual therapy. Groups provide ample opportunities to learn new social skills through modeling and rehearsing the skills in the group setting. Group therapy settings help to cultivate ***self-disclosure***—communicating personal problems with group members. The clients derive social support, feel that they are being accepted and valued by others. They come to realize that there are others who are suffering from similar problems and that their problems are neither unique nor serious compared to other members. Clients learn to relate to others adaptively and constructively. They gain self-knowledge by observing others and the therapist and come to know what motivates their behavior. Group therapy also offers an opportunity for clients to observe how their behavior affects others and to receive relevant feedback. Clients observe how others approach problems and learn to apply the same principles to solve their own problems. Since many of human problems and conflicts occur in the social context, group therapy is ideally suited not only to highlight and reveal the nature of a person's conflicts and maladjustments, but to offer corrective influences.

All therapies discussed above can be conducted in the group format. Clients are generally screened before being admitted to the therapy group to ensure that they can participate effectively in group processes and that they do not disrupt the group as a whole. The therapist always includes in the group some senior members to serve as models for identification, stimulate hope and offer practical advice and suggestions that have helped them to improve their condition. Group therapy is being widely used in several settings other than psychological clinics. It is used in managerial circles to alleviate stress and to bring about improved human relations. The training group (T-group), encounter group and sensitivity training group are popular in the organizational settings. Group therapy is extensively used in the treatment of alcoholism. ***Alcoholics Anonymous***, which is one of the famous self-help groups, uses group therapy as an effective method of inducing alcohol abstinence.

Family Therapy

Family therapy began with the observation that many clients who had shown marked improvement in individual therapy had a relapse when they returned home and began interacting with members of their families. This observation led to an important discovery in the area of psychotherapy, namely, that the psychological disturbance exhibited by the client may reflect dysfunctional relationships within the family system and that permanent recovery in the client may require that the entire family system be the focus of therapy. This is echoed in an oft-repeated statement: "Admit the patient and treat his family." In addition to the issue mentioned above, there are other problems that a family therapist may have to address. Some of the core problems in the family concern the inability to resolve conflicts make important decisions or solve problems. There may be rigid or chaotic organization in the family without agreed-upon responsibilities for members. In some closely knit families, there may be loss of individuality among members. It is difficult for closely knit families to change with changing circumstance. In other families, the members have little contact with or concern for each other. There may be disagreement among members regarding child-rearing practices.

Family therapy provides a valuable forum for airing hostilities, reviewing emotional ties and dealing with crises. The family therapist, therefore, may be called upon to help the family members understand how the family functions and how its unique pattern of interactions contribute to conflicts and to the problems of one or more members of the family. Family therapists view the family as a "system". The systems theory defines influences as mutual and causality as circular. The symptoms of a defective family system are said to take different forms in different members of the system. One or the other member cannot improve the family without understanding the conflicts that are to be found in the interactions of the family members. Each member has to contribute to the resolution of the problems. A family that functions poorly cannot adjust to change because its mechanisms are either inflexible or ineffectual. Therefore, it is imperative that the family therapist considers the family as a "whole." He follows a theoretical orientation that has come to be called ***systems therapy,*** which starts from the premise that no client is an island. A client's symptoms occur in a larger context or system (the family) and any change in one part of the system will affect the rest of the system. The systems therapy refers to the client as the "identified patient," but its target is the system, the real "patient" that requires treatment. Systems therapy focuses on a family's structure, communication pattern and power relationships. The therapist takes an active part by using techniques such as reframing (a new way of conceptualizing the problem) and validation (the therapist conveying his understanding of the client's feelings and wishes).

Marital Therapy

Marital therapy overlaps with family therapy, but has somewhat different roots. While family therapy involves helping the family to receive and live with a patient returning from a mental hospital, marital therapy developed in response to a large number of clients seeking assistance with couple's problems. Married life is not as smooth as it is reported to be. The so called 'happy married life,' some say, is an illusion. The incidence of divorce, separation and estrangement are on the rise all over the world. Couples seek marital therapy because they are troubled by their relationship or because they are contemplating divorce or separation. By seeing the therapist together, the partners can easily identify problems and alter the ways they relate to each other. The main advantage of couple's therapy is that the therapist, as an impartial observer, can easily witness the couple's interactions instead of hearing about them in a secondhand and perhaps one-sided report. Family therapy may be undertaken by psychodynamic, humanistic, behavioral or cognitive therapists. Regardless of the approach, the therapists focus on specific issues such as helping to couples increase communication, express feelings, help each other and enjoy shared experiences.

Research has shown that happily married couples differ from distressed ones in several ways: they talk more to one another; keep channels of communication open; show more sensitivity to each other's opinions, needs feelings and are more skilled in solving problems. An important trend in contemporary family therapy is the emphasis on "acceptance." The happy couples and those who profit from marital therapy make a decision to *accept* those aspects of the partner's behavior that are difficult to change. What cannot be cured must be endured. For instance, you do not expect a socially introverted person to become an out-going extrovert overnight. The best way is to accept him as he/she is. Therefore, the therapist helps couples to accept those traits of the partner that seem unlikely to change. This reduces frustration, decreases the demands on the other spouse and allows the couple to focus and enjoy the positive aspects of their relationships. The emphasis in marital therapy is on acceptance training and research has shown that this emphasis results in improved treatment outcomes.

EVALUATION OF PSYCHOTHERAPY

We have reviewed in the sections above some of the major forms of psychological treatments that are currently in use. According to one report, there are over 400 psychotherapies for adults and about 200 for children and adolescents. These are used to treat some 300 different kinds of psychological disorder. Then the question arises: Which therapy works best? Or, does psychotherapy work at all? Several groups of people such as patients and their families, clinical practitioners and researchers want to know about the effectiveness of psychotherapy. In fact, the much more complex question that needs answer is: *Which types of therapy administered by which kinds of therapists to which kinds of patients having which kinds of problems produce which kinds of effects?* After more than half a century of research involving hundreds of studies, this complex question is still not satisfactorily answered. But it is an important question that demands an answer. Selecting and applying the most appropriate therapy is vital in human terms.

British psychologist Hans Eysenck (1952) made a frontal attack on the effectiveness of psychotherapeutic procedures. After reviewing available data, he asserted that the rate of **spontaneous remission**—recovering from psychological disorders without any treatment—was as high as the success rates reported by psychotherapists. That is, troubled people who receive psychotherapy are no more likely to improve than are those who go untreated. He also reported that the outcome data were based on therapists, evaluations of their clients' improvement and it is possible that it could be biased by the therapists' needs to see themselves as competent and successful. Eysenck's conclusions sparked a fierce uproar among clinicians; but more importantly, it has triggered a healthy trend in psychotherapy research of using more sophisticated and powerful methods for evaluating the outcome of psychotherapy.

Research Methods in Psychotherapy

Conducting research in psychotherapy is not easy because of the number and nature of variables that cannot be controlled as is done in experimental research. The nature of interactions between the therapist and the client varies infinitely between and within therapies. The outcome measures vary enormously. Generally, gains in therapy are estimated based on therapist's evaluation, client's report and informants' opinion and psychological measurements taken before and after therapy on relevant aspects of functioning. Unfortunately, each of these sources has its own limitations. Keeping these difficulties in mind, let us examine some of the methods used to evaluate the effectiveness of psychotherapy. One of the age old methods in evaluating psychotherapy is the case study. Sigmund Freud made monumental discoveries in psychotherapy using only individual case studies. If objective data is collected and recorded throughout and following therapy, case study can be an important source of information to evaluate the treatment. But conservative researchers assert that conclusions drawn from case study cannot be generalized. If multiple case studies of clients who have received similar treatment are available, it can be a useful source of information.

Several researchers have employed survey research to study the effectiveness of psychotherapy. A large number of people who have received therapy can be contacted and their experience in therapy obtained. For example, Seligman (1995) contacted a random sample of 184,000 subscribers to a periodical *Consumer Reports* (CR) and obtained information about certain mental health issues from 22,000 respondents. Of these, 35 percent reported that they had a mental health problem; 40 percent of this group reported they had sought professional help from a psychologist, psychiatrist, social worker or marriage counselor. A majority of respondents reported that they have improved as a result of therapy and they were satisfied with the outcome. Clients also reported that they were more satisfied with the treatment from psychologists, psychiatrists and social workers than with marriage counselors. Seligman concluded that "CR has provided empirical validation of the effectiveness of therapy."

Randomized Clinical Trials

Some researchers have used a refined research procedure called ***Randomized Clinical Trials (RCT)***, in which clients who are suffering from a well-defined disorder, and who are similar in other variables that might affect response to treatment, are randomly assigned to either an experimental group that receives treatment or to a control group. The control group may be either a no treatment group (one that waits for treatment) or placebo control group (receiving a treatment that is not expected to work). The placebo condition is used to control for client expectations of improvement and for being seen by a therapist (for ethical reasons the control group clients are given the option of receiving the real treatment later). Carl Rogers and his associates (Rogers and Dymond, 1954) have used this procedure to study the effectiveness of client-centered therapy. In another research design, clients are randomly assigned to two treatment conditions, one that is being studied and another that has proven effective for that disorder. If the new treatment used on the experimental group is found to be at least as effective as the established treatment, then its value is supported.

To standardize the research on treatment, a committee appointed by the American Psychological Association (APA) recommended issuing a manual containing procedures that therapists have to follow exactly, and evaluating therapists' compliance with these procedures by observing them or taping their sessions. These recommendations aim to ensure that clients in a particular treatment condition are truly receiving the same kind of therapy. The committee also recommended that at least some of the measures of improvement be behavioral in nature. Further, to minimize experimenter bias in evaluating change during interviews or observations following treatment, interviewers and observers should not know whether a given client was in the control group or the experimental group. Finally, the committee insisted that therapists collect follow-up data to know the long-lasting effects of therapy. For example, follow-up studies of treating depression have shown that drug treatment yields quick results, while psychotherapy is more effective in the long run. In psychotherapy, it is found that clients learn specific skills, which they can apply in life after therapy ended; also the chances of relapse were fewer.

Using the rigorous criteria mentioned above, another APA task force identified certain ***Empirically Supported Treatments (EST)***—also called empirically validated treatments or 'evidence-based treatments'—that had been demonstrated, in several independent studies, to be efficacious in treating specific disorders. The therapies thus identified were cognitive and behavioral in nature. It was found that cognitive therapies were good for treating depression and exposure therapies for anxiety disorders. Unfortunately, this applies to situations where the patient is suffering from only one DSM-diagnosed disorder. But 30 to 50 percent of cases who seek treatment do not fit into a DSM category. Many have more than one disorder. In using EST, up to 70 percent cases had to be excluded because they had additional disorders.

Factors Affecting the Outcome of Therapy

Later, researchers have focused on empirically supported treatment principles that predict therapeutic outcome apart from empirically supported treatments. Several principles pertaining to patient variables, therapist variables, diagnostic type or treatment strategies were identified. The APA task force on empirically supported principles has identified variables that make a difference within each of these categories. Among the patient variables, three factors that were identified are the client's openness to therapy, self-relatedness, and nature of the problem. Openness refers to the clients' general willingness to participate in therapy and take the risks required to change themselves. Self-relatedness refers to the client's ability to experience and understand internal states, such as thoughts and feelings, to be attuned to the processes that go on in their relationship with their therapist, and to apply what they learn in therapy to life outside the clinic. The third client factor is the nature of the problem and its degree of fit with the therapy being used (the EST for the disorder). For example, phobias may respond well when exposure or desensitization techniques are used whereas, psychodynamic, humanistic or cognitive techniques are useful when the aim is to search for self-discovery or meaning in life.

Among therapist variables, the most important one is the relationship between the client and the therapist. Rogers emphasized the importance of qualities such as genuineness on the part of the therapist, unconditional positive regard for the client as a person, and the therapist's ability to experience the inner world of the client (empathy) as if it is his/her own. Rogers believed that these were the necessary and sufficient conditions for effective therapeutic changes in the client. When these conditions are not present or when there are hostile exchanges between the therapist and the client, the result may be deterioration in the client's condition. Apart from relationship variables, there are other therapist variables such as technique variables that make a difference in therapeutic success. For example, the therapist must be skilled and knowledgeable in selecting and implementing the appropriate technique for each client and situation. Studies have revealed that the correctness of the interpretations made by the psychoanalyst is related to more positive treatment outcome. An effective therapist must be capable of adjusting his technique to the special needs of the client.

After an intensive search, experts have identified some common factors shared by diverse forms of therapy that might contribute to therapeutic success. Common factors are curative aspects of therapy common to all types of treatments; for example, just going to and being in therapy provides hope, an opportunity to express pent up emotions in a supportive atmosphere, unconditional support, advice, explanation, understanding of one's difficulties and an opportunity to experiment with new behaviors and thoughts. Client's faith in the therapist, the belief that therapy will be helpful in solving problems, and increase in optimism and self-efficacy are other common factors. Several researchers have shown that emotional expression (verbally or in writing) during therapy—talking about one's fear, worry, anxiety, disappointment, sadness and despair or writing about one's experiences—has a positive effect on the client. It is as if the act of deliberately processing the emotional experience with a therapist transforms the experience into a less upsetting event. In contrast to common factors, there are specific factors—these are aspects that relate to the particular type of therapy employed. Clients nowadays do not ask whether therapy is helpful; they ask whether one type of therapy is better than another for treating a particular disorder. For example, with obsessive compulsive disorder (OCD), exposure with response prevention is a specific factor and this is the most important factor bringing improvement.

In recent times, researchers have used an advanced statistical technique called '**meta-analysis**' to assess the gains from psychotherapy. In the meta-analysis researchers combine the statistical results of many studies to arrive at an overall conclusion. Generally, they compute an effect size statistic, which tells what percentage of clients who received therapy had a more favorable outcome than that of the average control clients who did not receive the treatment. One such study (Smith and Glass, 1977) combined 375 studies of psychotherapy involving 25,000 clients and 25,000 control participants. The results indicated that the average therapy client had a more favorable outcome than the untreated cases. Smith and Glass dispute Eysenck's conclusion, maintaining that therapies do indeed have effects beyond spontaneous remission. Other meta-analytic studies support this conclusion. These researchers have also concluded that psychodynamic, client-centered, and behavioral approaches were quite similar in their effectiveness. But this conclusion has been challenged by other researchers who maintain that dumping together studies involving different kinds of clinical problems may mask differential effectiveness, that is, the fact that specific therapies might be highly effective for treating some disorders, but not others. However, the importance of these common factors and other specific factors such as therapeutic techniques in clinical practice are still unclear. The complexities of conducting research in psychotherapy are formidable; in spite of decades of research on the efficacy of therapy techniques, we are not in a position to make unequivocal statements about psychotherapy. In this context, the words of British psychotherapy researcher Isaac Marks (2002) is relevant: "Little is known about which treatment components produce improvement, how they do so and why they do not help all sufferers."

In summary, research on psychotherapy shows that, overall, those who receive some type of psychotherapy fare better than those who do not receive any treatment and that certain types of psychotherapy are more effective with certain disorders than with others. No single form of therapy works best on all problems. The gains of psychotherapy are found to exert their positive influence even after the therapy ends. On the other hand, psychotherapy does not work for everyone; it is reported that 10 percent of people show no improvement or actually their problems worsen after treatment.

RECENT ADVANCES IN PSYCHOTHERAPY

In recent years, psychotherapy is becoming eclectic; therapists are moving away from treatment based on single theoretical orientation such as psychodynamic, humanistic, cognitive, or behavioral. They use techniques derived from several orientations. Therapists' integrating of specific techniques without regard for an overarching theory has come to be known as ***technical eclecticism***. This integrative approach uses new techniques based on research findings rather than theoretical formulations. The therapists focus on the clinical needs of a particular client at a specific point of time in the treatment. They adopt the techniques used by other orientations when necessary. They offer help, listen to the client and suggest new ways of thinking about problems; employ specific techniques for a given disorder. Two clients suffering from the same disorder may receive different integrative treatments from the same therapist, depending on factors other than a diagnosis—such as family problems, client's preference for a specific type of (directive versus non-directive) treatment and other issues.

Computerized Treatment

Computer technology is gradually entering into the field of psychotherapy. Brief treatment aimed at reducing symptoms, using palmtop devices and other software is picking up. Palmtop devices are used for portable self-monitoring by clients; they are signaled to take drugs at the appropriate time, or to engage in specified therapeutic activity such as deep breathing or muscular relaxation. Software for facilitating behavior therapy techniques, such as exposure, cognitive therapy or cognitive restructuring has been tried. Internet is being used to offer individual therapy and even group therapy. The therapy conducted through e-mail is sometimes called '***cybertherapy***'. This therapy is believed to be helpful for people who do not have ready access to professional services, such as those living in remote rural areas, those suffering from disabling medical conditions in addition to psychological ailments, those who are concerned with privacy, and those who are hesitant or embarrassed to seek psychological help. Although, not many people are seeking online therapy today, it is expected to grow in the near future with the development of inexpensive, high quality two way video links.

Some therapists are critical about cybertherapy. They assert that psychotherapy is an interpersonal activity, in which the relationship between the therapist and client plays an important role and cybertherapy devoid of such a relationship may not be effective. The multitude of non-verbal cues (facial expressions, body language, emotional responsiveness, tone of voice) that occur during therapy are absent in cybertherapy. Confidentiality and privacy cannot be guaranteed on the internet; no one is able to guarantee that highly personal information shared on the web will not be open to computer hackers. The person offering treatment may not be professionally trained; anyone can call him- or her-self a therapist and offer therapy. The client may misrepresent himself easily than they could in face-to-face interaction. Finally, there are no large scale researches to support the effectiveness of online therapy. In spite of these limitations, cybertherapy in one form or another is likely to become a common option for several people seeking psychological help in the coming years.

BIOMEDICAL APPROACHES TO TREATMENT

When you have a headache, you take an analgesic and the problem disappears (at least temporarily). When you have appendicitis, you undergo surgery to get relief from the problem. Similarly, can we not treat the psychological disorders using some kind of medical or surgical treatment? The answer is "yes". It is known that certain biological conditions contribute to psychological disorders. Then, why not treat the body to cure the mind? Today, biomedical approaches are extensively used as an alternative (or in addition) to psychological treatment. Recent advances in brain research have led to tremendous progress in biomedical treatments in the form of drug treatment, electrical treatment and surgical treatment.

Psychopharmacology

The use of drugs in the treatment of psychological disorders falls under the new field known as **psychopharmacology**, a field that investigates the effect of drugs on cognitions, emotions and behavior. During the last few decades, increased knowledge about brain functions and neurotransmitters has led to enormous progress in the field of psychopharmacology. A number of **psychotropic drugs** have been developed to treat certain disorders, which were previously considered untreatable. The drugs that act on the brain are called '**psychoactive drugs**' or 'mind-altering' drugs. The commonly used psychotropic drugs fall into four categories:

1. Antipsychotic drugs.
2. Antidepressant drugs.
3. Antianxiety drugs.
4. Antimanic drugs.

Experts advise that these drugs are to be used in conjunction with psychotherapy for better results. In the following sections, we discuss the uses of some of these drugs in the treatment of psychological disorders.

Box 16.5: Commonly Used Antipsychotic Drugs

Drug Class	*Generic Name*	*Trade Name*
Conventional (first generation)	Chlorpromazine	Thorazine
	Perphenazine	Trilafon
	Molindone	Moban
	Thiothixene	Navane
	Trifluoperazine	Stelazine
	Haloperidol	Haldol
	Fluphenazine	Prolixin
Atypical (second generation)	Clozapine	Clozaril
	Risperidone	Risperdal
	Olanzapine	Zyprexa
	Quetiapine	Seroquel
	Ziprasidone	Geodon
	Aripiprazole	Abilify

Antipsychotic Drugs

A group of drugs called '**antipsychotic' drugs** (also known as **neuroleptic drugs**) is used in the treatment of schizophrenia and psychotic mood disorders. These drugs substantially reduce the intensity of psychotic symptoms, but it is doubtful whether they can cure the illness as such. It is well established that antipsychotic drugs have significant impact on the positive symptoms of schizophrenia such as hallucinations and delusions. They do this by blocking dopamine receptors. Studies have found that nearly 60 percent of patients with schizophrenia, treated with traditional antipsychotic drugs (such as chlorpromazine, perphenazine, molindone, fluphenazine, etc.) improve within 6 weeks compared to only about 20 percent of those treated with a placebo. These drugs are also useful in alleviating psychotic symptoms such as mania, psychotic depression and schizoaffective disorders. Box 16.5 for a list of commonly prescribed antipsychotic drugs.

But one important limitation of these drugs is their side effects. Prolonged use of these medications can cause **tardive dyskinesia,** an irreversible motor disorder characterized by involuntary movements of lips, tongue, jaws, extremities (smacking of the lips and display of facial grimaces) and other symptoms. Because the movement-related side effects are less common with atypical antipsychotic drugs, such as clozapine, risperidone, olanzapine, these are now preferred in the treatment of schizophrenia. In addition, these second generation drugs are found to reduce both positive and negative symptoms in schizophrenic patients. But, prolonged use of these neuroleptic drugs is also reported to have other types of side effects such as weight gain. Pharmacological treatment administered soon after the first psychotic episode is associated with better prognosis compared to treatment begun later.

Antidepressant Drugs

At present five groups of **antidepressant drugs** are prescribed in the treatment of depression. These are ***selective serotonin reuptake inhibitors (SSRI), serotonin and norepinephrine reuptake inhibitors (SNRI), tricyclics, monoamine oxidase inhibitors (MAOI)*** and atypical drugs. Box 16.6 details a list of antidepressants that are commonly prescribed.

As in the case of antipsychotic drugs, the antidepressants are classified into two groups: the classical or first generation antidepressants and the second generation

Box 16.6: Commonly Prescribed Antidepressant Drugs

Drug Class	*Generic Name*	*Trade Name*
Tricyclics	Amitriptyline	Elavil
	Clomipramine	Anafranil
	Desipramine	Norpramin
	Doxepin	Sinequan
	Imipramine	Tofranil
	Nortriptyline	Aventyl
	Trimipramine	Surmontil
MAOI	Phenelzine	Nardil
	Tranylcypromine	Parnate
	Isocarboxazid	Marplan
SSRI	Fluoxetine	Prozac
	Sertraline	Zoloft
	Paroxetine	Paxil
	Fluvoxamine	Luvox
	Citalopram	Celexa
	Escitalopram	Lexapro
SNRI	Venlafaxine	Effexor
	Reboxetine	Vestra
Atypical	Nefazodone	Serzone
	Trazodone	Desyrel
	Mirtazapine	Remeron
	Bupropion	Wellbutrin

depressants. The first generation depressants such as tricyclics and the MAOIs that were discovered first have been replaced by second generation drugs such as SSRIs. The tricyclics and MAOIs increase the activity of neurotransmitters serotonin and norepinephrine (the lowered activity level of these neurotransmitters in brain regions is related to the symptoms of depression). The tricyclic antidepressants (TCAs) operate to inhibit the reuptake of excitatory transmitters into the presynaptic neurons, allowing them to continue stimulating postsynaptic neurons. Although the MAOIs were the first antidepressants to be developed in the 1950s, they are used infrequently nowadays. MAOIs inhibit the activity of monoamine oxidase, an enzyme that breaks down the monoamine neurotransmitters in the synapse. The MAOIs have more severe side effects than the tricyclics. They cause dangerous elevations in blood pressure when taken with certain foods such as cheese and some types of wine. Nevertheless, MAOIs are used in certain cases of atypical depression that does not respond well to other classes of antidepressants.

Many patients refuse to take the first generation depressants because of their side effects. The SSRIs were developed to reduce the side effects. SSRIs are chemically unrelated to tricyclics and MAOIs. As the name suggests, SSRIs selectively inhibit the reuptake of serotonin only. They are generally not fatal in overdose as the tricyclics can be. However, SSRIs also have some side effects. Several patients who take Prozac, the most widely prescribed antidepressant, report nervousness, insomnia, nausea, diarrhea, sweating, joints pain, diminished sexual interest and difficulty with orgasm. But the side effects of SSRIs are mild when compared with tricyclics, and in addition, SSRIs reduce depression symptoms more rapidly. They also reduce the anxiety symptoms associated with depression. Because they have fewer side effects and are safer and easier to take, SSRIs are gradually replacing tricyclics in recent years.

Serotonin and norepinephrine reuptake inhibitors (SNRIs), such as venlafaxine (Effexor), block the reuptake of both norepinephrine and serotonin. The side effects resemble those of SSRIs, but are relatively safe in overdose. Patients who do not respond to other antidepressants respond well to these drugs. Several other drugs have been developed in recent times. For instance, trazodone (Desyrel) is not lethal when taken in overdose. It specifically inhibits the reuptake of serotonin. But its sedating property is a limiting factor. In rare cases, it is found to produce priapism (prolonged erection of the penis in the absence of sexual stimulation). Bupropion (Wellbutrin) does not block reuptake of serotonin or norepinephrine, but it seems to increase noradrenergic function in some other ways. One advantage of this drug is that it does not inhibit sexual activities. Nefazodone (Serzone) inhibits the reuptake of both serotonin and norepinephrine, does not cause insomnia and does not reduce sexual drive. Even here, the combination of psychotherapy and drug treatment appears to yield better recovery rates.

Antianxiety Drugs

The **antianxiety drugs** also called anxiolytic drugs are used extensively all over the world to reduce anxiety. It is reported that more than 15 percent of Americans between the ages of 16 and 74 use drugs such as Valium, Ativan, Xanax and others (the drug class called benzodiazepines). These drugs reduce anxiety and agitation and at higher doses induce sleep. Benzodiazepines and related anxiolytic drugs work by enhancing the activity of GABA receptors. The GABA is an inhibitory neurotransmitter that plays an important role in the way the human brain inhibits anxiety in stressful situations. The benzodiazepines appear to enhance GABA activity in certain areas of the brain known to be implicated in anxiety such as the limbic system. Antianxiety drugs are used in a variety of situations in which tension and anxiety are significant components. Sometimes, these drugs are used in combination with psychotherapy to help clients cope successfully with problematic situations. A temporary relief from anxiety may allow a client to enter anxiety-arousing situations and learn to cope more effectively with them. But one problem with these drugs is that patients can become psychologically and physiologically dependent on them and show withdrawal symptoms when the drugs are discontinued. Therefore, the clients have to be weaned from the drug carefully. Also, the relapse rates are high when the drug is discontinued.

A new antianxiety drug buspirone (Buspar) that is completely unrelated to the benzodiazepine group was released during the 1960s. It is supposed to act in complex ways on serotonergic functioning rather than on GABA and found to be as effective as benzodiazepines in treating general anxiety disorders. Buspar has low potential for abuse and does not cause withdrawal symptoms and has no sedative effects. The disadvantage is it takes 2 to 4 weeks to act and hence not very useful in acute anxiety states. A list of common antianxiety drugs is given in Box 16.7.

Antimanic Drugs (Mood Stabilizers)

Lithium, a mineral salt, has been used successfully in the treatment of bipolar disorders. About 70 to 80 percent of patients having a manic state show marked improvement after 2 to 3 weeks of taking lithium.

Lithium and drugs similar to it have a quality that sets them apart from other drugs. They prevent future episodes of bipolar disorders. Many patients who have had episodes of bipolar disorders in the past can prevent the recurrence of their symptoms by taking a daily dose of lithium. The drug is toxic and the dosage must be carefully controlled. There are some side effects such as weight gain, gastrointestinal problems, fatigue, tremor, dizziness, slurred speech and ataxia (loss of coordination of voluntary muscles). How lithium acts in the body is not known. Drugs such as valproic acid (Depakote) and carbamazepine (Tegretol)

Box 16.7: Commonly Prescribed Antianxiety Drugs

Drug Class	*Generic Name*	*Trade Name*
Benzo-diazepines	Alprazolam	Xanax
	Clonazepam	Klonopin
	Diazepam	Valium
	Lorazepam	Ativan
	Oxazepam	Serax
	Clorazepate	Tranxene
	Chlordiazep-oxide	Librium
Other	Buspirone	Buspar

are reported to be effective in reducing manic episodes, but they are not effective in treating depressive phases of bipolar disorders. These drugs also have side effects and careful monitoring of patients is required. Abilify, an antipsychotic drug is now being used in the treatment of bipolar disorders.

Electroconvulsive Therapy

Using convulsions to treat mental disorders goes back to a Swiss physician Paracelsus (1493–1591) who induced mental patients to drink camphor until they experienced convulsions. However, it is the Hungarian physician Ladislas von Meduna who is regarded as the originator of shock treatment. Meduna thought (erroneously) that schizophrenia rarely occurred in people with epilepsy, and that the two were incompatible, and hence speculated that one might be able to cure schizophrenia by inducing convulsions. First, he used camphor and later a drug called Metrazol to induce convulsions in schizophrenic patients. During 1930s, Sakel injected insulin to produce convulsions. Then in 1938, two Italian physicians Ugo Cerletti and Lucio Bini produced convulsion by passing an electric current through a patient's head. This method known as **Electroconvulsive Therapy (ECT)** became highly popular and still is in several parts of the world.

In the eyes of the public, ECT is a horrible, painful, primitive form of treatment. Several law suits have been brought against the use of shock treatment on patients who cannot give their consent. Despite all the misconceptions and distaste in the minds of people, ECT is a safe, effective and important form of treatment. In fact, it is the only form of treatment for severely depressed and suicidal patients. Depressed pregnant woman for whom administering antidepressant drugs may be risky and the elderly who cannot take antidepressants because of their medical conditions, ECT is the preferred treatment. Properly administered, ECT does not cause any structural damage to the brain. Studies have shown that ECT is also effective in the treatment of manic disorders. But surprisingly, no one knows how ECT works.

In the early applications of ECT, a wide-awake patient was strapped to a table, electrodes were attached to the patient's scalp and a current of roughly 100 volts was applied to the brain producing violent convulsions and loss of consciousness. Sometimes, the convulsions were so violent that patients fractured their arms or legs. But today, administering ECT is simpler than extracting a tooth. Generally, ECT is administered in two ways. In bilateral ECT, electrodes are placed on either side of the head and constant current of brief electrical pulses, either high or low intensity, are passed from one side of the head to the other for up to 1.5 seconds. In unilateral ECT, current is passed to one side of the brain, usually the right side (non-dominant side). Anesthetics allow the patient to sleep through the procedure and muscle relaxants are used to prevent the violent contractions. If you were to observe a patient receiving ECT today, all that you might see would be a small twitch of the hand or toes and a slight facial grimace, perhaps, as the convulsions occurred. After the ECT, the patient has amnesia for the period immediately preceding the therapy and is usually somewhat confused for the next hour or so. Sometimes, there may be a slight headache and muscle pain. Normally, a treatment series consists of fewer than a dozen sessions; occasionally one may need more. With repeated treatments, usually administered three times weekly, the patient gradually becomes deteriorated, a state that usually clears after termination of treatments. Bilateral ECT is more effective than the unilateral ECT, but the former is associated with some cognitive side effects and memory disturbance for about 3 months after ECT ends. It is advised to start with unilateral procedure and then change over to bilateral one.

Still, there are several critics of ECT. Some note that despite the positive outcome in depression, the relapse rate is very high, perhaps 85 percent. In some cases, permanent memory loss is reported. Repeated treatment may cause some brain damage. The effectiveness of the treatment in schizophrenia is doubtful and it cannot relieve anxiety. After reviewing the pros and cons, American Psychiatric Association concluded that ECT should be regarded as a useful treatment for major depression in patients who cannot take or do not respond to medication.

Recently a new treatment called '*transcranial magnetic stimulation* (TMS)' is being tried. In this procedure, an electromagnetic coil placed on the scalp transmits pulses of high intensity magnetism to the brain in short bursts lasting 100 to 200 microseconds. The TMS has varying effects depending on the exact location of the coil on the head and the frequency of the pulses. The TMS is found to be effective in treating depressive patients who have not responded to medication. The most common short-term side effect experienced by five to twenty percent of patients is a slight headache. Even in this case, it is not known how exactly the procedure works on the brain. More research is needed before TMS can be declared a proper form of treatment.

Psychosurgery

A surgical procedure that removes or destroys some brain tissues to relieve symptoms of psychological disorders is called '**psychosurgery**'. In fact, the term psychosurgery is a misnomer; it should be called 'neurosurgery'. Whatever the name, it is the least preferred biomedical treatment. In the 1930s, before the advent of antipsychotic drugs, a Portuguese surgeon António Egas Moniz (1874–1955) reported that severing the nerve tracts that connect the frontal lobes with subcortical areas of the brain involved in emotion resulted in the calming of violent psychotic patients. The operation, often called '**prefrontal lobotomy**' or 'leukotomy', eliminated emotional input from the limbic system into the areas of the brain connected with cognitive functions such as reasoning and planning. During the 1930s and 1940s several thousands of patients underwent this treatment. Moniz received the 1949 Nobel Prize for his discovery along with Swiss physiologist Walter Hess (it is reported that Moniz was later shot by a former patient). Walter Freeman developed a modified form of lobotomy, which involved inserting a sharp-edged instrument through the eye socket into the brain to cut the targeted nerve tracts.

Psychosurgery often did improve the patient's behavior, but there were several negative side effects. There were instances of remission of symptoms. Some suffered personality changes. Patient's behavior became bland, colorless and unemotional; others became aggressive and several were unable to control their impulses. Often the patients died. For these reasons, psychosurgery was branded as unethical and became nearly obsolete. With the advent of antipsychotic drugs, psychosurgical procedures became rare. Nowadays, the treatment is used as a last resort for patients who have not responded for all other forms of treatment and are experiencing severe disabling symptoms. Modern techniques (such as **cingulotomy**) involve the selective destruction of minute areas of the brain and the treatment is used in severe cases of obsessive-compulsive disorders.

MEDICATION OR PSYCHOTHERAPY, WHICH IS MORE EFFECTIVE?

Finally, one question remains: Which form of treatment, psychological or biological, is more effective in the treatment of psychological disorders? There is no answer that is unequivocal. Available evidence suggests that psychological treatments are useful in handling cases that do not involve severe psychopathology. Psychotherapies are not only less effective in treating serious disorders such as schizophrenia, but also in handling some emotional disorders, alcoholism and drug abuse. However, psychotherapy is found to be useful when combined with biomedical forms of treatments. The value of psychotherapies lies in helping the patient deal realistically with problems of day-to-day living. For example, social skill training has been used effectively to help patients to adjust better to hospital or community settings.

Psychopharmacological drugs have helped many individuals who would otherwise require hospitalization. These drugs have led to earlier discharge of hospitalized patients. They make the hospital climate comfortable for both patients and staff. Nevertheless, several issues arise in the use of psychotropic drugs. Antidepressant drugs produce dramatic improvement in people suffering from depression and have become the drugs of choice for these disorders. When compared with no-treatment conditions, the effect of antidepressant drugs is quite impressive. But when placebo controls are introduced in randomized clinical trials, the picture can change dramatically. If patients receiving a placebo simply believe that they are receiving antidepressant medication (ADM), they frequently show improvement that rivals drug effects. Several studies have shown insignificant difference in improvement between the placebo and drug groups. Researchers are questioning whether the benefits achieved through ADM outweigh possible costs. The results of ongoing studies of the efficacy, side effects and cost/benefit aspects of ADM have to be firmly established.

Antipsychotic drugs are used extensively in treating schizophrenia. It is widely accepted that these drugs are effective, particularly in the short-term. However, a substantial percentage of patients relapse and a moderate percentage become chronic. As mentioned earlier, the risk of tardive dyskinesia with a cumulative dose and duration of treatment cannot be dismissed. Antianxiety drugs should be used for limited periods; otherwise there is the risk of developing drug dependence. The ECT is often helpful for severe depression, but the side effects and ethical considerations have made its use less common. Of course, psychosurgery is hardly ever used today.

In short, the research on the efficacy or effectiveness of various treatments does not necessarily apply to a particular individual. For any particular person with a given disorder, one type of treatment may be more effective than another, which in turn may be more effective than medication. The opposite may be true for someone else with apparently identical symptoms. Medication or psychological treatment often seems to be equally effective in treatment of disorders like depression, but combined treatment have more advantages for some patients. One study reported that providing cognitive therapy along with antidepressant medication resulted in reduction of relapse rate compared to patients who received only medication. Another study found that a family therapy intervention combined with drug therapy for hospitalized bipolar disorder patients yielded better results than for drug therapy alone. It appears multimodal therapy that combines different approaches to clinical intervention is a better way of treatment for several disorders including drug abuse, borderline personality disorder, anxiety disorders and schizophrenia. Both psychological and biological treatments affect brain functioning in ways that can change disordered thoughts, emotions and behavior. Only, they may operate differently to produce the same changes.

An important factor to remember is that drug treatments, however effective in modifying some maladjusted behavior in the short-term, do not provide a permanent cure for the disorder. They suppress symptoms, but do not teach the client coping and problem solving skills to deal with stressful life situations. They may even prevent people from taking steps to confront the real causes of their problems. Many therapists believe that a major benefit of psychological treatment is their potential not only to help clients deal with current problems but also to increase their personal resources to deal with future problems. Therefore, it is advisable to take into consideration all factors—biological, psychological and environmental—while attempting therapeutic behavioral change.

COMMUNITY MENTAL HEALTH CENTERS

During the last several years, mental patients are being treated in institutional settings. There are many states run as well as private institutions. Although, there are some high quality institutions, which provide enriched facilities such as drug therapy, psychotherapy, social, educational and recreational programs, many of the state run hospitals do not and often cannot offer such services. Patients in these hospitals may receive drugs, but few of them receive psychological help. Often the hospitals are overcrowded, mismanaged understaffed and underfinanced. Patients live in relatively impoverished, unstimulating social environment. They provide little more than minimal custodial care. Utmost, they provide an escape from the stresses and demands of the outside world. Many patients admitted to these institutions sink into a chronic "sick role." Passive dependence and crazy behavior among patients are not only tolerated but expected. The patients lose self-confidence, motivation and skills needed to return and adapt to the outside world. When discharged, they have little chance of surviving outside the hospital.

In order to avoid these tragic consequences, a new approach to the treatment of psychological disorders has emerged during the last quarter of the 20th century. This is often referred to as ***deinstitutionalization movement*** or ***community mental health movement***, which attempts to transfer the primary focus of treatment from mental hospitals to the community. During the 1960s, the US Congress passed the Community Mental Health Act to provide for the establishment of one mental health center for every 50,000 people. Community mental health centers were designed to provide outpatient psychotherapy and drug treatment so that patients can remain in their normal, social and work environments. The centers were allowed to arrange for a short -term hospital stay, when patients become disturbed. The community mental health centers may engage in providing information about drugs to schools or educating police personnel on how to deal with mentally disturbed people in the community.

The idea of community treatment is a good one, because it allows patients to remain in their social and work environments, and receive treatment with minimal disruption of their lives. Unfortunately, the goals of community mental health movement have not been met. Community treatment requires the availability of expert mental health care in community clinics, halfway houses, sheltered workshops and other community facilities. When these facilities are available deinstitutionalization works. But many communities have never been able to fund the needed facilities. When community mental centers are ill equipped, discharged patients live in undesirable neighborhood, are socially isolated and receive little professional help. See what happened in the developed countries. During 1980s, funds to community centers were cut in the US. As a result, many patients discharged from the hospital came to the communities that were ill prepared to care for their needs. This gave rise to rehospitalization. It is said that nearly ¾th of all hospital admissions involved formerly hospitalized patients. What started as a worthy attempt of moving people out of mental institutions into the community ended in dumping them into a community that was ill prepared to support. Discharged patients became homeless and some of them started engaging in illegal activities such as robbery. Deinstitutionalization can be a boon to personal development if those discharged from the hospitals have a good place to live, sufficient social support and get needed professional help.

PREVENTION OF PSYCHOLOGICAL DISORDERS

You have all heard statements such as "Prevention is better than cure," and "An ounce of prevention is worth a pound of cure." Then the question arises: Can psychological disorders be prevented? If there is scientific information about the cause, course and effect of behavioral disorders, they can be prevented. But as you have seen in this chapter, our knowledge about mental disorders is sketchy. Therefore, we are really not sure of the steps to be taken to achieve the goal of preventing behavioral dysfunctions. Even when we know some of the steps, the society is not willing to take the needed steps. Vaguely it is said that prevention of physical or mental disorder can take place on three levels: primary prevention, secondary prevention and tertiary prevention:

1. ***Primary prevention*** aims at the general reduction of new cases of disorders and it is applicable to everyone in a given population.
2. ***Secondary prevention*** is directed toward a subgroup of the population that is at a higher than average risk for developing a psychological disturbance.
3. ***Tertiary prevention*** focuses on people who are already suffering from some disorder.

These three types of prevention were derived from public health strategies used for understanding and controlling infectious physical diseases and were believed to provide a useful perspective in the mental health area as well. Recently, the proposals were renamed as ***universal interventions, selective interventions*** and ***indicated interventions***.

Universal Interventions

Universal interventions target all members of the general population for the purpose of preventing the development of psychological disturbances. It is done in two ways:

1. Changing conditions that can cause or contribute to psychological disorders.
2. Introducing conditions that foster positive mental health.

The aim is to eradicate the risk factors and establish protective factors. These activities can take place at three levels: biological, psychological and sociocultural strategies. ***Biological strategies*** include efforts to improve physical well-being through good food, exercise and healthy habits, which in turn contribute to physical health. It is hoped that healthy body fosters a healthy mind. ***Psychological strategies*** aim at helping people to inculcate effective skills to solve problems of life, learn to express emotions constructively and to develop satisfying interpersonal relations. In addition, people may be helped to develop an identity for themselves as individual persons and face effectively the problems that occur at various stages of life such as adolescence, adulthood, middle and old age. All these cannot be done successfully without a supportive community. Individual and society cannot be separated. Healthy individuals create a healthy society and healthy society gives rise to healthy individuals. ***Sociocultural strategies*** include a broad spectrum of measures, such as universal public education, socioeconomic planning and ensuring adequate health care for all.

Selective Interventions

Selective interventions are directed toward subgroups that are considered at risk of developing mental disorders. Today, many of our youngsters are exposed to a vibrant environment consisting of attractive television advertising, unhealthy peer influence and negative parental role models. These and other factors encourage youngsters indirectly to take to drugs, alcohol, undesirable sex practices and antisocial behavior, which in turn predispose them to develop behavior disorders. Intervention programs identify high-risk teenagers and take special measures to see that they do not engage in activities such as unsafe sex, or develop drug-based habits. For example, drug abuse can be prevented by interdicting and reducing the supply of drugs, providing treatment for those who have already developed drug problems and alerting citizens to the issues surrounding abuse of alcohol and drugs. Children may be taught the dangers of these unhealthy habits in schools. Teachers, administrators and parents may have to be trained to identify and counter problems with alcohol and drugs. School-based interventions have proved to be effective in preventing and reducing aggressive behavior in children.

Indicated Intervention

Indicated interventions target those at higher risk, people who exhibit some symptoms of a disorder, but not the full-blown disorder. These interventions emphasize the early detection and prompt treatment of maladaptive tendencies in the individual's family and community settings to prevent long-term psychological consequences. For example, someone with minor symptoms of schizophrenia may be advised to take small doses of antipsychotic drugs. It is found that such interventions are in fact effective. Community mental health centers and hospitals can offer indicated interventions.

In short, people may become vulnerable to psychological disorders due to personal factors, situational factors or both. Therefore, it is advisable to approach prevention from two angles. From the personal side, we may emphasize competency-focused prevention and from the environmental side, the situation-focused prevention.

The competency-focused prevention (CFP) can be designed to increase personal resources and coping skills. These programs may help people to strengthen their resistance to stress by improving their social and vocational competencies, enhancing self-confidence and developing strong social relations.

Situation-focused prevention (SFP) can be directed to either reducing or eradicating the environmental causes of dysfunctional behavior or improving situational factors that help prevent the development of disorders. Reduction of familial tensions, improved social relations and a sense of belongingness in the community, organizational climates devoid of conflicts and proper educational facilities for children, have been found to prevent the occurrence of behavioral disorders.

At present, neither the society nor the administrative agencies is showing genuine interest in preventing mental disorders. It may be because we are not sure of the causes of these disorders. Even when the causes are known, we are not sure of the interventions that will succeed in eliminating them. This requires careful research into which type of programs are most effective in preventing which type of problems, in which type of people. Further, the effects of preventive measures cannot be seen immediately; it may be years before we see them. The effects cannot be objectively measured. As a consequence, it is difficult to convince the funding agencies about the effectiveness of preventive measures. Therefore, prevention of mental disorders and fostering mental health remain a challenge to researchers working in the field of psychopathology.

Chapter Summary

Treatment of mental disorders generally falls into two categories: psychological procedures and biomedical techniques. Psychological treatment (psychotherapy) is aimed at reducing troublesome behavior, changing maladaptive behavior, minimizing environmental stress, improving interpersonal competencies, resolving personal conflicts, reducing negative emotions, modifying inaccurate assumptions about self and others and fostering a positive self-image. There are several psychological techniques including psychodynamic, behavioristic, humanistic, cognitive and group approaches.

Psychodynamic procedures are derived from psychoanalysis developed by Freud. Freud's psychoanalytic treatment was directed to help patients achieve insight into their unconscious dynamics that underlie psychological impairments so that they can deal adaptively with their problems. The analyst employed free association, dream interpretation and dealt with resistance and transference. Psychoanalysis was time consuming and costly. Psychodynamic procedures are modified versions of Freudian technique; these are brief and less costly. Therapists focus on the current problems of clients instead of dwelling deep into unconscious childhood experiences as the causes of the present problems. Nowadays, psychoanalytically based procedures, specially designed to improve the client's social and interpersonal skills are being widely used.

Behavioristic therapies try to change maladaptive behavior employing techniques based on principles of learning. One group of behavior therapies is based on Pavlov's classical conditioning procedures. This group includes techniques such as exposure therapy, systematic desensitization and aversion therapy. In exposure therapy, the client is exposed to the threatening (conditioned) stimulus and is prevented from exhibiting avoidance responses, thus leading to extinction. Exposure may be provided *in vivo*, through imagination or through virtual reality. Desensitization procedures are designed to countercondition a response to anxiety-arousing stimuli that is incompatible with anxiety, such as relaxation. Systematic desensitization procedures were popularized by Joseph Wolpe in the treatment of phobia and other anxiety disorders. Aversion therapy is used to establish a conditioned aversion response to a stimulus that triggers the undesirable behavior. A second group of behavior therapy makes use of operant conditioning principles such as reinforcement and punishment. The token economy is a positive reinforcement program designed to strengthen healthy behaviors. Punishment has been used to reduce self-destructive behaviors in disturbed children. Modeling is an important component of social skill training programs, which helps clients learn and rehearse the more useful behavior.

The humanistic therapies are designed to help clients gain insight into their self-worth and value as human beings. Prominent humanistic therapies are Rogers' client-centered therapy and Perls' Gestalt therapy. Client-centered therapy emphasizes three important therapist characteristics that are said to be necessary and sufficient to bring about personality change. These are unconditional positive regard toward the client, empathic understanding of the inner world of the client, and communicating this understanding to the client. It is believed that the supportive environment provided by the therapist enables the client to make accurate self-exploration, which helps in self-acceptance and acceptance of the environment. The goal of Gestalt therapy is to remove blockages to clients' awareness of the wholeness of the immediate experience by making them more aware of their feelings and the ways in which they interact with others. In Gestalt therapy, the clients are actively encouraged (even forced) to express their feelings openly. The assumption is that through fully understanding and overtly expressing oneself as a whole person, one can take responsibility for the feelings and change them for the better.

Cognitive therapies are designed to remove irrational beliefs and negative thoughts that are at the root of psychological impairments. Among cognitive therapies, the two popular forms are Ellis' rational emotive behavior therapy (REBT) and Beck's cognitive therapy (CT). Both procedures focus on discovering and changing maladaptive belief systems and logical errors in thinking that underlie maladaptive behaviors and inappropriate emotional expressions. These techniques are used to treat a wide variety of clinical conditions ranging from depression to anger management. There is evidence to show that REBT and CT are effective in the treatment of a variety of psychological disturbances. Psychotherapy today shows a growing trend toward eclecticism—the combination of various theoretical perspectives and the development of new, more effective therapeutic procedures. Clinicians prefer multimodal therapies.

Contd...

Contd...

Group therapy provides a number of advantages to clients; such as providing opportunities for developing close interpersonal relationships, gaining insight into how to interact with others and how they are perceived by others. Clients can observe how others approach problems in their life. Family therapy assumes that the individual's problems are often reflections of a dysfunctional family system and such systems should be treated as a unit. Marital therapies help couples improve their communications and resolve difficulties in their relationships.

There is no unanimity regarding the effectiveness of psychotherapy. Eysenck asserted that the rate of improvement due to psychotherapy is not more than spontaneous remission. However, recent surveys indicate that clients are helped by psychotherapy and there is improvement in their conditions. Meta-analysis of treatment outcome studies found more improvement in therapy clients and little difference in effectiveness among various therapies. Research suggests that three sets of factors affect the outcome of treatment: client characteristics, therapist characteristics and therapy techniques. Client variables contributing to therapeutic success are openness, self-relatedness and a good match between the nature of the problem and the kind of therapy offered. The relationship between the client and the therapist is the most important determinant of therapeutic success. Factors common to many therapies, such as faith in the therapist, an unthreatening environment for self-exploration and the ability to try out new behaviors, contribute to therapeutic outcome. For female clients, whether the therapist is a man or woman seems less important to the outcome than gender sensitivity.

Drugs have revolutionized the treatment of psychological disorders. Medication and psychotherapy in combination hasten the relief from symptoms. Drug treatments exist for anxiety, schizophrenia and mood disorders. Anxiolytic medications work through their effect on the GABA system to decrease anxiety. The most commonly used antipsychotic drugs are the atypical neuroleptics. These improve patients' conditions and have fewer side effects. Some drugs have undesirable side effects and patients often develop an addiction to the drugs. All of them affect neurotransmission within the brain and they work on specific classes of neurotransmitters. ECT is used less frequently now than in the past and its safety has been increased. The ECT is used primarily to treat severe depression, particularly with patients who exhibit suicidal tendencies. Although ECT can cause some short-term cognitive disturbances, on the whole, it is safe when administered properly. Psychosurgery has become more precise, still it is used as the last resort. Studies have shown that successful therapeutic treatments, whether involving psychotherapy or drugs, are associated with similar alterations of brain functioning.

The introduction of drug therapies that normalize disturbed behavior, as well as the concerns about the deterioration of the life skills during hospitalization, has helped stimulate a move toward deinstitutionalization—the treatment of mental patients in their communities. Deinstitutionalization can work when adequate community treatment is provided. Unfortunately, many communities are unable to fund the needed facilities, resulting in a revolving door of release and rehospitalization. It has created a new generation of homeless people who live on the streets and do not receive needed treatment.

Mental health professionals not only try to cure psychological disorders, but also to prevent them or at least to reduce their severity. Prevention programs may be primary, secondary or tertiary. They may be situation-based or competency-focused, depending on whether they are directed at changing environmental conditions or personal factors. Primary prevention aims at reduction of incidence of disorders in the population. Secondary prevention concentrates on people who are at risk of developing disorders. Tertiary prevention is aimed at people who are suffering from psychological disorders. Thus, we can think of prevention at three levels. There are universal interventions that include biological, psychological and sociocultural strategies to reduce the long-term consequences of having had a disorder; selective interventions that are directed toward reducing the possibility of disorder and fostering positive mental health among those at risk of developing a disorder and indicated interventions that attempt to reduce the impact or duration of a problem that is already there.

Unfortunately, not enough is being done, either by public or private bodies, in the field of prevention of psychological disorders. There are several reasons for this impasse. One of them is that experts are not sure of the causes or cures of mental disorders. Secondly, preventive measures take a long time to become effective and the funding agencies have no patience to wait; they want immediate results. Thirdly, people are not as much worried about mental disorders as they do about physical illness; they tolerate psychological disturbances. Fortunately, it is good to see nowadays that international bodies, such as World Health Organization and World Federation for Mental Health, are focusing on mental health issues worldwide.

(Contd.)

Glossary

ABC model of attitude The assumption that each attitude is composed of affect (emotion), behavior and cognition.

Abnormal behavior Any deviant form of behavior that is detrimental to an individual or/ and the group.

Abnormal psychology Area of psychology concerned with the study of causes, cures and prevention of maladaptive behavior.

Absolute limen (threshold) The magnitude of a stimulus that is just enough for an observer to detect its presence at least 50 percent of time; it is also called 'absolute threshold'.

Absolute refractory period The brief interval of time during which the active neuron is absolutely unresponsive to any stimulation, no matter how intense.

Abstinence Refraining from, sex, alcohol and/or other forms of drugs.

Abstinence violation effect A response to a lapse in which an individual blames oneself and comes to the conclusion that he/she is incapable of resisting from engaging in risky acts.

Accommodation The process by which the lens in the eye changes its shape to focus images more clearly on the retina. In Piaget's theory, the process of creating new schemas or modifying existing ones to account for new experiences; changing the cognitive structure to accommodate new information.

Acetylcholine (ACh) An excitatory neurotransmitter found in a variety of locations such as neuromuscular junctions of all skeletal muscles, the ganglia of autonomic nervous system and diffusely throughout the brain.

Achievement motivation A drive possessed by all people in varying degrees to achieve something difficult, to succeed, master, organize ideas or people and to excel oneself and surpass others.

Achievement test A test that measures the degree of proficiency already attained in some specific skill or ability, usually in a school subject.

Acting out A defense mechanism in which an individual reduces anxiety, hostility or any other unpleasant feeling by permitting its expression in overt behavior.

Action potential A change from negative to positive charge in a nerve cell resulting in a nerve impulse.

Activation level A general state of an organism varying from extreme alertness to deep sleep.

Note: Items given in italics are main entries.

Actor-observer effect An overall tendency to attribute the causes of our own behavior to situational factors and the causes of other people's behavior to internal factors or dispositions.

Act psychology A system of psychology proposed by Franz Brentano, which regards psychological phenomena as the acts of a person. The acts are mental processes and are to be studied through phenomenological observation. Brentano studied acts such as sensing, feeling and judging. Act psychology was opposed to Wundt's psychology of contents.

Actualizing tendency In Rogers' theory, the basic tendency to actualize, maintain and enhance the experiencing organism; it moves the person constructively in the direction of fulfillment and wholeness.

Acute stress disorder The disorder that occurs within 4 weeks after a traumatic event and lasts for at least 2 days and a maximum of 4 weeks.

Addictive behavior Any behavior marked by a pathological craving for a substance (drug) or activity; for example, craving for alcohol, tobacco, cocaine or gambling.

Additive color mixture The mixture of lights (not paints). Two spotlights focused on the same spot yield additive mixture; colored sectors of paper rotated on a color wheel also yield an additive mixture.

Adjustment disorder A disorder in which an individual's response to a stressor is maladaptive and occurs within 3 months of the stressor.

Adler, Alfred (1870–1937) An early associate of Freud, who broke away from him and started a system called individual psychology. Adler emphasized the role of society in the development of personality and enriched psychology with concepts such as inferiority feeling, compensation, style of life and social interest. He founded a number a child guidance clinics in Vienna.

Adolescent egocentrism Excessive self-centered thinking found among children during their teenage years.

Adoption studies A research procedure in which adopted children are compared on some characteristics with their biological and adopted parents to determine the strength of the characteristic's genetic component.

Adrenal cortex Outer layer of adrenal gland, which secretes the adrenal steroids and other hormones.

Adrenal glands Endocrine glands located at the upper end of kidneys, which are made up of *adrenal cortex* and *adrenal medulla*.

Adrenaline Hormone secreted by adrenal medulla during emotional excitation, which causes bodily changes such as increase in blood sugar and a rise in blood pressure; also called 'epinephrine'.

Adrenal medulla The central core of adrenal glands, which secretes *adrenaline* (epinephrine) and noradrenaline (norepinephrine).

Adrenocorticotrophic hormone (ACTH) The hormone of the adenohypophysis that stimulates adrenal cortex to produce corticoids; it is also called 'corticotropin'.

Aerobic exercise Brisk activities such as walking, running, swimming and cycling that dramatically increase oxygen consumption over an extended period of time.

Affect Emotion, mood or feeling.

Afferent code The pattern of neural activity that occurs in the central and peripheral nervous system; the pattern corresponds to various aspects of the impinging external stimuli.

Affiliation motivation Desire to be with people, to please and win their affection, enjoy their company and cooperate with them.

Afterimage The image that remains after a stimulus is removed from a sense modality.

Aggression Any behavior ranging from verbal criticism to physical assault that is directed toward an object or person, including self, with the intention to hurt or injure the target.

Agitation Marked restlessness and psychomotor excitement.

Agonist A drug that increases or mimics the activity of a neurotransmitter.

Agoraphobia Fear of being in places or situations where a panic attack may occur and from which escape would be difficult or embarrassing or in which help would be unavailable in the event that some mishap occurred. One suffering from agoraphobia tends to avoid public places out of fear that a panic attack may occur.

A-ha A term used to indicate the emergence of insight in learning.

AIDS Acquired immunodeficiency syndrome; a disease, which gradually weakens and disables the immune system.

Alarm stage First stage of the general adaptation syndrome (GAS), during which an organism mobilizes the defenses to cope with the stressful situation.

Alcoholism An addiction marked by excessive dependence on alcohol to such an extent that it seriously endangers the body and interferes with the person's life adjustments.

Alcohol myopia Inability to think of possible undesirable consequences of behavior when one is under the influence of alcohol intoxication; it is a kind of shortsightedness caused by inability to pay attention to as much information as when sober.

Algorithm In problem solving, a set of rules or a formula using which a problem can be solved more or less mechanically.

Alienation Lack or loss of relationship with others characterized by loneliness, helplessness and a sense of meaninglessness.

All or none law The principle, which states that a nerve impulse is either evoked in full strength or not evoked at all.

Allostatic load The stress carried by the body to maintain equilibrium; maintaining equilibrium within a comfortable range through biological changes has a cost—cumulative wear and tear. As the number or intensity of stressors increases the allostatic load also increases. Allostatic load is determined by environmental demands, genetic predisposition, past experience with stressors and life style.

Alter identity In a patient suffering from dissociative identity disorder, personality other than the host (original) personality.

Alternate forms reliability Similarity of scores on the two forms of the same test administered to the same group of persons; the similarity is estimated in the form of a correlation coefficient.

Altruistic behavior The behavior that implies unselfish concern for the welfare of others even when it sometimes involves risk for the individual who behaves that way.

Alzheimer's disease A rare irreversible brain disorder whose prominent symptoms are loss of memory, confused thinking, impaired judgment, withdrawal and progressive mental deterioration.

Ambivalent attachment An attachment pattern in which the child becomes anxious when the caregiver leaves, is upset during the caregiver's absence, but both seeks and resists contact with him or her after return.

Amnesia Any loss of memory, partial or total; a person may forget his/her own identity and may not recognize familiar people and places.

Amniocentesis A technique for diagnosing fetal abnormalities involving examination of extracted fetal cells from the amniotic sac of pregnant women.

Amphetamines Drugs that produce a psychologically stimulating and energizing effect.

Amygdala A collection of almond-shaped nuclei, which lie in front of the hippocampus in the limbic system of the human brain. Amygdala is implicated in the regulation of emotion, especially fear.

Amyotrophic lateral sclerosis (ALS) An incurable degenerative disease of the nervous system.

Anal stage In Freud's theory of psychosexual development, the second stage that occurs about the age of 1 to 3 years; during this period, pleasure is derived physically by stimulation of anal area and psychologically from parental rewards and attention during toilet training. Anal stage is divided into two parts: the anal expulsive stage during which the pleasure is derived from defecation and the anal retentive stage in which the pleasure comes by withholding the feces. Anal fixation has important implications for later personality development. For example, anal expulsive personality is characterized by messiness, lack of self-discipline and carelessness. Anal retentive personality is characterized by perfectionism, excessive need for neatness and punctuality.

Anal triad Three bipolar traits: miserliness-over generosity, stubbornness-acquiescence and orderliness-sloppiness, which develop as a consequence of anal fixation.

Analytical psychology Carl Jung's system of psychology that minimizes the role of sexuality, aggression, childhood experience and emphasizes instead religious, mystical and inherited racial factors (archetypes) in the formation and functioning of personality; the major stress of Jung's psychology is on the preparation for the future.

Androgens Male sex hormones, which are responsible for the development and maintenance of male characteristics such as beard growth and masculine voice. These hormones (principally, but not exclusively testosterone) are produced by the testes.

Angell, James Rowland (1869–1949) American psychologist who molded the functionalistic movement started by William James and John Dewey into a working school, and incidentally made the department of psychology at Chicago University the most important and influential place. Later, as President of Yale University, he was instrumental in starting the Yale Institute of Human Relations that nourished several eminent psychologists who conducted groundbreaking researches.

Angiotensin A substance that circulates with blood and is believed to trigger thirst.

Anhedonia A condition characterized by lack of ability to enjoy things and the pleasures of life and loss of interest in living; it is a symptom depression.

Animism Tendency to attribute life to inanimate objects such as clouds, plants, or anything that moved.

Anorexia nervosa A severe eating disorder in which people refuse to eat because of the fear of becoming fat.

Antabuse Any drug that is used in the treatment of alcoholism; for example, disulfiram causes violent vomiting when followed by ingestion of alcohol and prevents the immediate return to drinking.

Antagonist A drug that inhibits or decreases the activity of a neurotransmitter.

Anterograde amnesia Loss or impairment of the ability to form or store information in memory for events following an accident, trauma or shock.

Antianxiety drugs The drugs that are primarily used to alleviate anxiety.

Antibodies Substances circulating in the blood, which are coded for detection of and binding to a particular antigen.

Anticathexis The use of psychic energy by the ego to oppose, inhibit or delay a dangerous or immoral cathexis.

Anticipatory nausea and vomiting (ANV) Conditioned nausea and vomiting that occurs when cancer patients are exposed to stimuli associated with their treatment.

Antidepressant drugs The drugs that are primarily used to elevate mood and relieve depression.

Antidiuretic hormone (ADH) Hormone (vasopressin) secreted by posterior pituitary gland that signals the kidney to reabsorb water into the bloodstream instead of secreting it as urine.

Antigen A foreign body, such as a virus or bacteria or an internal disorder (a tumor) that can trigger an immune response.

Antimanic drugs (mood stabilizes) Drugs such as lithium used in the treatment of bipolar disorders.

Antipsychotic drugs Medicines that alleviate or decrease the intensity of psychotic symptoms such as delusions and hallucinations.

Antisocial personality disorder One of the personality disorders characterized by continued violation of societal rules; the individuals display no regard for the moral and ethical principles and the rights of others.

Anxiety A vague, unpleasant emotional state characterized by intense fear and physiological arousal.

Anxiety disorders A group of psychological disorders in which *anxiety* and related symptoms are at the core impairing the person's day-to-day life. Basically, the anxiety is excessive and inappropriate to the situation.

Aphasia Loss or impairment of the ability to use language—reading, writing, speaking. It may result from brain injury or disease.

Approach-approach conflict A conflict in which an individual is attracted at the same time by two incompatible, but equally attractive (positive) goals.

Approach-avoidance conflict A conflict in which an individual is both attracted and repelled by the same goal.

Aptitude tests Psychological tests that measure an individual's potential ability; such tests indicate whether a person can profit from training in an occupation or skill.

Archetypes Jung's term for universal thought forms, inherited from past generations that predispose people to apprehend the world in particular ways. Archetypes are said to be the results of oft repeated experiences of humanity and residing in the collective unconscious. The major archetypes studied by Jung include anima, animus, persona, shadow, self, mother, father, husband, wife, child, the wise old man, energy and God.

Aristotle (384–322 BC) One of the greatest Greek thinkers known for his contributions to the field of physical and biological sciences, politics, esthetics, logic, metaphysics and psychology; he believed that sensory experience to be the basis of all knowledge. Many historians rate Aristotle as the greatest intellectual ever lived.

Army General Classification Test A group test of intelligence developed during World War II to classify army recruits according to their ability to learn military duties. The test consists of three types of items: vocabulary, arithmetic and block counting.

Arteriosclerosis It is a condition in which the walls of the coronary arteries (or others) thicken, harden and lose their elasticity.

Artificialism A term used by Piaget to refer to children's tendency to attribute the occurrence of natural phenomena, such as sun or rain, to artificial causes or to human intentions.

Assertiveness therapy A technique of behavior therapy used to help people to become more assertive in their interpersonal interactions.

Assimilation In Piaget's theory, the process of making new information part of already existing schema or framework or the use of existing schema to identify and classify new information; in short, assimilation is the process of integrating new information into a set of already existing information.

Association areas The areas of the cerebral cortex that do not have sensory or motor functions, but are involved in the processing of neural activities that underlie higher mental activities such as perception, thinking, reasoning, language and judgment.

Associationism One of the earliest theoretical perspectives in psychology, which made association of ideas the fundamental principle of mental life. Association of ideas was the major concern of British philosophers such as Locke, Berkeley, Hume, Hartley, James Mill and JS Mill.

Associative network The view that long-term memory is organized as a huge network of associated ideas and concepts.

Asthenic A body type proposed by Kretschmer referring to slight, slender, long-boned people who are prone to develop schizoid personality.

Atherosclerosis A disease condition in which fatty, fibrous plaques narrow the opening of an artery, threatening blood supply to the heart, brain or other vital organs.

Athletic One of the body types proposed by Kretschmer that is strong and sturdy with a predisposition more toward schizophrenic than the manic depressive type of adjustment.

Atrophy Wasting away or shrinking of bodily organs.

Attachment An affectional bond between an infant and the primary caregiver; it is reflected in such behaviors as following the caregiver and crying when the care giver is absent.

Attention The focal activity of consciousness leading to heightened awareness toward a limited range of stimuli.

Attention deficit/hyperactivity disorder (ADHD) A childhood disorder characterized by difficulties that interfere with task-oriented behavior; prominent characteristics are impulsivity, excessive motor activity, difficulties in sustaining attention.

Attitude An evaluative tendency (positive or negative) toward objects, persons and/or events. Attitude is the extensively researched topic in social psychology.

Attribution The process by which we attribute causes and meanings to other people's behavior, our own behavior and to environmental events.

Audition The act of hearing.

Auditory area The sensory area in the temporal lobe of the brain involved in hearing.

Auditory nerve The VIII cranial nerve that transmits auditory information to the brain.

Auditory perception Perceiving the direction and distance of the source of sound stimuli.

Authoritarian parents The parents who emphasize control and obedience in bringing up children; they are generally cold, unresponsive and rejecting. Their children tend to have low self-esteem, perform poorly in school and are less popular with their peers.

Authoritarian submission An authoritarian personality trait that emphasizes the need for unquestioning, blind submission to a dominant leader or source of authority.

Authoritative parents The parents who combine respect for a child's individuality with an effort to instill social values in child rearing. They are also controlling, but warm, caring and supportive. Such parents establish clear rules and consistently reward their children when the rules are complied with. Their children tend to have high self-esteem, achieve good grades in school and show fewer conduct problems.

Autism A developmental disorder characterized by lack of normal social interaction, impaired imagination and communication and restricted range of abilities and interests. The person will be absorbed in fantasy exclusively without any interest in reality. It was first believed to be a symptom of schizophrenia, but autism is now seen in other conditions such as senile psychosis, Kanner's syndrome (early infantile autism) and some cases of depression.

Autoclitic behavior Skinner's term for behavior that provides a grammatical framework for verbal behavior.

Autoerotic stages The early stages of psychosexual development during which the child derives pleasure by stimulating his/her own erogenous body parts.

Autonomic nervous system (ANS) The branch of the peripheral nervous system that stimulates the body's involuntary muscles and internal organs; it consists primarily of ganglia connected with the brain stem and the spinal cord. ANS is subdivided into sympathetic and parasympathetic systems.

Autonomic reactivity An individual's characteristic degree of emotional reactivity to stress.

Autonomous morality stage A stage of moral development during which intentionality replaces the consequences of an act as the basis for moral judgment (Piaget).

Autonomy A need to get free, to shake off restraint and break out of confinement.

Autosomes The 22 pairs of human chromosomes other than the sex chromosomes.

Availability heuristic A strategy (heuristic) for making judgments on the basis of how easily some information can be brought to mind. Information that can be readily remembered is viewed as more prevalent or important than information that cannot be remembered.

Aversion therapy See *Aversive conditioning*.

Aversive conditioning A therapeutic technique of systematically and repeatedly pairing an aversive stimulus (an electric shock) with the occurrence of thoughts, feelings or behaviors that a client considers undesirable and wishes to eliminate; same as aversive therapy.

Aversive stimulus Any unpleasant stimulus that induces an avoidance reaction.

Avoidance-avoidance conflict A conflict in which a person is caught between two negative goals ("devil and deep sea"). As an individual tries to avoid one, he will be closer to the other and vice versa.

Avoidance learning An organism's learning a response to avoid an unpleasant stimulus.

Avoidant attachment A kind of attachment in which, the child neither cries when separated from the primary caregiver nor seeks contact with him or her after return.

Avoidant personality disorder A personality disorder characterized by extreme inhibition and introversion, hypersensitivity to criticism and rejection, limited social interaction, and low esteem.

Axon An extension from the cell body of the neuron that carries nerve impulses away from the cell body to other neurons.

Backward conditioning Presenting the conditioned stimulus after the unconditioned stimulus; little or no conditioning occurs from such pairing.

Bandura, Albert (born 1925) Canadian-born American psychologist well known for his social cognitive approach in psychology; he explains behavior in terms of continuous reciprocal interaction between cognitive, behavioral, and environmental determinants. His conception of humans neither casts people into the role of powerless objects controlled by environmental forces nor free agents who can become whatever they choose. Both people and their environment are reciprocal determinants of each other.

Barbiturates Drugs that act as depressants to calm the individual and induce sleep.

Base rate The normal frequency of occurrence of something.

Base rate fallacy In making judgments, people tend to ignore or underscore base rate information, which is information about how prevalent something is in general. This is a common phenomenon; for example, people are afraid to make an airplane journey despite the much higher base rate of accidents on roads than in the skies.

Basic anxiety The feeling of being alone in an unfriendly and threatening world. According to Horney, basic anxiety includes three basic components: helplessness, aggressiveness and detachment. Basic anxiety is the product of pathogenic social influence during childhood, notably parental errors and therefore is wholly avoidable.

Basilar membrane A membrane within the cochlea supporting the organ of Corti in the ear. Movements of the basilar membrane stimulate the hair cells of the organ of Corti producing the neural effects of auditory stimulation.

Basket nerve endings Afferent nerve endings surrounding the roots of body hair, which respond to touch on the hair.

Beck, Aaron Tomkin (born 1921) An American psychiatrist who developed an insight-focused treatment procedure called cognitive therapy, which emphasizes changing people's negative thoughts and maladaptive beliefs. Beck assumes that to understand the nature of an emotional episode or disturbance, it is essential to focus on the cognitive content of an individual's reaction to the upsetting event or stream of thoughts. The goal of cognitive therapy is to change the way people think by using their automatic thoughts to reach the core schemata and begin to introduce the idea of restructuring the schemata. This is done by encouraging clients to gather and weigh the evidence in support of their beliefs.

Behavior-outcome expectation The subjective likelihood that a particular consequence will occur after a particular response in a given situation.

Behavioral activation system (BAS) A neural system in the brain that is activated by cues indicating potential reward and positive need gratification; activity of this neural system causes an individual to begin or to increase movement toward positive goals in anticipation of pleasure.

Behavioral activation treatment A therapy for depression that engages clients in life activities designed to increase positive reinforcement in their lives.

Behavioral inhibition system (BIS) A neural system in the brain, which responds to stimuli that signals potential pain, absence of reward and punishment; activity in this system produces fear, inhibition and avoidance behaviors.

Behavioral neuroscience A field within psychology that studies brain activities underlying behavior and experience.

Behavioral signatures A term used to refer to consistent ways of responding in particular classes of situations.

Behavior genetics A field of study engaged in investigating genetic basis of individual difference in psychological functioning.

Behavior modification Therapeutic techniques based on learning principles, especially operant conditioning.

Behavior therapy Therapeutic techniques developed based on the principles of learning.

Being values In Maslow's writings, growth-oriented needs whose purpose is to extend individual's experience and enrich life.

Bell, Sir Charles (1774–1842) British physiologist who demonstrated that sensory nerves enter the posterior (dorsal) roots of the spinal cord and the motor nerves emerge from the anterior (ventral) roots. See *Bell-Magendie law*.

Bell-Magendie law The principle that the ventral roots of the spinal cord are motor and the dorsal roots are sensory. The law was enunciated by Bell in 1811 and Magendie in 1822 and hence the name Bell-Magendie law.

Bereavement The emotional reactions (depression accompanied by poor appetite, sleeplessness and sense of worthlessness) experienced after the death of a loved one.

Bestiality A perverted form of sexual behavior involving sexual contact between humans and animals.

Big Five Factors See *Big Five Factors Model*.

Bilingualism The simultaneous learning or use of two languages during childhood.

Binet, Alfred (1857–1911) French psychologist who developed (along with Theodore Simon) the first test of intelligence; Binet was the father of experimental psychology in France.

Binet-Simon Scale of Intelligence The first successful intelligence test developed in 1905, which had items grouped in age levels. The test served as a forerunner for several other intelligence tests.

Binge-eating disorder A form of non-purging bulimia nervosa whereby binging (uncontrolled overeating) is not accompanied by inappropriate compensatory behavior (purging) to limit weight gain.

Binge eating/purging type An eating disorder in which a person overeats and later purges because of the fear of overweight.

Binocular (retinal) disparity The binocular depth perception cue produced by the projection of slightly different images of an object on the retina of the two eyes.

Binocular cues of depth perception Cues for depth perception that involve both the eyes such as retinal (binocular) disparity and convergence.

Biological amnesia Memory loss caused by some kind of damage to the brain tissue; also called 'organic amnesia'.

Biopsychosocial model The model of mental disorders that emphasizes the interacting roles of biological, psychological and sociocultural factors in the causation of psychopathology.

Bipolar cells A layer of cells in the retina that transfers excitation from rods and cones to ganglion cells of the optic nerve.

Bipolar disorders Mood disorders in which a person experiences both manic and depressive episodes. In *bipolar I disorder* the person experiences both manic and major depressive episodes. In *bipolar* II *disorder* a person experiences both hypomanic and major depressive episodes.

Bipolar factors In studies of personality, traits that can be described as varying between two opposite poles. For example, introversion-extraversion is a bipolar factor.

Bipolar I disorder See *Bipolar disorders.*

Bipolar II disorder See *Bipolar disorders.*

Bisexuals Persons who are attracted sexually to both males and females.

Blind spot A small insensitive area in the retina near the fovea where the nerve fibers from the ganglion cells join together to form the optic nerve; it is also called 'optic disk'.

Body dysmorphic disorder A somatoform disorder in which the patient is preoccupied with an imagined defect in appearance. The patient's commonly complain of wrinkles, skin spots, excessive body hair and shape of the nose.

Body language Cues provided by the position, posture, gesture and movement of body or body parts; such non-language cues often provide information about a person's inner feelings, emotional states and likes or dislikes toward others.

Borderline personality disorder One of the personality disorders characterized by unstable behavior, affect, personal identity and interpersonal relationships.

Bottom-up processing Name given to cognitive processing that begins with the analysis of stimulus elements and work up to the brain's integration of them into a unified perception.

Brainstem Structures lying near the core of the brain between the spinal cord and the cerebrum; the structures that constitute brainstem are the medulla, pons and the midbrain.

Brentano, Franz (1838–1917) A German philosopher, psychologist and priest, who is regarded as the father of phenomenology and act psychology; Brentano exerted profound influence upon some of his students, such as Carl Stumpf, Anton Marty, Edmund Husserl and Alexius Meinong, who distinguished themselves in psychology.

Brightness A dimension of color that describes its nearness in brilliance to white (as contrasted with black); a bright color reflects more light than a dark one.

Brightness constancy A perceptual tendency to see a familiar object as of the same brightness regardless of light and shadow that change its stimulus properties.

Broca, Paul (1824–1880) French physiologist, surgeon and anthropologist who discovered the area of articulate speech production in the vicinity of the third frontal convolution in the left hemisphere of the brain in 1861. The area has come to be called *'Broca's area'*.

Broca's aphasia Partial or total loss of ability to produce language presumed to be due to damage to the Broca's area.

Broca's area A cortical area involved in the processing of language functions. The area is located in the inferior frontal gyrus of the left-hemisphere for a left-handed person (on rare occasion it is found in the corresponding area on the right).

Bulimia nervosa Eating disorder characterized by repeated episodes of binge eating followed by misuse of laxatives and self-induced vomiting.

Burnout A state of physical and psychological exhaustion produced by long-term exposure to an emotionally demanding (organizational) situation.

Bystander apathy Total indifference and lack of concern on the part of individuals who watch an emergency; it is failure to help a stranger in need or distress.

Bystander effect Research finding that people are much less likely to help in an emergency (or indeed to take action of any sort) when they are with others than when they are alone. Being with others sometimes results in the group members defining the situation as less critical than they would if they were alone. Being with others also diffuses the responsibility for helping and reduces the speed of responding. See *Diffusion of responsibility*.

Bystander intervention Helping a stranger in distress; psychologists have studied factors affecting whether or not a person will be helped by others nearby.

Cannon, Walter B (1871–1945) American physiologist, who made significant contributions to the physiology of hunger and thirst, proposed a theory of emotion and introduced the concept of homeostasis.

Cannon-Bard theory of emotion A theory of emotion which proposed that both physiological and emotional arousals occur simultaneously and are produced by the same nerve stimulus.

Cardinal trait In GW Allport's theory, an extremely strong characteristic that plays an important role in shaping an individual's total personality; later Allport called it cardinal disposition.

Carr, Harvey (1873–1954) One of the leaders of functionalism, who along with JR Angell, made the department of psychology at Chicago University one of the best in the United States of America. During his tenure, some 130 students earned their doctorates in psychology.

Case study Detailed study of a single individual, group or event.

Castration anxiety In Freud's theory, a boy's fear that he will be emasculated by his father as a punishment for his libidinal attachment to his mother; it occurs during the latter part of phallic stage. The castration anxiety helps in the resolution of *Oedipus complex*.

Castration complex The counterpart of male castration anxiety in female is penis envy (see this entry). Freud included both these phenomena (castration anxiety and penis envy) collectively under castration complex.

Catatonic schizophrenia A subtype of schizophrenia marked by alternating agitated excitement and stuporous states.

Cathexis In Freudian theory, the term refers to investing of libidinal energy in an object, person or activity.

Cattell, James McKeen (1860–1944) One of the early American students of Wundt, Cattell founded the psychological laboratory in Pennsylvania University in 1889. Later he joined Columbia University where he trained a number of psychologists, such as EL Thorndike, EK Strong and several others. He founded Psychological Review, an important journal of psychology in 1894, and started Psychological Corporation in 1921. Cattell coined the term "mental test" and was a pioneer in the study of individual differences.

Cattell, Raymond B (1905–1998) British-American psychologist, who proposed an influential theory of personality and a theory of intelligence, both based on factor analysis. He was the author of several psychological tests and books.

Causalgia Severe burning pain (not caused by heat) associated with nerve injury; the pain occurs after a wound has healed and damaged nerves have regenerated.

Cell body The integral life-supporting **component of a** neuron; also called 'soma', it contains the nucleus and other related structures. When the cell body is damaged the whole neuron dies.

Cellular dehydration thirst The thirst drive triggered by loss of water in the cells.

Centering In Piaget's theory of cognitive development, the tendency of preoperational children to focus on one aspect of a situation and neglect others; also called 'centration'.

Central executive In the Baddeley model of memory, the component of working memory that controls the processing of information; it is responsible for coordinating the other subsystems in the working memory, receiving and processing stored information and filtering out distracting thoughts.

Central fissure A *fissure* of each cerebral hemisphere that separates the frontal lobe from the parietal lobe; it is also called fissure of Rolando.

Central nervous system In vertebrates, the brain and the spinal cord and their associated neural processes.

Central route (processing) Interpretation of information that is characterized by thoughtful consideration of the issues and arguments used to persuade.

Central traits In GW Allport's theory, characteristics that are important in shaping personality, but not as pervasive as *cardinal traits*; also called central disposition.

Centroid technique A technique of factor analysis used by Thurstone to determine the factors that constitute complex constructs such as personality or intelligence.

Cephalocaudal sequence A principle stating that development proceeds in a head-to-tail direction; upper parts of the body develop before the lower parts.

Cerebellum A large structure of the *hindbrain* that mediates postural responses to input from the vestibular senses, muscle spindles and the cerebral cortex.

Cerebral cortex The surface covering of grey matter that forms the outermost layer of the *cerebrum*.

Cerebrotonic One of the three components of temperament proposed by Sheldon. A cerebrotonic is restrained, self-conscious and fearful.

Cerebrum The largest structure of the brain consisting two hemispheres separated by the longitudinal fissure and connected by three cerebral commissures. It is involved in the processing and interpretation of sensory input, control over voluntary motor activity, planning and executing of action, thinking, reasoning and consciousness.

Chaining In operant conditioning, establishing a sequence of responses by reinforcing each response that leads to the performance of the next response.

Child sexual abuse Sexual activity involving a child and an adult person.

Choleric According to Hippocrates, a person who is irritable, touchy and easily angered.

Chromosomes Small paired particles (coils of DNA) found in the cells of the body. Chromosomes carry the *genes*, the ultimate genetic determiners. In humans there are 46 chromosomes, arranged in 23 pairs.

Chronological age (CA) Age from birth.

Chunking Organization of learning material in such a way as to include more information per unit; combining individual items into larger units of meaning.

Cingulotomy A form of psychosurgery in which certain selected fibers in the cingulate cortex are severed to provide relief from symptoms to patients suffering from severe bipolar and obsessive-compulsive (anxiety) disorders.

Clairvoyance A term in parapsychology referring to the extrasensory perception of objects or events in the past, present or future.

Classical conditioning A simple form of learning (first demonstrated by Pavlov) in which a previously neutral stimulus (conditioned stimulus) when paired with another stimulus (unconditioned stimulus), which naturally elicits a response (unconditioned response) several times, acquires the capacity to elicit the response similar to unconditioned response; this response is called 'conditioned response'.

Client-centered therapy Humanistic psychotherapy developed by Rogers; it assumes that a client's inherent potential for growth will be released when unconditional positive regard in a non-threatening warm atmosphere is offered. The therapy involves non-judgmental listening and reflecting to the client his own feelings.

Clinical psychology A branch of psychology concerned with the diagnosis and treatment of psychological problems without using drugs.

Cochlea A snail-shaped bony structure in the inner ear where sound is translated into nerve impulses. Cochlea is a bony cavity containing three fluid-filled canals (the scala vestibuli, scala tympani and scala media). The canals are separated from each other by the Reissner's membrane and the basilar membrane.

Cognition A broad term used to refer to such higher mental activities as remembering, conceiving, thinking, reasoning, problem solving and in short, information processing.

Cognitive-affective personality system (CAPS) A theory in which personality is defined in terms of the cognitive-affective person variables and the interaction among them. According to CAPS theory, how a person behaves depends on many factors, including the features of the situation, how these features are encoded, the expectancies and beliefs that are activated, the goals that are relevant, the emotions that might occur and the plans and the self-regulatory processes that help determine the behavior.

Cognitive appraisal The process of making judgments about situations, personal capabilities, likely consequences and personal meaning of consequences; that is, the interpretations and meanings that are attached to sensory stimuli, which influence what emotions are evoked and how we deal with them.

Cognitive behaviorism A behavioral approach proposed by Bandura that incorporates cognitive concepts, suggesting that the environment influences our behavior by affecting our thoughts and giving us information.

Cognitive behavior therapy A form of therapy that combines behavioral techniques such as gradual exposure, with cognitive techniques that focus on challenging and correcting faulty ways of thinking.

Cognitive dissonance A state of internal tension brought about by conflicting attitudes and behavior.

Cognitive dissonance theory Festinger's theory, which suggests that people are motivated to resolve discrepancies between their attitudes and behavior.

Cognitive map A mental representation of the spatial layout of an area (such as a maze).

Cognitive neuroscience An area of psychology that is interested in the study of brain processes underlying mental activities.

Cognitive perspective Approach to psychology that considers human beings as rational information processors and problem solvers; its main focus is mental processes that influence behavior.

Cognitive psychology An area of psychology that is engaged in the study of higher mental processes such as memory, attention, perception, thinking, reasoning and planning.

Cognitive relaxation A state of mental rest and relaxation produced by meditation or similar techniques.

Cognitive restructuring A stress-reduction procedure involving attempts to detect, dispute and change maladaptive or irrational thoughts that produce negative emotions.

Cohesiveness The tendency of members of a group to stick together or to be united.

Cohorts Group of people born in the same year.

Collective unconscious According to Jung, a part of the unconscious that consists of racial memories an individual inherits from subhuman and human ancestors; it is the home of archetypes, which are the major determinants of behavior.

Collectivism A cultural characteristic that emphasizes the good of the group rather than the individual goals.

Color constancy The tendency for a colored object to look the same under wide variations in lighting conditions and viewing conditions.

Communicator credibility The extent to which the audience views the communicator as trustworthy based on his/her expertise.

Community psychology An area of psychology that emphasizes the improvement of the welfare of community members and their quality of life.

Comorbidity The simultaneous existence of two or more disorders.

Companionate love A love relationship characterized by commitment and intimacy; it indicates an individual's concern for the well-being of the partner.

Comparative psychology An area of psychology engaged in the study of subhuman species for the purpose of determining the similarities and differences of behavior among them.

Compliance Conforming behavior that occurs in response to a direct request from others.

Compulsion Uncontrollable urge to repeat an act often triggered by an obsessive thought or image.

Computerized axial tomography (CAT) A non-invasive technique of studying brain; narrow beams of X-rays are passed repeatedly through the brain tissues and the results are analyzed and combined by a computer to provide pictures of brain structures from many different angles.

Concept An abstract idea derived from the grouping of objects in terms of some common property.

Concordance A term used in genetics to denote the likelihood that two people (a twin pair) possess or lack a particular characteristic.

Concrete operational stage The third stage in Piaget's theory of cognitive development (7 to 12 years of age) during which children can perform basic cognitive operations concerning problems that involve tangible objects and events.

Concurrent validity One of the types of validity determined by comparing (correlating the scores of) a new test with another test that has been established as measuring similar psychological operations.

Conditioned aversion 1) An acquired dislike of and negative reaction toward something (such as a food). 2) A behavior therapy technique in which the presence of an inappropriate, gratifying stimulus such as alcohol is paired with a negative effect such as nausea or shock.

Conditioned response (CR) A response that is established by pairing it with a neutral (unconditioned) stimulus that previously elicited a similar response.

Conditioned stimulus (CS) A neutral stimulus that has been paired with an unconditioned stimulus to bring about a response formerly produced only by the unconditioned stimulus.

Conditions of worth Internalized standards of self-worth developed from conditional positive regard received from others.

Conduct disorder A psychiatric disorder referring to an individual's chronic and habitual maladaptive behavior. People with conduct disorder have no regard for the rights of others and they violate important social norms.

Conduction deafness The deafness resulting from failure in the transmission of sound waves to the cochlea.

Cones The photoreceptors in the retina that mediate color vision.

Confederate An accomplice of the experimenter who poses as a participant in the experiment, but behaves in ways predetermined by the experimenter.

Confirmation bias The tendency to seek and accept information that we like instead of critically examining it.

Conflict A psychological condition produced when two or more incompatible motives are aroused simultaneously.

Conformity The tendency to agree with the behavior or opinion of the group; generally we tend to fall in line with others.

Confounding When two variables in an experiment vary together in such a way that the effects of one cannot be separated from the effects of the other, confounding is said to occur. Any variable that systematically varies with the independent variable is called 'confounding variable'.

Congruence In Rogers' theory of personality, symbolizing in consciousness accurately organismic experience; compare with *incongruence*.

Conjugal love The love between husband and wife.

Consciousness Awareness of what is happening around us; consciousness involves selective attention to our sensations, thoughts and feelings.

Consensus The extent to which actions by one person are also shown by others.

Conservation In Piaget's theory, phenomenon of perceiving the basic properties of objects (mass or quantity) as remaining the same even though their outward appearance has changed.

Consistency The extent to which an individual responds to a given stimulus or situation in the same way on different occasions.

Constant Anything that does not vary or is not permitted to vary.

Construct validity Establishing that a specific test measures the construct (such as for example, emotional intelligence) that it is designed to measure. Unlike other validities, there are no objective measures of construct validity. It involves a set of procedures for evaluating the degree to which the test items capture the hypothetical quality or trait the test is designed to measure.

Consumer psychology A branch of applied social psychology dealing with the principles and motives underlying people's buying behavior.

Contact comforts The infant's innate tendency to derive pleasure from contact with another body, especially the mother or primary caregiver.

Content In Rorschach, a category of response based on the content of the blot.

Content validity Determining the validity of a test based on the extent to which the items represent the population of items from which they are selected.

Context-dependent memory The phenomenon that it is easier to remember material in the same environment where it was originally learned.

Continuous reinforcement A schedule of reinforcement in which every response of particular type the organism makes is reinforced.

Contraprepared behavior Responses which, for a certain organism, is almost impossible to learn; compare with *prepared behavior*.

Control group A group in an experiment that is matched with the experimental group in all possible respects except that it is not exposed to the independent variable.

Convergence The turning of the eyes inward to focus on an object that is being viewed binocularly; it is an effective binocular cue for depth perception.

Convergent thinking The thinking concerned with a particular end result in which the thinker gathers information relevant to the problem and then proceeds by reasoning to solve the problem.

Conversion disorder Psychiatric condition in which a person suddenly suffers from serious symptoms such as loss of skin sensation, blindness or paralysis that have no physiological basis.

Coping self-efficacy Belief of an individual pertaining to his/her own ability to cope with stress.

Corpus callosum A broad band of myelinated nerve fibers that connect the right and left hemispheres; corpus callosum allows the two hemispheres to communicate with each other.

Correlation See *Correlation coefficient*.

Correlational research A research procedure in which there is no manipulation of the independent variable; only, two or more dependent variables are measured to identify the possible relationship between them.

Correlation coefficient A number that expresses the degree and direction of the relationship between two variables. The value of the correlation coefficient may range from – 1 to + 1. When it is – 1, it indicates perfect negative correlation; that is, the increases in one variable are systematically associated with decreases in the other. When it is + 1, it indicates perfect positive correlation; that is, the increases in one are systematically associated with the increases in the other. When the coefficient is zero, it means that the changes in one are unrelated to the changes in the other. There are a number of different procedures to calculate the coefficient depending on the nature of the data. The most often used statistic is the Pearson's product-moment correlation coefficient, whose symbol is r. When there is a relationship, it can be used for making predictions about the expected value of one variable given the known value of the other. The stronger the relationship, the greater the confidence in the accuracy of prediction.

Counterconditioning The process of conditioning an incompatible response to a particular stimulus to eliminate an undesirable response; it is a procedure commonly used in systematic desensitization.

Countertransference In psychoanalysis, an unconscious displacement of emotion by the analyst to the patient; countertransference tends to interfere with therapy.

Creative thinking Mental processes that lead to answers, solutions, ideas, artistic forms or scientific theories that are unique and novel.

Creativity Creating something new and useful.

Criterion-related validity The extent to which a psychological test score correlates with some non-test behavior (criterion) assumed to be influenced by the construct measured by the test.

Criterion A standard against which a test score is evaluated.

Critical period A stage in the development during which the organism is optimally ready to learn certain response patterns. Exposure to certain stimuli is required during the critical period for normal growth to occur.

Cross-cultural psychology A branch of psychology concerned with the comparative study of behavior across cultures and subcultures.

Cross-gender identification Identifying with a member of the opposite sex by adopting the dress, hair style, speech and gesture.

Cross-sectional method Study of samples of different ages or developmental levels at one point of time.

Crystallized intelligence According to RB Cattell, the type of intelligence involved in applying what has already been learned.

Culture The shared beliefs, customs, values, traditions and expectations about the appropriate ways to behave in certain situations prevalent in a society; the way a certain society lives.

Cutaneous sense Receptors located just beneath the surface of the skin serving the sensations of pressure, pain, cold and warmth.

Cyclothymic disorder Mild mood disorder characterized by cyclical periods of hypomania and depressive episodes.

Dark adaptation The process of adjusting of the eyes for low intensities of illumination; the totally dark adapted eye will be one million times as sensitive as the normally illuminated eye.

Death instinct In psychoanalysis, one of the two groups of instincts that is at the root of aggression and destruction, including self-destruction; Freud called it '*Thanatos*'.

Debriefing Informing the participants of an experiment what it was all about and when necessary, revealing any deception that might have been an element in the study.

Decay theory A theory of forgetting that learned material leaves a trace in the brain, which in the long run, will disappear unless it is kept alive by use.

Decentering In Piaget's theory, the ability to think simultaneously about several aspects of a situation; compare with *centering*.

Decibel (dB) A logarithmic measure of sound intensity. A whisper is approximately 10 decibels; a conversation 60 decibels and the thunder about 120 decibels.

Declarative memory The memory for factual knowledge; it consists of two subcategories: *episodic memory*, which is memory for personal events and *semantic memory*, which is memory for knowledge of general facts and language.

Deductive reasoning A logical operation, which proceeds from the general to the particular; reasoning from a general principle to a specific case.

Deep structure In linguistics, a layer of meaning that underlies the surface layer of a sentence as given by the actual words.

Defense mechanisms Unconscious strategies used by the ego to cope up with and protect from anxiety and traumatic experience; the commonly used defense mechanisms are repression, rationalization and projection.

Deindividuation A state of increased anonymity; under such state the individual may behave in disinhibited manner, especially when in group.

Deinstitutionalization A policy intended to reduce the number of patients in mental hospitals by shifting them from inpatient care to community based outpatient facilities.

Delayed conditioning A classical conditioning procedure in which the conditioned stimulus begins several seconds or more before the onset of the unconditioned stimulus and continues with it until the response occurs.

Delayed reinforcement Offering reward long after the response was emitted.

Delusion A false belief opposed to reality, but maintained in spite of logical persuasion and strong evidence to the contrary.

Demand characteristics Cues inadvertently provided by the researcher during an experiment concerning the purpose of the study or the behavior expected from participants. The term refers to *confounding* features in a study that contaminate the results.

Dementia A generalized deterioration of psychological operations such as memory, understanding, judgment, and emotional functions due to organic brain disease. Dementia is commonly seen among cases of encephalitis, senility, cerebral arteriosclerosis, syphilitic infection, etc.

Dendrites Extensions of the cell body of a neuron that receive excitations or inhibitions from other neurons.

Denial A defense mechanism in which an individual defends himself against anxiety by denying the existence of the threatening stimulus itself or refuse to believe in the threat.

Deoxyribonucleic acid (DNA) A large chemical compound in genes, which is the basis for all heredity and carrying of genetic information.

Dependence 1) In social psychology, a tendency to rely on others. 2) In psychopathology, a strong, compelling desire or craving for a drug; dependence may be psychological or physiological.

Dependent variable A variable measured by the experimenter in an investigation; a change caused by the independent variable.

Depressants Drugs that reduce neural activity, bring down the level of arousal and decrease feelings of anxiety and tension.

Depressive cognitive triad A pattern of negative evaluations of the self, the world and the future often found among depressed people.

Depth perception The perception of the distance of an object from the observer; perception of the world in three dimensions.

Descartes, Rene (1596–1650) French philosopher and mathematician who, in many ways, symbolizes the transition in human thought from the Renaissance to Modern period. Descartes is often called 'the father of modern philosophy'. He laid the foundation for analytical geometry, which is named Cartesian geometry in his honor. He asserted that body and mind are separate, but interact with each other thus becoming a dualist and an interactionist in the realm of mind-body relationship. He wrote about psychological issues such as emotions, visual perception and reflex action. Some call him the first physiological psychologist.

Descriptive statistics Statistical procedures used to describe, organize and summarize data collected in a study. The most generally used statistics are *measures of central tendency* (mean, median and mode) and *measures of variability* (standard deviation, average deviation and range).

Determinants One of the major scoring categories in Rorschach referring to the perceived features of the inkblot such as form, movement, color or shading that precipitate the response of the test taker.

Developmental psychology A branch of psychology that studies the physical, psychological and social changes in the individual from conception to death. It is also called 'life span development'.

Deviation IQ One type of IQ calculated as a standard score with a mean of 100 and a standard deviation of 15 (in Wechsler scales) or 16 (in Stanford-Binet) to correspond approximately to the traditional IQ.

Dewey, John (1859–1952) American philosopher and educationist who sparked functionalism as a definite movement in psychology and attacked psychological molecularism and reductionism of behaviorism; Dewey asserted that the study of the organism as a whole functioning in its environment should be the proper subject matter of psychology.

Diathesis-stress model A theory of psychopathology postulating that mental disorders result from the interaction of constitutional predisposition and environmental stress.

Dichromats People who suffer from either red-green or yellow-blue color blindness.

Difference limen (DL) The minimal difference in magnitude of energy needed to detect a difference between two stimuli. In practice, it is a difference that can be detected in 50 percent of the time; also called difference threshold or 'differential threshold'.

Differential Aptitude Tests (DAT) A battery of tests designed to measure a wide range of functions such as verbal reasoning, numerical ability, abstract reasoning, space relations, mechanical reasoning, clerical speed and accuracy and spelling and sentence usage.

Diffusion of responsibility Diffusion of one's sense of responsibility in helping others who are in need owing to the presence of many other people, all of whom may be viewed as potentially responsible for helping. It is one of the causes of the *bystander apathy*.

Directed thinking The type of thinking directed toward the solution of a problem or creating something new.

Discrimination 1) In social psychology any behavior characterized by denial of rights and privileges to others solely on the basis of their membership in a disapproved group. 2) In conditioning, the occurrence of a conditioned response to one stimulus, but not another.

Discriminative stimulus In operant conditioning, a stimulus that signals that a particular response will be reinforced.

Disorganized schizophrenia A type of schizophrenia in which the patient exhibits incoherent speech, disorganized thought, inappropriate affect and severe disintegration of personality. Earlier, it was called 'hebephrenic schizophrenia'.

Displacement A defense mechanism in which psychic energy is shifted from the original object to a substitute that is less threatening.

Dissociative amnesia (psychogenic amnesia) A sudden inability to remember one's own identity and in certain cases, one's past life, but without forgetting basic habits and skills.

Dissociative disorders Psychiatric conditions involving a disruption in an individual's sense of personal identity or memory.

Dissociative fugue A dissociative disorder in which the person is not only amnesic for some or all aspects of his/her past life, but also departs from home surroundings and lives in a different place.

Dissociative identity disorder (DID) A dissociative disorder in which a person exhibits at least two or more identities or personality states that alternate in some way in taking control of behavior; formerly called multiple personality disorder.

Distinctiveness The extent to which an individual responds in a similar manner to different stimuli or different situations.

Distraction-conflict theory A theory suggesting that *social facilitation* stems from conflict produced when people attempt simultaneously to pay attention to other persons and the task being performed.

Distributed practice A method of learning in which study time is distributed across several sessions at different times as opposed to a single session of massed practice.

Divergent thinking A type of creative thinking that is directed toward producing more than one possible new solutions rather than a single correct solution to a problem.

Dizygotic twins The twins produced by the simultaneous fertilization of two separate eggs (ova) by two separate sperms; also called 'fraternal twins'.

Doctrine of specific nerve energies Johannes Muller's theory that each sensory nerve, no matter how it is stimulated, releases an energy specific to that nerve; for example, if an eye is stimulated with a mechanical stimulus, it produces visual sensation only.

Door-in-the-face technique A procedure of gaining compliance in which you begin with a large request and when this is refused, retreat to a smaller one (the one you actually desired all along).

Dopamine A neurotransmitter of the catecholamine family that has both excitatory and inhibitory functions depending on the pathway and the properties of the postsynaptic receptors. Dopamine has been implicated in a number of functions such as attention, learning, movement and a number of neuropsychiatric disorders. Decrease of dopamine is associated with rigidity, poor balance and akinesia of Parkinson's disease.

Dopamine hypothesis The hypothesis that schizophrenia is the result of an excessive dopamine activity in certain synaptic sites.

Double-depletion hypothesis An assumption that thirst and drinking are caused by cellular dehydration and hypovolemia.

Double aspectism A metaphysical point of view proposed by Spinoza, which states that mental and bodily activities are two aspects of the same occurrence.

Double bind hypothesis A term used by anthropologist Gregory Bateson to characterize a situation confronting a person who is receiving contradictory messages from another powerful person. For example, when a child shows affection toward mother, she exhibits lack of warmth, but when the child pulls back, she complains that the child has no love for her. Thus, the child receives contradictory messages and is caught in a double bind. It was assumed to be one of the etiological factors of schizophrenia.

Double blind situation (procedure) An experimental condition in which neither the participant nor the experimenter knows which treatment the participant is receiving.

Down syndrome A form of mental retardation induced by three chromosomes instead of the usual two in the 21st pair (trisomy-21). The afflicted child is characterized by flat skull, stubby fingers, an unusual pattern of skin folds on the palms of the hands and the soles of the feet and a fissured tongue.

Dream analysis A psychoanalytic technique in which the contents of dreams are analyzed to unearth the unconscious factors underlying a psychological disturbance.

Drive-reduction theory A theory, which states that a motivated sequence of behavior can best be explained as moving from an aversive state of heightened tension (drive) to a goal state in which the drive is reduced. Psychologists Hull as well as Thorndike used drive in their theories of learning.

Drive Internal condition that directs an organism toward a specific goal; a drive generally involves biological rather than psychological urge.

Drive theory of aggression A theory that views aggression as stemming from particular environmental conditions that serve to arouse a strong motive to engage in harm-producing behavior.

Drive theory of social facilitation A theory suggesting that the mere presence of others is arousing and increases the tendency to perform dominant responses (responses one is most likely to make in a given situation; these responses may be either correct or incorrect).

DSM Abbreviation for the Diagnostic and Statistical Manual of Mental Disorders, developed by American Psychiatric Association as a guide to diagnose psychological disorders; it has been revised several times and the one that is now in use is DSM-IV-TR.

Dual coding (hypothesis) A point of view that human memory is composed of two coding systems, one based on visual-imagery process and another on a verbal coding process.

Dualism The philosophical system of mind and body relationship that accepts the separate and the real existence of mental events and material entities.

Dyspareunia A sexual disorder marked by recurrent pain during intercourse; it may occur in both sexes.

Dysthymia A mood disorder characterized by depression of moderate intensity that lasts for a long duration of time, but does not disrupt the individual's functioning as a major depression does.

Echoic behavior Repeating someone else's verbal utterances.

Echoic memory A sensory store for holding a mental representation of a sound for a few seconds after it registers in the ear.

Eclecticism An approach to psychotherapy that makes use of principles of various other therapeutic procedures.

Ectomorphic One of the three body types in Sheldon's theory; an ectomorph is a person whose body is thin with large skin surfaces relative to weight.

Ego In Freudian theory, the executive arm of personality; ego mediates between the instinctive cravings of the Id, the prohibitions of superego and the dictates of external reality.

Ego cathexis In psychoanalysis, the investing of psychic energy within the domain of the ego.

Egocentrism In Piaget's theory, the tendency to see the world from one's own perspective; it includes an inability to consider another person's point of view.

Eidetic memory A vivid and persistent mental representation of visual image; it is often called photographic memory.

Elaboration likelihood model A model proposing two routes to persuasion and attitude change: *central route* (focusing on the message) and *peripheral route* (focusing on extraneous factors).

Elaborative rehearsal The process of focusing on the meaning of information and/or relating it to other things that are already known.

Electra complex The female version of the Oedipus complex in which a girl child experiences erotic feelings toward her father along with a hatred toward the mother. Freud did not use the term; he only used the term feminine Oedipus complex to refer to the condition among girls.

Electroconvulsive therapy (ECT) A form of treatment for mental disorders in which high voltage electric current is passed briefly through the skull producing epileptic-like convulsion; the treatment has been found to be effective in the treatment of depression.

Electroencephalography (EEG) A graphical record of brain's electrical activity obtained by placing electrodes on the scalp and measuring the brain wave impulses.

Embryo The developing organism during the 2nd and 8th week after conception.

Embryonic stage The second stage of prenatal development lasting from 2nd to 8th week characterized by the rapid development of major body organs.

Emotional intelligence Skills underlying the accurate understanding, assessment, evaluation, expression and regulation of emotions in oneself and others.

Empathic joy hypothesis A theory of prosocial behavior stating that we are motivated to help because of the joy we get when we know that somebody is happy and we are responsible for that.

Empathy-altruism hypothesis An assertion that true altruism exists and that it is produced by the capacity to show *empathy* toward the person who is in need of help.

Empathy Capacity to experience another person's emotions and feelings as if they are your own; according to Rogers, empathy is an essential factor in therapeutic success.

Empirical approach An approach to test construction in which the items are selected based on their capacity to differentiate between two groups that are known to differ on a particular personality variable. The approach has been used in the construction of Minnesota Multiphasic Personality Inventory (MMPI).

Empirically supported treatments (ESTs) Psychotherapeutic techniques that have been shown to be effective in controlled clinical trials.

Empiricism A philosophical point of view, which asserts that all knowledge is derived from experience, especially sensory experience.

Empty chair technique A technique used by Gestalt therapists wherein an internal dialogue occurs between two opposing aspects (the top dog and the underdog) of his/her personality.

The client sits in one chair and converses with his imagined part of the self (the top dog) on the other chair, and then goes to the other chair and talks to the person (underdog) in the first chair. The exercise helps the client to accept that portion of his personality which was denied all along and resolve the conflict between the two.

Empty nest syndrome A negative emotional state experienced by parents, when children grow up and leave home.

Encoding Storing information in memory by translating it into a neural code that the brain can understand.

Encoding specificity principle A principle which states that memory is enhanced when the conditions present during retrieval are similar to those that were present at the time of encoding.

Endocrine system In human body, the system of ductless glands that secrete hormones to the blood stream directly and thereby influence several functions.

Endomorphic component One of the three components of physique proposed by Sheldon; it comprises of the prominence of intestines and other visceral organs including prominent abdomen as in the obese individual.

Endorphins Opiates produced in the brain and throughout the body that function like neurotransmitters to reduce pain sensations.

Engram A hypothesized neural change thought to be responsible for memory.

Environmental psychology An area of psychology engaged in investigating the relationship between the living environment (the physical world) and behavior.

Episodic buffer The component of working memory, which provides a temporary storage space where information from long-term memory and from phonological loop and/or visuospatial sketchpad can be integrated, manipulated and made available for conscious awareness.

Episodic memory The memory for spatial and temporal aspects of an individual's experience; these are mostly autobiographical in nature; that is, memory for where, when and how certain things were done.

Equilibration Piaget's term for the tendency to seek a stable balance among cognitive elements.

Erogenous zone Area of the body that is capable of producing pleasurable sensations when stimulated. Freud has included mouth, anus and genitals under erogenous zones.

Eros In psychoanalytic theory, the name given to *life instincts*.

Erotomania An excessive preoccupation with sex in thought, speech and action.

Escape learning A form of learning in which the organism learns to perform a behavior to terminate an aversive stimulus.

Estrogen Female sex hormone produced by follicles of the ovary; estrogen influences the sex drive and is also partially responsible for the growth of secondary sex characteristics.

Evaluation apprehension Concern over being evaluated by others; such concern can increase arousal and so contribute to social facilitation.

Evolutionary psychology A branch of psychology that applies Darwin's principles of natural selection and survival of fittest to individual behavior; evolutionary psychologists propose that we are born with tendencies that guide our thinking and behavior. The innate mechanisms that are acquired through natural selection from our ancestors help us in solving several of adaptive problems.

Exhaustion stage The third stage of Selye's general adaptation syndrome (GAS) in which the organism experiences depletion of bodily resources to deal with stressors.

Exhibitionism A paraphilia characterized by exposing one's genitals to unsuspecting others.

Existentialism A philosophical movement that emphasizes man's responsibility for himself and becoming the person he should be. It is concerned with man's existence in the world, his freedom to choose life goals and the search for meaning in life. Existentialism has influenced some thinkers in the areas of psychology, psychiatry, and literature.

Expectancy effects When an experimenter's preconceived notions about how participants should behave are subtly communicated to the participants and in turn, affect the participants' behavior, expectancy effects are said to be operating. This is an instance of *experimenter bias and similar to* concepts such as *demand characteristics and self-fulfilling prophecy.*

Experimental group A group of participants in a study which receives a non-zero level of the independent variable.

Experimental neurosis A neurotic-like behavior produced in animals by inescapable conflicts in the laboratory.

Experimental psychology A branch of psychology that studies behavior in controlled laboratory conditions.

Experimenter bias The behavior of the experimenter influencing the results of the study; such bias results because of two factors: *expectancy effects* and uneven treatment of participants across treatments.

Explicit memory Intentional or conscious recollection of what has been learned; when people use the term memory, they generally mean explicit memory. It is a rough synonym for *declarative memory*.

Ex post facto research A kind of research conducted after the experimental effects have already taken place; for example, studying the effect of some natural calamity (accidents, floods, fires) after it has occurred.

Exposure therapy Behavior therapy technique designed to extinguish the anxiety by exposing persons to anxiety-arousing stimuli or situations while preventing the escape behavior.

Expressed emotion Negative communication involving excessive criticism or emotional overinvolvement expressed by members of family directed toward a patient.

External auditory meatus Canal from the external ear to the tympanic membrane.

External validity The extent to which the results of a study can be generalized beyond the limited sample that is being investigated.

Extinction The decrease in frequency and eventual disappearance of a conditioned response.

Extraneous variable Any variable that is not systematically manipulated in an experiment, but that may still affect the behavior that is being investigated.

Extrasensory perception (ESP) Any perception that occurs without the involvement of any of the sense receptors; ESP is the subject of investigation in parapsychology.

Extraversion-introversion A personality trait that can be described as varying between two opposite ends (extraversion and introversion). Earlier, introversion and extraversion were thought of as representing two independent types of personality, but nowadays introversion and extraversion are considered as two poles of the same personality dimension.

Extrinsic motivation Any motivation that is triggered by external rewards, such as money, recognition and respect from others.

Extroversion An attitude, first described by Jung, characterized by interest in the external world of people and objects; it is the attitude of an outward going person. Today it is thought of as one pole of a bipolar factor, extraversion-introversion.

Eysenck, Hans J (1916–1997) A British clinical psychologist well-known for his contribution to the fields of personality, behavior therapy and clinical psychology.

Eysenck Personality Questionnaire Personality inventory developed by Hans Eysenck and Sybil Eysenck to study extraversion-introversion, neuroticism and psychoticism.

Facial feedback hypothesis The assumption that awareness of one's facial expression is a primary ingredient in the experience of emotions. It is hypothesized that mimicking facial movements associated with a particular emotion will produce the corresponding emotional state.

Factor analysis A statistical procedure that analyzes complex psychological constructs, such as intelligence or personality, into the constituent components. It is a technique of reducing a large number of measures to a small number of factors using correlation among the measures. The factors themselves may be oblique (correlated) or orthogonal (uncorrelated) to each other.

Faculty psychology A discredited theory that mental processes can be divided into separate specialized abilities, which can be developed by regular exercises in the same way that muscles are strengthened by regular exercise.

False consensus effect The tendency to assume that others think and behave like us to a greater extent than is actually true.

Family therapy Psychotherapy with the family members as a group instead of treating an individual with a problem belonging to the family; the emphasis is on interpersonal relationships within the family.

Fear of success The hypothesized fear on the part of women that success will be accompanied by loss of femininity.

Fechner, Gustav Theodor (1801–1887) German physicist, philosopher and psychologist who founded psychophysics, the exact science of functional relations between mind and body. Psychologists remember him as the one who gave them a set of experimental procedures called psychophysical methods.

Female orgasmic disorder Female sexual disorder characterized by absence of orgasm or persistent delay or difficulty in achieving orgasm after normal sexual excitation phase.

Female sexual arousal disorder A type of sexual dysfunction among women involving inability or difficulty in becoming sexually aroused after all forms of erotic stimulation.

Feminist therapy Psychotherapy designed to solve problems facing women; it strives to help women achieve greater self-determination and self-actualization.

Feral children Young children reared in forests (social isolation) by animals.

Fetal alcohol syndrome A pattern of symptoms observed among children born to alcoholic mothers; the typical characteristics are facial or limb irregularity, reduced body weight and behavioral abnormality.

Fetal stage The final stage of prenatal development lasting from 8th week after conception to the time of birth.

Fetishism A paraphilia in which an individual derives sexual gratification from non-sexual objects (handkerchief, panties, hair, etc.) that symbolize the person to whom they belong.

Fetus An organism in the later stages of prenatal development. In humans, from the 3rd month of pregnancy to birth is called the fetal stage.

Fight-or-flight response The response pattern that prepares the organism to fight or run away from a threatening or dangerous situation. The responses include a rise in blood pressure, heart rate, respiration rate and blood sugar level; there is also increased palmar sweating and muscle tension.

Figure-ground relations Perceptual organization in which the focal stimulus is seen as the figure against a background formed of all other stimuli.

Filial love The love of parents or caregivers toward the children.

FI scallop A shape of the graph of cumulative responses typically produced by an organism on fixed interval schedules of reinforcement; there will be relatively few responses immediately after reinforcement, with the number increasing dramatically towards the end of the interval.

Fissure Large, deep fold or groove on the cerebral cortex.

Five Factors Model A contemporary trait model of personality consisting of five factorially derived dimensions of personality—openness, conscientiousness, extroversion, agreeableness and neuroticism (OCEAN).

Fixation According to psychoanalysis, the attachment of libido to an earlier psychosexual stage to which a person regresses when faced with some crises in later life.

Fixed-interval (FI) schedule Reinforcing the first correct response occurring after a specified interval of time measured from the delivery of the preceding reinforcement; for example reinforcing after every 30 seconds.

Fixed-ratio (FR) schedule Reinforcing the last of a specified number of correct responses counted from the preceding reinforcement; for example, reinforcing every 10th response.

Flashbulb memories Emotionally charged memories of an event that are vivid and appear like a snapshot.

Flourens, Pierre (1794–1867) French physiologist who localized psychological and motor functions in various parts of the brain; Flourens' discovery is recognized as a landmark in the history of neurophysiology.

Fluid intelligence According to RB Cattell, the ability to process information, reason and solve problems; this ability is related to biological growth and does not depend on formal learning.

Foot-in-the-door technique A method of obtaining compliance in which a person makes a small request first and when that is conceded goes on to make a larger request.

Forebrain Brain structures above the midbrain including thalamus, hypothalamus, limbic system and the cerebral hemispheres; forebrain is involved in higher-order sensory, motor and cognitive functions.

Forensic psychology The study of the relationship between psychology and law; it deals with the role of the psychologist as an expert witness, the reliability of eyewitness testimony and the jury selection process.

Formal operational stage According to Piaget, the period in which an individual is able to think logically about problems and solve them systematically; people at this stage can formulate hypotheses and test them using data thoughtfully and logically.

Fovea A small area in the central part of the retina that is packed with cones; it is the most sensitive part of retina for visual details and color.

Fragile X syndrome A genetic disorder caused by a weakness in the X chromosome; the affected male will have large testicles, poor speech and mental retardation; affected females are subclinical.

Fraternal love The love toward brothers, sisters and friends.

Free association In Freudian analysis, the procedure of freely talking about all that comes to the mind without bothering about its relevance or irrelevance.

Free nerve endings Afferent nerve endings that are believed to be the receptors for pain.

Frequency theory of hearing An auditory theory, which maintains that the number of nerve impulses sent to the brain by the hair cells of the cochlea corresponds to the frequency of the sound wave; the theory holds good only for low frequencies.

Freud, Sigmund (1856–1939) The founder of psychoanalysis, a school of psychology that emphasizes the role of unconscious motives (instinctual forces such as sex and aggression) in the determination of human behavior and personality. Freud's influence on psychology and psychiatry is immense. His ideas are being both eulogized and severely criticized even today.

Fromm Erich (1900–1980) One of the neo-Freudians who agreed more with Adler and Horney than with Freud; Fromm emphasized the role of social forces in shaping personality; he believed that humans, paradoxically, by achieving more freedom from nature and social systems, have become more lonely, isolated insignificant and this pathological condition can be removed by creating a healthy society.

Frontal lobe Portion of the cerebrum that lies in front of the precentral gyrus; this part of the brain controls higher mental process such as reasoning and thinking.

Frotteurism A paraphilia in which an individual derives sexual gratification by touching or rubbing against an unwilling person. The act (frottage) usually takes place in crowded places.

Frustration-aggression hypothesis A proposition which assumes that frustration always leads to aggression and that aggression is always produced by frustration. Although the assumption appears intuitively correct, it does not hold true in all situations.

Frustration The emotional state when a goal-directed behavior is blocked.

Fully functioning person A concept proposed by Rogers to a psychologically healthy person: such persons are free from conditions of worth, congruent, spontaneous, creative; in short they are self-actualizing people.

Functional autonomy A controversial concept introduced by GW Allport, which states that adult motives are self-sustaining contemporary systems growing out of antecedent systems, but functionally independent of them. Not all motives are functionally autonomous.

Functional fixedness In problem solving situations, a tendency to think in terms of the customary use of an object, which interferes with its use in novel situations and ways.

Functionalism An early school of American psychology, which emphasized the functions of consciousness and behavior in helping organisms to adjust to their environment.

Fundamental attribution error Tendency to underestimate the influence of external situational factors and overestimate the role of personal factors in explaining other people's behavior.

Galvanic skin response (GSR) A measure of the electrical response of the skin as measured by a galvanometer. The measure is used as an indication of emotional arousal.

Gamete A reproductive cell, either a sperm or an egg in its mature state.

Gamma-aminobutyric acid (GABA) An amino acid that works like an inhibitory neurotransmitter in many sites of the central nervous system; GABA is implicated in Huntington's chorea and severe anxiety disorders.

Gate control theory A theory of pain asserting that there are gating mechanisms in the spinal cord and brain, which can increase or decrease the experience of pain by regulating the flow of pain impulses to the brain.

Gender constancy The belief that you are a boy or girl and will continue to be so permanently.

Gender dysphoria Persistent discomfort about one's biological sex and a feeling that the gender role is inappropriate.

Gender identity The psychological sense of maleness or femaleness; an individual's identification as being male or female.

Gender identity disorder Identification with the members of the opposite sex, discomfort with one's biological sex and a strong desire to change to the opposite sex.

Gender roles The cultural expectations imposed on boys and girls to behave in ways deemed appropriate for their gender; also called *sex-role stereotypes*.

Gender schema An organized set of beliefs and expectations (schema) that guide the way people process information about men and women in general.

General adaptation syndrome (GAS) The pattern of the body's response to stress proposed by Hans Selye; it is said to pass through three stages: *alarm*, *resistance* and *exhaustion*.

General factor (g) In Spearman's two-factor theory of intelligence, the central intellective component that takes part in almost all cognitive functions as opposed to specific factors that are specific to each task.

Generalized anxiety disorder A chronic state of diffuse anxiety that is not related to any specific object or event.

General paresis A mental disorder associated with syphilitic infection of the brain. Formerly, it was called general paresis of the insane (GPI).

Genes Biological structures within the chromosomes that contain the individual's genetic code.

Genital stage In Freudian theory of psychosexual development, the fifth and the final stage that begins around puberty heralding the emergence of mature sexuality; the person is now capable of developing appropriate relationship with parents and members of the opposite sex.

Genotype The genetic makeup of the individual, which may or may not be expressed in the phenotype.

Germinal stage First stage of prenatal development; it spans the period from fertilization through implantation.

Gestalt psychology A German School of psychology, which stood for the understanding of conscious experience as a whole without analyzing its elements. Gestalt psychologists have made enormous contributions to the fields of perception, learning and thinking.

Gestalt therapy Psychotherapy based on Gestalt principles developed by Perls. It emphasizes wholeness of the person and integration of thoughts feelings and behavior.

Gonadotrophic hormones The hormones produced by the anterior pituitary, which stimulate activity in the gonads. For example, follicle stimulating hormone, which stimulates the development of ovarian follicles and spermatogenesis.

Gonads A common name for glands producing sex hormones.

Group polarization The tendency of group members to shift toward a more extreme point of view than the one they initially held as a result of group discussion.

Groupthink The tendency of a highly cohesive group to think in an uncritical manner in making decisions because of an intense desire to reach unanimity; often groupthink has led to decisions with dangerous consequences, especially in the military.

Gustation The sense of smell.

Hall, Granville Stanley (1844–1924) An early promoter of psychology in the United States of America, Hall was a founder of laboratories, institutions and journals of psychology. He was the first to receive a doctorate in psychology in the USA, first American student of Wundt, first president of the American Psychological Association, which he founded and was the first president of Clark University. Hall introduced psychoanalysis to America by inviting Freud and Jung to Clark University to deliver lectures.

Hallucination Sensory experience occurring in the absence of any physical stimulation; hallucination is a major symptom in several psychological disorders.

Hardiness A personality dimension referring to an individual's stable way of responding to the stresses of life; hardiness involves commitment to work, having control over the outcomes and a sense of challenge in life.

Hassles Annoyances of daily life (like traffic jam) that produce stress.

Health psychology A branch of psychology engaged in the study of psychological factors involved in wellness and illness; its major goal is a deeper understanding of psychological processes as aids to improving physical health outcomes for individuals.

Helmholtz, Hermann LF, von (1821–1894) German scientist whose contributions in the area of nerve conduction, vision, audition and perception are unparalleled in the history of science.

Hering, Ewald (1834–1918) German physician who opposed the empirical approach in psychology and offered the nativistic viewpoint; his theory of color vision explains several phenomena that Helmholtz's theory failed to do.

Heritability The degree to which heredity accounts for variations in behavior or personality.

Heteronomous morality stage It is the first stage of moral development in which the child's behavior is determined by rules prescribed by others (parents and other elders). The stage up to the seventh year (Piaget).

Heuristics Procedures used for solving a problem; a heuristic reduces the possible range of solutions to a problem or the number of possible answers to a question. Algorithm guarantees finding of a solution to the problem, while heuristics do not.

Higher order conditioning Classical conditioning in which a conditioned stimulus from an earlier conditioning experiment is used as the unconditioned stimulus in a new conditioning situation.

Hindbrain In evolutionary terms, the oldest part of the brain situated just above the spinal cord; it consists of the medulla, pons and cerebellum.

Hippocampus A structure in the limbic system that plays an important part in memorization process; it resembles a sea horse in shape, hence the name hippocampus.

Homeostasis A term introduced by WB Cannon to refer to certain automatic biological processes triggered within an organism to retain steady states such as body temperature, body fluid level and their chemical composition. Psychologists have used the concept to explain how certain psychological steady states are regulated.

Hormic psychology A school of psychology proposed by William McDougall; it is concerned with goal-directed (purposive) behavior propelled instincts.

Hormones Chemicals secreted by endocrine glands; hormones travel in the bloodstream and affect several physiological and psychological activities.

Horney, Karen (1885–1952) German-born American neo-Freudian psychoanalyst who opposed several of the Freudian concepts, especially those concerning women; her views were nearer to Adler than to Freud. Horney was very influential through her books that could be head and understood by non-specialists.

Hostile aggression Behavior aimed at harming or injuring another organism who is motivated to avoid such treatment.

Hue The dimension of visual sensation corresponding chiefly to the wavelength of light; what we generally refer to as colors such as red, green, blue, yellow and so on.

Hull CL (1884–1952) American learning theorist who is known for his drive reduction theory; Hull wrote extensively on learning, while directing some classic works of others.

Human Genome Project An international cooperative venture that has mapped human chromosomes and identified roughly 35,000 genes in the human genome.

Humanistic psychology Approach to psychology that emphasizes the goodness of humans, their free will, freedom to choose and intrinsic capacity to actualize their potentialities.

Huntington's disease An inherited neurological disease characterized by progressive cognitive and muscular deterioration, finally leading to alteration in personality. The disease is caused by a dominant gene.

Hypnosis A trance-like psychological state of increased suggestibility induced in a cooperative individual.

Hypoactive sexual desire disorder A sexual dysfunction in which either a man or a woman shows little or no desire or interest in sexual activity.

Hypochondriasis A somatoform disorder characterized by preoccupation with imagined physical symptoms.

Hypomania Mild form of mania.

Hypothalamus A small, pea-shaped structure in the forebrain, which plays a key role in the regulation of body temperature, reproduction, emotion and motivation.

Hypothesis A precise statement about the outcome of an experiment; a tentative answer to the research problem.

Iconic memory A sensory store that holds a mental representation of a visual image for a fraction of a second.

Id In Freudian theory, the oldest and the most primitive part of personality, which is the store house of the entire psychic energy and the animal instincts; the Id consists of everything inherited by the individual. The contents of the id and its processes are obscure, unorganized and unconscious. It is irrational, amoral, timeless and is wholly governed by the pleasure principle. It needs immediate gratification of its instinctual urges.

Idealists The philosophers who believe that ultimate reality consists of ideas or perceptions and therefore is not physical.

Ideal self The self, one would like to be.

Identical twins The twins developing from the same zygote and having identical genes; also called *monozygotic twins*.

Identification Generally an ego defense mechanism in which a person identifies himself/herself with some person or institution, usually of an illustrious nature. In Freudian theory, the process by which a young child adopts characteristics and behaviors of the parent of the same sex.

Identity In Erikson's theory, an organized sense of self, consisting of goals, values and beliefs to which a person is committed.

Identity crisis In Erikson's theory, a stressful period in which serious self-examination of issues relating to personal values and direction in life are made.

Identity statuses Marcia's term for states of ego development that depend on the presence or absence of crisis or commitment.

Identity versus identity confusion In Erikson's theory of psychosocial development, the fifth stage in which an adolescent is passing through an *identity crisis* searching for personal identity.

Illusion In perception, a misrepresentation of the relations among presented stimuli so that what is perceived does not correspond to physical reality.

Imaginary audience The common belief among adolescents that they are the center of other people's attention.

Imitation The process of copying the behavior of others. See *Modeling*.

Immediate reinforcement Offering reward immediately after making a response.

Implicit memory Memories that influence behavior without conscious awareness; implicit memory can be tapped by priming.

Impression formation The process through which we combine various information about others into a unified picture of them.

Impression management The ways in which we select and control our behavior, as well as the situation in which it is displayed, in order to make a favorable impression on others.

Imprinting The formation of a strong bond between the newborn and the first moving object; a sudden biologically primed behavior such as an attachment that can be observed in certain species of animals.

Incentive An environmental stimulus that motivates behavior.

Incest Sexual relationship between family members such as a brother and sister or a parent and child that is prohibited universally by all societies.

Incongruence Improper symbolization of organismic experience in consciousness; a discrepancy between conscious self-experience and the total organismic experience.

Incubation In problem solving, a period of rest during which the problem solver suspends search for the solution, but after a while the solution appears.

Incus One of the three bones (ossicles) in the middle ear (looks like an anvil), which transmits vibrations from the eardrum to the cochlea. See also *Malleus* and *Stapes*.

Independent variable In an experiment, the variable that is under the control of and manipulated by the experimenter.

Individualism A cultural orientation that favors individual achievement over group goals; mostly found in Western cultures. Individualism contrasts with *collectivism*.

Individual psychology A neo-Freudian school started by Alfred Adler, which emphasized the role of social factors in the development of personality.

Inductive reasoning The reasoning that starts with a set of specific facts to draw a general principle; a logical operation, which proceeds from the individual to the general.

Indulgent parents The parents who exhibit warmth toward their children, but do not provide guidance and discipline; their children tend to become self-centered.

Industrial-organizational psychology (I-O psychology) A branch of psychology that applies psychological principles to the work-related issues and the organization in which work is done.

Industry versus inferiority Fourth stage in Erikson's theory in which the concern of the child is learning and moving ahead or feeling inadequate and experiencing inferiority.

Infancy Typically, the first year of life.

Infantile amnesia Inability to remember personal experiences that occurred during the first few years of life.

Inferential statistics Procedures used to make inferences about the population based on the study of sample utilizing the principles of probability.

Inferiority complex According to Adler, the feelings of inadequacy or inferiority among young children that influence the development of their personalities in later years.

Informational social influence Following other people driven by the belief that they have accurate knowledge and what they are saying or doing is 'right'.

Information processing approach (model) An approach to the study of cognitive development that emphasizes observation and analysis of mental processes in handling information.

Informed consent An ethical principle in psychological research, which states that participants in the study should be fully informed about the procedures, the benefits and the risks involved, the right to withdraw at any time and matters of confidentiality and privacy.

Ingratiation A strategy whereby you induce in others a liking for you so that they may comply with your request. It may include flattery, agreement with the person's opinion and doing some favors for the target.

In-group A group to which we belong, with which we identify and from which we tend to exclude others (the members of *out-group*); it is 'us' as opposed to 'they'.

In-group differentiation bias Thinking that members of in-group (us) are diverse and heterogeneous.

Initiative versus guilt In Erikson's theory, the third stage in which children try to balance the urge to pursue goals with moral reservations that may prevent carrying them out.

Insanity Legal term for mental disorder; the term implies lack of responsibility for one's acts and inability to manage one's affairs.

Insight 1) In Gestalt psychology, a sudden perception of an important relationship or a solution to a problem. 2) In psychoanalysis becoming aware of the unconscious dynamics underlying maladjusted behavior.

Insomnia A disorder of sleep characterized by an inability to fall asleep or stay asleep.

Instinctive drift A tendency for instinctive behavior to override conditioning procedures, thus making it difficult to establish or maintain a conditioned response; the phenomenon was observed by two of Skinner's students, while they were trying to train animals.

Instincts Innate behavior patterns that are not products of learning.

Instrumental aggression Aggressive behavior used as a means to achieve a goal.

Intelligence The ability to learn, to think and plan effectively and deal adaptively with the environment.

Intelligence quotient (IQ) An index of intelligence obtained by dividing mental age (MA) by chronological age (CA) and multiplying by 100. IQ = MA/CA × 100.

Interactionism A theory of mind and body relationship, which states that body and mind are separate entities, but the two interact with and influence each other.

Interference theory The theory stating that what we learn is interfered by the material learned earlier to or later than the material we are learning now.

Intermittent reinforcement Schedules of reinforcement in which some of the responses made go unreinforced; also called partial reinforcement.

Internal-External (IE) Scale A test developed by Julian B Rotter to assess internality versus externality. Internality refers to an expectancy that one's outcomes are under personal control and externality to expectancy that the outcomes are controlled by environmental factors.

Internal motivation Behaviors that appear to be entirely self-motivated.

Internal validity The degree to which an experimental treatment produces clear-cut causal relationship. Internal validity will be high in the absence of confounding variable effects.

Interneurons Connecting neurons in the brain, which are neither sensory nor motor. They perform integrative or associative functions in the nervous system.

Interpersonal therapy A form of therapy designed to foster interpersonal skills and relationships in clients.

Interquartile range A measure of dispersion based on the middle 50 percent of a frequency distribution, that is, between the 25th and 75th percentiles (between the first quartile and the third quartile).

Interstitial cell-stimulating hormone (ICSH) The hormone which stimulates secretion of estrogen and ovulation.

Intimacy versus isolation Erikson's sixth stage in which young adults either make a commitment to others or face a possible sense of isolation and self-absorption.

Intrinsic motivation Engaging in an activity simply because it is interesting and enjoyable and not for any reward or reinforcement.

Irreversibility Piaget's term for a preoperational child's inability to reverse the direction of a sequence of events to their starting point.

James, William (1842–1910) An American philosopher and psychologist who first offered a course in psychology and started a psychological laboratory at Harvard; he wrote the first textbook of psychology that became a landmark in the history of psychology. Some of his students like Hall, Thorndike, and Woodworth became stalwarts in American psychology.

James-Lange theory of emotion A controversial theory of emotion, which states that emotions result from perception of bodily changes.

Jung, Carl Gustav (1875–1961) An early associate of Freud, Jung dissociated from him and started a new school of psychoanalysis called Analytical Psychology. His theory of personality and psychotherapy influenced thinkers in and outside of psychology. Jung was a prolific writer and his writings fill some twenty volumes. Several of his concepts such as collective unconscious, archetypes, introversion and extraversion have influenced psychological thought all over the world.

Just noticeable difference (jnd) The difference between two stimuli on some attribute that can be just noticed.

Kierkegaard, Soren (1813–1855) A Danish philosopher and theologian who is regarded as the founder of *existentialism*.

Kinesthesis The sense of body movement and movement of body parts; kinesthesis include muscle sense, joint sense and tendon sense.

Klinefelter's syndrome An abnormality caused by a chromosomal anomaly (trisomy XXY); a boy with trisomy XXY, although physically male, will have marked feminine characteristics. The condition is also associated with mental retardation.

Knowledge acquisition components In Sternberg's triarchic theory of intelligence, the ability that allows people to learn from experience, store information in memory and integrate new learning with previously acquired information.

Koffka, Kurt (1886–1941) German psychologist who introduced Gestalt psychology to Americans through his scholarly books in English language.

Kohlberg, Lawrence (1927–1987) American psychologist and educator who proposed an influential theory of moral development.

Kohler, Wolfgang (1887–1967) Gestalt psychologist who made seminal contributions to the field of learning through his experiments on insight learning among apes.

Korsakoff syndrome A psychotic state caused by chronic alcohol abuse; it is characterized by memory loss for current events and polyneuritis.

Kulpe, Oswald (1862–1915) A student of Wundt who disagreed with his teacher and started the Würzburg school of psychology, which investigated higher mental processes including thinking. Wundt had said that higher mental processes like thinking cannot be studied in the laboratory. Kulpe and his students belied Wundt's conviction and became famous for their studies in thought processes such as imageless thought, conscious attitudes, determining tendencies, and set.

Labyrinthine sense See *Static sense*.

Lactogenic hormone A hormone secreted by the anterior pituitary responsible for the onset and maintenance of lactation in mammals after the birth of the young; also called prolactin or luteotropic hormone.

Language acquisition device (LAD) An innate, biologically-based mechanism that helps language acquisition; the concept was proposed by linguist Chomsky.

Language acquisition support system (LASS) Social learning opportunities involved in learning a language.

Latency stage In Freudian theory of psychosexual development, the period between the end of phallic stage and the beginning of puberty, during which sexual interest is believed to be dormant.

Latent learning The learning that has taken place, but not yet manifested itself as a performance; the phenomenon of latent learning has been amply demonstrated by laboratory experiments.

Lateral fissure The deep fissure between temporal lobe and parietal lobes of each cerebral hemisphere; it is also called fissure of Sylvius.

Lateral hypothalamus A part of the hypothalamus that is believed to be involved in initiating eating; when this part is removed, an animal refuses to eat.

Lateralization Degree of localization of specific mental functions on one or the other side (hemisphere) of the brain.

Law of effect An important law of learning, first proposed by Thorndike, which states that a stimulus-response connection will be strengthened if it is followed by satisfying consequence and weakened if followed by an annoying state; the law was revised later and only the former proposition was retained.

Learned helplessness A concept proposed by Seligman, which says that if people are unable to control some events in life, they develop a sense of helplessness that leads to depression.

Learning A relatively permanent change in an organism's behavior that occurs as a result of experience; changes brought about by maturation, disease or drugs do not qualify to be called learning.

Leibniz GW (1646–1716) A German philosopher and mathematician who proposed that body and mind are separate, they do not interact and only run in parallel courses. This view is called psychophysical parallelism. Leibniz founded differential calculus, an important branch of mathematics.

Lens The crystalline structure behind the pupil of the eye that focuses light rays on the retina.

Levels of processing The idea that the more deeply the information is processed, the better it will be remembered.

Libido A term used by Freud to refer to the energy that propels sex. Later analysts like Jung used the term to refer to general psychological energy.

Life instincts In psychoanalytic theory, one of the two groups of instincts which cater to the survival of the individual; Freud named it *eros* after the Greek god of love.

Limbic system A group of interconnected subcortical structures including anterior thalamus, part of hypothalamus, septum, hippocampus and amygdala the limbic system structures are assumed to plan important role in memory, emotion and motivation.

Linguistic relativity hypothesis The assumption made by linguist Benjamin Whorf asserting that the language we speak determines the way we think and perceive.

Linguistics The study of the origins, structure and development of language.

Locke, John (1632–1704) British philosopher who developed the empirical theory of knowledge; Locke asserted that the mind of a newborn baby is an empty tablet (*tabula rasa*), and sensory experience writes on it. Thus, Locke as an empiricist denied the existence of innate ideas. He introduced the concept of associationism that played an important role in later psychological theorizing.

Locus of control The term used to refer to the perceived source of control over one's behavior. It is measured along a dimension running from high internal to high external using a test called *Internal-External (IE)* Scale developed by JB Rotter. Internals are those who tend to take responsibility for their own actions and to view themselves as having control over their destinies and the externals are those who tend to see control as residing elsewhere and to attribute success or failure to outside forces.

Long-term memory (LTM) The relatively permanent component of memory system, as opposed to short-term memory (STM).

Longitudinal fissure The fissure that divides the brain into right and left hemispheres.

Longitudinal method A method of research in which a sample of cohorts is studied repeatedly over an extended period of time to observe developmental changes.

Luteinizing hormone Same as *prolactin* or *lactogen*.

Magnetic resonance imaging (MRI) A procedure to scan brain structure, which produces detailed images of living tissues based on the tissue's response to a magnetic field. Functional MRI (fMRI) can be used to study brain functions.

Mainstreaming The practice (in the USA) of placing children with special needs in a regular classroom environment.

Maintenance rehearsal Rote repetition of information to retain it in memory.

Major depressive disorders Severe mood disorder characterized by only major depressive episodes.

Male erectile disorder Sexual disorder in which a male cannot achieve and maintain penile erection sufficient enough for gratification.

Male orgasmic disorder Inability to achieve orgasm and ejaculate after normal sexual excitement.

Malleus One of the three bones of the middle ear; an ossicle, which is also called the hammer.

Mand A verbal command that is reinforced when the listener carries out the command; for example, the mand "come here," is reinforced when the person comes toward you.

Mania Emotional state characterized by euphoria, psychomotor overactivity and rush of thought.

Marital therapy Counseling couples who are experiencing interpersonal conflicts; therapy involves meeting both husband and wife and discussing the importance of mutual need gratification, social role expectation and communication pattern.

Maslow, Abraham (1908–1970) One of the leaders of humanistic psychology, Maslow is known for his holistic-dynamic approach to psychological issues, a theory of motives, and the study of self-actualization.

Massed practice Learning situation in which study time is restricted to one single, lengthy session as opposed to distributed practice.

Masturbation Deriving sexual gratification by self-stimulation; often called 'solitary sex'.

Materialism A philosophical viewpoint which asserts that matter is truth and mind is a fiction; the view holds that matter secrets the mind.

Maturation The biological unfolding of the organism according to the underlying genetic code.

Maximizing inclusive fitness An evolutionary theory, which states that we tend to enhance the reproductive odds of those who share our genes.

McDougall, William (1871–1938) British psychologist and founder of hormic psychology, McDougall emphasized the purposive and goal directed nature of the behavior; he wrote extensively and his book on social psychology was a landmark publication. His concept of instinct was severely criticized by sociologists and psychologists. McDougall taught at Oxford and Harvard Universities.

Mean The most often used measure of central tendency; it is the arithmetic average of the scores.

Means-ends analysis A problem-solving process in which one examines the difference between the present situation and a solution situation and continues to perform operations until no difference is noticed.

Measures of central tendency Measures such as mean, median and mode, computed from data; these represent the general magnitude of the scores in the distribution.

Measures of dispersion Measures such as standard deviation, average deviation and range, computed from data; these represent the variability of the scores in the distribution; also called *measures of variability*.

Measures of variability See *Measures of dispersion*.

Median The middle most value in a frequency distribution.

Medical model A view assuming that psychological disorders are produced by specific causes and the cure is possible by removing the root cause. This is the disease model prevalent in the medical field.

Medulla oblongata The posterior part of the hindbrain that controls vital functions including respiration and heartbeat.

Meissner corpuscles Pressure receptors situated in hairless areas of skin.

Melancholic One of Kretschmer's personality types in which the person is cognitively oriented and depressed.

Melatonin A hormone of the pineal gland that is implicated in facilitating sleep and relaxation.

Memory The cognitive process that allows us to register, store and retrieve information.

Memory codes Mental representations of information or stimulus.

Menarche Onset of menstruation; the first menstruation.

Menopause The time of life at which menstruation stops.

Menstrual synchrony The tendency among women living together to menstruate more or less at the same time.

Mental age An index of intelligence used by Binet; it refers to the age at which an individual passes all the items meant for the average person of that age. When a 5-year-old child X passes all the items meant for the average child of five, X's mental age is 5.

Mental image A representation of the stimulus that occurs in the brain rather than from external sensory input.

Mental set A tendency to stick to old ways of solving problems instead of trying new ones that are available.

Mere exposure effect The tendency to develop a liking for a person or an object you see every day.

Mesomorph One of the three body types in Sheldon's theory; a mesomorph is one whose body is strong and well-muscled.

Meta-analysis A special statistical technique in which the results of different investigations are combined to draw general conclusions.

Metacognition Knowledge of one's own cognitive processes underlying thinking.

Method of loci Visualizing images of things to be memorized on an orderly arrangement of locations.

Midbrain The middle of the three divisions of the brain containing centers that play important role in regulating vision, audition, attention and consciousness; it is also called mesencephalon.

Midlife crisis Stressful experience precipitated by the review and re-evaluation of one's own past typically occurring in the early to mid forties.

Minnesota Multiphasic Personality Inventory (MMPI) A widely used multi-item personality inventory, whose items were selected using the *empirical approach* of comparing various psychiatric groups with a normal sample.

Misinformation effect The distortion of memory by introducing misleading postevent information.

Mixed episodes A condition in which a person exhibits symptoms of both full-blown manic episode and major depressive episode for at least one week, whether the symptoms are intermixed or alternate rapidly every few days.

Mnemonic devices Strategies used to improve memory.

Mode The most frequently occurring score in a frequency distribution.

Modeling A procedure in which a participant observes another person perform some behavior and then attempts to imitate that behavior. It is an instance of social learning.

Monism A philosophical point of view, which states that there is only one reality. Materialists believe that matter exists and all mental events are reducible to physical events in the brain. Idealists assert that only the mind exists and everything including the physical world is the result of human consciousness.

Monists See *Monism*.

Monochromats People suffering from total color blindness.

Monocular cues Depth cues that require only one eye; the cues are linear perspective, texture, clarity, overlap, shadow and size of the object.

Monozygotic twins The twins resulting from the spontaneous splitting of a fertilized zygote. Such twins will be of the same sex and are generally called *identical twins*.

Mood-congruent memory The tendency to remember events or information that are congruent (similar to or identical with) with our current mood.

Mood disorders Psychological disorders whose main symptom is depression or mania or both alternating.

Moral anxiety In psychoanalysis, anxiety deriving from the prohibitions of the superego.

Morpheme The smallest meaningful unit in a given language.

Motivation The psychological state of an organism that activates and energizes goal-directed behavior.

Motor areas The cortical areas in the rear portion of the frontal lobe (at the precentral gyrus) that controls voluntary movements in the opposite side of the body.

Motor neurons Nerve cells that carry information from the brain and spinal cord to muscles and glands.

Müller, Johannes (1801–1858) Müller who is recognized as the father of modern experimental physiology is important for psychology also. He is believed to have said that no one can be psychologist unless he is a physiologist.

Myelin sheath A fatty insulating substance covering the axons of some neurons; myelin sheath increases the speed of neural transmission.

Myers-Briggs Type Indicator An inventory designed to measure personality types proposed by Carl Jung.

Narcissism Exaggerated interest in self; self-love.

Narcissistic personality disorder A disturbed personality characterized by an exaggerated sense of self-importance.

Narcolepsy A disorder of sleep characterized by sudden and uncontrollable attacks of sleep during waking hours.

Narcotics Drugs that induce relaxation and reduce pain.

Nativism A philosophical orientation in psychology that stresses the genetic, inherited influences on behavior over the acquired, experiential influences (*empiricism*).

Naturalistic observation An observational procedure in which participants are observed in their natural habitat. The observer remains unobtrusive without interfering with natural activities of the participants being observed.

Natural selection As a primary mechanism of evolution, the term refers to the assumption that traits contributing to an organism's survival are the ones that are most likely to be passed on to the next generation. In simple terms, characteristics that increase the likelihood of survival and reproduction are preserved in the gene pool and thereby become more common in a species over time.

Nature-nurture issues The issues pertaining to the degree to which heredity and environment influence behavior and development.

Need for achievement (nAch) A tendency to work hard to reach a goal, accomplish something difficult and compete with a standard of excellence.

Need for affiliation (nAff) The desire to seek interpersonal relationships and to make and retain friendship.

Need for positive regard In Rogers' theory of personality, an innate need to be positively evaluated by significant others.

Need for power (nPow) A need to seek and exercise power.

Need for self-regard Rogers' term referring to a psychological need of a person to feel positively about himself or herself.

Negative punishment A type of punishment in which a response is weakened by the removal of pleasant stimulus; for example, a mother telling a child "Don't talk to me," when the child misbehaves. See *Response cost*.

Negative reinforcement Reinforcing a response by removing an aversive stimulus; for example, giving an analgesic when one is suffering from pain.

Negative state relief model A theory of prosocial behavior stating that when we are experiencing a negative emotion, we are motivated to help others as a way of getting relief from such an emotional state.

Negative symptoms Schizophrenic symptoms such as inappropriate emotional expressions (e.g. apathy), speech disturbances or lack of interpersonal relations (e.g. withdrawal), which affect normal functioning of the individual.

Neglecting parents The parents who provide neither warmth nor rules nor guidance; their children tend to be impulsive and aggressive, score poorly in school and exhibit poor social relationship with peers.

Neo-Freudians Some of the followers of Freud who disagreed with him on several issues and later developed modified systems of psychoanalysis.

NEO-PI A personality inventory designed to assess the *Big Five factors*.

Neonate A newborn child.

Nerve deafness One type of deafness resulting from any neurological impairment of the auditory receptors in the cochlea or the auditory nerve.

Neuralgia A painful condition in the absence of any apparent tissue damage, but in which pain can be provoked by minimal stimulation.

Neuroleptic drugs A synonym for antipsychotic drugs.

Neurons Nerve cells that constitute the building blocks of nervous system; generally a neuron consists of the cell body, axon and dendrites.

Neurotic anxiety One of the three types of anxiety postulated by Freud; it refers to the vague fear that derives from irrational, amoral, instinctual urges of the Id.

Neuroticism One of the factorially derived dimensions of personality; it indicates a proneness to experience anxiety, anger, depression, impulsiveness and self-consciousness.

Neurotransmitters Chemicals that are released into a synapse by the presynaptic neuron to help transport nerve impulse from one nerve cell to another.

Nietzsche, Friedrich Wilhelm (1844–1900) A German philosopher who was a subtle observer of human nature; Nietzsche influenced philosophy, psychology, and literature. Even before Freud, Nietzsche emphasized the influence of sexual and unconscious factors on human thought and behavior. He is believed to have coined the term "Id" as a representative of irrational forces of unconscious.

Non-common effects In the *theory of correspondent inference*, the effects produced by one behavioral choice, but not by an alternative choice.

Non-sense syllables Items consisting of two consonants with a vowel in between, which are extensively used in the study of rote memorization.

Non-verbal communication Certain ways of communication between individuals that do not involve spoken words. It consists of unspoken body language, facial expressions and eye contact.

Noradrenaline Hormone secreted by adrenal medulla that functions as neurotransmitter and produces psychophysiological changes characteristic of emotional excitement; it is also called norepinephrine.

Normal probability curve An important bell-shaped distribution in statistics; several scores on human characteristics (such as intelligence) are distributed normally.

Normative social influence Conformity induced by the desire to gain social acceptance and avoid social rejection.

Norm of reciprocity A social norm stating that we should help those who helped us.

Norm of social responsibility A social norm stating that we should help others and contribute toward social welfare.

Norms 1) Standards with which individual scores are compared. 2) Unwritten rules in a society that specify what behavior is desirable and accepted and what must be avoided.

Nucleus The central body within a cell that contains the basic mechanism for cell growth, repair and reproduction.

Null hypothesis The hypothesis of no difference; it proposes that the observed difference between two or more samples is due to chance and that the independent variable had no effect on the dependent variable.

Obedience Acting in accordance with rules or orders; it is form of social influence about which psychologists have made startling discoveries. For instance, Stanley Milgram demonstrated that people have tendency to obey the commands of authority figures.

Object cathexis Freud's term for investing psychic energy in an object. Object here may be a person or part of a person or an image of either. Objects are required to satisfy the instinctual urges.

Object permanence The understanding that an object continues to exist even when it is out of sight. It is a critical aspect in a child's cognitive development.

Observational learning A type of learning by observing other's behavior and its consequences. This form of learning, called social learning or modeling, is an important construct in Albert Bandura's writings.

Obsession Persistent and recurrent intrusive thoughts, images or impulses that a person experiences as disturbing and inappropriate, but has difficulty in controlling.

Obsessive-compulsive disorders (OCD) An anxiety disorder characterized by persistent intrusion of undesirable thoughts (obsessions) or/and an uncontrollable urge to engage in non-adaptive acts (compulsions). An individual engages in compulsive behaviors to neutralize the anxiety associated with obsessive thoughts.

Occipital lobe The posterior lobe of cerebral hemispheres chiefly connected with vision.

Oedipus complex A central concept in Freud's theory, which implicates a child's erotic desire toward parent of opposite sex with a concomitant hatred toward the parent of the same sex. That is, boys are prone to love their mothers and dislike fathers and girls to love their fathers and dislike mothers. The name is derived from the main character of a Greek drama by Sophocles.

Olfaction The sense of smell.

Olfactory bulb A structure in the forebrain that receives input from olfactory receptors in the nose.

Olfactory epithelium Two patches of mucous membrane located at the top of the nasal passageways that contain the receptors for the sense of smell.

Operant A response that operates on the environment to produce a consequence that determines whether the response is retained or removed.

Operant conditioning A form of learning proposed by Skinner. According to Skinner the consequence of making a response determines the fate of response; if a response is followed by a positive consequence (reward), the likelihood of its occurrence increases and if it is followed by negative consequence (punishment), the probability of its occurrence decreases.

Operant discrimination Occurring of an operant response to a particular antecedent stimulus, but not to another antecedent stimulus.

Operant extinction Weakening and finally termination of a previously reinforced response by not offering reinforcement.

Operant generalization Occurring of an operant response to a new antecedent stimulus similar to the original antecedent stimulus.

Operant level The rate at which an operant is emitted prior to reinforcement.

Operational definition Defining a concept in terms of the specific procedures used to produce or measure it.

Opiates Drugs containing opium or opium derivatives; morphine, codeine and heroin are opiates.

Oppositional defiant disorder A childhood disorder characterized by persistent acts of aggression or antisocial behavior; it occurs approximately around the 6th year.

Optic nerve The nerve (bundle of ganglion axons) that carries information from the visual receptor to the visual area of the brain via thalamus. It is the second cranial nerve.

Oral stage In Freud's theory, the first psychosexual stage in which the child derives erotic pleasure from the stimulation of mouth and lips (principally by sucking and biting); the stage occurs during the first 18 months of the child's life. According to Freud, oral fixation has important influence on adult personality.

Organ of Corti The auditory receptor of the inner ear that rests on the basilar membrane; it is involved in the transduction of the fluid movements in the cochlea into auditory nerve impulses.

Orgasm The peak of sexual excitement associated with rhythmic contraction of muscles in the genital organ.

Ossicles The three bony structures in the middle ear (*malleus, incus, stapes*) that conduct the sound vibrations from eardrum to oval window.

Out-group A group comprised of any and all persons not in one's in-group; also called "they-group."

Out-group homogeneity bias The tendency of members of in-group to assume that there is a greater similarity among the members of out-groups than there actually is.

Oval window The membrane in the wall of *cochlea* to which the stapes is attached.

Ovulation The release of an egg from the ovary.

Ovum The single female egg cell or gamete.

Pacinian corpuscles Specialized nerve endings in the skin believed to be the receptors for pressure.

Panic disorders Anxiety disorders characterized by repeated, sudden attacks of panic, often accompanied by anxiety about having another one.

Pansexualism A point of view that all human behavior can be explained in terms of sexuality, a criticism attributed to Freudian theories.

Parallel distributed processing model A neural network model of memorization in which each item in memory is represented by a particular pattern of distributed yet interconnected nodes that are activated simultaneously; that is, they operate in parallel.

Paranoid personality disorder A condition marked by pervasive suspiciousness and distrust of others.

Paranoid schizophrenia A type of schizophrenia in which the person exhibits suspiciousness, difficulties in interpersonal relationships and absurd illogical delusions.

Paraphilias Deviant patterns of sexual behaviors employing unusual objects, rituals or situations for gratification. *Exhibitionism, fetishism, voyeurism, transvestism and bestiality* are paraphilias.

Parapsychology The discipline engaged in the study of paranormal phenomena such as telepathy, clairvoyance, and psychokinesis.

Parasympathetic nervous system A branch of autonomic nervous system that is active during the relaxed state of the organism and engaged in conservation of energy.

Parental love The love of children toward parents and elders.

Parietal lobe A major area of the brain located at the top rear between the frontal and occipital lobes. Parietal lobes are involved in processing bodily sensations.

Parkinson's disease A progressive neurological disease characterized by a mask-like, expressionless face, loss of sensorimotor coordination, inability to initiate action, rigidity and coarse tremors. The condition is named after James Parkinson who described it.

Partial reinforcement See *Intermittent reinforcement.*

Passionate love A form of love characterized by intense emotional arousal and a craving for the partner.

Pavlov, Ivan Petrovich (1849–1936) Nobel Prize winning Russian physiologist who revolutionized psychology through the discovery of conditioning phenomenon; conditioned reflex became the cornerstone on which the influential school of behaviorism was built.

Peak experience A term used by Maslow for mystical, transcendent, awe-inspiring experiences representing the highest and healthiest functions of the human mind; a characteristic of some of the self-actualizers.

Pedophilia A sexual deviation in which an adult engages in sexual relationship with a child.

Penis envy During the *phallic stage*, the desire of girls to have a penis just like boys. Penis envy causes *Oedipus complex* in girls.

Perception A complex higher mental process in which sensory input is organized, integrated and interpreted to create a meaningful representation of the world.

Perceptual constancies The tendency to perceive shape, size, color or brightness of objects as they are in spite of the changing stimulus conditions; for example, a white sheet of paper in a dark room is seen as white in spite of the fact that the amount of light falling on it has changed enormously (brightness constancy).

Peripheral nervous system The part of the nervous system that connects the spinal cord and brain with sensory organs, muscles and glands. It is made up of long axons and dendrites branching out from the spinal cord and brain; it includes autonomic nervous system and somatic system.

Peripheral route (processing) Interpretation of message taking into consideration the details related to the source of the message (the speaker's traits, the emotional appeal, etc.), rather than scrutinizing the nature of the message itself.

Personal fables The common belief among adolescents that their feelings and experiences cannot possibly be understood by others and that they are personally invulnerable to harm.

Personality The enduring organization of characteristics that distinguishes one person from the other; a pattern of traits that makes a person unique.

Personality disorders A group of disorders characterized by inflexible, maladaptive personality traits that make it difficult for the person to function effectively in society.

Personal unconscious In Jung's theory of personality, the part of the unconscious that contains an individual's repressed memories and experiences.

Person-centered therapy An alternative term for *client-centered therapy.*

Personology Murray's theory of personality; Murray suggested that psychology may be called personology because the study of personality is the beginning and end of psychology.

Phallic stage In Freud's theory, the third of the psychosexual stages (around third year) during which the child derives erotic pleasure by manipulating the genitals; it is the period in which Oedipus conflict occurs.

Phantom limb pain Experience of pain arising from a limb that has been amputated.

Phenomenology A philosophical approach emphasizing the role of immediate experience in understanding human behavior.

Phenotype The observed structural and functional characteristics of an individual; phenotypes result from an interaction between genotype and the environment.

Pheromones Chemicals emitted by animals to communicate sexual receptivity or alarm and also to mark out their territory.

Phi-phenomenon The perceptual experience of apparent movement, which can occur while viewing two lights flashing on and off in sequence; if the interval between the two lights is around 150 milliseconds, then one perceives movement of the light from the first location to the second. It is a stroboscopic movement in its simplest form.

Phobia Persistent and excessive fear of objects and situations, which are generally not fear-producing.

Phobic disorders The disorders characterized by persistent, disproportionate and irrational fear (phobias) of some specific object or situation that presents little or no danger.

Phoneme The smallest unit of sound in a language; it serves to distinguish utterances from one another.

Phonetics The study of production, perception and transcription of speech sounds (phones).

Phonological loop The speech-based part of working memory that allows for the verbal rehearsal of sounds or words.

Phonology The study of the smallest units of the sound called phonemes.

Photopigments Protein molecules in rods and cones whose chemical reactions during absorption of light produce visual nerve impulses.

Physiological psychology A branch of psychology that studies the neurophysiological bases of behavior.

Piaget, Jean (1896–1980) A well-known Swiss developmental psychologist who proposed a very influential theory of cognitive development.

Pinna The fleshy outer part of the external ear.

Pituitary gland Endocrine gland attached to the base of the brain; it is often called the master gland because it regulates the functioning of all other endocrine glands. It has two parts; anterior pituitary (adenohypophysis) and posterior pituitary (neurohypophysis). The adenohypophysis secretes somatotropic hormone (STH), which regulates growth; adrenocorticotropic hormone (ACTH), which regulates the activity of adrenal cortex; thyrotropic hormone, which regulates the functioning of the thyroid gland; gonadotropic hormones including follicle-stimulating hormone (FSH), which stimulates ovarian follicles in females and spermatogenesis in males; luteinizing hormone (LH) or interstitial cell-stimulating hormone (ICSH), which along with FSH stimulates secretion of estrogens and ovulation and lactogenic hormone (prolactin), which controls milk production in mature mammary glands. Neurohypophysis secretes the antidiuretic hormone (ADH), which controls metabolism, vasopressin which induces contraction of smooth muscles of blood vessels and oxytocin, which strengthens uterine contractions and the milk-ejecting functions of the mammary glands.

Placebo An inert substance that has no significant effect on the organism; it is given as false treatment.

Placebo effect A change in behavior that occurs because of the expectation or belief that one is receiving a treatment.

Place theory of hearing Theory stating that different areas of the basilar membrane respond to different frequencies of the sound wave.

Plato (427–347 BC) A great philosopher and political thinker, Plato was a student of Socrates and teacher of Aristotle. He held that body and mind were different entities and this concept of dualism has influenced later thinking about the relationship between body and mind.

Pleasure principle The principle governing the functioning of the Id, which needs immediate gratification.

Polygenic transmission A number of genes working together to produce a phenotypic characteristic.

Polygraph An instrument that measures multiple physiological functions such as blood pressure, heart rate, galvanic skin response and respiration rate.

Pons A structure in the brain stem involved in sleep and dreaming.

Population The entire set of individuals about whom a researcher wants to draw conclusions based on the study made on a subset (sample) of the same.

Positive psychology A new emerging subfield of psychology emphasizing the study of human strength, assets, fulfillment, virtues and optimal living rather than weaknesses and deficits.

Positive punishment Reduction of occurrence of response by the application of an aversive stimulus (positive punisher).

Positive reinforcement Strengthening the occurrence of a response by providing with a reward.

Positive symptoms Schizophrenic symptoms such as delusions, hallucinations and disorders of thought and speech; these are called positive because they are added to an individual's normal repertoire of behavior.

Positron-emission tomography A scanning technique that measures metabolic processes to appraise how well an organ is functioning.

Post-traumatic stress disorder (PTSD) An anxiety disorder that follows an extreme traumatic event; the person suffering from PTSD re-experiences the traumatic event, avoids the memories of the event, and exhibits persistent arousal.

Postconventional level In Kohlberg's theory of moral development, a stage in which moral judgments are made based on well-thought-of, internalized moral principles.

Practical intelligence The type of intelligence needed for overall successful living.

Pragmatics Knowledge about how to use a language such as choice of proper words, intonation, knowledge of the intentions of the speaker and how to produce an effective speech response.

Precognition The paranormal (psi) phenomenon referring to the ability to know the future events.

Preconventional level In Kohlberg's theory of moral development, a stage in which moral judgment is made based on anticipated reward or punishment.

Predictive validity A type of validity indicating the extent to which the test scores are predictive of actual performance.

Prefrontal cortex The area of the frontal lobe (anterior part of frontal lobe) involved in self-awareness, planning and executive functions.

Prefrontal lobotomy A surgical procedure in which connections between frontal lobes of the brain and other centers were severed resulting in permanent changes in brain and behavior; the procedure is not in use nowadays.

Prejudice Negative or positive attitudes toward people based on their membership of a group.

Premature ejaculation Recurrent onset of ejaculation of semen and orgasm during intercourse with minimum of sexual arousal.

Preoperational stage In Piaget's theory of cognitive development, the stage in which children can represent the world symbolically through words and images, but cannot understand basic mental operations or rules.

Prepared behavior Responses, which can be learned (conditioned) easily by certain organisms. Compare with *contraprepared behavior* and *unprepared behavior*.

Primacy effect People's tendency to attach more importance to information received first during impression formation about others.

Primary drive Any drive that arises from an inner physiological state of an organism such as hunger, thirst, sex, etc.

Primary gain According to Freudian theory, it is the goal achieved by conversion symptoms: keeping unconscious conflicts out of awareness.

Primary mental abilities Seven basic mental abilities that Thurstone believed constitute intelligence.

Primary process In Freudian theory, the way the Id obtains immediate need gratification and discharges tension using motor activities and hallucinations of desired objects.

Primary reinforcer A reinforcer that satisfies a biological (primary) drive such as hunger.

Priming A phenomenon in which exposure to a stimulus later makes it easier to recall that same or similar stimulus; in memorization, the activation of one word or idea by another word or idea.

Proactive interference The interference of material previously learned with material currently being learned.

Problem-focused coping Dealing with stress by direct confrontation and mastery over a stressful situation.

Problem solving The processes involved in the solution of a problem; it is rule-guided, motivated behavior directed toward solution of a problem.

Procedural memory The memory for habitual motor skills, such as driving a car that have become automatic; also called non-declarative memory. Some people consider implicit memory as a rough synonym for procedural memory.

Programmed learning A learning procedure proposed by Skinner in which the information is presented to the learner in small steps, immediate feedback is given indicating whether the material was learned properly and the learner is permitted to determine the pace with which he/she goes through the material.

Projection In classical psychoanalytic theory, a defense mechanism in which one ascribes one's own traits, impulses and wishes (usually undesirable ones) onto another person.

Projective tests Personality tests in which standardized, unstructured stimuli (such as inkblots) are used to elicit responses from which inferences are made about a person. It is believed that people project internal feelings onto the ambiguous stimuli.

Proprium A term coined by GW Allport to refer to various components and functions of self-concept; Allport included seven aspects of self-including self-image, self-identity, self-esteem, rational thinking, cognitive style and bodily self under the proprium; the term was coined to clear the confusion in the repeated use of the terms self and ego.

Prosocial behavior Helping people in an emergency without anticipating anything in return.

Prospective memory Remembering something to be done in future.

Prototype The most representative (typical) examples of a concept. For example, dog is a prototype for the concept animal.

Proximodistal sequence The progression of physical and motor development from the center of the body toward the periphery; for example, the child masters the shoulder movements before he could control the hand and finger movements.

Psi phenomenon The special paranormal ability believed to be possessed by some people who perform well in experiments of extrasensory perception (ESP) and psychokinesis.

Psychiatrist A medical doctor specializing in the treatment of mental disorders.

Psychiatry The specialty area of medicine studying the diagnosis, treatment, and prevention of psychological disorders. The activities of psychiatrists overlap with those of clinical psychologists except that the latter do not prescribe drugs.

Psychic energy The hypothetical fuel (energy) that powers mental activities.

Psychoactive drugs (substances) Chemicals that affect behavior and consciousness or mental functioning.

Psychoanalysis Freudian system of psychology that emphasizes unconscious dynamics and infantile experiences in the determining of behavior; it is also the name for a form of treatment of psychological disorders.

Psychodynamic therapy Therapeutic procedures based on modified forms of psychoanalytic treatment; the therapy is based on the assumption that the primary factors causing psychological disorders are unresolved unconscious conflicts.

Psychokinesis The alleged psychic capacity (psi) to move objects without using physical force.

Psycholinguistics The special area that studies the psychological aspects of language.

Psychological amnesia Selective memory loss for events that occur after a traumatic experience.

Psychology The science of behavior and mental processes.

Psychometric methods Statistical methods used in the measurement of psychological processes.

Psychoneuroimmunology (PNI) A field of study that examines the relationships among the psychological factors, the immune system and the functions of the brain in the causation of illness and wellness.

Psychopharmacology Science of determining the drugs that are effective in the treatment of psychological disorders and how they work.

Psychophysical parallelism A theory of mind-body relationship, which states that the mind and body are different (dualism) entities, they do not interact and run on parallel courses giving the appearance of interaction.

Psychophysics The study of the relationship between stimuli and sensory experience.

Psychophysiological disorder Physical disorders that are caused by psychological factors; earlier these were called psychosomatic disorders.

Psychosexual stages In psychoanalytic theory, the developmental stages through which every human child passes; Freud discusses five stages namely, oral, anal, phallic, latency and genital phases. The experiences in these stages have immense bearing on the development of personality.

Psychosocial development Erikson's characterization of personality development, which stresses the interaction between a person and the social environment; the theory proposes that every human being passes through eight stages of psychosocial development from childhood to old age. They can be regarded as an extension and elaboration of Freud's theory of psychosexual development.

Psychosurgery A surgery of the brain conducted to reduce the severity of mental symptoms; lobotomy and leukotomy were the procedures used. Nowadays the psychosurgery is rarely used if ever.

Psychotherapy Psychological procedures used to treat mental and behavioral disorders.

Psychoticism One of the dimensions of personality proposed by Eysenck; psychoticism subsumes a continuum from normal behavior through criminal and psychopathic behavior to schizophrenia and other psychotic states in which contact is lost with reality and there is severely disturbed cognition, emotion and behavior.

Psychotropic drugs Psychiatric drugs used in the treatment of psychological disorders.

Puberty The developmental stage marked by rapid biological changes including sexual maturity.

Punisher Any act, event or stimulus that operates to terminate the occurrence of response.

Punishment Any stimulus that weakens the probability of occurrence of a response.

Purposivism A system of psychology proposed by William McDougall, which asserted that behavior is goal-directed.

Pyknic One of the three body types described by Kretschmer as fatty and plum.

Q-sort An assessment technique in which a person is given a set of personality relevant adjectives or statements and asked to put them into piles ranging from least characteristic to most characteristic of him/her or another person. Often the number of items to be put into piles is restricted to obtain a normal distribution. The items are given weights according to the pile into which they are put. The method is mostly used to assess self-constructs.

Quartile deviation See *Interquartile range*.

Racial unconscious An alternative term for *collective unconscious*.

Random sample A group of people selected from a population in such a way that each member of the population has an equal chance of being selected. It is assumed that such sample will be representative of the population.

Range The simplest measure of variability indicating the difference between the highest and the lowest scores in a distribution.

Rape Having forced sexual gratification with another person; may use a threat or coercion.

Rational emotive behavior therapy (REBT) One of the forms of psychotherapy developed by Ellis that attempts to change a person's maladaptive belief system into a more realistic, rational set of views.

Rationalism The philosophical approach put forward by Plato in which reason is given the highest place as a means of getting at the truth.

Rationalization An ego-defense mechanism that involves offering of possible explanation rather than the real explanation for behaviors including failures or unworthy acts.

Rational theoretical approach An approach to test construction in which the items are selected based on a theory of the construct that one intends to measure.

Reactance A negative emotional and cognitive reaction shown when there are attempts to curtail one's freedom or change attitude.

Reaction formation Ego-defense mechanism in which an unacceptable idea or wish is first repressed and its opposite is given expression in consciousness. For example, a person with criminal tendency may strive to become lawgiver or a judge in a law court.

Realism The ability to recognize that the objective world exists apart from oneself. According to Piaget this cognitive ability emerges around the age of 7 years.

Realistic conflict theory A theory maintaining that competition for limited resources is the cause of prejudice.

Reality anxiety Fear of really dangerous things existing in the external environment. This is what we generally call fear.

Reality principle The governing principle of the ego whose aim is inhibiting the discharge of excitation (the Id impulses) until appropriate object in the environment that satisfies the need is discovered. In Freudian psychology, reality principle tries to postpone immediate gratification of the Id wishes until suitable object is available.

Reasoning The process of logical (inferential) thinking or problem solving employing general principles.

Recency effect The tendency to remember information received (learned) recently.

Reciprocal determinism Bandura's belief that there are two way causal relationships between a person's cognition, behavior, and environment.

Referred pain The sensation of pain in a location other than the one affected.

Reflex action Automatic, inborn responses triggered by specific stimuli; in psychoanalytic theory the way the Id impulses are satisfied.

Refractory period In the sexual response cycle, the temporary period following the resolution stage during which the male cannot be sexually aroused.

Regression In psychoanalytic theory, a defense mechanism in which an individual, usually when under stress, reverts to behavior characteristic of an earlier stage of development.

Rehearsal The repetition of information in short-term memory for retaining it for longer duration.

Reinforcement Increasing the probability of occurrence of a response by a stimulus (a reward) that follows the response.

Reissner's membrane The membrane that separates scala vestibuli from the scala media in the cochlea.

Relapse prevention A therapeutic procedure designed to teach coping skills, increase self-efficiency and counter the abstinence violation effect, thus reducing the likelihood of relapse.

Relaxation response A method of relaxation for stress management developed by cardiologist Herbert Benson; the technique combines muscle relaxation in a comfortable position, a passive attitude, a quiet environment and a repetitive sound. The client sits with closed eyes for about 20 minutes chanting a simple word (such as 'one'). It is similar to transcendental meditation (TM) popularized by Maharishi Mahesh Yogi.

Relearning method A procedure for testing retention by comparing the number of trials needed to learn material with the number of trials needed to relearn the material at a later date. Suppose one took ten trials to learn a list of nonsense syllables initially and takes only five trials to relearn a second time. The saving is 50 percent (5/10 × 100). The method developed by Ebbinghaus is also called 'the saving method'.

Reliability An index determined to see whether a measuring tool (for example, a psychological test) produces the same result when used multiple times; an index of consistency of the measuring tool.

Remote behavior sampling A method to collect samples of behavior from clients as they live their daily lives.

Replication Repeating a study to determine whether the same results as in the original one can be obtained.

Representativeness heuristic A strategy for making judgments based on the extent to which current stimuli or events resemble ones we consider typical.

Repression A basic defense mechanism, which pushes all painful and anxiety-arousing information into the unconscious.

Residual schizophrenia A term used to refer to people who have experienced a schizophrenic episode from which they have recovered enough to not show prominent symptoms, but are still exhibiting some mild signs of the disorder.

Resistance In Freudian therapy a stage in which the clients start refusing to free associate, absent from therapy, and do not follow the instructions of the therapist; they do this because they want to protect themselves from anxiety-producing material that is surfacing during therapy.

Resistance stage The second stage in the general adaptation syndrome (GAS) in which an organism attempts to take action to avoid, overcome or adapt to stressor.

Resolution stage The interval following orgasm during which the male's body returns to its normal state, reversing the changes produced by sexual arousal.

Response cost A type of punishment in which a response is weakened by removing the pleasant stimulus the subject was enjoying; it is something like removing a privilege, withholding an increment, etc. It is also called 'negative punishment' or 'punishment by removal'.

Resting state The state of a nerve cell in which there is a negative electrical charge across the membrane within the nerve cell.

Reticular formation The part of the brain from the medulla through the pons consisting of groups of nerve cells that can immediately activate other parts of the brain to produce general arousal.

Retina The photosensitive part at the back of the eye that converts the electromagnetic energy into information that the brain can understand.

Retrieval Accessing information stored in the long-term memory; the act of recalling.

Retroactive interference The interference caused by recently learned material in recalling earlier learned material.

Retrograde amnesia Loss of memory for events prior to the amnesia-producing trauma.

Reuptake The reabsorption of a substance, such as a neurotransmitter, by the presynaptic neuron so that it does not stimulate the postsynaptic neuron.

Reversibility The property of a series of operations such that reversing their order restores the original state. In Piaget's theory, it is an indication that the child has understood the principle of conservation.

Risky shift A laboratory finding stating that people are willing to take risky decisions after participating in a group discussion than before. Later studies have shown that whether the risky shift occurs or not depends on the importance of the issue to the group.

Rods Photoreceptors in the retina that are active during low illumination; rods are not involved in color sensation.

Rogers CR (1902–1987) An American psychotherapist and personality theorist, Rogers was a leading figure, along with Maslow, in advancing the humanistic psychology movement. He is known as the founder of client-centered counseling, which is being practiced all over the world.

Romanticism A philosophical view that emphasizes the uniqueness of each person and values irrationality much more than rationality. The view asserts that people can and should trust their natural impulses.

Rorschach Inkblot Test A projective test developed by a Swiss psychiatrist Hermann Rorschach; the test consists of ten cards containing inkblots to which participants respond. The responses are scored according to standard procedures and the participant's personality is inferred from the pattern of scores.

Rotter, Julian Bernard (1916–2014) An American psychologist who along with Bandura developed social learning theory: some of the tests Rotter developed such as Internal-External Scale (I-E Scale), and a measure of interpersonal trust have initiated a good deal of research.

Rousseau, Jean-Jacques (1712–1778) Considered the founder of romanticism, Rousseau believed that human nature is basically good and that the best society is one in which people subjugate their individual will to the general will. He is said to have influenced the development of humanistic viewpoints in psychology.

Sample A small number of individuals drawn from a large population for including in research.

Sampling error The difference between the characteristics of a sample and the population from which it was drawn.

Sampling with replacement Sampling in which the selected elements are placed back in the population so that they are available for further sampling.

Saturation The color dimension which refers to the purity or richness of color.

Saving method *See Relearning method.*

Scaffolding Temporary support provided by elders to help a child master a task (Vygotsky).

Schedules of reinforcement Programs of continuous or intermittent reinforcement including interval schedules and ratio schedules and various combinations thereof, presented to subjects who are learning operants. The four major types of schedules are fixed interval, variable interval, fixed ratio and variable ratio.

Schema An organized pattern of information in mind (a mental framework) about some aspect of the environment, which determines the way in which new information is interpreted, assimilated and stored in memory.

Schizophrenia A group of severe psychotic disorders involving impairments in perceiving (hallucinations), thinking (delusions), emotion (apathy), communication (speech), and behavior.

Schools of psychology Groups of psychologists with common assumptions, problems and methods about human behavior; important schools that once flourished were structuralism, functionalism, behaviorism, psychoanalysis, Gestalt psychology and so on. All the schools were absorbed by the general stream of psychology. Today we have only perspectives, but no schools in psychology.

Scientific explanation A tentative explanation for a phenomenon based on objective observation and logic and subject to empirical test.

Scientific method The method of enquiry used by scientists to understand and explain the phenomena in the universe. It involves observing phenomena, developing hypotheses, empirically testing the hypotheses, revising and refining the hypothesis in the light of the results and finally developing a theory.

Secondary drive Acquired drive such as desire for prestige, power, money, etc. Generally, it is assumed that secondary drives are acquired because of their association with a primary drive.

Secondary gain Sympathy gained by becoming sick.

Secondary process In Freud's theory, mental functioning that is conscious, rational and logical. Secondary processes are conceptually linked with the ego and the reality principle.

Secondary reinforcer A stimulus that acquires reinforcing properties by being associated with a primary reinforcer; for example, money is a secondary reinforcer.

Secondary trait In GW Allport's theory, a characteristic that is more limited in its occurrence, less crucial to a description of personality and more focalized in the responses it leads to, as well as the stimuli to which it is appropriate.

Self-actualization In humanistic theories, a sovereign motive that impels people to become what they can become.

Self-concept A descriptive and evaluative picture humans have about themselves. Humanists, especially Rogers, emphasized the importance of self-concept in their theoretical formulations.

Self-efficacy A conviction that one can perform the necessary acts to produce the desired result; Bandura has initiated extensive research on the concept of self-efficacy.

Self-esteem The positive value an individual attaches to his/her self-concept.

Self-fulfilling prophecy The finding that people can make others act as they expect them to act without even being aware that they are doing so; it is also called 'the Rosenthal effect'.

Self-love An accurate understanding and appreciation of oneself.

Self-presentation Techniques designed to create a favorable impression of ourselves in others.

Self-serving bias The tendency to take credit for our successes and to explain away our failures; blaming the situation for one's failure.

Self See *Self-concept*.

Semantic memory Simply put, memory for meaning. Generally, the term refers to factual knowledge about words, concepts and the rules for using them in language stored in long-term memory.

Semantics The linguistic rules for connecting symbols in language to what they represent; that is, the rules governing the meaning of words and sentences.

Semicircular canals The three semicircular membranous structures in the inner ear that are sensory receptors for detecting body movements.

Senile dementia A form of mental disorder caused in part by degenerative brain changes during old age.

Sensation The process by which stimuli from the external world are detected, converted into nerve impulses, and communicated to the brain.

Sensation Seeking Scale A test designed to assess an individual's need to engage in novel experiences.

Sensitive period An optimal age range at which certain experiences occur for normal development.

Sensorimotor stage In Piaget's theory, a period (from birth to 2 years) during which the children understand their world through sensory and motor activities.

Sensory areas Sites in the brain that receive sensory input; for example, visual area in the occipital lobe.

Sensory memory The initial, momentary storage of information in memory lasting only for a fraction of a second, but long enough to be recognized.

Sensory neurons Specialized neurons that carry information from various parts of the body to the brain; these are also called 'afferent neurons'.

Sensory registers Subsystems of sensory memory, which are the initial processors of information.

Separation anxiety (disorder) A childhood disorder marked by unrealistic fears, over-reaction, self-consciousness, nightmares and chronic anxiety, when there is a threat of separation.

Sequential design A research procedure, which involves testing repeatedly several age cohorts as they grow older. It combines both cross-sectional and longitudinal designs.

Seriation Arrangement of things in a series in consecutive order; a cognitive achievement in Piaget's theory.

Serotonin An inhibitive neurotransmitter found in the central nervous system; serotonin is implicated in several functions such as sleep, pain and depression.

Set point A biologically determined standard around which body weight is regulated.

Sex-role stereotypes See *Gender roles*.

Sex chromosome The chromosome, which determines the sex of the zygote; in humans the 23rd pair of chromosomes.

Sex typing Treating people differentially based on their sex.

Sexual abuse Sexual gratification involving physical or psychological coercion and without the consent of the partner.

Sexual aversion disorder A condition in which an individual shows extreme aversion to, and avoidance of, all genital sexual contact with a partner.

Sexual dysfunction An impairment either in the desire for sexual gratification or in the ability to achieve it.

Sexual masochism Deriving sexual stimulation and gratification by experiencing pain inflicted by the partner.

Sexual orientation An individual's sexual and emotional preference for either men or women.

Sexual response cycle A physiological response pattern occurring during sexual arousal; Masters and Johnson have found four basic phases: excitement, plateau, orgasm and resolution.

Sexual sadism Deriving sexual gratification by inflicting pain (physical and/or psychological) on a sexual partner.

Shape constancy Perceiving an object in its actual shape in spite of changes in the viewing conditions.

Shaping Form of operant conditioning in which the behavior of an organism is shaped; first all responses resembling the desired one are reinforced and later only close approximations and finally, only the correct response. See *Successive approximation*.

Short-term memory (STM) A hypothesized memory store that holds limited amount of information for a short period.

Simple random sampling A sampling procedure in which every member of a population has an equal chance of being selected for a sample and in which the sampling is done on a purely random basis.

Simulation A laboratory research procedure in which an attempt is made to recreate as closely as possible a real world event.

Sixteen Personality Factor Test (16 PF) A personality inventory developed by RB Cattell to measure 16 components of personality obtained through factor analysis.

Size constancy Perceiving an object in its actual size in spite of changes in the viewing conditions. An approaching car is perceived as of a constant size although its image on your retina is becoming bigger and bigger as it approaches you.

Skinner, Burrhus Frederic (1904–1990) A famous behaviorist who believed that psychology should study the functional relationship between environmental events such as reinforcement contingencies and behavior. In addition to an influential theory of learning, Skinner's creative products are Skinner box, teaching machine used in programmed learning, and an air crib used in raising children. He wrote a novel, Walden II, which describes how his views can be applied to living.

Skinner box A test chamber usually consisting of a grid floor, lever, light and food cup used in operant conditioning experiments.

Social cognition The way in which we process, store and later remember information about other people or ourselves.

Social cognitive theory An approach to the study of personality proposed by Bandura and Mischel, which emphasizes the role of social learning, cognitive processes and self-regulation.

Social comparison Comparing one's characteristics (abilities, skills and opinion) with those of other people.

Social compensation Increased effort put in by one or more members of a group to compensate for *social loafing* on the part of one or more others.

Social decision schemes Rules relating to the initial distribution of member views regarding final group decisions.

Social desirability Tendency or inclination to behave in socially approved ways so as to appear socially desirable to others.

Social facilitation Effects upon task performance resulting from the presence of others.

Social identity theory A theory of prejudice stating that prejudice stems from a need to enhance self-esteem.

Socialization The process by which culture is transmitted to members of society.

Social learning theory An approach to the study of personality, which emphasizes the role of *observational learning* or modeling in the development of personality.

Social loafing The tendency of people to put in less effort when working in a group than when working alone.

Social norms Expected standards of how people should behave in a group.

Social perception The process with which we form impressions, make judgments, develop attitudes and in short, understand the people around us. Social perception involves attribution and impression formation.

Social phobia Inappropriate and intense fear of social situations such as public speaking, eating with others, etc.; these possibly result from the fear of being evaluated by others.

Social rules Guidelines indicating how people should behave in social situations.

Sociocultural perspective An approach to the study of psychology, which emphasizes the importance of culture and social environment in explaining similarities and differences in human behavior.

Socrates (469–399 BC) The great Greek philosopher who devised the method of sharpening truth and exposing ignorance and falsehood in a dialogue; Socrates emphasized the importance of knowing about one's own self with the famous dictum 'Know thyself'.

Somatic nervous system The branch of peripheral nervous system, which carries information from sense receptors to the brain and the brain's instructions to the voluntary muscles.

Somatization disorders Psychiatric disorders exhibiting multiple complaints of physical ailments that are inadequately explained by independent findings of physical illness or injury. The condition begins around 30 years of age and continues for several years leading to medical treatment.

Somatoform disorders Psychological difficulties that manifest in the form of physical ailments that have no physiological or neurological basis.

Somatosensory area Cortical area located in the front portion of the parietal lobe that receives sensory input from the opposite side of the body.

Somatotonic One who is characterized by an extreme desire for muscular activity and need for assertiveness; one of the temperament in Sheldon's theory.

Somatotrophic hormone A hormone of the anterior pituitary that controls body growth; also called somatotrophin.

Somesthetic senses The skin senses, kinesthesis and internal sensitivity taken collectively.

Source traits In RB Cattell's theory, basic elements of personality that are not apparent in observed behavior, but are inferred from the underlying relationships among *surface traits*.

Spearman CE (1863–1945) British psychologist regarded as the founder of the factor school of psychology and the author of *two-factor theory of intelligence*; he was a student of Wundt and successor to McDougall at London University.

Specific factor (s) One of the factors in Spearman's two-factor theory along with the general factor (g); while the general factor is common to all tasks (tests), specific factor is specific to each task or test.

Specific phobia Persistent fear of specific objects such as animals, blood, narrow places, height, etc. These fears are irrational and disproportionate to the stimulus.

Sperm Male reproductive cell (*gamete*).

Spinal cord Mass of soft nervous and supporting tissues contained within the vertebral column; almost all nerves to and from the brain pass through the spinal cord.

Split-brain studies Research associated with split-brain surgery in which the fibers connecting the two hemispheres are severed for the purpose of studying the functions associated with each hemisphere.

Split-half reliability Establishing the reliability of a test by correlating the scores on one-half of the test with the other half.

Spontaneous recovery In conditioning, the returning of the conditioned response after it has been extinguished.

Spontaneous remission Spontaneous disappearance of symptoms of a disorder without treatment.

Standard deviation A statistic that indicates the spread or variability of scores in a distribution.

Stapes One of the three bones (ossicles) in the middle ear, which looks like a stirrup.

State-dependent memory The increase in the ability to recall information when the internal state of the person matches his/her original state during learning.

Statistic A value summarizing a characteristic of a sample and theoretically reflecting the population from which the sample was drawn. For example, the arithmetic mean is a statistic.

Statistics The branch of mathematics which deals with collecting, classifying and analyzing data.

Stereotype Cognitive framework that strongly influences the processing of incoming social information: sweeping generalizations about a group of people as sharing certain traits without sufficient evidence. For example, the British are conservative, Americans are practical, French are romantic and Indians are philosophical.

Stereotype threat The anxiety created by the perceived possibility that one's behavior will confirm a negative stereotype about one's group.

Stern, Wilhelm (1871–1938) German philosopher and psychologist who introduced the concept of intelligence quotient (IQ) into psychology; his system is called 'personalistic psychology' and he defined psychology as the science of person as having experience or as capable of having experience.

Stimulus discrimination Learning to respond differently to different stimuli that may have some similarities; for example, responding differently to a circle and an ellipse.

Stimulus generalization The spread of conditioned response to other stimuli which are similar to but not identical with the conditioned stimulus.

Storage The retention of information in memory.

Stranger anxiety Distress exhibited by children during the second half of the 1st year when they are faced with strange people and places.

Strange situation A procedure developed by Mary Ainsworth to assess infant attachment to the mother, consisting of a series of brief separations and reunions with the mother in a playroom situation.

Stratified random sample A sampling procedure in which the population is divided into segments (strata) and subjects are randomly sampled from each segment. It helps to ensure that the full population is properly represented.

Stress Any condition, internal or external, which disturbs the dynamic equilibrium of an organism's body system making strong demands on the organism and inducing a number of neuropsychological responses to deal with the situation.

Stress inoculation training A form of cognitive training given to manage stress; it occurs in three steps: conceptualization, skill acquisition and rehearsal and application.

Stressor A stress-provoking stimulus.

Stress response The pattern of cognitive, behavioral and physiological reactions made under stress; these may be faulty, maladaptive and pathological involving feelings of tension and panic or task-oriented involving objective appraisal of the situation to handle it effectively.

Striving for superiority In Adler's theory, an innate urge for perfection, conquest or a final goal toward which all humans move giving consistency and unity to personality.

Structure of intellect model A model of intelligence proposed by Guilford along three dimensions: *operations, contents and products*. The model proposes that there are 120 different varieties of intellectual functions.

Style of life A recurrent theme in Adler's theory, style of life is the idiographic principle that explains the uniqueness of the person. Everyone has a style of life that is unique determining how he/she perceives, thinks and acts in life.

Subgoal analysis A heuristic in which people attack a large problem by formulating intermediate goals toward a solution.

Subjective well-being (SWB) The overall degree of contentment and happiness with one's life.

Sublimation An ego-defense mechanism in which the frustrated expression of sexual energy is directed toward a noble substitutive activity; for example, an unmarried woman who wants a child may start an orphanage.

Substance abuse Maladaptive behavior centered on the regular use of a substance such as a drug or alcohol.

Substance dependence A severe form of substance use disorder involving physiological dependence on the substance, tolerance, withdrawal and compulsive drug use.

Successive approximation Reinforcing only those responses that become increasingly similar to the response that is finally desired; a process used in *shaping*.

Sudden infant death syndrome (SIDS) The sudden and unexplained death of infants that usually occurs when they are sleeping in their cribs; SIDS is often called 'crib death'.

Superego In Freudian theory, the moral component of personality; it consists of two subdivisions: *conscience* and *ego ideal*.

Superstitious behavior In Skinner's system, any behavior acquired through coincidental association of a response and reinforcement.

Surface structure In linguistics, the sequence of elements (phonemes, words and phrases) that comprise an actual message as written or spoken.

Surface traits Cattell's term for personality traits at the surface level that can be inferred from observation of behavior; compare with *source traits*.

Survey research The use of surveys generally carried out using questionnaires, polls or other sampling techniques to assess public opinion about certain issues.

Sympathetic nervous system A division of autonomic nervous system that is active in emergency situations, preparing the individual to face the threat either by fight or flight.

Synapse The site of communication between the axon of one neuron and the dendrites of another neuron.

Syntax The rules that indicate how words and phrases are combined to form sentences.

Systematic desensitization A behavior therapy technique in which counterconditioning is used to eliminate anxiety; it is done by teaching the client to relax while in the presence of an anxiety-provoking stimulus, a response that is incompatible with anxiety-producing conditioned stimulus.

Szasz, Thomas Stephen (1920) Hungarian-born American psychiatrist who is well-known for the anti-psychiatry movement; he asserted that "Mental illness is a myth," and wrote a book with the same title.

Tabula rasa A Latin term, which means 'blank tablet'. The term refers to a philosophical view that the human mind of a newborn child is an empty sheet of paper and on which learning and experience are written to constitute what we call the mind. Aristotle was the first to hold this view, but British empiricists, especially John Locke, popularized it.

Tact Skinner's term for verbal behavior of naming objects and events; such behavior results in reinforcement when things are named correctly.

Tardive dyskinesia An Irreversible neurological disorder that may occur as a side effect when certain antipsychotic drugs are administered; the side effects may occur months or even years after the drug has been started or stopped. The symptoms include involuntary movements of tongue, lips, jaw and extremities.

Taste buds Chemical receptors for taste on the tongue and the in the roof and the back of the mouth, which are sensitive to the qualities of sweet, sour, salt, and bitterness.

Telepathy A claimed form extrasensory perception (ESP) in which what is perceived depends upon thought transference from one person to another.

Temperament Biologically based pattern of exhibiting behavior and emotion.

Temporal lobe Portion of the cerebrum on each side of the hemispheres below the lateral fissure and in front of the occipital lobe; temporal lobes are involved in processing auditory information.

Teratogens Substances that can harm a developing fetus and cause birth defects.

Terminal buttons Small bulges at the end of axons of a neuron that release neurotransmitters to send messages to other neurons.

Test-retest reliability Similarity of scores on the same test administered to the same group of persons on two different occasions; a correlation coefficient between the two sets of scores is taken as an index of reliability.

Testis determining factor (TDF) gene A gene in the Y chromosome that triggers male sexual development.

Testosterone Primary testicular hormone in men, which accelerates tissue growth, causes maturation of male genitals and the production of sperm. It stimulates the development of secondary sex characteristics. Small quantities of testosterone are produced by the adrenal glands in both men and women.

Thalamus A pair of egg-shaped mass of nuclei in the forebrain that operate as a relay center for sensory input. It is often called the 'brain's sensory switch board'.

Thanatos In Freudian theory, the death instinct that is responsible for human destructive and aggressive tendencies; it may be directed toward self as well as others.

Thematic Apperception Test (TAT) A projective test, which makes use of stories, told about a series of ambiguous pictures presented to participants. The personality characteristics are inferred from the stories.

Theory A set of assumptions about the causes of a phenomenon (for example, in psychology, learning) and the rules that specify how the causes operate. A theory is subjected to empirical test and retained, revised or rejected depending on the results.

Theory of correspondent inference The Jones and Davis theory of attribution, which explains how we use others behavior as a basis for inferring their stable personality traits.

Theory of mind A person's set of beliefs about the mind and the ability to understand other people's mental processes.

Thorndike, Edward Lee (1874–1949) American psychologist who offered the psychological world the first miniature system of learning that proved to have profound influence on the course of learning theory for the next half century.

Thurstone, Louis Leon (1887–1955) An outstanding psychometrician of his time, Thurstone's main contributions are in the area of application of statistical methods to psychological problems. He developed the centroid method of factor analysis, established *primary mental abilities* and constructed tests to measure them. Thurstone's law of comparative judgment in psychophysics provided the basis for psychological scaling and he was the first to measure attitudes using the method of equal-appearing intervals. He was the President of American Psychological Association in 1933.

Thyroid gland Paired endocrine glands located at the neck that secrete the growth hormone thyroxin.

Thyrotropic hormone A hormone of the anterior pituitary that stimulates thyroid to produce thyroxin.

Thyroxin Thyroid hormone that governs the metabolic rate of all cells of the body.

Tip of the tongue (TOT) phenomenon The experience of inability to recall a word or name when one is quite sure that he/she knows it.

Titchener, Edward Bradford (1867–1927) British-American psychologist who is often called the Dean of Experimental Psychology in America. Titchener was a student of Wundt and epitomized Wundtian system in America. However, his system called structuralism did not survive in America.

Token economy A behavior therapy technique in which desirable activities are reinforced with tokens that can later be exchanged for other goods and services that the person wants.

Tolerance Need for increased amount of drug or substance to achieve the required effect.

Top-down processing Interpreting sensory input in the light of existing knowledge, concepts, ideas and expectations.

Traits An enduring characteristic that can be used to explain regularities in behavior.

Transduction The process of translating physical stimuli impinging on the sense receptors into nerve impulses.

Transductive thinking In Piaget's theory, the term refers to the tendency of the child during the preoperational period to mentally link particular phenomena to see whether or not there is a causal relationship.

Transference (neurosis) In psychoanalysis, a situation in which the patient develops an inappropriate affectional attachment toward the analyst.

Transfer of learning Transfer of learned skills from one situation to another.

Transformational grammar A linguistic theory, which states that when a person wants to communicate something the words are mentally represented in the deep structure. By using *transformation rules* the deep structure is converted into the *surface structure,* what is actually expressed.

Transformation rules The rules guiding the conversion of the deep structure into sur*face structure.*

Transsexualism Identification with members of the opposite sex along with a strong desire to change to the opposite sex; some of them do change their sex. In most cases, it is a gender identity disorder.

Transvestic fetishism A paraphilia in which a person has a recurrent urge to dress like a member of the opposite sex to attain sexual gratification.

Trauma-dissociation theory A theory proposed to explain *dissociative identity disorder* as a defense against a childhood trauma.

Trial and error learning Thorndike's early proposition that learning consists of gradual elimination of ineffectual responses and strengthening of useful responses step by step; the view is more or less discarded.

Triangular theory of love Sternberg's assertion that various forms of love result from different combinations of three basic factors; intimacy, commitment and passion.

Triarchic theory of intelligence Sternberg's view that intelligence consists of three forms of mental ability: analytical, practical and creative.

Trichromats People with normal color vision .They can see all the three sets (red-green, yellow-blue, block-white) of colors.

Trisomy-21 See *Down syndrome.*

t-test An inferential statistic used to evaluate the reliability of the difference between two means. There are different versions of the test for different research designs, such as between-subjects and within-subjects.

Turner's syndrome A condition in woman caused by a missing X chromosome (45 instead of the normal 46). It is characterized by short stature and missing ovary.

Two-factor theory of emotion Schachter and Singer's theory, which maintains that the intensity of physiological arousal determines perceived intensity of emotion, whereas our appraisal of environmental cues (cognitive factor) tells us what emotion we are experiencing.

Two-point threshold The minimum distance between two stimuli on skin at which they are perceived as two rather than one.

Two factor theory of intelligence Spearman's theory which states that intelligence consists of a general factor (g) that partakes all tests and a specific factor (s) that is specific to each test.

Tympanic membrane The eardrum; also called 'tympanum'.

Type A behavior pattern Behavior characterized by excessive drive, competition, a sense of urgency, ambition and a desire to excel; this type of behavior is associated with high incidence of coronary disease.

Type B behavior pattern Behavior marked by relaxation, easygoing approach, lack of intense ambition and a tendency for self-reflection.

Ultrasound imaging A procedure to detect the outline and the movement of the fetus; it helps in determining whether the pregnancy is proceeding normally.

Unconditional positive regard An attitude communicated by a counselor toward a client; it is marked by the unqualified acceptance of the client that conveys to the client his/her intrinsic worth. In client-centered therapy, it is a necessary condition for therapeutic change.

Unconditioned response (UCR) An innate reflexive response to a stimulus (unconditioned stimulus) such as salivating at the sight of food.

Unconditioned stimulus (UCS) A stimulus that automatically elicits a particular response (unconditioned response); for example, contraction of the pupil when there is bright light.

Unconscious In Freud's psychology, a large portion of the mind containing materials that the individual is not aware of. According to Freud a vast amount of mental activity is unconscious.

Unipolar disorders Mood disorders that exhibit only depressive episodes as opposed to *bipolar disorders*.

Universal grammar A hypothesized set of basic grammatical rules assumed to be fundamental to all natural languages.

Unprepared behavior Responses, which can be easily acquired by some animals when specific learning procedures are employed.

Vaginismus Involuntary spasm of the muscles at the entrance to the vagina that prevents penetration and intercourse; it is also called 'vaginism'.

Validity The extent to which a measuring tool (for example, an intelligence test) measures what it was designed to measure.

Variability The spread or dispersion of scores in a distribution.

Variable Any quantity or quality that can take on a range of values.

Variable interval (VI) schedule A schedule of reinforcement in which the organism's response is reinforced based on an average, but varying time intervals following the last reinforced response.

Variable ratio (VR) schedule A schedule of reinforcement in which the organism's response is reinforced based on an average, but a variable number of responses.

Variance A statistic obtained by averaging the squared deviations of each score from the mean; it is the square of standard deviation.

Vasopressin A hormone secreted by the posterior pituitary gland that raises the blood pressure by causing peripheral vasoconstriction; it is also called 'antidiuretic hormone (ADH)' because it controls the water retention mechanism in the organism.

Ventromedial hypothalamus A part of the hypothalamus believed to be involved in regulating satiety feelings. When this part is removed, the animal overeats and gains body weight.

Vestibular sacs Two small sacs in the inner ear that respond to gravity and provide information about the orientation of the head.

Vestibular canal See *Cochlea.*

Vestibular sense The sense of body orientation or equilibrium; it tells whether you are in an upright or horizontal position and regain equilibrium when you are pushed.

Viscerotonic One of the three temperaments in Sheldon's theory; a viscerotonic is sociable, loving and relaxed.

Visual cliff An experimental device designed to study depth perception in infants and animals; it consists of a large box with a heavy glass top and a narrow board across the center of the glass. One half of the surface below the glass is a short drop (the shallow side), while the other is a drop of several feet (the deeper side). The participant is placed at the midpoint and must crawl to one of the two sides to get off. Most participants refuse to crawl to the deeper side indicating the ability to see depth.

Visuospatial sketchpad The storage buffer for visual-spatial material held in working (short-term) memory.

Voyeurism Deriving sexual pleasure by watching clandestinely someone who is disrobing or others engaged in intercourse; a person engaged in voyeurism is often called 'Peeping Tom.'

Vulnerability-stress model A model that attempts to explain psychological disorders as resulting from predisposing biological or psychological factors (vulnerabilities) that are triggered by stress.

Vulnerability A combination of factors that predisposes an individual toward a disease.

Watson, John Broadus (1878–1958) Founder of behaviorism, Watson declared that all behavior including thinking and emotion are learned. He was an extreme environmentalist and discarded all subjective concepts such as mind and consciousness that cannot be objectively observed.

Weber, Ernst Heinrich (1795–1878) German physiologist and anatomist who is known for his work in tactile sensation and a law relating to just noticeable difference which has become famous as Weber's law.

Weber's law A psychophysical law stating that small equally perceptible increments in response (R) correspond to proportional increments in stimulus (S). That is, as R increases by a small constant amount δR, S must make a certain percentage increase. In equation form the law is written $\delta S = KS$, where δS is any increment in S corresponding to a defined unitary change in R and K is the ratio of the increment to S. K is a constant for any given observer and a given stimulus continuum under a given set of conditions. If we divide the equation through by S, we get the more common form of statement of Weber's law $\delta S/S = K$. The constant K is often called 'Weber ratio'.

Wechsler, D (1896–1981) A Rumanian-American psychologist who developed intelligence tests that are in use all over the world; three of his tests are Wechsler Adult Intelligence Scale (WAIS), Wechsler Intelligence Scale for Children (WISC) and Wechsler Preschool and Primary School Scale of Intelligence (WPPSI) among others.

Wernicke's area An area of the left temporal lobe that is believed to be involved in speech comprehension.

Wertheimer, Max (1880–1943) One of the founders of the Gestalt school of psychology; in addition to demonstrating the factors associated with apparent motion (phi phenomenon), Wertheimer did seminal work on productive thinking.

Withdrawal symptoms A pattern of compensatory responses that occur when a drug is discontinued from a drug-dependent person; these are often physiological reactions opposite to those that had been produced by the drug. The common symptoms are tremors, sweating and tension.

Working memory A hypothetical memory system that is believed to temporarily store information, actively processes it and supports other cognitive functions; some researchers use the term as equivalent to short-term memory.

Wundt, Wilhelm (1832–1920) German physiologist, philosopher, and psychologist who founded the first official experimental psychology laboratory at Leipzig University in the year 1879; Wundt trained some of the great psychologists such as GS Hall, McKeen Cattell EB, Titchener, Frank Angell, Judd, Witmer, Warren, Stratton, Kraepelin, Lehmann, Meumann, Kulpe and a host of others. Although what he taught and wrote in the name of psychology did not last long, the fact remains that he was responsible for establishing psychology as a scientific discipline.

X chromosome Sex determining chromosome; all female reproductive cells (gametes) contain X chromosomes and if the fertilized ovum receives an X chromosome from the male, the offspring will be female.

XYY syndrome An observation that males having an extra Y chromosome are prone to outburst of violence. Recent researches doubt the validity of such a phenomenon.

Y chromosome Sex determining chromosome contained in male gametes; when it combines with a female gamete, which always contains an X, the offspring will be male (XY).

Yerkes-Dodson law A principle stating that there is an optimal level of arousal for performing any activity and too much or too little arousal produces inferior performance.

Young, Thomas (1773–1829) A British physicist who formulated a theory of color vision, which has come to be known Young-Helmholtz theory of color vision.

Young-Helmholtz theory of color vision A theory of color vision that postulates three basic color receptors one for red, another for green and a third for blue; the theory explains some, but not all, of the phenomena of color sensation.

Zone of proximal development A term used by Vygotsky referring to the difference between what children can do alone by themselves and what they can do with help.

Zygote A single-celled living being resulting from fertilization (in humans, combining of sperm and ovum).

Bibliography

Adamson RE (1952). Functional fixedness as related to problem solving: A repetition of three experiments. Journal of Experimental Psychology, 44, 288-291.

Ader R (2001). Psychoneuroimmunology. Current Directions in Psychological Science, 10, 94-98.

Adorno TW, Frenkel-Brunswick E, Levinson DJ and Sanford RN (1950). The authoritarian personality. New York: Harper & Row.

Ainsworth MDS, Blehar MC, Waters E and Wall S (1978). Patterns of attachment: A psychological study of the strange situation. Hillsdale, NJ: Erlbaum.

Ajzen I (1991). The theory of planned behavior. Organizational Behavior and Human Decision Processes, 50, 179-211.

Allport GW (1937). Personality: A psychological interpretation. New York: Henry Holt & Company.

Allport GW (1961). Pattern and growth in personality. New York: Holt.

Arnett JJ (2001). Conceptions of the transition to adulthood: Perspectives from adolescence through midlife. Journal of Adult Development, 8, 133-143.

Asch SE (1946). Forming impressions of personality. Journal of Abnormal and Social Psychology, 41, 258-290.

Asch SE (1951). Effects of group pressure upon the modification and distortion of judgment. In H Guetzkow (Ed). Groups, leadership, and men. Pittsburgh: Carnegie Press.

Atkinson RC, Shiffrin RM (1968). Human memory: A proposed system and its control processes. In KW Spence and JT Spence (Eds). The psychology of learning and motivation. Vol. 2, 80-95. New York: Academic Press.

Ayllon T and Azrin NH (1968). The token economy: A motivational system for therapy and rehabilitation. New York: Appleton-Century-Crofts.

Babich FR, Jacobson AL, Bubash, Suzanne and Jacobson, Ann. (1965). Transfer of a response to naïve rats by injection of ribonucleic acid extracted from trained rats. Science, 149, 656-657.

Baddeley AD (1992). Working memory. Science, 255, 556-559.

Baltes PB (1987). Theoretical propositions of life-span development psychology: On the dynamics between growth and decline. Developmental Psychology, 23(5), 611-626.

Bandura A (1965). Influence of models' reinforcement contingencies on the acquisition of imitated responses. Journal of Personality and Social Psychology, 1, 589-595.

Bandura A (1973). Aggression: A social learning analysis. Englewood Cliffs, NJ: Prentice Hall.

Bandura A (1986). Social foundations of thought and action: A social cognitive theory. Englewood Cliffs, NJ: Prentice-Hall.

Bandura A (1997). Self-efficacy: The exercise of control. New York: WH Freeman.

Bandura A (1999). Social cognitive theory of personality. In D Cervone and Y Shoda (Eds). The coherence of personality. New York: Guilford Press.

Baron RS (1986). Distraction-conflict theory: Progress and problems. In L Berkowitz (Ed). Advances in experimental social psychology. Vol. 20, New York: Academic Press.

Bartlett FC (1932). Remembering: An experimental and social study. London: Cambridge University Press.

Batson CD and Olson KC (1991). Current status of the empathy-altruism hypothesis. In MS Clark (Ed). Prosocial behavior. Newbury Park, CA: Sage.

Batson CD, Ahmad N and Stocks EL (2004). Benefits and liabilities of empathy-induced altruism. In AG Miller (Ed). The social psychology of good and evil. New York: Guilford Press.

Baumeister RF and Leary MR (1995). The need to belong: Desire for interpersonal attachments as a fundamental human motivation. Psychological Bulletin, 117, 497-529.

Baumrind D (1967). Child care practices anteceding three patterns of preschool behavior. Genetic Psychology Monographs, 75, 43-88.

Beck AT (1976). Cognitive therapy and emotional disorders. New York: International Universities Press.

Bem DJ (1972). Self-perception theory. In L Berkowitz (Ed). Advances in experimental social psychology. Vol. 6. New York: Academic Press.

Benson H, Beary JF and Carol MP (1974). The relaxation response. Psychiatry, 17, 37-46.

Berkoweitz L (1993). Aggression: Its causes, consequences, and control. New York: McGraw-Hill.

Berlyne D (1967). Arousal and reinforcement. In D Levine (Ed). Nebraska symposium on motivation. Lincoln: University of Nebraska Press.

Biondi M and Zannino L (1997). Psychological stress, neuroimmunomodulation, and susceptibility to infectious diseases in animals and man: A review. Psychotherapy and Psychosomatics, 66, 3-26.

Bowlby J (1969). Attachment and loss. Vol. 1. Attachment, New York: Basic Books.

Breland K and Breland M (1961). The misbehavior of organisms. American Psychologist, 16, 681-684.

Brown SL, Nesse RM, Vinokur AD and Smith DM (2003). Providing social support may be more beneficial than receiving it: Results from a prospective study of mortality. Psychological Science, 14, 320-327.

Buss A and Plomin R (1975). A temperament theory of personality development. New York: Wiley.

Buss A and Plomin R (1984). Temperament: Early developing personality traits. Hillsdale, NJ: Erlbaum.

Cameron J and Pierce WD (1994). Reinforcement, reward, and intrinsic motivation: A meta-analysis. Review of Educational Research, 64, 363-423.

Cannon WB (1932). The wisdom of the body. New York: Norton.

Carroll JB (1993). Human cognitive abilities: A survey of factor-analytic studies. New York: Cambridge University Press.

Carson RC, Butcher JN, Mineka S and Hooley JM (2007). Abnormal psychology (13th Edition). New Delhi: Pearson Education, Inc.

Cattell RB (1950). Personality: A systematic, theoretical, and factual study. New York: McGraw-Hill.

Cattell RB (1971). Abilities: Their growth, structure, and action. Boston: Houghton Mifflin.

Chang EC (1996). Cultural differences in optimism, pessimism, and coping: Predictors of subsequent adjustment in American and Caucasian American college students. Journal Counseling Psychology, 43, 113-123.

Chen C, Greenberger E, Lester J, Dong Q and Guo MS (1998). A cross-cultural study of family and peer correlates of adolescent misconduct. Developmental Psychology, 34, 770-781.

Chess S and Thomas A (1996). Temperament: Theory and practice. New York: Brunner/Mazel.

Chomsky N (1972). Language and mind. New York: Harcourt.

Cohen F and Lazarus RS (1979). Coping with the stress of illness. In GC Stone, F Cohen and NE Adler (Eds). Health psychology: A handbook. San Francisco, CA: Jossey-Boss.

Cohen S and Herbert TB (1996). Health psychology: Psychological factors and physical disease from the perspective of human psychoneuroimmunology. Annual Review of Psychology, 47, 113-142.

Costa PT Jr and McCrae RR (1988). Personality in adulthood: A six-year longitudinal study of self-reports and spouse ratings on the NEO Personality Inventory. Journal of Personality and Social Psychology, 54, 853-863.

Darley JM and Latané B (1968). By stander intervention in emergencies: Diffusion of responsibility. Journal of Personality and Social Psychology, 8, 377-383.

Darwin CR (1872) The expressions of emotions in man and animals. London: John Murray.

Davidson RJ (1994). Complexities in the search for emotion-specific physiology. In P Ekman and RJ Davidson (Eds). The nature of emotion. New York: Oxford University Press.

Deci EL (1975). Intrinsic motivation. New York: Plenum Press.

Deci EL and Ryan RM (1985). Intrinsic motivation and self-determination in human behavior. New York: Plenum Press.

Deci EL and Ryan RM (2002). Handbook of self-determination theory research. Rochester, NY: University of Rochester Press.

DeFleur ML and Westie FR (1958). Verbal attitudes and overt acts: An experiment on the salience of attitudes. American Sociological Review, 23, 667-673.

Diener E (2000). Subjective well-being: The science of happiness and proposal for national index. American Psychologist, 53, 34-43.

Diener E and Seligman M (2004). Beyond money: Toward an economy of well-being. Psychological Science in the Public Interest. 5, 1-31.

Dollard J, Doob LW, Miller NE Mowrer OH and Sears RR (1939). Frustration and aggression. New Haven, CT: Yale University Press.

Dollard J and Miller NE (1950). Personality and psychotherapy: An analysis in terms of learning, thinking, and culture. New York: McGraw-Hill.

Dutton DG and Aron AP (1974). Some evidence for heightened sexual attraction under conditions of high anxiety. Journal of personality and Social Psychology, 30, 510-570.

Eagly AH and Chaiken S (1995). Attitude strength, attitude structure, and resistance to change. In RE Petty and JA Krosnick (Eds). Attitude strength: Antecedents and consequences. Mahwah, NJ: Erlbaum.

Ekman P (1972). Universals and cultural differences in facial expression of emotions. In J Cole (Ed). Darwin and facial expression: A century of research in review (pp. 169-222). New York: Academic Press.

Elkind D (1967). Egocentrism in adolescence. Child Development, 38, 1025-1034.

Ellis A (1962). Reason and emotion in psychotherapy. New York: Lyle Stuart.

Erikson EH (1950). Childhood and society. New York: Norton.

Erikson EH (1968). Identity: Youth and crisis. New York: Norton.

Eysenck HJ (1952). The effects of psychotherapy: An evaluation. Journal of Consulting Psychology, 16, 319-324.

Eysenck HJ, Eysenck MW (1985). Personality and individual differences: A natural science approach. New York: Plenum.

Eysenck HJ and Eysenck SBG (1975). Manual for the Eysenck Personality Questionnaire. London: Hodder & Stoughton.

Feldman RS (1997). Essentials of understanding psychology (3rd Edition). New York: McGraw-Hill.

Feldman RS (2002). Understanding psychology (6th Edition). New York: McGraw-Hill.

Festinger L (1954). A theory of social comparison processes. Human Relations, 2, 117-140.

Festinger L (1957). A theory of cognitive dissonance. Stanford, CA: Stanford University Press.

Festinger L and Carlsmith JM (1959). Cognitive consequences of forced compliance. Journal of Abnormal and Social Psychology, 58, 203-210.

Flynn JR (1999). Searching for justice: The discovery of IQ gains over time. American Psychologist, 54, 5-20.

Franks DD and Smith TS (Eds) (1999). Mind, Brain, and Society: Toward a neurosociology of emotion. Vol. 5. Stamford, CT: Jai Press.

Freud A (1946). The ego and the mechanisms of defense. New York: International Universities Press.

Fromm E (1956). The art of loving. New York: Bantam.

Fuligni AJ (1998). Authority, autonomy, and parent-adolescent conflict and cohesion: A study of adolescents from Mexican, Chinese, Filipino, and European backgrounds. Developmental Psychology, 34, 782-792.

Gardner H (2000). Multiple intelligences: The theory in practice. New York: Basic Books.

Gesell A (1948). Studies in child development. New York: Harper & Row.

Gibson E and Walk RD (1960). The visual cliff. Scientific American, 202, 80-92.

Gilligan C (1982). In a different voice: Psychological theory and woman's development. Cambridge, MA: Harvard University Press.

Gough HG (1975). California Psychological Inventory manual (Review Edition). Palo Alto, CA: Consulting Psychologists Press.

Gray JA (1991). Neural systems, emotions, and personality. In J Madden IV (Ed). Neurobiology of learning, emotion, and affect. New York: Raven Press.

Guilford JP (1959). Three faces of intellect. American Psychologist, 14, 469-479.

Guilford JP (1967). The nature of human intelligence. New York: McGraw-Hill.

Hall GS (1904). Adolescence. Vols. 1 and 2. New York: Appleton-Century-Crofts.

Hammen C (1991). Depression runs in families: The social context of risk and resilience in children of depressed mothers. New York: Springer-Veerlag.

Harlow HF (1958). The nature of love. The American Psychologist, 13, 673-685.

Harlow HF and Zimmerman RR (1959). Affectional responses in the infant monkeys. Science, 130, 421-432.

Haskell WL, Alderman EL, Fair JM, et al (1994). Effects of intensive multiple risk factor reduction on coronary atherosclerosis and clinical cardiac events in men and women with coronary artery disease. Circulation, 89, 975-990.

Heider F (1958). The psychology of interpersonal relations. New York: Wiley.

Hergenhahn BR (2001). An introduction to the history of psychology (4th Edition). Belmont, CA: Wadsworth/Thomson Learning.

Hernstein RJ and Murray C (1994). The bell curve: Intelligence and class structure in American life. New York: Free press.

Hilgard ER and Bower GH (1975). Theories of learning (4th Edition). Englewood Cliffs, NJ: Prentice Hall.

Hilgard ER, Atkinson RC and Atkinson RL (1975). Psychology (6th Edition). New Delhi: Oxford & IBH Publishing Co.

Hobson CJ, Kamen J, Szostek J, Nethercut CM, et al (1998). Stressful life events: A revision and update of the Social Readjustment Rating Scale. International Journal of Stress Management, 5, 123.

Holmes TH and Rahe RH (1967). The Social Readjustment Rating Scale. Journal of Psychosomatic Research, 11, 213-218.

Horn JL and Cattell RB (1966). Refinement and test of the theory of fluid and crystallized general intelligences. Journal of Educational Psychology, 57, 253-270.

House JS, Landis KR and Umberson D (1988). Social relationships and health. Science, 241, 540-545.

Hovland C, Janis I and Kelly HH (1953). Communication and persuasion. New Haven, CT: Yale University Press.

Hull CL (1943). Principles of behavior: An introduction to behavior theory. New York: Appleton-Century.

Izard CE (1971). The face of emotion. New York: Appleton-Century-Crofts.

Izard CE (1977). Human emotions. New York: Plenum Press.

Izard CE (1989). The structure and functions of emotions: Implications for cognition, motivation, and personality. In JS Cohen (Ed). The G Stanley Hall Lecture Series. Vol. 9. Washington, DC: American Psychological Association.

Jacobson E (1938). Progressive relaxation. Chicago: University of Chicago Press.

James W (1890). The principles of psychology. New York: Holt.

Janis IL (1982). Groupthink (2nd Edition). Boston: Houghton Mifflin.

Jenson AR (1969). How much can we boost IQ and scholastic achievement? Harvard Educational Review, 39, 1-123.

Jersild AT and Holms FB (1935). Children's fears. New York: Teachers College Press.

Jones EE and Davis KE (1965). From acts to disposition: The attribution process in person perception. In L Berkowitz (Ed). Advances in experimental social psychology. Vol. 2, pp. 219-266. New York: Academic Press.

Jones EE and Nisbett RE (1971). The actor and the observer: Divergent perceptions of the causes of behavior. Morristown. NJ: General Learning Press.

Jones MC (1924). A laboratory study of fear: The case of Peter. Pedagogical Seminary, 31, 308-315.

Kagan J, Reznick S and Snidman N (1988). Biological basis of childhood shyness. Science, 240, 167-171.

Kahneman D, Tversky A (1973). On the psychology of prediction. Psychological Review, 80, 237-251.

Kanner AD, Coyne JC, Schaefer C and Lazarus RS (1981). Comparison of two modes of stress measurement: Daily hassles and uplifts versus major life events. Journal of Behavioral Medicine, 4, 1-13.

Kanner L (1943). Autistic disturbance of affective contact. Nervous child, 12, 17-50.

Kelley HH (1950). The warm-cold variable in first impression of persons. Journal of Personality and Social Psychology, 431-439.

Kelley HH (1972). Attribution in social interaction. In EE Jones, et al (Eds). Attribution: Perceiving the causes of behavior. Morristown. NJ: General Learning Press.

Kelly G (1955). The psychology of personal constructs. New York: Norton.

Kelly GF (2001). Sexuality today: The human perspective (5th Edition). Boston: McGraw-Hill.

Kerlinger FN (1973). Foundations of behavioral research. New York: Holt Rinehart and Winston.

Kessler RC, McGonagle KA, Zhao S, Nelson CB, et al (1994). Lifetime and 12-month prevalence of DSM-III-R psychiatric disorders in the United States. Archives of General Psychiatry, 51, 8-19.

Kimble GA (1961). Hilgard and Marquis' leaning and conditioning (2nd Edition). Englewood Cliffs, NJ: Prentice Hall.

Koch S (1933). "Psychology" or "the psychological studies?" American Psychologist, 48, 902-904.

Kohlberg L (1963). The development of children's orientation toward a moral order: I. Sequence in the development of moral thought. Human Development, 6, 11-33.

Kohlberg L (1969). Stages in the development of moral thought and action. New York: Holt, Rinehart & Winston.

Kohlberg L (1981). Essays in moral development. San Francisco: Harper and Row.

Kinsey AC, Pomeroy WB and Martin CE (1948). Sexual behavior in the human male. Philadelphia Saunders.

Kinsey AC, Pomeroy WB, Martin CE and Gebhard PH (1953). Sexual behavior in the human female. Philadelphia: Saunders.

Kleinginna PR and Kleinginna AM (1981). A categorized list of emotion definitions, with suggestions for a consensual definition. Motivation and Emotion, 5, 345-379.

Kluckhohn C and Murray HA (1953). Personality formation: the determinants. In C Kluckhohn, HA Murray and DM Schneider (Eds). Personality in nature, culture, and society. New York: Knopf.

Kobasa SC (1979). Stressful life events, personality, and health: An inquiry into hardiness. Journal of Personality and Social Psychology, 37, 1-11.

Kobasa SC, Maddi SR and Kahn S (1982). Hardiness and health: S prospective study. Journal of Personality and Social Psychology, 42, 168-177.

Kohler W (1925). The mentality of apes (English translation). New York: Harcourt.

Kosslyn SM and Rosenberg RS (2005). Psychology in context. Pearson Education, Inc (Indian Edition).

Kottak CP (2000). Cultural anthropology (8th Edition). Boston: McGraw Hill.

Kübler-Ross E (1969). On death and dying. New York: Macmillan.

LaPiere RT (1934). Attitude and actions. Social Forces, 13, 230-237.

Larson R and Buss DM (2002). Personality psychology: Domains of knowledge about human nature. Boston: McGraw-Hill.

Laumann EO, Gagnon JH, Michael RT and Michaels S (1994). The social organization of sexuality: Sexual practice in the United States. Chicago: University of Chicago Press.

Lazarus AA (1989). The practice of multimodal therapy. Baltimore: Johns Hopkins University press.

Lazarus RS (1991). Progress on a cognitive-motivational-relational theory of emotion. American Psychologist, 46, 819-834.

Leeper RW (1970). The motivational and perceptual properties of emotions as indicating their fundamental character and role. In MB Arnold (Ed). Feelings and emotions: The Loyola Symposium. New York: Academic Ptess.

Le Doux JE and Pelps EA. Emotional networks in the brain. In M Lewis and JM Haviland-Jones (Eds). Handbook of emotions (2nd Edition). New York: Guilford Press.

Lepper MR, Greene D and Nisbett RE (1973). Undermining children's intrinsic interest with external reward: A test of the "overjustification" hypothesis. Journal of Personality and Social Psychology, 28, 129-137.

Levenson RW (1994). The search for autonomic specificity. In P Ekmanand, RJ Davidson (Eds). The nature of emotions: Fundamental questions. New York: Oxford University Press.

Levinson DJ, Darow CN, Klein EB, Levinson MH and McKee B (1978). The seasons of a man's life, New York: Knopf.

Levinson DJ (1986). A conception of adult development. American Psychologist, 41, 313.

Liberman A and Chaiken S (1992). Defensive processing of personally relevant health messages. Personality and Social Psychology Bulletin, 18, 669-679.

Lobel M, DeVincent CJ, Kaminer A and Mayer BA (2000). The impact of prenatal maternal stress and optimistic disposition on birth outcomes in medically high-risk women. Health Psychology, 19, 544-553.

Luchins AS and Luchins EH (1959). Rigidity of behavior. Eugene, OR: University of Oregon Press.

Maddi SR and Khoshaba DM (1994). Hardiness and mental health. Journal of Personality Assessment, 63, 265-274.

Marcia JE (1966). Development and validation of ego identity status. Journal of Personality and Social Psychology, 3, 551-558.

Marks IM (2002). The maturing of psychotherapy: Some brief psychotherapies help anxiety/depressive disorders but mechanisms of action are unclear. British Journal of Psychiatry, 180, 200-2004.

Maslow AH (1954). Motivation and personality. New York: Harper.

Maslow AH (1970). Motivation and personality (2nd Edition). New York: Harper & Row.

Maslow AH (1971). The farther reaches of human nature. New York: Viking.

Masters WH and Johnson V (1966). Human sexual response. London: Churchill.

Mayer JD, Salovey P and Caruso DR (2004). Emotional intelligence: Theory, findings and implications. Psychological Inquiry, 15, 197-215.

McCrae RR and Costa PT (2003). Personality in adulthood: A Five-Factor Theory perspective. New York: Guilford Press.

McClelland DC, Atkinson JW, Clark RA and Lowell EL (1953). The achievement motive. New York: Appleton-Century-Crofts.

McDougall W (1908). Introduction to social psychology. London: Methuen.

Meichenbaum D (1977). Cognitive behavior modification: An integrative approach. New York: Plenum.

Meichenbaum D (1985). Stress inoculation training. New York: Pergamon Press.

Meltzoff AN (2002). Elements of a developmental theory of imitation. In AN Meltzoff, N Andrew, and W Prinz (Eds).The imitative mind: Development, evolution, and brain bases. Cambridge studies in cognitive perceptual development. New York: Cambridge University Press.

Melzack R and Wall PD (1965). Pain mechanisms: A theory. Science, 150, 971-979.

Melzack R (1999). From the gate to the neuromatrix. Pain, Suppl 6, 121-126.

Michael RT, Gagnon JH, Laumman EO and Kolata G (1994). Sex in America: A definitive survey. Boston: Little, Brown.

Milgram S (1974). Obedience to authority: An experimental view. New York: Harper & Row.

Miller GA (1956). The magical number seven, plus or minus two: some limits on our capacity for processing information. Psychological Review, 63, 81-97.

Miller JG (1984). Culture and development of everyday social explanation. Journal of Personality and Social Psychology, 46, 961-978.

Miller NE (1944). Experimental studies of conflict. In J McV Hunt (Ed). Personality and behavior disorders. Vol. 1. New York: Ronald Press.

Mischel W (1999). Personality coherence and dispositions in a cognitive-affective personality system (CAPS) approach. In D Cervone and Y Shoda (Eds). Coherence of personality. New York: Guilford Press.

Morgan GT, King RA, Weisz JR and Schopler J (1986). Introduction to psychology (7th Edition). New Delhi: Tata McGraw-Hill.

Morgan CD and Murray HA (1938). Thematic Apperception Test. In HA Murray, et al (1938). Explorations in personality: A clinical and experimental study of fifty men of college age. New York: Oxford University Press.

Murray HA, et al (1938). Explorations in personality: A clinical and experimental study of fifty men of college age. New York: Oxford University Press.

Nairne JS (2006). Psychology: The adaptive mind (4th Edition). Belmont CA: Thomson Wadsworth.

Nevid JS (2007). Psychology: Concepts and Applications. Boston: NY: Houghton Mifflin Company.

Paivio A (1969). Mental imagery in associative learning and memory. Psychological Review, 76, 241-263.

Pankspp J (2005). Basic affects and the instinctual emotion system of the brain: The primordial sources of sadness, joy and seeking. In ADR Manstead, NH Frijda, AH Fischer and K Oatley (Eds). Feelings and emotions. The Amsterdam Symposium. New York: Cambridge University Press.

Passer MW and Smith RE (2007). Psychology: The science of mind and behavior. New Delhi: Tata McGraw-Hill.

Paulus PB (Ed) (1989). Psychology of influence (2nd Edition). Hillside, NJ: Erlbaum.

Pennebaker JW (1997). Opening up: The healing power of expressing emotions (Review Edition). New York: Guilford Press.

Pettigrew TF and Tropp LR (2000). Does intergroup contact reduce prejudice: Recent meta-analytic findings. In S Oskamp (Ed). Reducing prejudice and discrimination: The Claremont Symposium on Applied Social Psychology. Mahwah, NJ: Erlbaum.

Petty RE and Cacioppo JT (1986). Communication and persuasion: Central and peripheral routes to attitude change. New York: Springer-Verlag.

Piaget J (1932). The moral judgment of the child. New York: Harcourt Brace.

Piaget J (1970). Piaget's theory. In PH Mussen (Ed). Carmichael's manual of child psychology. Vol. 1. New York: Wiley.

Pinker S (2000). Language as an adaptation to the cognitive niche. In M Christianson and S Kirby (Eds). Language evolution: Reports from the research frontier. New York: Oxford University press.

Plutchik R (1980). Emotion: A psychoevolutionary synthesis. New York: Harper & Row.

Plutchik R (1994). Psychology of emotion. Reading, MA: Addison-Wesley.

Prochaska JO and DiClemete CC (1984). The transtheoretical approach: Crossing traditional boundaries of therapy. Illinois: Down Jones-Irwin.

Prochaska JO, Johnson S and Lee P (1998). The transtheoretical model of behavior change. In SA Shumaker and EB Schron (Eds). The handbook of health behavior change (2nd Edition). New York Springer.

Putnam FW (1989). Diagnosis and treatment of multiple personality disorder. New York: Guilford Press.

Rachman S (1998). Anxiety. Mahwah, NJ: Erlbaum.

Renner MJ and Mackin RS (1998). A life stress instrument for classroom use. Teaching of Psychology, 25, 46-48.

Resnick SM, Pham DL, Kraut MS, Zonderman AB and Davatzikos C (2003). Longitudinal magnetic resonance imaging studies of older adults: A shrinking brain. Journal of Neuroscience, 23, 3295-3301.

Rogers CR (1951). Client-centered therapy: Its current practice, implications, and theory. Boston: Houghton Mifflin.

Rogers CR (1959). A theory of therapy, personality, and interpersonal relationships, as developed in the client-centered framework. In S Koch (Ed). Psychology: A study of a science. Vol. 3, pp.14-256. New York: McGraw-Hill.

Rogers CR (1961). On becoming a person. Boston: Houghton Mifflin.

Rogers CR and Dymond RF (Eds) (1954). Psychotherapy and personality change: Coordinated studies in the client-centered approach. Chicago: Chicago University Press.

Rorschach H (1924). Psychodiagnostics: A diagnostic test based on perception. New York: Grune & Stratton.

Rosenhan DL (1975). On being sane in insane places. Science, 179, 250-258.

Rosenthal R (1966). Experimenter effects in behavioral research. New York: Appleton-Century-Crofts.

Rosenthal R and Jacobsen L (1967). Pygmalion in the classroom: Self-fulfilling prophesies and teacher expectations. New York: Holt.

Rotter JB (1966). Generalized expectancies for internal versus external control of reinforcement. Psychological Monographs, 80 (Whole No. 609).

Ryan RM and Deci EL (2000). Intrinsic and extrinsic motivations: Classic definitions and new directions. Contemporary Educational Psychology, 25, 54-67.

Sarason IG and Sarason BR (1996). Abnormal psychology. New Delhi: Prentice-Hall of India.

Schaie KW (1994). The course of adult intellectual development. American Psychologist, 49, 304-313.

Schachter S and Singer JE (1962). Cognitive, social, and physiological determinants of emotional state. Psychological Review, 69, 379-399.

Schachter S and Wheeler L (1962). Epinephrine, chlorpromazine, and amusement. Journal of Abnormal and Social Psychology, 65, 121-128.

Scheier MF, Matthews KA, Owens JE, Schulz R, Bridges MW, Magovern GJ, et al (1999). Optimism and rehospitalization after coronary artery bypass graft surgery. Archives of Internal Medicine, 159, 829-935.

Searcy E, Eisenberg N (1992). Defensiveness in response aid from a sibling. Journal personality and Social Psychology, 62, 422-433.

Seligman MEP (1970). On the generality of the laws of learning. Psychological Review, 77, 406-418.

Seligman MEP (1995). The effectiveness of psychotherapy. The Consumer Reports study. American Psychologist, 50, 965-974.

Seligman MEP (2002). Authentic happiness: Using the new positive psychology to realize your potential for lasting fulfillment. New York: Free Press.

Selye H (1976). The stress of life. New York: McGraw Hill.

Sherif M, Harvey OJ, White BJ, Hood WE and Sherif CW (1961). Intergroup conflict and cooperation: The Robbers Cave experiment. Norman, OK: Institute of Group Relations.

Shweder RA, Mahapatra M and Miller JG (1990). Culture and moral development. In JW Stigler, RA Shweder and G Herdt (Eds). Cultural Psychology. New York: Cambridge University Press.

Skinner BF (1938). The behavior of organisms: an experimental analysis. New York: Appleton Century-Crofts.

Skinner BF (1953). Science and human behavior. New York: Macmillan.

Skinner BF (1957). Verbal behavior. New York: Prentice Hall.

Skinner BF (1971). Beyond freedom and dignity. New York: Knopf.

Skinner BF (1989). The origins of cognitive thought. American Psychologist, 44, 13-18.

Sloan D and Marx D (2004). A closer examination of the structured written disclosure procedure. Journal of Consulting and Clinical Psychology, 72, 165-175.

Slovic P, Eischoff B and Lichenstein S (1976). Cognitive processes and social risk taking. In JS Carroll and JW Payne (Eds). Cognition and social behavior. Mahwah, NJ: Erlbaum.

Smith ML and Glass GV (1977). Meta-analysis of psychotherapy outcome studies. American Psychologist, 32, 752-760.

Smith RE, Smoll FL and Ptacek JT (1990). Conjunctive moderator variables in vulnerability and resiliency research: Life stress, social support, and coping skills, and adolescent sport injuries. Journal of Personality and Social Psychology, 58, 360-370.

Snarey JR (1985). Cross-cultural universality of social-moral development: A critical review of Kohlbergian research. Psychological Bulletin, 97, 202-232.

Snarey JR (1995). In a communitarian voice: The sociological expansion of Kohlbergian theory, research, and practice. In WM Kurtines and JL Gewirtz (Eds). Moral development: An introduction. Boston: Allyn & Bacon.

Speisman J, Lazarus RL, Mordkoff A and Davidson L (1964). Experimental reduction of stress based on ego-defense theory. Journal of Abnormal and Social Psychology, 68, 367-380.

Spearman CE (1927). The abilities of man. London: Macmillan.

Sperling G (1960). The information available in brief visual presentations. Psychological Monographs, 74 (Whole No. 11).

Spiegler MD and Guevremont DC (2003). Contemporary behavior therapy. Belmont, CA: Wadsworth.

Stagner R and Solley CM (1970). Basic psychology: A perceptual-homeostatic approach. New York: McGraw Hill.

Stark E (1989, May). Teen sex: Not for love. Psychology Today, 10-11.

Steele CM (1997). A threat in the air: How stereotypes shape intellectual identity and performance. American Psychologist, 52, 613-629.

Sternbach RA (1968). Pain: A psychological analysis. New York Academic Press.

Sternberg RJ (1986). A triangular theory of love. Psychological Review, 93, 119-135.

Sternberg RJ (2004). Culture and intelligence. American Psychologist, 59, 325-338.

Super DE (1957). The psychology of careers. New York: Harper and Row.

Swindle R, Heller K, Prescosolido B and Kikuzawa S (2000). Responses to nervous breakdowns in America over a 40-year period. American Psychologist, 55, 740-749.

Szasz TS (1961). The myth of mental illness. New York: Harper & Row.

Szasz TS and Hollender MH (1956). A contribution to the philosophy of medicine: The basic models of the doctor-patient relationship. Archives of internal medicine, 97, 585-592.

Taylor JA (1953). A personality scale of manifest anxiety. Journal of Abnormal Psychology, 48, 285-290.

Tellegen A, Lykken DT, Bouchard TJ, Wilcox KJ, Segal NL and Rich S (1988). Personality similarity in twins reared apart and together. Journal of Personality and Social Psychology, 54, 1031-1039.

Terman LM and Merrill MA (1972). Stanford-Binet Intelligence Scale (3rd Edition) form L-M. Boston: Houghton Mifflin.

Thorndike EL, Hagen E and Sattler J (1986). Stanford-Binet (4th Edition). Chicago: Riverside Press.

Thurstone LL (1938). Primary mental abilities. Chicago: University of Chicago Press.

Tomkins SS (1970). Affect as a primary motivational system. In MB Arnold (Ed), Feelings and emotions: The Loyola Symposium. New York: Academic Press.

Tomkins SS (1981). The quest for primary motives: Biography and autobiography of an idea. Journal of Personality and Social Psychology, 41, 306-329.

Tomkins SS (1991). Affect, imagery, and consciousness. New York: Springer-Verlag.

Torrey EF, Bowler A, Taylor E and Gottesman II (1994). Schizophrenia and manic-depressive disorder. New York: Basic Books.

Triandis HC (2001). Individualism-collectivism and personality. Journal of Personality, 69, 907-924.

Tryon RC (1940). Studies in individual differences in maze ability: VII. The specific components of maze ability, and a general theory of psychological components. Journal of Comparative Psychology, 30, 283-335.

Tversky A and Kahneman D (1987). Rational choice and the framing of decisions. In R Hogarth and M Reder (Eds). Rational choice: the contrast between economics and psychology. Chicago: University of Chicago Press.

Vaughan C and Leff J (1976). The measurement of expressed emotion in the families of psychiatric patients. British Journal of Social and Clinical Psychology, 15, 157-165.

Vernon PE (1950). The structure of human abilities. London: Methuen.

Vygotsky LS (1978). Mind in society: The development of higher psychological processes. Cambridge, MA: Harvard University Press (Original work was published in 1935).

Walker LJ and Taylor JH (1991). Family interactions and the development of moral reasoning. Child Development, 62, 254-283.

Ward WC, Kogan N and Pankove E (1972). Incentive effects in children's creativity. Child Development, 43, 669-677.

Watson JB (1924). Behaviorism. New York: People's Institute.

Watson JB and Rayner R (1920). Conditioned emotional reactions. Journal of Experimental Psychology, 3, 1-14.

Wechsler D (1975). Intelligence defined and undefined. American Psychologist, 30, 135-139.

Wegner DM and Pennebaker JW (1993). Changing our minds: An introduction to mental control. In DM Wegner and JW Pennebaker (Eds). Handbook of mental control. Englewood Cliffs, NJ: Prentice Hall.

Welsh GS (1975). Creativity and intelligence: A personality approach. Chapel Hill, NC: Institute for Research in Social Science, University of North Carolina at Chapel Hill.

Weissman MM, Bland RC, Canino GJ, et al (1996). Cross-national epidemiology of major depression and bipolar disorders. Journal of American Medical Association, 276, 293-99.

White RW (1959). Motivation reconsidered: The concept of competence. Psychological Review, 66, 297-333.

White KM, Hogg MA, Terry DJ (2002). Improving attitude behavior correspondence through exposure to normative support from a salient in group. Basic and Applied Social Psychology, 24, 91-103.

Whorf BL (1956). Science and linguistics. In JB Carroll (Ed). Language thought and reality: Selected writings of Benjamin Lee Whorf. Cambridge, MA: MIT Press.

Wicker AW (1969). Attitudes versus actions: The relationship of verbal and overt behavioral responses to attitude objects. Journal of Social Issues, 25, 41-78.

Winter DG (1973). The power motive. New York: Free Press.

Wolpe J (1958). Psychotherapy by reciprocal inhibition. Stanford, CA: Stanford University Press.

Wolpe J (1990). The practice of behavior therapy (4th Edition). Elmsford, NY: Pergamon Press.

Zajonc RB (1965). Social facilitation. Science, 149, 269-274.

Zinovieva IL (2001). Why do people work if they are not paid? An example from Eastern Europe. In DR Denison (Ed). Managing organizational change in transition economics. Mahwah, NJ: Erlbaum.

Zuckerman M (1978) Sensation seeking. In H London and JE Exner Jr (Eds). Dimensions of personality. New York: Wiley.

Zuckerman M, Hall JA, DeFrank RS and Rosenthal R (1976). Encoding and decoding of spontaneous and posed facial expressions. Journal of Personality and Social Psychology, 34, 966-977.

Zubin J and Spring B (1977). Vulnerability: New view of schizophrenia. Journal of Abnormal Psychology, 86, 103-126.

Index

Page numbers followed by *f* refer to figure and *t* refer to table

C

D

G

H

Q

R

S

V

W

X

Y

Z